Cancer
SOURCEBOOK
Third Edition

Health Reference Series

Third Edition

Cancer
SOURCEBOOK

Basic Consumer Health Information about Major Forms and Stages of Cancer, Featuring Facts about Primary and Secondary Tumors of the Respiratory, Nervous, Lymphatic, Circulatory, Skeletal, and Gastrointestinal Systems, and Specific Organs:

Along with Statistical and Demographic Data, Treatment Options, Strategies for Coping, a Glossary, and a Directory of Sources for Additional Help and Information

Edited by
Edward J. Prucha

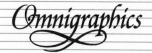

Omnigraphics

615 Griswold Street • Detroit, MI 48226

Bibliographic Note

Because this page cannot legibly accommodate all the copyright notices, the Bibliographic Note portion of the Preface constitutes an extension of the copyright notice.

Beginning with books published in 1999, each volume of the *Health Reference Series* on a new topic will be individually titled and called a "First Edition." Subsequent updates will carry sequential edition numbers. To help avoid confusion and to provide maximum flexibility in our ability to respond to informational needs, the practice of consecutively numbering each volume will be discontinued.

Edited by Edward J. Prucha

Health Reference Series

Karen Bellenir, *Series Editor*
Peter D. Dresser, *Managing Editor*
Joan Margeson, *Research Associate*
Dawn Matthews, *Verification Assistant*
Margaret Mary Missar, *Research Coordinator*
Jenifer Swanson, *Research Associate*
EdIndex, Services for Publishers, *Indexers*

Omnigraphics, Inc.

Matthew P. Barbour, *Vice President, Operations*
Laurie Lanzen Harris, *Vice President, Editorial Director*
Kevin Hayes, *Production Coordinator*
Thomas J. Murphy, *Vice President, Finance and Comptroller*
Peter E. Ruffner, *Senior Vice President*
Jane J. Steele, *Marketing Consultant*

Frederick G. Ruffner, Jr., Publisher

©2000, Omnigraphics, Inc.

Library of Congress Cataloging-in-Publication Data

Cancer sourcebook : basic consumer health information about major forms and stages of cancer, featuring facts about primary and secondary tumors of the respiratory, nervous lymphatic, circulatory, skeletal, and gastrointestinal systems, and specific organs, along with statistical and demographic data, treatment options, strategies for coping, a glossary, and directory of sources for additional help and information / edited by Edward J. Prucha.-- 3rd ed.
    p. cm.
Includes bibliographical references and index.
ISBN 0-7808-0227-6 (lib. bdg. : alk. paper)
    1. Cancer--Popular works. 2. Cancer--Handbooks, manuals, etc. I. Prucha, Edward J.

RC263 .C294 2000
616.99'4--dc21

00-036307

∞

Table of Contents

Cancers of the Gastrointestinal and Urinary Tracts

Lymphomas and Blood Cell Cancers

Endocrine Cancers

Part IV: Cancer Prevention and Research

Part V: Coping Strategies

Part VI: Additional Help and Information

Preface

About This Book

The American Cancer Society estimates that about 1.25 million new cancer cases are diagnosed annually. Although cancer is responsible for one out of every five deaths in the United States, survival rates have steadily improved. Consumer education, more valuable diagnostic procedures, and better treatments have all played important roles in increasing the five year survival rate for all cancers to more than 50 percent. New information on cancers and cancer treatment, however, can be confusing and sometimes questionable.

This Third Edition of Omnigraphics' *Cancer Sourcebook*, provides up-to-date, clear, concise, and reliable facts from government agencies and professional organizations. It offers descriptions of the major forms and stages of cancers affecting specific organs and the respiratory, nervous, lymphatic, circulatory, skeletal, and gastrointestinal systems. It provides facts about treatments, side effects, alternative therapies, clinical trials, and coping strageties. A glossary of terms will help readers discuss their concerns with health care providers, and a directory of organizations able to provide assistance will guide readers who need additional help or information.

Other books in the *Health Reference Series* provide additional information on specific types of cancer:

- *Pediatric Cancer Sourcebook* describes cancers that occur most commonly in children;

ix

- *Cancer Sourcebook for Women* provides information about cancers that primarily affect the female reproductive organs;

- *Breast Cancer Sourcebook* gives the reader in-depth information about the disease and the side effects of treatment, preventive measures, and a list of additional resources.

How to Use This Book

This book is divided into parts and chapters. Parts focus on broad areas of interest. Chapters are devoted to single topics within a part.

Part I: Introduction provides general cancer information and a question and answer chapter about common concerns.

Part II: Types of Cancer contains detailed information on a wide variety of cancers, including head and neck cancers; lung cancers; cancers of the gastrointestinal and urinary tracts; lymphomas and blood cell cancers; endocrine cancers; skin cancers; bone, marrow, and connective tissure cancers; and other types of cancers.

Part III: Treatments and Therapies provides detailed information for the cancer patient and family regarding various treatment methods for cancer. In addition to mainstream treatment with chemotherapy, radiation therapy, and bone marrow transplantation, it contains a descriptive listing of chemotherapy drugs, information about marijuana for side effects of treatments, and a chapter on alternative medicine.

Part IV: Coping Strategies includes helpful information on diet, pain, fatigue, depression, sexuality, and other coping issues that the cancer patient will find useful.

Part V: Additional Help and Information contains an extensive glossary of terms that the cancer patient might hear during discussions of the disease and a directory of cancer organizations for further information.

Bibliographic Note

This volume contains documents and excerpts from publications issued by the following U.S. government agencies: National Institute of Health (NIH); National Cancer Institute (NCI); U. S. Department of Health and Human Services (DHHS); Public Health Service (PHS);

National Institutes of Mental Health (NIMH); and the Agency for Health Care Policy and Research (AHCPR).

In addition, this volume contains copyrighted documents from the following organizations or journals: *The Johns Hopkins Medical Letter*; *Journal of the National Cancer Institute*; *Cancer Nursing*; Oncology Nursing Society, and Tirgan Oncology Associates.

Full citation information is provided on the first page of each chapter. Every effort has been made to secure all necessary rights to reprint the copyrighted material. If any omissions have been made, please contact Omnigraphics to make corrections for future editions.

Acknowledgements

In addition to the organizations listed above that provided the material presented in this volume, special thanks are due to series editor Karen Bellenir for her unswerving instincts, researchers Joan Margeson and Margaret Mary Missar, permissions specialist Maria Franklin, verification assistant Dawn Matthews, and document engineer Bruce Bellenir. The index was prepared by members of EdIndex, Services for Publishers.

Note from the Editor

This book is part of Omnigraphics' *Health Reference Series*. The series provides basic consumer health information about a broad range of medical concerns. It is not intended to serve as a tool for diagnosing illness, in prescribing treatments, or as a substitute for the physician/patient relationship. All persons concerned about medical symptoms or the possibility of disease are encouraged to seek professional care from an appropriate health care provider.

Our Advisory Board

The *Health Reference Series* is reviewed by an Advisory Board comprised of librarians from public, academic, and medical libraries. We would like to thank the following board members for providing guidance to the development of this series:

Dr. Lynda Baker,
Associate Professor of Library and Information Science
Wayne State University, Detroit, MI

Nancy Bulgarelli
William Beaumont Hospital Library, Royal Oak, MI

Karen Imarasio
Bloomfield Township Public Library, Bloomfield Township, MI

Karen Morgan
Mardigian Library, University of Michigan-Dearborn,
Dearborn, MI

Rosemary Orlando
St. Clair Shores Public Library, St. Clair Shores, MI

Health Reference Series *Update Policy*

The inaugural book in the *Health Reference Series* was the first edition of *Cancer Sourcebook* published in 1992. Since then, the *Series* has been enthusiastically received by librarians and in the medical community. In order to maintain the standard of providing high-quality health information for the lay person, the editorial staff at Omnigraphics felt it was necessary to implement a policy of updating volumes when warranted.

Medical researchers have been making tremendous strides, and it is the purpose of the *Health Reference Series* to stay current with the most recent advances. Each decision to update a volume will be made on an individual basis. Some of the considerations will include how much new information is available and the feedback we receive from people who use the books. If there is a topic you would like to see added to the update list, or an area of medical concern you feel has not been adequately addressed, please write to:

Editor
Health Reference Series
Omnigraphics, Inc.
615 Griswold Street
Detroit, MI 48226

The commitment to providing on-going coverage of important medical developments has also led to some format changes in the *Health Reference Series*. Beginning with books published in 1999, each volume on a new topic will be individually titled and called a "First Edition." Subsequent updates will carry sequential edition numbers. To help avoid confusion and to provide maximum flexibility in our ability to respond to informational needs, the practice of consecutively numbering each volume has been discontinued.

Part One

Introduction

Chapter 1

Cancer: An Overview

What You Need to Know about Cancer

This chapter from the National Cancer Institute (NCI) will give you some important information about cancer. It describes some of the warning signs of cancer and stresses the importance of early detection. It also explains how this disease is diagnosed and treated and has information to help you deal with cancer if it affects you or someone you know. This chapter also lists some possible causes of cancer and suggests ways to avoid many of them.

Our publications cannot answer every question you may have about cancer. They cannot take the place of talks with doctors, nurses, and other members of the health care team. We hope our information will help with those talks.

Researchers continue to look for better ways to diagnose and treat cancer, and our knowledge is growing. For up-to-date information about cancer, call the NCI-supported Cancer Information Service (CIS) toll free at 1-800-4-CANCER (1-800-422-6237).

What Is Cancer?

Cancer is a group of more than 100 different diseases. Cancer occurs when cells become abnormal and keep dividing and forming more cells without control or order.

What You Need to Know about Cancer, NIH Publication No. 98-1563, updated September 1999.

All organs of the body are made up of cells. Normally, cells divide to produce more cells only when the body needs them. This orderly process helps keep us healthy.

If cells keep dividing when new cells are not needed, a mass of tissue forms. This mass of extra tissue, called a growth or tumor, can be benign or malignant.

- Benign tumors are not cancer. They can usually be removed and, in most cases, they do not come back. Most important, cells from benign tumors do not spread to other parts of the body. Benign tumors are rarely a threat to life.

- Malignant tumors are cancer. Cancer cells can invade and damage nearby tissues and organs. Also, cancer cells can break away from a malignant tumor and enter the bloodstream or the lymphatic system. This is how cancer spreads from the original (primary) tumor to form new tumors in other parts of the body. The spread of cancer is called metastasis.

Most cancers are named for the type of cell or the organ in which they begin. When cancer spreads, the new tumor has the same kind of abnormal cells and the same name as the primary tumor. For example, if lung cancer spreads to the liver, the cancer cells in the liver are lung cancer cells. The disease is called metastatic lung cancer (it is not liver cancer).

Early Detection

In many cases, the sooner cancer is diagnosed and treated, the better a person's chance for a full recovery. If you develop cancer, you can improve the chance that it will be detected early if you have regular medical checkups and do certain self-exams. Often a doctor can find early cancer during a physical exam or with routine tests even if a person has no symptoms. Some important medical exams, tests, and self-exams are discussed on the next pages. The doctor may suggest other exams for people who are at increased risk for cancer.

Ask your doctor about your cancer risk, about problems to watch for, and about a schedule of regular checkups. The doctor's advice will be based on your age, medical history, and other risk factors. The doctor also can help you learn about self-exams. (More information and free booklets about self-exams are available from the Cancer Information Service.

Many local health departments have information about cancer screening or early detection programs. The Cancer Information Service also can tell you about such programs.

Exams for Both Men and Women

Skin. The doctor should examine your skin during regular check-ups for signs of skin cancer. You should also check regularly for new growths, sores that do not heal, changes in the size, shape, or color of any moles, or any other changes on the skin. Warning signs like these should be reported to the doctor right away.

Colon and Rectum. Beginning at age 50, you should have a yearly fecal occult blood test. This test is a check for hidden (occult) blood in the stool. A small amount of stool is placed on a plastic slide or on special paper. It may be tested in the doctor's office or sent to a lab. This test is done because cancer of the colon and rectum may cause bleeding. However, noncancerous conditions may also cause bleeding, so having blood in the stool does not necessarily mean a person has cancer. If blood is found, the doctor orders more tests to help make a diagnosis.

To check for cancer of the rectum, the doctor inserts a gloved finger into the rectum and feels for any bumps or abnormal areas. A digital rectal exam should be done during regular checkups.

Every 3 to 5 years after age 50, you should have sigmoidoscopy. In this exam, the doctor uses a thin, flexible tube with a light to look inside the rectum and colon for abnormal areas.

Mouth. Your doctor and dentist should examine your mouth at regular visits. Also, by looking in a mirror, you can check inside your mouth for changes in the color of the lips, gums, tongue, or inner cheeks, and for scabs, cracks, sores, white patches, swelling, or bleeding. It is often possible to see or feel changes in the mouth that might be cancer or a condition that might lead to cancer. Any symptoms in your mouth should be checked by a doctor or dentist. Oral exams are especially important for people who use alcohol or tobacco products and for anyone over age 50.

Exams for Men

Prostate. Men over age 40 should have a yearly digital rectal exam to check the prostate gland for hard or lumpy areas. The doctor feels the prostate through the wall of the rectum.

Testicles. Testicular cancer occurs most often between ages 15 and 34. Most of these cancers are found by men themselves, often by doing a testicular self exam. If you find a lump or notice another change, such as heaviness, swelling, unusual tenderness, or pain, you should see your doctor. Also, the doctor should examine the testicles as part of regular medical checkups.

Exams for Women

Breast. When breast cancer is found early, a woman has more treatment choices and a good chance of complete recovery. So it is important that breast cancer be detected as early as possible. The National Cancer Institute encourages women to take an active part in early detection. They should talk to their doctor about this disease, the symptoms to watch for, and an appropriate schedule of checkups. Women should ask their doctor about:

- Mammograms (x-rays of the breast),

- Breast exams by a doctor or nurse, and

- Breast self-examination (BSE).

A mammogram can often show tumors or changes in the breast before they can be felt or cause symptoms. However, we know mammograms cannot find every abnormal area in the breast. This is especially true in the breasts of young women. Another important step in early detection is for women to have their breasts examined regularly by a doctor or a nurse.

Between visits to the doctor, women should examine their breasts every month. By doing BSE, women learn what looks and feels normal for their breasts, and they are more likely to find a change. Any changes should be reported to the doctor. Most breast lumps are not cancer, but only a doctor can make a diagnosis.

Cervix. Regular pelvic exams and Pap tests are important to detect early cancer of the cervix. In a pelvic exam, the doctor feels the uterus, vagina, ovaries, fallopian tubes, bladder, and rectum for any change in size or shape.

For the Pap test, a sample of cells is collected from the upper vagina and cervix with a small brush or a flat wooden stick. The sample is placed on a glass slide and checked under a microscope for cancer or other abnormal cells.

Women should start having a Pap test every year after they turn 18 or become sexually active. If the results are normal for 3 or more years in a row, a woman may have this test less often, based on her doctor's advice.

Symptoms of Cancer

You should see your doctor for regular checkups and not wait for problems to occur. But you should also know that the following symptoms may be associated with cancer: changes in bowel or bladder habits, a sore that does not heal, unusual bleeding or discharge, thickening or lump in the breast or any other part of the body, indigestion or difficulty swallowing, obvious change in a wart or mole, or nagging cough or hoarseness. These symptoms are not always a sign of cancer. They can also be caused by less serious conditions. Only a doctor can make a diagnosis. It is important to see a doctor if you have any of these symptoms. Don't wait to feel pain: Early cancer usually does not cause pain.

Diagnosis

If you have a sign or symptom that might mean cancer, the doctor will do a physical exam and ask about your medical history. In addition, the doctor usually orders various tests and exams. These may include imaging procedures, which produce pictures of areas inside the body; endoscopy, which allows the doctor to look directly inside certain organs; and laboratory tests. In most cases, the doctor also orders a biopsy, a procedure in which a sample of tissue is removed. A pathologist examines the tissue under a microscope to check for cancer cells.

Imaging

Images of areas inside the body help the doctor tell whether a tumor is present. These images can be made in several ways. In many cases, the doctor uses a special dye so that certain organs show up better on film. The dye may be swallowed or put into the body through a needle or a tube.

X-rays are the most common way doctors make pictures of the inside of the body. In a special kind of x-ray imaging, a CT or CAT scan uses a computer linked to an x-ray machine to make a series of detailed pictures.

In radionuclide scanning, the patient swallows or is given an injection of a mildly radioactive substance. A machine (scanner) measures radioactivity levels in certain organs and prints a picture on paper or film. By looking at the amount of radioactivity in the organs, the doctor can find abnormal areas.

Ultrasonography is another procedure for viewing the inside of the body. High-frequency sound waves that cannot be heard by humans enter the body and bounce back. Their echoes produce a picture called a sonogram. These pictures are shown on a monitor like a TV screen and can be printed on paper.

In MRI, a powerful magnet linked to a computer is used to make detailed pictures of areas in the body. These pictures are viewed on a monitor and can also be printed.

Endoscopy

Endoscopy allows the doctor to look into the body through a thin, lighted tube called an endoscope. The exam is named for the organ involved (for example, colonoscopy to look inside the colon). During the exam, the doctor may collect tissue or cells for closer examination.

Laboratory Tests

Although no single test can be used to diagnose cancer, laboratory tests such as blood and urine tests give the doctor important information. If cancer is present, lab work may show the effects of the disease on the body. In some cases, special tests are used to measure the amount of certain substances in the blood, urine, other body fluids, or tumor tissue. The levels of these substances may become abnormal when certain kinds of cancer are present.

Biopsy

The physical exam, imaging, endoscopy, and lab tests can show that something abnormal is present, but a biopsy is the only sure way to know whether the problem is cancer. In a biopsy, the doctor removes a sample of tissue from the abnormal area or may remove the whole tumor. A pathologist examines the tissue under a microscope. If cancer is present, the pathologist can usually tell what kind of cancer it is and may be able to judge whether the cells are likely to grow slowly or quickly.

Staging

When cancer is found, the patient's doctor needs to know the stage, or extent, of the disease to plan the best treatment. The doctor may order various tests and exams to find out whether the cancer has spread and, if so, what parts of the body are affected. In some cases, lymph nodes near the tumor are removed and checked for cancer cells. If cancer cells are found in the lymph nodes, it may mean that the cancer has spread to other organs.

Treatment

Cancer is treated with surgery, radiation therapy, chemotherapy, hormone therapy, or biological therapy. Patients with cancer are often treated by a team of specialists, which may include a medical oncologist (specialist in cancer treatment), a surgeon, a radiation oncologist (specialist in radiation therapy), and others. The doctors may decide to use one treatment method or a combination of methods. The choice of treatment depends on the type and location of the cancer, the stage of the disease, the patient's age and general health, and other factors.

Some cancer patients take part in a clinical trial (research study) using new treatment methods. Such studies are designed to improve cancer treatment.

Getting a Second Opinion

Before starting treatment, the patient may want another doctor to review the diagnosis and treatment plan. Some insurance companies require a second opinion; others may pay for a second opinion if the patient requests it. There are a number of ways to find specialists to consult for a second opinion:

- The patient's doctor may suggest a specialist for a second opinion.

- The Cancer Information Service, at 1-800-4-CANCER, can tell callers about treatment facilities, including cancer centers and other programs in their area supported by the National Cancer Institute.

- Patients can get the names of doctors from their local medical society, a nearby hospital, or a medical school.

Preparing for Treatment

Many people with cancer want to learn all they can about their disease and their treatment choices so they can take an active part in decisions about their medical care. Often, it helps to make a list of questions to ask the doctor. Patients may take notes or, with the doctor's consent, tape record the discussion. Some patients also find it helps to have a family member or friend with them when they talk with the doctor to take part in the discussion, to take notes, or just to listen.

When a person is diagnosed with cancer, shock and stress are natural reactions. These feelings may make it difficult to think of every question to ask the doctor. Patients may find it hard to remember everything the doctor says. They should not feel they need to ask all their questions or remember all the answers at one time. They will have other chances for the doctor to explain things that are not clear and to ask for more information.

Here are some questions a patient may want to ask the doctor:

- What is my diagnosis?
- What is the stage of the disease?
- What are my treatment choices? Which do you recommend for me? Why?
- What are the chances that the treatment will be successful?
- Would a clinical trial be appropriate for me?
- What are the risks and possible side effects for each treatment?
- How long will treatment last?
- Will I have to change my normal activities?
- What is the treatment likely to cost?

Methods of Treatment

Surgery. Surgery is local treatment to remove the tumor. Tissue around the tumor and nearby lymph nodes may also be removed during the operation.

Radiation Therapy. In radiation therapy (also called radiotherapy), high-energy rays are used to damage cancer cells and stop them from growing and dividing. Like surgery, radiation therapy is a local treatment; it can affect cancer cells only in the treated area. Radiation may come from a machine (external radiation). It also may come from an implant (a small container of radioactive material) placed directly into or near the tumor (internal radiation). Some patients get both kinds of radiation therapy.

External radiation therapy is usually given on an outpatient basis in a hospital or clinic 5 days a week for several weeks. Patients are not radioactive during or after the treatment.

For internal radiation therapy, the patient stays in the hospital for a few days. The implant may be temporary or permanent. Because the level of radiation is highest during the hospital stay, patients may not be able to have visitors or may have visitors only for a short time. Once an implant is removed, there is no radioactivity in the body. The amount of radiation in a permanent implant goes down to a safe level before the patient leaves the hospital.

Chemotherapy. Treatment with drugs to kill cancer cells is called chemotherapy. Most anticancer drugs are injected into a vein (IV) or a muscle; some are given by mouth. Chemotherapy is systemic treatment, meaning that the drugs flow through the bloodstream to nearly every part of the body.

Often, patients who need many doses of IV chemotherapy receive the drugs through a catheter (a thin flexible tube). One end of the catheter is placed in a large vein in the chest. The other end is outside the body or attached to a small device just under the skin. Anticancer drugs are given through the catheter. This can make chemotherapy more comfortable for the patient. Patients and their families are shown how to care for the catheter and keep it clean. For some types of cancer, doctors are studying whether it helps to put anticancer drugs directly into the affected area.

Chemotherapy is generally given in cycles: A treatment period is followed by a recovery period, then another treatment period, and so on. Usually a patient has chemotherapy as an outpatient—at the hospital, at the doctor's office, or at home. However, depending on which drugs are given and the patient's general health, the patient may need to stay in the hospital for a short time.

Hormone Therapy. Some types of cancer, including most breast and prostate cancers, depend on hormones to grow. For this reason, doctors may recommend therapy that prevents cancer cells from getting or using the hormones they need. Sometimes, the patient has surgery to remove organs (such as the ovaries or testicles) that make the hormones; in other cases, the doctor uses drugs to stop hormone production or change the way hormones work. Like chemotherapy, hormone therapy is a systemic treatment; it affects cells throughout the body.

Biological Therapy. Biological therapy (also called immunotherapy) is a form of treatment that uses the body's natural ability (immune system) to fight infection and disease or to protect the body from some of the side effects of treatment. Monoclonal antibodies, interferon, interleukin-2 (IL-2), and several types of colony stimulating factors (CSF, GM-CSF, G-CSF) are forms of biological therapy.

Side Effects of Cancer Treatment

It is hard to limit the effects of treatment so that only cancer cells are removed or destroyed. Because treatment also damages healthy cells and tissues, it often causes unpleasant side effects.

The side effects of cancer treatment vary. They depend mainly on the type and extent of the treatment. Also, each person reacts differently. Doctors try to plan the patient's therapy to keep side effects to a minimum and they can help with any problems that occur.

Surgery. The side effects of surgery depend on the location of the tumor, the type of operation, the patient's general health, and other factors. Although patients are often uncomfortable during the first few days after surgery, this pain can be controlled with medicine. Patients should feel free to discuss pain relief with the doctor or nurse. It is also common for patients to feel tired or weak for a while. The length of time it takes to recover from an operation varies for each patient.

Radiation Therapy. With radiation therapy, the side effects depend on the treatment dose and the part of the body that is treated. The most common side effects are tiredness, skin reactions (such as a rash or redness) in the treated area, and loss of appetite. Radiation therapy also may cause a decrease in the number of white blood cells, cells that help protect the body against infection.

Although the side effects of radiation therapy can be unpleasant, the doctor can usually treat or control them. It also helps to know that, in most cases, they are not permanent.

Chemotherapy. The side effects of chemotherapy depend mainly on the drugs and the doses the patient receives. Generally, anticancer drugs affect cells that divide rapidly. These include blood cells, which fight infection, help the blood to clot, or carry oxygen to all parts of the body. When blood cells are affected by anticancer drugs, patients are more likely to get infections, may bruise or bleed easily, and may have less energy. Cells that line the digestive tract also divide rapidly. As a result of chemotherapy, patients may have side effects, such as loss of appetite, nausea and vomiting, hair loss, or mouth sores. For some patients, the doctor may prescribe medicine to help with side effects, especially with nausea and vomiting. Usually, these side effects gradually go away during the recovery period or after treatment stops.

Hair loss, another side effect of chemotherapy, is a major concern for many patients. Some chemotherapy drugs only cause the hair to thin out, while others may result in the loss of all body hair. Patients may feel better if they decide how to handle hair loss before starting treatment.

In some men and women, chemotherapy drugs cause changes that may result in a loss of fertility (the ability to have children). Loss of fertility may be temporary or permanent depending on the drugs used and the patient's age. For men, sperm banking before treatment may be a choice. Women's menstrual periods may stop, and they may have hot flashes and vaginal dryness. Periods are more likely to return in young women.

In some cases, bone marrow transplantation and peripheral stem cell support are used to replace tissue that forms blood cells when that tissue has been destroyed by the effects of chemotherapy or radiation therapy.

Hormone Therapy. Hormone therapy can cause a number of side effects. Patients may have nausea and vomiting, swelling or weight gain, and, in some cases, hot flashes. In women, hormone therapy also may cause interrupted menstrual periods, vaginal dryness, and, sometimes, loss of fertility. Hormone therapy in men may cause impotence, loss of sexual desire, or loss of fertility. These changes may be temporary, long lasting, or permanent.

Biological Therapy. The side effects of biological therapy depend on the type of treatment. Often, these treatments cause flu-like symptoms such as chills, fever, muscle aches, weakness, loss of appetite, nausea, vomiting, and diarrhea. Some patients get a rash, and some bleed or bruise easily. In addition, interleukin therapy can cause swelling. Depending on how severe these problems are, patients may need to stay in the hospital during treatment. These side effects are usually short-term; they gradually go away after treatment stops.

Doctors and nurses can explain the side effects of cancer treatment and help with any problems that occur. The National Cancer Institute booklets *Radiation Therapy and You* and *Chemotherapy and You* also have helpful information about cancer treatment and coping with side effects.

Nutrition for Cancer Patients

Some patients lose their appetite and find it hard to eat well. In addition, the common side effects of treatment, such as nausea, vomiting, or mouth sores, can make it difficult to eat. For some patients, foods taste different. Also, people may not feel like eating when they are uncomfortable or tired.

Eating well means getting enough calories and protein to help prevent weight loss and regain strength. Patients who eat well during cancer treatment often feel better and have more energy. In addition, they may be better able to handle the side effects of treatment.

Doctors, nurses, and dietitians can offer advice for healthy eating during cancer treatment. Patients and their families also may want to read the National Cancer Institute booklet *Eating Hints for Cancer Patients*, which contains many useful suggestions.

Clinical Trials

When laboratory research shows that a new treatment method has promise, cancer patients can receive the treatment in carefully controlled trials. These trials are designed to find out whether the new approach is both safe and effective and to answer scientific questions. Often, clinical trials compare a new treatment with a standard approach so that doctors can learn which is more effective.

Researchers also look for ways to reduce the side effects of treatment and improve the quality of patients' lives. Patients who take part in clinical trials make an important contribution to medical science. These patients take certain risks, but they also may have the first chance to benefit from improved treatment methods.

Clinical trials offer important options for many patients. Cancer patients who are interested in taking part in a clinical trial should talk with their doctor. They may want to read *Taking Part in Clinical Trials: What Cancer Patients Need To Know*, a booklet that explains treatment studies and outlines some of their possible benefits and risks.

One way to learn about clinical trials is through PDQ, a computerized resource developed by the National Cancer Institute. PDQ contains information about cancer treatment and about clinical trials in progress all over the country. The Cancer Information Service can provide PDQ information to doctors, patients, and the public.

Support for Cancer Patients

Living with a serious disease is difficult. Cancer patients and those who care about them face many problems and challenges. Coping with these problems is often easier when people have helpful information and support services.

Cancer patients may worry about holding their job, caring for their family, or keeping up daily activities. Worries about tests, treatments, hospital stays, and medical bills are also common. Doctors, nurses, and other members of the health care team can answer questions about treatment, working, or daily activities. Meeting with a social worker, counselor, or member of the clergy also can be helpful to patients who want to talk about their feelings or discuss their concerns about the future or about personal relationships.

Friends and relatives, especially those who have had personal experience with cancer, can be very supportive. Also, it helps many patients to meet with others who are facing problems like theirs. Cancer patients often get together in support groups, where they can share what they have learned about cancer and its treatment and about coping with the disease. It is important to keep in mind, however, that each patient is different. Treatments and ways of dealing with cancer that work for one person may not be right for another—even if both have the same kind of cancer. It is always a good idea to discuss the advice of friends and family members with the doctor.

Often, a social worker at the hospital or clinic can suggest groups that help with rehabilitation, emotional support, financial aid, transportation, or home care. The American Cancer Society has many services for patients and families. Local offices of the American Cancer Society are listed in the white pages of the telephone directory.

In addition, the public library has many books and articles on living with cancer. The Cancer Information Service also has information on local resources.

What the Future Holds

Researchers are finding better ways to detect and treat cancer, and the chance of recovery keeps improving. Still, it is natural for patients to be concerned about their future.

Sometimes patients use statistics to try to figure out their chance of being cured. It is important to remember, however, that statistics are averages based on large numbers of patients. They cannot be used to predict what will happen to a particular patient because no two patients are alike. The doctor who takes care of the patient is in the best position to discuss the chance of recovery (prognosis). Patients should feel free to ask the doctor about their prognosis, but they should keep in mind that not even the doctor knows exactly what will happen. Doctors often talk about surviving cancer, or they may use the term remission rather than cure. Even though many cancer patients are cured, doctors use these terms because the disease may recur.

Causes and Prevention of Cancer

The number of new cases of cancer in the United States is going up each year. People of all ages get cancer, but nearly all types are more common in middle-aged and elderly people than in young people. Skin cancer is the most common type of cancer for both men and women. The next most common type among men is prostate cancer; among women, it is breast cancer. Lung cancer, however, is the leading cause of death from cancer for both men and women in the United States. Brain cancer and leukemia are the most common cancers in children and young adults.

The more we can learn about what causes cancer, the more likely we are to find ways to prevent it. Scientists study patterns of cancer in the population to look for factors that affect the risk of developing this disease. In the laboratory, they explore possible causes of cancer and try to determine what actually happens when normal cells become cancerous.

Our current understanding of the causes of cancer is incomplete, but it is clear that cancer is not caused by an injury, such as a bump or bruise. And although being infected with certain viruses may increase the risk of some types of cancer, cancer is not contagious; no one can "catch" cancer from another person.

Cancer develops gradually as a result of a complex mix of factors related to environment, lifestyle, and heredity. Scientists have identified many risk factors that increase the chance of getting cancer. They estimate that about 80 percent of all cancers are related to the use of tobacco products, to what we eat and drink, or, to a lesser extent, to exposure to radiation or cancer-causing agents (carcinogens) in the environment and the workplace. Some people are more sensitive than others to factors that can cause cancer.

16

Many risk factors can be avoided. Others, such as inherited risk factors, are unavoidable. It is helpful to be aware of them, but it is also important to keep in mind that not everyone with a particular risk factor for cancer actually gets the disease; in fact, most do not. People at risk can help protect themselves by avoiding risk factors where possible and by getting regular checkups so that, if cancer develops, it is likely to be found early.

These are some of the factors that are known to increase the risk of cancer:

Tobacco. Tobacco causes cancer. In fact, smoking tobacco, using "smokeless" tobacco, and being regularly exposed to environmental tobacco smoke without actually smoking are responsible for one-third of all cancer deaths in the United States each year. Tobacco use is the most preventable cause of death in this country.

Smoking accounts for more than 85 percent of all lung cancer deaths. If you smoke, your risk of getting lung cancer is affected by the number and type of cigarettes you smoke and how long you have been smoking. Overall, for those who smoke one pack a day, the chance of getting lung cancer is about 10 times greater than for nonsmokers. Smokers are also more likely than nonsmokers to develop several other types of cancer (such as oral cancer and cancers of the larynx, esophagus, pancreas, bladder, kidney, and cervix). The risk of cancer begins to decrease when a smoker quits, and the risk continues to decline gradually each year after quitting.

The use of smokeless tobacco (chewing tobacco and snuff) causes cancer of the mouth and throat. Precancerous conditions, or tissue changes that may lead to cancer, begin to go away after a person stops using smokeless tobacco.

Exposure to environmental tobacco smoke, also called involuntary smoking, increases the risk of lung cancer for nonsmokers. The risk goes up 30 percent or more for a nonsmoking spouse of a person who smokes. Involuntary smoking causes about 3,000 lung cancer deaths in this country each year.

If you use tobacco in any form and you need help quitting, talk with your doctor or dentist, or join a smoking cessation group sponsored by a local hospital or voluntary organization. For information on such groups or other programs, call the Cancer Information Service or the American Cancer Society.

Diet. Your choice of foods may affect your chance of developing cancer. Evidence points to a link between a high-fat diet and certain cancers, such as cancer of the breast, colon, uterus, and prostate. Being seriously overweight appears to be linked to increased rates of cancer of the prostate, pancreas, uterus, colon, and ovary, and to breast cancer in older women. On the other hand, studies suggest that foods containing fiber and certain nutrients help protect us against some types of cancer.

You may be able to reduce your cancer risk by making some simple food choices. Try to have a varied, well balanced diet that includes generous amounts of foods that are high in fiber, vitamins, and minerals. At the same time, try to cut down on fatty foods. You should eat five servings of fruits and vegetables each day, choose more whole-grain breads and cereals, and cut down on eggs, high-fat meat, high-fat dairy products (such as whole milk, butter, and most cheeses), salad dressings, margarine, and cooking oils.

Sunlight. Ultraviolet radiation from the sun and from other sources (such as sunlamps and tanning booths) damages the skin and can cause skin cancer. Repeated exposure to ultraviolet radiation increases the risk of skin cancer, especially if you have fair skin or freckle easily. The sun's ultraviolet rays are strongest during the summer from about 11 a.m. to about 3 p.m. (daylight saving time). The risk is greatest at this time, when the sun is high overhead and shadows are short. As a rule, it is best to avoid the sun when your shadow is shorter than you are.

Protective clothing, such as a hat and long sleeves, can help block the sun's harmful rays. You can also use sunscreens to help protect yourself. Sunscreens are rated in strength according to their SPF (sun protection factor), which ranges from 2 to 30 and higher. Those rated 15 to 30 block most of the sun's harmful rays.

Alcohol. Drinking large amounts of alcohol increases the risk of cancer of the mouth, throat, esophagus, and larynx. (People who smoke cigarettes and drink alcohol have an especially high risk of getting these cancers.) Alcohol can damage the liver and increase the risk of liver cancer. Some studies suggest that drinking alcohol also increases the risk of breast cancer. So if you drink at all, do so in moderation—not more than one or two drinks a day.

Radiation. Exposure to large doses of radiation from medical x-rays can increase the risk of cancer. X-rays used for diagnosis expose you to very little radiation and the benefits nearly always outweigh the risks.

However, repeated exposure can be harmful, so it is a good idea to talk with your doctor or dentist about the need for each x-ray and ask about the use of shields to protect other parts of your body.

Before 1950, x-rays were used to treat noncancerous conditions (such as an enlarged thymus, enlarged tonsils and adenoids, ringworm of the scalp, and acne) in children and young adults. People who have received radiation to the head and neck have a higher-than-average risk of developing thyroid cancer years later. People with a history of such treatments should report it to their doctor and should have a careful exam of the neck every I or 2 years.

Chemicals and other substances in the workplace. Being exposed to substances such as metals, dust, chemicals, or pesticides at work can increase the risk of cancer. Asbestos, nickel, cadmium, uranium, radon, vinyl chloride, benzidene, and benzene are well known examples of carcinogens in the workplace. These may act alone or along with another carcinogen, such as cigarette smoke. For example, inhaling asbestos fibers increases the risk of lung diseases, including cancer, and the cancer risk is especially high for asbestos workers who smoke. It is important to follow work and safety rules to avoid contact with dangerous materials.

Hormone replacement therapy. Many women use estrogen therapy to control the hot flashes, vaginal dryness, and osteoporosis (thinning of the bones) that may occur during menopause. However, studies show that estrogen use increases the risk of cancer of the uterus. Other studies suggest an increased risk of breast cancer among women who have used high doses of estrogen or have used estrogen for a long time. At the same time, taking estrogen may reduce the risk of heart disease and osteoporosis.

The risk of uterine cancer appears to be less when progesterone is used with estrogen than when estrogen is used alone. But some scientists are concerned that the addition of progesterone may also increase the risk of breast cancer.

Researchers are still studying and finding new information about the risks and benefits of taking replacement hormones. A woman considering hormone replacement therapy should discuss these issues with her doctor.

Diethylstilbestrol (DES). DES is a form of estrogen that doctors prescribed from the early 1940s until 1971 to try to prevent miscarriage. In some daughters of women who were given DES during pregnancy, the uterus, vagina, and cervix do not develop normally. DES-exposed daughters also have an increased chance of developing abnormal cells (dysplasia) in the cervix and vagina. In addition, a rare type of vaginal and cervical cancer has been found in a small number of DES-exposed daughters. Women who took DES during pregnancy may have a slightly increased risk of developing breast cancer. DES-exposed mothers and daughters should tell their doctor about this exposure. DES daughters should have regular special pelvic exams by a doctor familiar with conditions related to DES.

Exposure to DES before birth does not appear to increase the risk of cancer in DES-exposed sons; however, reproductive and urinary system problems may occur. These men should tell the doctor and should have regular medical checkups.

Close relatives with certain types of cancer. A small number of cancers (including melanoma and cancers of the breast, ovary, and colon) tend to occur more often in some families than in the rest of the population. It is not always clear whether a pattern of cancer in a family is due to heredity, factors in the family's environment, or chance. Still, if close relatives have been affected by cancer, it is important to let your doctor know this and then follow the doctor's advice about cancer prevention and checkups to detect problems early.

Resources

Information about cancer is available from many sources, including the ones listed below. You may wish to check for additional information at your local library or bookstore and from support groups in your community.

Cancer Information Service

The Cancer Information Service, a program of the National Cancer Institute, is a nationwide telephone service for cancer patients and their families and friends, the public, and health care professionals. The staff can answer questions in English or Spanish and can send free printed material on cancer prevention, early detection and self-exams, specific types of cancer, cancer treatment, and living with cancer. They also know about local resources and services. One toll-free number, 1-800-4-CANCER (1-800-422-6237), connects callers with the office that serves their area.

American Cancer Society

The American Cancer Society is a voluntary organization with a national office and local units all over the country. It supports research, conducts educational programs, and offers many services to patients and their families. It also provides free booklets about cancer. To obtain information about services and activities in local areas, call the Society's toll-free number, 1-800-ACS-2345 (1-800-227-2345), or the number listed under American Cancer Society in the white pages of the telephone book.

Chapter 2

Questions and Answers about Cancer

Important Questions

1. What is cancer?

Cancer is a group of many different diseases that have some important things in common. Cancer affects our cells, the body's basic unit of life.

To understand cancer, it is helpful to know how normal cells become cancerous. The body is made up of many types of cells. Normally, cells grow, divide, and produce more cells to keep the body healthy and functioning properly. Sometimes, however, the process goes astray—cells keep dividing when new cells are not needed. The mass of extra cells forms a growth or tumor. Some types of cells are more prone to abnormal growth than others. Tumors can be benign or malignant.

Benign tumors are not cancer. They often can be removed and, in most cases, they do not come back. Cells in benign tumors do not spread to other parts of the body. Most important, benign tumors are rarely a threat to life.

Malignant tumors are cancer. Cells in malignant tumors are abnormal and divide without control or order. These cancer cells can invade and destroy the tissue around them. Cancer cells can also

---

This Chapter is comprised of two documents: "Questions and Answers About Cancer," June 1998; and "Understanding Prognosis and Cancer Statistics," June 1997. Both are National Cancer Institute Fact Sheets.

break away from a malignant tumor and enter the bloodstream or lymphatic system vessels (the two systems of vessels that bathe and feed all of the body's organs). This process, called metastasis, is how cancer spreads from the original tumor to form new tumors in other parts of the body.

2. What are some of the common signs and symptoms of cancer?

Cancer can cause a variety of symptoms. These are some of them:

- Change in bowel or bladder habits,
- A sore that does not heal,
- Unusual bleeding or discharge,
- Thickening or lump in the breast or any other part of the body,
- Indigestion or difficulty swallowing,
- Obvious change in a wart or mole,
- Nagging cough or hoarseness.

When these or other symptoms occur, they are not sure signs of cancer. Symptoms may be caused by infections, benign tumors, or other problems. It is important to see a doctor if you have any of these symptoms or if you are concerned about other changes in your body or the way you feel. Only a doctor can make a diagnosis. Don't wait to feel pain: Early cancer usually does not cause pain.

If symptoms occur, the doctor may order various tests and/or a biopsy. A biopsy is the most reliable way to know whether a medical problem is cancer. During a biopsy, the doctor removes a sample of tissue from the abnormal area. The tissue is then examined under a microscope to check for cancer cells.

3. How is cancer treated?

Cancer may be treated with surgery, radiation therapy, chemotherapy, hormone therapy, or biological therapy. The doctor may use one method or a combination of methods. The choice of treatment depends on the type and location of the cancer, whether the disease has spread, the patient's age and general health, and other factors.

An important option for people with cancer is to take part in clinical trials. Doctors conduct clinical trials to learn about the effectiveness and side effects of new treatments. Through research, doctors learn new ways to treat cancer that may be more effective than the standard therapy. In some studies, all patients receive the new treatment. In others, doctors compare different therapies by giving the new treatment to one group of patients and the standard therapy to another group. Research like this has led to significant advances in the treatment of cancer. People who take part in these studies have the first chance to benefit from treatments that have shown promise. They also make an important contribution to medical science.

4. Can cancer be prevented?

Cancer develops gradually as a result of a complex mix of factors related to environment, lifestyle, and heredity. Scientists have identified many factors that increase the chance of getting cancer. Some people are more sensitive than others to factors that can cause cancer.

Many cases of cancer can be prevented by not using tobacco products, avoiding harmful rays of the sun, and choosing foods with less fat and more fiber. In addition, alcohol and exposure to certain chemicals and/or radiation may increase a person's risk of developing cancer.

Many risk factors can be avoided. Others, such as inherited factors, are unavoidable. It is helpful to be aware of them, but it is also important to keep in mind that not everyone with a particular risk factor for cancer actually gets the disease; in fact, most do not. People who have an increased likelihood of getting cancer can help protect themselves by avoiding risk factors where possible and by getting regular checkups so that, if cancer develops, it is likely to be found early. Treatment is likely to be more effective when cancer is detected early.

Understanding Prognosis and Cancer Statistics

It is natural for anyone facing cancer to be concerned about what the future holds. Understanding the nature of cancer and what to expect can help patients and their loved ones plan treatment, anticipate lifestyle changes, and make quality of life and financial decisions. Cancer patients frequently ask their doctor or search on their own for statistics to answer the question, "What is my prognosis?"

Prognosis is a prediction of the future course and outcome of a disease and an indication of the likelihood of recovery from that disease. However, it is only a prediction. When doctors discuss a patient's prognosis, they are attempting to project what is likely to occur for that individual patient. The doctor may speak of a favorable prognosis, if the cancer is expected to respond well to treatment, or an unfavorable prognosis, if the cancer is likely to be difficult to control.

A cancer patient's prognosis can be affected by many factors, particularly the type of cancer the patient has, the stage of the cancer (the extent to which the cancer has metastasized, or spread), or its grade (how aggressive the cancer is or how closely the cancer resembles normal tissue). Other factors that may also affect a person's prognosis include the patient's age and general health or the effectiveness of treatment.

Statistics are also used by the doctor to help estimate prognosis. Survival statistics indicate how many people with a certain type and stage of cancer survive the disease. The 5-year survival rates are the most common measure used. They measure the effect of the cancer over a 5 year period of time. Survival rates include persons who survive 5 years after diagnosis, whether in remission, disease-free, or under treatment. It is important to understand that statistics alone cannot be used to predict what will happen to a particular patient because no two patients are exactly alike.

Patients and their loved ones face many uncertainties when dealing with cancer. For some, coping is easier if they know the statistics; for others, statistical information is confusing, fearful, and too impersonal to be of use. The doctor who is most familiar with the patient's situation is in the best position to discuss a patient's prognosis and to help interpret what the statistics may mean for them.

If patients or their loved ones feel they want to know prognostic information, they should talk with the doctor. At the same time, it is important for patients to understand that even the doctor cannot tell them exactly what to expect; in fact, a patient's prognosis may change over time if the cancer progresses, or if treatment is successful.

Seeking prognosis information and understanding statistics can help some patients reduce their fears as they learn more about what their prognosis means for them. It is a personal decision and the patient's choice about how much information to accept and how to deal with it.

National Cancer Institute Information Resources

You may want more information for yourself, your family, and your doctor. The following National Cancer Institute (NCI) services are available to help you.

Telephone

Cancer Information Service (CIS) Provides accurate, up-to-date information on cancer to patients and their families, health professionals, and the general public. Information specialists translate the latest scientific information into understandable language and respond in English, Spanish, or on TTY equipment. Toll-free: 1-800-4-CANCER (1-800-422-6237). TTY: 1-800-332-8615

Internet

These web sites may be useful:

http://www.nci.nih.gov—NCI's primary web site; contains information about the Institute and its programs. Also includes news, upcoming events, educational materials, and publications for patients, the public, and the mass media on http://rex.nci.nih.gov.

http://cancernet.nci.nih.gov—CancerNet; contains material for health professionals, patients, and the public, including information from PDQ about cancer treatment, screening, prevention, supportive care, and clinical trials, and CANCERLIT, a bibliographic database.

http://cancertrials.nci.nih.gov—CancerTrials; NCI's comprehensive clinical trials information center for patients, health professionals, and the public. Includes information on understanding trials, deciding whether to participate in trials, finding specific trials, plus research news and other resources.

E-mail

CancerMail. Includes NCI information about cancer treatment, screening, prevention, and supportive care. To obtain a contents list, send e-mail to cancermail@icicc.nci.nih.gov with the word "help" in the body of the message.

Fax

CancerFax. Includes NCI information about cancer treatment, screening, prevention, and supportive care. To obtain a contents list, dial 301-402-5874 from a fax machine hand set and follow the recorded instructions.

Part Two

Types of Cancer

Chapter 3

Brain Tumors

Each year more than 17,000 people in the United States find out they have a brain tumor. The National Cancer Institute (NCI) has written this chapter to help patients and their families and friends better understand brain tumors. We also hope others will read it to learn more about these tumors.

This chapter describes the symptoms, diagnosis, and treatment of brain tumors. Other NCI publications about cancer, its treatment, and living with the disease are listed below in the section entitled "Other Booklets." We know that booklets cannot answer every question about brain tumors. They cannot take the place of talks with doctors, nurses, and other members of the health care team, but we hope our information will help with these talks.

The Brain

Together, the brain and spinal cord form the central nervous system. This complex system is part of everything we do. It controls the things we choose to do—like walk and talk—and the things our body does automatically like breathe and digest food. The central nervous system is also involved with our senses—seeing, hearing, touching, tasting, and smelling—as well as our emotions, thoughts, and memory.

What You Need To Know About Brain Tumors, National Cancer Institute (NCI) Publication 98-1558, September 1998.

The Brain and Spinal Cord

The brain is a soft, spongy mass of nerve cells and supportive tissue. It has three major parts: the cerebrum, the cerebellum, and the brain stem. The parts work together, but each has special functions.

The cerebrum, the largest part of the brain, fills most of the upper skull. It has two halves called the left and right cerebral hemispheres. The cerebrum uses information from our senses to tell us what's going on around us and tells our body how to respond. The right hemisphere controls the muscles on the left side of the body, and the left hemisphere controls the muscles on the right side of the body. This part of the brain also controls speech and emotions as well as reading, thinking, and learning.

The cerebellum, under the cerebrum at the back of the brain, controls balance and complex actions like walking and talking.

The brain stem connects the brain with the spinal cord. It controls hunger and thirst and some of the most basic body functions, such as body temperature, blood pressure, and breathing.

The brain is protected by the bones of the skull and by a covering of three thin membranes called meninges. The brain is also cushioned and protected by cerebrospinal fluid. This watery fluid is produced by special cells in the four hollow spaces in the brain, called ventricles. It flows through the ventricles and in spaces between the meninges. Cerebrospinal fluid also brings nutrients from the blood to the brain and removes waste products from the brain.

Spaces that Contain Cerebrospinal Fluid

The spinal cord is made up of bundles of nerve fibers. It runs down from the brain through a canal in the center of the bones of the spine. These bones protect the spinal cord. Like the brain, the spinal cord is covered by the meninges and cushioned by cerebrospinal fluid.

Spinal nerves connect the brain with the nerves in most parts of the body. Other nerves go directly from the brain to the eyes, ears, and other parts of the head. This network of nerves carries messages back and forth between the brain and the rest of the body.

About Brain Tumors

The body is made up of many types of cells. Each type of cell has special functions. Most cells in the body grow and then divide in an orderly way to form new cells as they are needed to keep the body healthy and working properly. When cells lose the ability to control their growth, they divide too often and without any order. The extra cells form a mass of tissue called a tumor. Tumors are benign or malignant.

- Benign brain tumors do not contain cancer cells. Usually these tumors can be removed, and they are not likely to recur. Benign brain tumors have clear borders. Although they do not invade nearby tissue, they can press on sensitive areas of the brain and cause symptoms.

- Malignant brain tumors contain cancer cells. They interfere with vital functions and are life threatening. Malignant brain tumors are likely to grow rapidly and crowd or invade the tissue around them. Like a plant, these tumors may put out "roots" that grow into healthy brain tissue. If a malignant tumor remains compact and does not have roots, it is said to be encapsulated. When an otherwise benign tumor is located in a vital area of the brain and interferes with vital functions, it may be considered malignant (even though it contains no cancer cells).

Doctors refer to some brain tumors by grade—from low grade (grade I) to high grade (grade IV). The grade of a tumor refers to the way the cells look under a microscope. Cells from higher grade tumors are more abnormal looking and generally grow faster than cells from lower grade tumors; higher grade tumors are more malignant than lower grade tumors.

Possible Causes

The causes of brain tumors are not known. Researchers are trying to solve this problem. The more they can find out about the causes of brain tumors, the better the chances of finding ways to prevent them. Doctors cannot explain why one person gets a brain tumor and another doesn't, but they do know that no one can "catch" a brain tumor from another person. Brain tumors are not contagious.

Although brain tumors can occur at any age, studies show that they are most common in two age groups. The first group is children 3 to 12 years old; the second is adults 40 to 70 years old.

By studying large numbers of patients, researchers have found certain risk factors that increase a person's chance of developing a brain tumor. People with these risk factors have a higher than average risk of getting a brain tumor. For example, studies show that some types of brain tumors are more frequent among workers in certain industries, such as oil refining, rubber manufacturing, and drug manufacturing. Other studies have shown that chemists and embalmers have a higher incidence of brain tumors. Researchers also are looking at exposure to viruses as a possible cause. Because brain tumors sometimes occur in several members of the same family, researchers are studying families with a history of brain tumors to see whether heredity is a cause. At this time, scientists do not believe that head injuries cause brain tumors to develop.

In most cases, patients with a brain tumor have no clear risk factors. The disease is probably the result of several factors acting together.

Primary Brain Tumors

Tumors that begin in brain tissue are known as primary brain tumors. (Secondary tumors that develop when cancer spreads to the brain are discussed below.) Primary brain tumors are classified by the type of tissue in which they begin. The most common brain tumors are gliomas, which begin in the glial (supportive) tissue. There are several types of gliomas:

- Astrocytomas arise from small, star-shaped cells called astrocytes. They may grow anywhere in the brain or spinal cord. In adults, astrocytomas most often arise in the cerebrum. In children, they occur in the brain stem, the cerebrum, and the cerebellum. A grade III astrocytoma is sometimes called an anaplastic astrocytoma. A grade IV astrocytoma is usually called glioblastoma multiforme.

- Brain stem gliomas occur in the lowest, stemlike part of the brain. The brain stem controls many vital functions. Tumors in this area generally cannot be removed. Most brain stem gliomas are high-grade astrocytomas.

- Ependymomas usually develop in the lining of the ventricles. They also may occur in the spinal cord. Although these tumors can develop at any age, they are most common in childhood and adolescence.

- Oligodendrogliomas arise in the cells that produce myelin, the fatty covering that protects nerves. These tumors usually arise in the cerebrum. They grow slowly and usually do not spread into surrounding brain tissue. Oligodendrogliomas are rare. They occur most often in middle-aged adults but have been found in people of all ages.

There are other types of brain tumors that do not begin in glial tissue. Some of the most common are described below:

- Medulloblastomas were once thought to develop from glial cells. However, recent research suggests that these tumors develop from primitive (developing) nerve cells that normally do not remain in the body after birth. For this reason, medulloblastomas are sometimes called primitive neuroectodermal tumors (PNET). Most medulloblastomas arise in the cerebellum; however, they may occur in other areas as well. These tumors occur most often in children and are more common in boys than in girls.

- Meningiomas grow from the meninges. They are usually benign. Because these tumors grow very slowly, the brain may be able to adjust to their presence; meningiomas often grow quite large before they cause symptoms. They occur most often in women between 30 and 50 years of age.

- Schwannomas are benign tumors that begin in Schwann cells, which produce the myelin that protects the acoustic nerve—the nerve of hearing. Acoustic neuromas are a type of schwannoma. They occur mainly in adults. These tumors affect women twice as often as men.

- Craniopharyngiomas develop in the region of the pituitary gland near the hypothalamus. They are usually benign; however, they are sometimes considered malignant because they can press on or damage the hypothalamus and affect vital functions. These tumors occur most often in children and adolescents.

- Germ cell tumors arise from primitive (developing) sex cells, or germ cells. The most frequent type of germ cell tumor in the brain is the germinoma.

- Pineal region tumors occur in or around the pineal gland, a tiny organ near the center of the brain. The tumor can be slow growing (pineocytoma) or fast growing (pineoblastoma). The pineal region is very difficult to reach, and these tumors often cannot be removed.

Secondary Brain Tumors

Metastasis is the spread of cancer. Cancer that begins in other parts of the body may spread to the brain and cause secondary tumors. These tumors are not the same as primary brain tumors. Cancer that spreads to the brain is the same disease and has the same name as the original (primary) cancer. For example, if lung cancer spreads to the brain, the disease is called metastatic lung cancer because the cells in the secondary tumor resemble abnormal lung cells, not abnormal brain cells.

Treatment for secondary brain tumors depends on where the cancer started and the extent of the spread, as well as other factors, including the patient's age, general health, and response to previous treatment.

Symptoms of Brain Tumors

The symptoms of brain tumors depend mainly on their size and their location in the brain. Symptoms are caused by damage to vital tissue and by pressure on the brain as the tumor grows within the limited space in the skull. They also may be caused by swelling and a buildup of fluid around the tumor, a condition called edema. Symptoms also may be due to hydrocephalus, which occurs when the tumor blocks the flow of cerebrospinal fluid and causes it to build up in the ventricles. If a brain tumor grows very slowly, its symptoms may appear so gradually that they are overlooked for a long time.

The most frequent symptoms of brain tumors include:

- Headaches that tend to be worse in the morning and ease during the day,
- Seizures (convulsions),
- Nausea or vomiting,
- Weakness or loss of feeling in the arms or legs,
- Stumbling or lack of coordination in walking (ataxic gait),
- Abnormal eye movements or changes in vision,
- Drowsiness,
- Changes in personality or memory, and
- Changes in speech.

These symptoms may be caused by brain tumors or by other problems. Only a doctor can tell for sure.

Diagnosis

To find the cause of a person's symptoms, the doctor asks about the patient's personal and family medical history and does a complete physical examination. In addition to checking general signs of health, the doctor does a neurologic exam. This includes checks for alertness, muscle strength, coordination, reflexes, and response to pain. The doctor also examines the eyes to check for swelling caused by a tumor pressing on the nerve that connects the eye and the brain.

Depending on the results of the physical and neurologic examinations, the doctor may request one or both of the following:

- A CT (or CAT) scan is a series of detailed pictures of the brain. The pictures are created by a computer linked to an x-ray machine. In some cases, a special dye is injected into a vein before the scan. The dye helps to show differences in the tissues of the brain.

- MRI (magnetic resonance imaging) gives pictures of the brain, using a powerful magnet linked to a computer. MRI is especially useful in diagnosing brain tumors because it can "see" through the bones of the skull to the tissue underneath. A special dye may be used to enhance the likelihood of detecting a brain tumor.

The doctor also may request other tests:

- A skull x-ray can show changes in the bones of the skull caused by a tumor. It can also show calcium deposits, which are present in some types of brain tumors.

- In a brain scan, areas of abnormal growth in the brain are revealed and recorded on special film. A small amount of a radioactive material is injected into a vein. This dye is absorbed by the tumor, and the growth shows up on the film. (The radiation leaves the body within 6 hours and is not dangerous.)

- An angiogram, or arteriogram, is a series of x-rays taken after a special dye is injected into an artery (usually in the area where the abdomen joins the top of the leg). The dye, which flows through the blood vessels of the brain, can be seen on the x-rays. These x-rays can show the tumor and the blood vessels that lead to it.

37

- A myelogram is an x-ray of the spine. A special dye is injected into the cerebrospinal fluid in the spine, and the patient is tilted to allow the dye to mix with the fluid. This test may be done when the doctor suspects a tumor in the spinal cord.

Treatment

Treatment for a brain tumor depends on a number of factors. Among these are the type, location, and size of the tumor, as well as the patient's age and general health. Treatment methods and schedules often vary for children and adults. The doctor develops a treatment plan to fit each patient's needs.

The patient's doctor may want to discuss the case with other doctors who treat brain tumors. Also, the patient may want to talk with the doctor about taking part in a research study of new treatment methods. Such studies, called clinical trials, are discussed below.

Many patients want to learn all they can about their disease and their treatment choices so they can take an active part in decisions about their medical care. A person with a brain tumor will have many questions, and the doctor is the best person to answer them. Most patients want to know what kind of tumor they have, how it can be treated, how effective the treatment is likely to be, and how much it's likely to cost. Here are some important questions to ask the doctor:

- What type of treatment will I receive?
- What are the expected benefits of treatment?
- What are the risks and possible side effects of treatment?
- What can be done about side effects?
- Would a clinical trial be appropriate for me?
- Will I need to change my normal activities? For how long?
- How often will I need to have checkups ?

Many people find it helpful to make a list of their questions before they see the doctor. Taking notes can make it easier to remember what the doctor says. Some patients also find that it helps to have a family member or friend with them when they talk with the doctor—either to take part in the discussion or just to listen.

Patients and their families have a lot to learn about brain tumors and their treatment. They should not feel that they need to understand everything the first time they hear it. They will have other chances to ask the doctor to explain things that are not clear.

Planning Treatment

Decisions about treatment for brain tumors are complex. Before starting treatment, the patient might want a second doctor to review the diagnosis and treatment plan. There are several ways to find a doctor to consult:

- The patient's doctor may be able to suggest a doctor who specializes in treating brain tumors.

- The Cancer Information Service, at 1-800-4-CANCER, can tell callers about cancer centers and other NCI-supported programs in their area.

- Patients can get the names of specialists from their local medical society, a nearby hospital or cancer center, or a medical school.

Treatment Methods

Brain tumors are treated with surgery, radiation therapy, and chemotherapy. Depending on the patient's needs, several methods may be used. The patient may be referred to doctors who specialize in different kinds of treatment and work together as a team. This medical team often includes a neurosurgeon, a medical oncologist, a radiation oncologist, a nurse, a dietitian, and a social worker. The patient also might work with a physical therapist, an occupational therapist, and a speech therapist.

Before treatment begins, most patients are given steroids, which are drugs that relieve swelling (edema). They also may be given anticonvulsant medicine to prevent or control seizures. If hydrocephalus is present, the patient may need a shunt to drain the cerebrospinal fluid. A shunt is a long, thin tube placed in a ventricle of the brain and then threaded under the skin to another part of the body, usually the abdomen. It works like a drainpipe: excess fluid is carried away from the brain and is absorbed in the abdomen. (In some cases, the fluid is drained into the heart.)

Surgery is the usual treatment for most brain tumors. To remove a brain tumor, a neurosurgeon makes an opening in the skull. This operation is called a craniotomy.

Whenever possible, the surgeon attempts to remove the entire tumor. However, if the tumor cannot be completely removed without damaging vital brain tissue, the doctor removes as much of the tumor as possible. Partial removal helps to relieve symptoms by reducing pressure on the brain and reduces the amount of tumor to be treated by radiation therapy or chemotherapy.

Some tumors cannot be removed. In such cases, the doctor may do only a biopsy. A small piece of the tumor is removed so that a pathologist can examine it under a microscope to determine the type of cells it contains. This helps the doctor decide which treatment to use.

Sometimes, a biopsy is done with a needle. Doctors use a special headframe (like a halo) and CT scans or MRI to pinpoint the exact location of the tumor. The surgeon makes a small hole in the skull and then guides a needle to the tumor. (Using this technique to do a biopsy or for treatment is called stereotaxis.)

Radiation therapy (also called radiotherapy) is the use of high powered rays to damage cancer cells and stop them from growing. It is often used to destroy tumor tissue that cannot be removed with surgery or to kill cancer cells that may remain after surgery. Radiation therapy is also used when surgery is not possible.

Radiation therapy may be given in two ways. External radiation comes from a large machine. Generally, external radiation treatments are given 5 days a week for several weeks. The treatment schedule depends on the type and size of the tumor and the age of the patient. Giving the total dose of radiation over an extended period helps to protect healthy tissue in the area of the tumor.

Radiation can also come from radioactive materials placed directly in the tumor (implant radiation therapy). Depending on the material used, the implant may be left in the brain for a short time or permanently. Implants lose a little radioactivity each day. The patient stays in the hospital for several days while the radiation is most active.

External radiation may be directed just to the tumor and the tissue close to it or, less often, to the entire brain. (Sometimes the radiation is also directed to the spinal cord.) When the whole brain is treated, the patient often receives an extra dose of radiation to the area of the tumor. This boost can come from external radiation or from an implant.

Stereotactic radiosurgery is another way to treat brain tumors. Doctors use the techniques described above to pinpoint the exact location of the tumor. Treatment is given in just one session; high-energy rays are aimed at the tumor from many angles. In this way, a high dose of radiation reaches the tumor without damaging other brain tissue. (This use of radiation therapy is sometimes called the gamma knife.)

Chemotherapy is the use of drugs to kill cancer cells. The doctor may use just one drug or a combination, usually giving the drugs by mouth or by injection into a blood vessel or muscle. Intrathecal chemotherapy involves injecting the drugs into the cerebrospinal fluid.

Chemotherapy is usually given in cycles: a treatment period followed by a recovery period, then another treatment period, and so on. Patients often do not need to stay in the hospital for treatment. Most drugs can be given in the doctor's office or the outpatient clinic of a hospital. However, depending on the drugs used, the way they are given, and the patient's general health, a short hospital stay may be necessary.

Clinical Trials

Researchers are looking for treatment methods that are more effective against brain tumors and have fewer side effects. When laboratory research shows that a new method has promise, doctors use it to treat cancer patients in clinical trials. These trials are designed to answer scientific questions and to find out whether the new approach is both safe and effective. Patients who take part in clinical trials make an important contribution to medical science and may have the first chance to benefit from improved treatment methods.

Many clinical trials of new treatments for brain tumors are under way. Doctors are studying new types and schedules of radiation therapy, new anticancer drugs, new drug combinations, and combinations of chemotherapy and radiation.

Scientists are trying to increase the effectiveness of radiation therapy by giving treatments twice a day instead of once. Also, they are studying drugs called radiosensitizers. These drugs make the cancer cells more sensitive to radiation. Another method under study is hyperthermia, in which the tumor is heated to increase the effect of radiation therapy.

Many drugs cannot reach brain cells because of the blood-brain barrier, a network of blood vessels and cells that filters blood going to the brain. Researchers continue to look for new drugs that will pass through the blood brain barrier. Studies are under way using different techniques to temporarily disrupt the barrier so that drugs can reach the tumor.

In other studies, scientists are exploring new ways to give the drugs. Drugs may be injected into an artery leading to the brain or may be put directly into the ventricles. Doctors also are studying the effectiveness of placing tiny wafers containing anticancer drugs directly into the tumor. (The wafers dissolve over time.)

Researchers are also testing the use of very high doses of anticancer drugs. Because these higher doses may damage healthy bone marrow, doctors combine this treatment with bone marrow transplantation to replace the marrow that has been destroyed.

Biological therapy is a new way of treating brain tumors that is currently under study. This type of treatment is an attempt to improve the way the body's immune system fights disease.

Patients interested in taking part in a clinical trial should discuss this option with their doctor. They may want to read *What Are Clinical Trials All About?*, an NCI booklet that explains some of the possible benefits and risks of treatment studies.

One way to learn about clinical trials is through PDQ, a computerized resource of cancer treatment information. Developed by NCI, PDQ contains an up-to-date list of trials in progress all over the country. Doctors can use a personal computer or the services of a medical library to get PDQ information. The Cancer Information Service, at 1-800-4-CANCER, is another source of PDQ information for doctors, patients, and the public.

Side Effects of Treatment

Cancer treatment often causes side effects. These side effects occur because treatment to destroy cancer cells damages some healthy cells as well.

The side effects of cancer treatment vary. They depend on the type of treatment used and on the area being treated. Also, each person reacts differently. Doctors try to plan the patient's therapy to keep side effects to a minimum. They also watch patients very carefully so they can help with any problems that occur.

A craniotomy is a major operation. The surgery may damage normal brain tissue, and edema may occur. Weakness, coordination problems, personality changes, and difficulty in speaking and thinking may result. Patients may also have seizures. In fact, for a short time after surgery, symptoms may be worse than before.

Most of the side effects of surgery lessen or disappear with time. Most of the side effects of radiation therapy go away soon after treatment is over. However, some side effects may occur or persist long after treatment is complete.

Some patients have nausea for several hours after treatment. Patients receiving radiation therapy may become very tired as treatment continues. Resting is important, but doctors usually advise their patients to try to stay reasonably active. Radiation therapy to the scalp causes most patients to lose their hair. When it grows back, the new hair is sometimes softer and may be a slightly different color. In some cases, hair loss is permanent.

Skin reactions in the treated area are common. The scalp and ears may be red, itchy, or dark; these areas may look and feel sunburned. The treated area should be exposed to the air as much as possible but should be protected from the sun. Patients should not wear anything on the head that might cause irritation. Good skin care is important at this time. The doctor may suggest certain kinds of soap or ointment, and patients should not use any other lotions or creams on the scalp without the doctor's advice.

Sometimes brain cells killed by radiation form a mass in the brain. The mass may look like a tumor and may cause similar symptoms, such as headaches, memory loss, or seizures. Doctors may suggest surgery or steroids to relieve these problems. About 4 to 8 weeks after radiation therapy, patients may become quite sleepy or lose their appetite. These symptoms may last several weeks, but they usually go away on their own. Still, patients should notify the doctor if they occur.

Children who have had radiation therapy for a brain tumor may have learning problems or partial loss of eyesight. If the pituitary gland is damaged, children may not grow or develop normally.

The side effects of chemotherapy depend on the drugs that are given. In general, anticancer drugs affect rapidly growing cells, such as blood cells that fight infection, cells that line the digestive tract, and cells in hair follicles. As a result, patients may have a lower resistance to infection, loss of appetite, nausea, vomiting, or mouth sores. Patients also may have less energy and may lose their hair. These side effects usually go away gradually after treatment stops.

Some anticancer drugs can cause infertility. Women taking certain anticancer drugs may have symptoms of menopause (hot flashes and vaginal dryness; periods may be irregular or stop). Some drugs used to treat children and teenagers may affect their ability to have children later in life.

Certain drugs used in the treatment of brain tumors may cause kidney damage. Patients are given large amounts of fluid while taking these drugs. Patients also may have tingling in the fingers, ringing in the ears, or difficulty hearing. These problems may not clear up after treatment stops.

Treatment with steroids to reduce swelling in the brain may cause increased appetite and weight gain. Swelling of the face and feet is common. Steroids can also cause restlessness, mood swings, burning indigestion, and acne. Patients should not stop using steroids or change their dose without consulting the doctor, however. The use of steroids must be stopped gradually to allow the body time to adjust.

Loss of appetite can be a problem for patients during therapy. People may not feel hungry when they are uncomfortable or tired. Some of the common side effects of cancer treatment, such as nausea and vomiting, can also make it hard to eat. Yet good nutrition is important because patients who eat well generally feel better and have more energy. In addition, they may be better able to withstand the side effects of treatment. Eating well means getting enough calories and protein to help prevent weight loss, regain strength, and rebuild normal tissues. Many patients find that eating several small meals and snacks during the day works better than trying to have three large meals.

Patients being treated for a brain tumor may develop a blood clot and inflammation in a vein, most often in the leg. This is called thrombophlebitis. A patient who notices swelling in the leg, leg pain, or redness in the leg should notify the doctor right away.

Doctors, nurses, and dietitians can explain the side effects of cancer treatment and can suggest ways to deal with them. In addition, the NCI booklets *Radiation Therapy and You*, *Chemotherapy and You*, and *Eating Hints* contain helpful information about cancer treatment and coping with side effects. *Young People With Cancer: A Handbook for Parents* provides information to help children handle the side effects of treatment.

Rehabilitation

Rehabilitation is a very important part of the treatment plan. The goals of rehabilitation depend on the patient's needs and how the tumor has affected his or her daily activities. The medical team makes every effort to help patients return to their normal activities as soon as possible.

Patients and their families may need to work with an occupational therapist to overcome any difficulty in activities of daily living, such as eating, dressing, bathing, and using the toilet. If an arm or leg is weak or paralyzed, or if a patient has problems with balance, physical therapy may be necessary. Speech therapy may be helpful for individuals having trouble speaking or expressing their thoughts. Speech therapists also work with patients who are having difficulty swallowing.

If special arrangements are necessary for school-age children, they should be made as soon as possible. Sometimes, children have tutors in the hospital or after they go home from the hospital. Children who have problems learning or remembering what they learn may need tutors or special classes when they return to school.

Followup Care

Regular followup is very important after treatment for a brain tumor. The doctor will check closely to be sure that the tumor has not returned. Checkups usually include general physical and neurologic exams. From time to time, the patient will have CT scans or MRI.

Patients who receive radiation therapy to large areas of the brain or certain anticancer drugs may have an increased risk of developing leukemia or a second tumor at a later time. Also, radiation that affects the eyes may lead to the development of cataracts. Patients should carefully follow their doctor's advice on health care and checkups. If any unusual health problem occurs, they should report it to the doctor as soon as it appears.

Living with a Brain Tumor

The diagnosis of a brain tumor can change the lives of patients and the people who care about them. These changes can be hard to handle. Patients and their families and friends may have many different and sometimes confusing emotions.

At times, patients and those close to them may feel frightened, angry, or depressed. These are normal reactions when people face a serious health problem. Most patients, including children and teenagers, find it helps to share their thoughts and feelings with loved ones. Sharing can help everyone feel more at ease and can open the way for others to show their concern and offer their support.

Worries about tests, treatments, hospital stays, rehabilitation, and medical bills are common. Parents may worry about whether their children will be able to take part in normal school or social activities. Doctors, nurses, social workers, and other members of the health care team may be able to calm fears and ease confusion. They also can provide information and suggest helpful resources.

Patients and their families are naturally concerned about what the future holds. Sometimes they use statistics to try to figure out whether the patient will be cured or how long he or she will live. It is important to remember, however, that statistics are averages based on large numbers of patients. They can't be used to predict what will happen to a certain patient because no two cancer patients are alike. The doctor who takes care of the patient and knows that person's medical history is in the best position to discuss the patient's outlook (prognosis).

People should feel free to ask the doctor about their prognosis, but it is important to keep in mind that not even the doctor can tell exactly what will happen. When doctors talk about recovering from a brain tumor, they may use the term remission rather than cure. Even though many people recover completely, doctors use this term because a brain tumor can recur.

Support for Cancer Patients

Living with a serious disease is not easy. Everyone involved faces many problems and challenges. Finding the strength to cope with these difficulties is easier when people have helpful information and support services.

The doctor can explain the disease and give advice about treatment, going back to work or school, or other activities. If patients want to discuss concerns about the future, family relationships, and finances, it also may help to talk with a nurse, social worker, counselor, or member of the clergy.

Friends and relatives who have had personal experience with cancer can be very supportive. Also, it helps many patients to meet and talk with other people who are facing problems like theirs. Cancer patients often get together in self-help and support groups, where they can share what they have learned about cancer and its treatment and about coping with the disease. In addition to groups for adults with cancer, special support groups for children or teens with cancer or for parents whose children have cancer are available in many cities. It's important to keep in mind, however, that each patient is different. Treatments and ways of dealing with cancer that work for one person may not be right for another even if they both have the same kind of cancer. It's always a good idea to discuss the advice of friends and family members with the doctor.

Often, a social worker at the hospital or clinic can suggest local and national groups that will help with rehabilitation, emotional support, financial aid, transportation, or home care. The American Cancer Society is one such group. This nonprofit organization has many services for patients and their families. More information about this resource can be found in the "Resources" section.

The American Brain Tumor Association is another organization that can help patients find support groups in local areas. Information about this resource can be found in the "Resources" section below.

Candlelighters Childhood Cancer Foundation sponsors support groups for parents of children with cancer. In some cities, the Foundation has special groups for children or teens with cancer, as well. Candlelighters is described below in the "Resources" section.

Information about other programs and services for cancer patients and their families is available through the Cancer Information Service. The toll-free number is 1-800-4-CANCER.

The public library is a good place to find books and articles on living with cancer. Cancer patients and their families can also find helpful suggestions in the NCI booklets listed in the "Other Booklets" section.

Resources

Information about brain tumors is available from many sources. Several are listed below. You also may wish to check for additional information at your local library or bookstore or from support groups in the community.

Cancer Information Service (CIS)

The Cancer Information Service, a program of the National Cancer Institute, provides a nationwide telephone service for cancer patients and their families and friends, the public, and health care professionals. The staff can answer questions and can send booklets about cancer. They also have information about local resources and services. One toll-free number, 1-800-4-CANCER (1-800-422-6237), connects callers with the office that serves their area. Spanish-speaking staff members are available.

American Cancer Society (ACS)
1599 Clifton Road, N.E.
Atlanta, GA 30329
1-800-ACS-2345

The American Cancer Society is a voluntary organization with a national office (at the above address) and local units all over the country. It supports research, conducts educational programs, and publishes booklets about cancer. It also offers many services to patients and their families. To obtain booklets or to learn about services and activities in local areas, call the Society's toll-free number, 1-800-ACS-2345 (1-800-227-2345), or the number listed under American Cancer Society in the white pages of the telephone book.

American Brain Tumor Association (ABTA)

3725 North Talman Avenue
Chicago, IL 60618
1-800-886-ABTA

The American Brain Tumor Association supports research on brain tumors and provides information to the public through booklets and newsletters. This organization also provides resource listings of doctors, treatment facilities, and support groups throughout the country.

Candlelighters Childhood Cancer Foundation (CCCF)

Suite 460
7910 Woodmont Avenue
Bethesda, MD 20814
1-800-366-CCCF

Candlelighters is a national organization of parents whose children have or have had cancer. It operates a patient information service and publishes newsletters for parents and young people. Local chapters sponsor family support groups.

National Institute of Neurological Disorders and Stroke (NINDS)

NINDS Information Center
Post Office Box 5801
Bethesda, MD 20824
1-800-352-9424

The National Institute of Neurological Disorders and Stroke, an agency of the Federal Government, supports research on brain tumors and other disorders that affect the brain and nervous system. The Information Center can send free printed materials on brain tumors.

Other Booklets

The National Cancer Institute booklets listed below are available free of charge by calling 1-800-4-CANCER (1-800-422-6237).

Booklets about Cancer and Its Treatment

- *Chemotherapy and You: A Guide to Self-Help During Treatment* *
- *Radiation Therapy and You: A Guide to Self-Help During Treatment* *
- *Eating Hints: Recipes and Tips for Better Nutrition During Cancer Treatment*
- *What Are Clinical Trials All About?* *
- *Questions and Answers About Pain Control* (also available from the American Cancer Society)

Booklets about Living With Cancer

- *Facing Forward: A Guide for Cancer Survivors* *
- *Taking Time: Support for People With Cancer and the People Who Care About Them*
- *When Cancer Recurs: Meeting the Challenge Again* *
- *Advanced Cancer: Living Each Day* *

* Reprinted in this volume: see Table of Contents

Chapter 4

Eye Cancer: Retinoblastoma

What Is Retinoblastoma?

Retinoblastoma is a malignant (cancerous) tumor of the retina. The retina is the thin nerve tissue that lines the back of the eye that senses light and forms images.

Although retinoblastoma may occur at any age, it most often occurs in younger children, usually before the age of 5 years. The tumor may be in one eye only or in both eyes. Retinoblastoma is usually confined to the eye and does not spread to nearby tissue or other parts of the body.

Retinoblastoma may be hereditary (runs in families) or nonhereditary. The hereditary form may be in one or both eyes. Most retinoblastoma occurring in only one eye is not hereditary; when the disease occurs in both eyes, it is always hereditary. Because of the hereditary factor, brothers and sisters of children with retinoblastoma may warrant examination to find out if they may develop the disease.

If your child has retinoblastoma, particularly the hereditary type, there is an increased chance that he or she may develop a second cancer in later years. Parents may therefore decide to continue taking their child for medical check-ups even after the cancer has been treated.

Your child's prognosis (chance of recovery and of retaining sight) and choice of treatment depend on the extent of the disease within and outside of the eye.

PDQ statement, National Cancer Institute, revised February 1999.

Stages of Retinoblastoma

Once retinoblastoma is found, more tests will be done to determine the size of the tumor and whether it has spread to surrounding tissue or to other parts of the body. This is called staging.

To plan treatment, your child's doctor needs to know the stage of disease. Although there are several staging systems currently available for retinoblastoma, for the purposes of treatment retinoblastoma is categorized into intraocular and extraocular disease.

Intraocular Retinoblastoma

Cancer is found in one or in both eyes but does not extend beyond the eye into the tissues around the eye or to other parts of the body.

Extraocular Retinoblastoma

The cancer has extended beyond the eye. It may be confined to the tissues around the eye, or it may have spread to other parts of the body.

Recurrent Retinoblastoma

Recurrent disease means that the cancer has come back (recurred) or progressed (continued to grow) after it has been treated. It may recur in the eye or elsewhere in the body.

How Retinoblastoma Is Treated

There are treatments for all children with retinoblastoma, and most children can be cured. The type of treatment given depends on the extent of the disease within the eye, whether the disease is in one or both eyes, and whether the disease has spread beyond the eye. Treatment options consider both cure and preservation of sight, and include the following:

- Enucleation: Surgery to remove the eye.

- Cryotherapy: The use of extreme cold to destroy cancer cells.

- Photocoagulation: The use of laser light to destroy blood vessels that feed the tumor.

- Internal or external-beam radiation therapy. Radiation therapy uses high-energy radiation from x-rays and other sources to kill cancer cells and shrink tumors. Radiation may come from a machine outside the body (external-beam radiation therapy) or may be administered by placing radioactive material into or very near the tumor (internal radiation therapy or brachytherapy).

- Chemotherapy is the use of drugs to kill cancer cells. Chemotherapy is called a systemic treatment because the drug enters the bloodstream, travels through the body, and can kill cancer cells throughout the body. Chemotherapy drugs may be taken by mouth or injected into a vein (intravenous) or a muscle. In children with retinoblastoma, chemotherapy drugs may be injected directly into the fluid that surrounds the brain and spinal cord (intrathecal chemotherapy).

Treatment by Stage

Your child may receive treatment that is considered standard based on its effectiveness in a number of patients in past studies, or you may choose to have your child take part in a clinical trial. Not all patients are cured with standard therapy and some standard treatments may have more side effects than are desired. For these reasons, clinical trials are designed to test new treatments and find better ways to treat children with cancer. Clinical trials are ongoing in many parts of the country for advanced stages of retinoblastoma. For more information, call the Cancer Information Service at 1-800-4-CANCER (1-800-422-6237); TTY at 1-800-332-8615.

Intraocular Retinoblastoma

Treatment depends on whether the cancer is in one or both eyes. If the cancer is in one eye, treatment may be one of the following:

- Surgery to remove the eye (enucleation) is used for large tumors when there is no expectation that useful vision can be preserved.

- External radiation therapy, photocoagulation, cryotherapy, or brachytherapy may be used with smaller tumors when there is potential for preservation of sight.

If the cancer is in both eyes, treatment may be one of the following:

- Surgery to remove the eye with the most cancer, and radiation therapy (with or without other types of treatment) to the other eye.

- Radiation therapy to both eyes if there is potential for vision in both eyes.

Extraocular Retinoblastoma

Treatment may be one of the following:

- Radiation therapy and/or intrathecal chemotherapy.
- Clinical trials are testing new combinations of chemotherapy drugs and new ways of administrating chemotherapy drugs.

Recurrent Retinoblastoma

Treatment depends on the site and extent of the recurrence (or progression). If the cancer comes back only in the eye, your child may have surgery or radiation therapy. If the cancer comes back outside of the eye, treatment depends of many factors and is based on individual concerns; you may want to have your child participate in a clinical trial.

To Learn More

To learn more about retinoblastoma, call the National Cancer Institute's Cancer Information Service at 1-800-4-CANCER (1-800-422-6237); TTY at 1-800-332-8615. The call is toll-free and a trained information specialist can answer your questions.

The Cancer Information Service can also send you booklets. The following booklets on childhood cancer may be helpful to you:

Young People with Cancer: A Handbook for Parents

Talking with Your Child About Cancer

Managing Your Child's Eating Problems During Cancer Treatment

When Someone in Your Family Has Cancer

The following general booklets on questions related to cancer may also be helpful:

Taking Time: Support for People with Cancer and the People Who Care About Them

What Are Clinical Trials All About?

Chemotherapy and You: A Guide to Self-Help During Treatment *

Radiation Therapy and You: A Guide to Self-Help During Treatment *

What You Need To Know About Cancer *

* Reprinted in this volume—see Table of Contents

There are many other places where material about cancer treatment and information about services are available. Check the hospital social service office for local and national agencies that help with finances, getting to and from treatment, care at home, and dealing with other problems. Write to the National Cancer Institute at this address:

National Cancer Institute
Office of Cancer Communications
31 Center Drive, MSC 2580
Bethesda, MD 20892-2580

Chapter 5

Eye Cancer: Intraocular Melanoma

What Is Intraocular Melanoma?

Intraocular melanoma, a rare cancer, is a disease in which cancer (malignant) cells are found in the part of the eye called the uvea. The uvea contains cells called melanocytes, which contain color. When these cells become cancerous, the cancer is called a melanoma. The uvea includes the iris (the colored part of the eye), the ciliary body (a muscle in the eye), and the choroid (a layer of tissue in the back of the eye). The iris opens and closes to change the amount of light entering the eye. The ciliary body changes the shape of the lens inside the eye so it can focus. The choroid layer is next to the retina, the part of the eye that makes a picture.

If there is melanoma that starts in the iris, it may look like a dark spot on the iris. If melanoma is in the ciliary body or the choroid, a person may have blurry vision or may have no symptoms, and the cancer may grow before it is noticed. Intraocular melanoma is usually found during a routine eye examination, when a doctor looks inside the eye with special lights and instruments.

The chance of recovery (prognosis) depends on the size and cell type of the cancer, where the cancer is in the eye, and whether the cancer has spread.

PDQ Statement, National Cancer Instutute, revised February 1998.

Stages of Intraocular Melanoma

Once intraocular melanoma is found (diagnosed), more tests will be done to find out exactly what kind of tumor the patient has and whether cancer cells have spread to other parts of the body. This is called staging. A doctor needs to know the stage to plan treatment. Intraocular melanoma is staged based on the area of the eye where the tumor is found and the size of the tumor.

Iris Melanoma

Intraocular melanomas of the iris occur in the front colored part of the eye. Iris melanomas usually grow slowly and do not usually spread to other parts of the body.

Ciliary Body and Choroid Melanoma, Small Size

Intraocular melanomas of the ciliary body and/or choroid occur in the back part of the eye. They are grouped by the size of the tumor.

Small size ciliary body or choroid melanoma is 2 to 3 millimeters or less thick.

Ciliary Body and Choroid Melanoma, Medium/Large Size

Intraocular melanomas of the ciliary body and/or choroid occur in the back part of the eye. They are grouped by the size of the tumor.

Medium/large size ciliary body or choroid melanoma is more than 2 to 3 millimeters thick.

Extraocular Extension Melanoma

The melanoma has spread outside the eye, to the nerve behind the eye (the optic nerve), or to the eye socket.

Recurrent Intraocular Melanoma

Recurrent disease means that the cancer has come back (recurred) after it has been treated.

How Intraocular Melanoma Is Treated

There are treatments for all patients with intraocular melanoma. In some cases a doctor may watch the patient carefully without treatment until the cancer begins to grow. When treatment is given, three types of treatment are commonly used:

- surgery (taking out the cancer)
- radiation therapy (using high-dose x-rays or other high-energy rays to kill cancer cells)
- photocoagulation (destroying blood vessels that feed the tumor)

Surgery is the most common treatment of intraocular melanoma. A doctor may remove the cancer using one of the following operations:

- Iridectomy removes only parts of the iris.
- Iridotrabeculectomy removes parts of the iris and the supporting tissues around the cornea, the clear layer covering the front of the eye.
- Iridocyclectomy removes parts of the iris and the ciliary body.
- Choroidectomy removes parts of the choroid.
- Enucleation removes the entire eye.

Radiation therapy uses x-rays or other high-energy rays to kill cancer cells and shrink tumors. Radiation may come from a machine outside the body (external beam radiation therapy) or from putting materials that contain radiation (radioisotopes) in the area where the cancer cells are found (internal radiation therapy). In intraocular melanoma, internal radiation may be put next to the eye using small implants called plaques. Radiation can be used alone or in combination with surgery.

Photocoagulation is a treatment that uses a tiny beam of light, usually from a laser, to destroy blood vessels and kill the tumor.

Treatment by Stage

The choice of treatment depends on where the cancer is in the eye, how far it has spread, and the patient's general health and age.

Standard treatment may be considered because of its effectiveness in patients in past studies, or participation in a clinical trial may be considered. Not all patients are cured with standard therapy and some standard treatments may have more side effects than are desired. For these reasons, clinical trials are designed to find the best ways to treat cancer patients and are based on the most up-to-date information. A large clinical trial is ongoing in many parts of the country for patients with intraocular melanoma. To learn more about clinical trials, call the Cancer Information Service at 1-800-4-CANCER (1-800-422-6237); TTY at 1-800-332-8615.

Iris Melanoma

If the tumor is small, there are no symptoms, and the tumor is not growing, treatment may not be needed. If the tumor begins to grow or if there are symptoms, treatment may be one of the following:

1. Surgery to remove parts of the iris (iridectomy).

2. Surgery to remove parts of the iris and the supporting tissues around the cornea (iridotrabeculectomy).

3. Surgery to remove parts of the iris and the ciliary body

4. Surgery to remove the eye (enucleation).

Ciliary Body and Choroid Melanoma, Small Size

If the tumor is small, there are no symptoms, and the tumor is not growing, treatment may not be needed. If the tumor begins to grow, or if there are symptoms, treatment may be one of the following:

1. Internal radiation therapy.

2. External beam radiation therapy.

3. Surgery to remove the tumor and part of the iris or choroid (iridocyclectomy or choroidectomy).

4. Surgery to remove the eye (enucleation).

5. External beam radiation therapy followed by enucleation.

Ciliary Body and Choroid Melanoma, Medium/Large Size

If the tumor is not growing, treatment may not be needed. If treatment is needed, it may be one of the following:

1. Internal radiation therapy.

2. External beam radiation therapy.

3. Surgery to remove the tumor and part of the iris or choroid (iridocyclectomy or choroidectomy).

4. Surgery to remove the eye (enucleation).

5. External beam radiation therapy followed by enucleation.

6. A clinical trial. A large trial is in progress in many parts of the country comparing standard treatments. Clinical trials are also testing new treatments.

Extraocular Extension Melanoma

Treatment may be one of the following:

1. Surgery to remove the eye and other tissues in the eye socket (orbital exenteration) with or without radiation therapy.

2. Surgery to remove the eye (enucleation) with or without radiation therapy.

Recurrent Intraocular Melanoma

Treatment will depend on the treatment the patient received before, the patient's age and health, where the cancer came back, and how far the cancer has spread. The patient may want to take part in a clinical trial.

To Learn More

To learn more about intraocular melanoma, call the National Cancer Institute's Cancer Information Service at 1-800-4-CANCER (1-800-422-6237); TTY at 1-800-332-8615. By dialing this toll-free number, trained information specialists can answer your questions.

The Cancer Information Service also has booklets about cancer that are available to the public and can be sent on request. The following general booklets on questions related to cancer may be helpful:

What You Need To Know About Cancer *

Taking Time: Support for People with Cancer and the People Who Care About Them

What Are Clinical Trials All About?

Radiation Therapy and You: A Guide to Self-Help During Treatment *

Eating Hints for Cancer Patients *

Advanced Cancer: Living Each Day *

When Cancer Recurs: Meeting the Challenge Again *

* Reprinted in this volume—see Table of Contents

There are other places where people can get material and information about cancer treatment and services. The social service office at a hospital can be checked for local and national agencies that help with getting information about finances, getting to and from treatment, getting care at home, and dealing with problems. For more information from the National Cancer Institute, please write to this address:

National Cancer Institute
Office of Cancer Communications
31 Center Drive, MSC 2580
Bethesda, MD 20892-2580

Chapter 6

Metastatic Squamous Neck Cancer

Metastatic Squamous Neck Cancer with Occult Primary

Cancer is a disease in which certain cells begin to divide too quickly and without any order. Cancer can spread to tissues and organs near the place where it started (called the primary site). Cancer cells can also spread through the bloodstream and the lymph system to other parts of the body to form new tumors. Cancer that started in one place, but has spread to another part of the body is called metastatic cancer.

Squamous cells line the outside of many body organs, including the mouth, nose, skin, throat, and lungs. Cancer can begin in the squamous cells and spread (metastasize) from its original site to the lymph nodes in the neck or around the collarbone. Lymph nodes are small bean-shaped structures that are found throughout the body. They produce and store infection-fighting cells. When the lymph nodes in the neck are found to contain squamous cell cancer, a doctor will try to find out where the cancer started (the primary tumor). If the doctor cannot find a primary tumor, the cancer is called a metastatic cancer with unseen (occult) primary.

A doctor should be seen if there is a lump or pain in the neck or throat that doesn't go away. If tissue that is not normal is found, the doctor will need to cut out a small piece and look at it under the microscope to see if there are any cancer cells. This is called a biopsy. If

PDQ Statement, National Cancer Instutute, revised March 1998.

the biopsy shows that a person has squamous cell cancer, the doctor will do many kinds of tests to see whether a primary site can be found. If the primary site cannot be found, the doctor will treat the cancer in the neck.

The chance of recovery (prognosis) depends on how many lymph nodes contain cancer, where the cancer is found in the neck, whether or not a primary tumor is found, and the patient's general state of health.

Stage Explanation

Once metastatic squamous neck cancer with occult primary is found, more tests will be done to find out how far the cancer cells have spread. This is called staging. A doctor needs to know the stage of the disease to plan treatment. The following stages are used for metastatic squamous neck cancer with occult primary:

Untreated

Untreated metastatic squamous neck cancer with occult primary means no treatment has been given for the cancer except to treat symptoms.

Recurrent

Recurrent disease means that the cancer has come back (recurred) after it has been treated. It may come back in the neck or in another part of the body.

Treatment Option Overview

There are treatments for all patients with metastatic squamous neck cancer with occult primary. Two kinds of treatment are used:

- surgery (taking out the cancer)
- radiation therapy (using high-dose x-rays or other high-energy rays to kill cancer cells)

Chemotherapy is being studied in clinical trials.

Surgery is a common treatment of metastatic neck cancer. A doctor may cut out the lymph nodes that contain cancer and some of the healthy lymph nodes around them (lymph node dissection).

Radiation therapy uses high-energy x-rays to kill cancer cells and shrink tumors. Radiation may come from a machine outside the body (external radiation therapy) or from putting materials that produce radiation (radioisotopes) through thin plastic tubes that are put into the area where the cancer cells are found (internal radiation therapy). External radiation to the thyroid or the pituitary gland may change the way the thyroid gland works. The doctor may wish to test the thyroid gland before and after therapy to make sure it is working properly.

Chemotherapy uses drugs to kill cancer cells. Chemotherapy may be taken by pill, or it may be put into the body by a needle in a vein or muscle. Chemotherapy is called a systemic treatment because the drug enters the bloodstream, travels through the body, and can kill cancer cells outside the neck.

Treatment by Stage

Treatment of metastatic squamous neck cancer with occult primary depends on how many lymph nodes contain cancer, whether or not an original (primary) tumor is found, and the patient's age and overall condition.

Standard treatment may be considered because of its effectiveness in patients in past studies, or participation in a clinical trial may be considered. Not all patients are cured with standard therapy and some standard treatments may have more side effects than are desired. For these reasons, clinical trials are designed to find better ways to treat cancer patients and are based on the most up-to-date information. Clinical trials are ongoing in some parts of the country for metastatic squamous neck cancer. To learn more about clinical trials, call the Cancer Information Service at 1-800-4-CANCER (1-800-422-6237); TTY at 1-800-332-8615.

Untreated Metastatic Squamous Neck Cancer with Occult Primary

Treatment may be one of the following:

1. Surgery to remove the lymph nodes in the neck (lymph node dissection).

2. Radiation therapy.

3. Radiation therapy plus surgery.

4. A clinical trial that includes chemotherapy, radiation therapy, and/or surgery.

Recurrent Metastatic Squamous Neck Cancer with Occult Primary

Treatment depends on the type of treatment the patient had before, where the cancer came back, and the patient's health. A patient may want to take part in a clinical trial of new treatments.

To Learn More

To learn more about metastatic squamous neck cancer with occult primary, call the National Cancer Institute's Cancer Information Service at 1-800-4-CANCER (1-800-422-6237); TTY at 1-800-332-8615. By dialing this toll-free number, trained information specialists can answer your questions.

The Cancer Information Service also has booklets about cancer that are available to the public and can be sent on request. The following general booklets on questions related to cancer may be helpful:

What You Need To Know About Cancer *

Taking Time: Support for People with Cancer and the People Who Care About Them

What Are Clinical Trials All About?

Chemotherapy and You: A Guide to Self-Help During Treatment *

Radiation Therapy and You: A Guide to Self-Help During Treatment *

Eating Hints for Cancer Patients *

Advanced Cancer: Living Each Day *

When Cancer Recurs: Meeting the Challenge Again *

* Reprinted in this volume—see Table of Contents

There are many other places where people can get material and information about cancer treatment and services. The social service office at a hospital can be checked for local and national agencies that help with getting information about finances, getting to and from treatment, getting care at home, and dealing with problems. For more information from the National Cancer Institute, please write to this address:

National Cancer Institute
Office of Cancer Communications
31 Center Drive, MSC 2580
Bethesda, MD 20892-2580

Chapter 7

Paranasal Sinus and Nasal Cavity Cancer

What Is Cancer of the Paranasal Sinus and Nasal Cavity?

Cancer of the paranasal sinus and nasal cavity is a disease in which cancer (malignant) cells are found in the tissues of the paranasal sinuses or nasal cavity. The paranasal sinuses are small hollow spaces around the nose. The sinuses are lined with cells that make mucus, which keeps the nose from drying out; the sinuses are also a space through which the voice can echo to make sounds when a person talks or sings. The nasal cavity is the passageway just behind the nose through which air passes on the way to the throat during breathing. The area inside the nose is called the nasal vestibule.

There are several paranasal sinuses, including the frontal sinuses above the nose, the maxillary sinuses in the upper part of either side of the upper jawbone, the ethmoid sinuses just behind either side of the upper nose, and the sphenoid sinus behind the ethmoid sinus in the center of the skull.

Cancer of the paranasal sinus and nasal cavity most commonly starts in the cells that line the oropharynx. Much less often, cancer of the paranasal sinus and nasal cavity starts in the color-making cells called melanocytes, and is called a melanoma. If the cancer starts in the muscle or connecting tissue, it is called a sarcoma. Another type of cancer that can occur here, but grows more slowly, is called an

PDQ Statement, National Cancer Institute, revised June 1998.

inverting papilloma. Cancers called midline granulomas may also occur in the paranasal sinuses or nasal cavity, and they cause the tissue around them to break down.

A doctor should be seen if the sinuses are blocked and don't clear, or if there is a sinus infection, bleeding through the nose, a lump or sore that doesn't heal inside the nose, frequent headaches or pain in the sinus region, swelling or other trouble with the eyes, pain in the upper teeth, or problems with dentures.

If there are symptoms, a doctor will examine the nose using a mirror and lights. The doctor may order a CT scan (a special x-ray that uses a computer) or an MRI scan (an x-ray-like procedure that uses magnetic energy) to make a picture of the inside of parts of the body. A special instrument (called a rhinoscope or a nasoscope) may be put into the nose to see inside. If tissue that is not normal is found, the doctor will need to cut out a small piece and look at it under the microscope to see if there are any cancer cells. This is called a biopsy. Sometimes the doctor will need to cut into the sinus to do a biopsy.

The chance of recovery (prognosis) depends on where the cancer is in the sinuses, whether the cancer is just in the area where it started or has spread to other tissues (the stage), and the patient's general state of health.

Stages of Cancer of the Paranasal Sinus and Nasal Cavity

Once cancer of the paranasal sinus and nasal cavity is found, more tests will be done to find out if cancer cells have spread to other parts of the body. This is called staging. A doctor needs to know the stage of the disease to plan treatment. There is no staging system for cancer of the nasal cavity or for some of the less common paranasal sinus cancers. The following stages are used for cancer of the maxillary sinus, the most common type of paranasal sinus cancer:

Stage I

The cancer is in only the maxillary sinus and has not destroyed any of the bone in the sinus. The cancer has not spread to lymph nodes in the area (lymph nodes are small bean-shaped structures that are found throughout the body; they produce and store infection-fighting cells).

Stage II

The cancer has begun to destroy the bones around the sinus, but has not spread to lymph nodes in the area.

Stage III

Either of the following may be true:

- The cancer has spread no further than the bones around the si-nus and to only one lymph node on the same side of the neck as the cancer. The lymph node that contains cancer measures no more than 3 centimeters (just over one inch).

- The cancer has spread to the cheek, the back of the maxillary sinus, the eye socket, or the ethmoid sinus in front of the maxil-lary sinus. The cancer may or may not have spread to one lymph node on the same side of the neck as the cancer.

Stage IV

Any of the following may be true:

- The cancer has spread to the eye or to other sinuses or places around the sinuses. The lymph nodes in the area may or may not contain cancer.

- The cancer is in only the sinuses or has spread to the areas around it. The cancer has spread to more than one lymph node on the same side of the neck as the cancer, to lymph nodes on one or both sides of the neck, or to any lymph node that mea-sures more than 6 centimeters (over 2 inches).

- The cancer has spread to other parts of the body.

Recurrent

Recurrent disease means that the cancer has come back (recurred) after it has been treated. It may come back in the paranasal sinuses or nasal cavity or in another part of the body.

How Cancer of the Paranasal Sinus and Nasal Cavity Is Treated

There are treatments for all patients with cancer of the paranasal sinus and nasal cavity. Three kinds of treatment are used:

- surgery (taking out the cancer)

- radiation therapy (using high-dose x-rays or other high-energy rays to kill cancer cells)

- chemotherapy (using drugs to kill cancer cells)

Surgery is commonly used to remove cancers of the paranasal sinus or nasal cavity. Depending on where the cancer is and how far it has spread, a doctor may need to cut out bone or tissue around the cancer. If cancer has spread to lymph nodes in the neck, the lymph nodes may be removed (lymph node dissection).

Radiation therapy is also a common treatment of cancer of the paranasal sinus and nasal cavity. Radiation therapy uses high-energy x-rays to kill cancer cells and shrink tumors. Radiation may come from a machine outside the body (external radiation therapy) or from putting materials that produce radiation (radioisotopes) through thin plastic tubes in the area where the cancer cells are found (internal radiation therapy). External radiation to the thyroid or the pituitary gland may change the way the thyroid gland works. The doctor may wish to test the thyroid gland before and after therapy to make sure it is working properly.

Chemotherapy uses drugs to kill cancer cells. Chemotherapy may be taken by pill, or it may be put into the body by a needle in a vein or muscle. Chemotherapy is called a systemic treatment because the drug enters the bloodstream, travels through the body, and can kill cancer cells throughout the body.

Because the paranasal sinuses and nasal cavity help in talking and breathing, and are close to the face, patients may need special help adjusting to the side effects of the cancer and its treatment. A doctor will consult with several kinds of doctors who can help determine the best treatment. Trained medical staff can also help in recovery from treatment. Patients may need plastic surgery if a large amount of tissue or bone around the paranasal sinuses or nasal cavity is taken out.

Treatment by Stage

Treatment of cancer of the paranasal sinus and nasal cavity depends on where the cancer is, the stage of the disease, and the patient's age and overall health.

Standard treatment may be considered because of its effectiveness in patients in past studies, or participation in a clinical trial may be considered. Not all patients are cured with standard therapy and some standard treatments may have more side effects than are desired. For these reasons, clinical trials are designed to find better ways to treat cancer patients and are based on the most up-to-date information.

Clinical trials are ongoing in some parts of the country for patients with cancer of the paranasal sinus and nasal cavity. To learn more about clinical trials, call the Cancer Information Service at 1-800-4-CANCER (1-800-422-6237); TTY at 1-800-332-8615.

Stage I

Treatment depends on the type of cancer and where the cancer is found.

If cancer is in the maxillary sinus, treatment will probably be surgery to remove the cancer. Radiation therapy may be given after surgery. If cancer is in the ethmoid sinus, treatment may be one of the following:

1. Radiation therapy if the cancer cannot be removed with surgery.

2. Surgery followed by radiation therapy.

If cancer is in the sphenoid sinus, treatment will probably be radiation therapy.

If cancer is in the nasal cavity, treatment may be surgery, radiation therapy, or both.

If the cancer is an inverting papilloma, treatment will probably be surgery.

If the cancer is a melanoma or sarcoma, treatment will probably be surgery. For certain types of sarcoma, surgery, radiation therapy, and chemotherapy may be given.

If the cancer is a midline granuloma, treatment will probably be radiation therapy.

If cancer is in the nose (nasal vestibule), treatment may be surgery or radiation therapy.

Stage II

Treatment depends on the type of cancer and where the cancer is found.

If cancer is in the maxillary sinus, treatment will probably be surgery to remove the cancer. Radiation therapy is given before or after surgery.

If cancer is in the ethmoid sinus, treatment may be one of the following:

1. External beam radiation therapy.

73

2. Surgery followed by radiation therapy.

If cancer is in the sphenoid sinus, treatment will probably be radiation therapy.

If cancer is in the nasal cavity, treatment may be surgery, radiation therapy, or both.

If the cancer is an inverting papilloma, treatment will probably be surgery. If the cancer comes back after surgery, patients may receive radiation therapy.

If the cancer is a melanoma or sarcoma, treatment will probably be surgery. For certain types of sarcoma, surgery, radiation therapy, and chemotherapy may be given.

If the cancer is a midline granuloma, treatment will probably be radiation therapy.

If the cancer is in the nose (nasal vestibule), treatment may be surgery or radiation therapy.

Stage III

Treatment depends on the type of cancer and where the cancer is found.

If cancer is in the maxillary sinus, treatment may be one of the following:

1. Surgery to remove the cancer. Radiation therapy is given before or after surgery.

2. A clinical trial of a special type of radiation therapy given before or after surgery.

3. A clinical trial of chemotherapy combined with radiation therapy.

If cancer is in the ethmoid sinus, treatment may be one of the following:

1. Surgery followed by radiation therapy.

2. A clinical trial of chemotherapy before surgery or radiation therapy.

3. A clinical trial of chemotherapy following surgery with or without radiation therapy.

4. A clinical trial of chemotherapy combined with radiation therapy.

If cancer is in the sphenoid sinus, treatment will probably be radiation therapy.

If cancer is in the nasal cavity, treatment may be one of the following:

1. Surgery.

2. Radiation therapy.

3. Surgery plus radiation therapy.

4. A clinical trial of chemotherapy before surgery or radiation therapy.

5. A clinical trial of chemotherapy following surgery with or without radiation therapy.

6. A clinical trial of chemotherapy combined with radiation therapy.

If the cancer is an inverting papilloma, treatment will probably be surgery. If the cancer comes back after surgery, patients may receive radiation therapy.

If the cancer is a melanoma or sarcoma, treatment will probably be surgery. Radiation therapy may be given if the cancer cannot be removed with surgery. For certain types of sarcoma, surgery, radiation therapy, and chemotherapy may be given.

If the cancer is a midline granuloma, treatment will probably be radiation therapy.

If the cancer is in the nose (nasal vestibule), treatment may be one of the following:

1. External beam and/or internal radiation therapy.

2. Surgery if the cancer comes back following treatment.

3. A clinical trial of chemotherapy before surgery or radiation therapy.

4. A clinical trial of chemotherapy following surgery with or without radiation therapy.

5. A clinical trial of chemotherapy combined with radiation therapy.

Stage IV

Treatment depends on the type of cancer and where the cancer is found.

If cancer is in the maxillary sinus, treatment will probably be one of the following:

1. Radiation therapy.

2. A clinical trial of chemotherapy before surgery or radiation therapy.

3. A clinical trial of chemotherapy following radiation therapy.

4. A clinical trial of chemotherapy combined with radiation therapy.

If cancer is in the ethmoid sinus, treatment may be one of the following:

1. Surgery followed by radiation therapy.

2. Radiation therapy followed by surgery.

3. A clinical trial of chemotherapy before surgery or radiation therapy.

4. A clinical trial of chemotherapy following surgery with or without radiation therapy.

5. A clinical trial of chemotherapy combined with radiation therapy.

If cancer is in the sphenoid sinus, treatment will probably be radiation therapy.

If cancer is in the nasal cavity, treatment may be one of the following:

1. Surgery.

2. Radiation therapy.

3. Surgery plus radiation therapy.

4. A clinical trial of chemotherapy before surgery or radiation therapy.

5. A clinical trial of chemotherapy following surgery with or without radiation therapy.

6. A clinical trial of chemotherapy combined with radiation therapy.

If the cancer is an inverting papilloma, treatment will probably be surgery. If the cancer comes back after surgery, patients may receive radiation therapy.

If the cancer is a melanoma or sarcoma, treatment will probably be surgery, if possible. Radiation therapy or chemotherapy may be given if the cancer cannot be removed with surgery.

If the cancer is a midline granuloma, treatment will probably be radiation therapy.

If the cancer is in the nose (nasal vestibule), treatment may be one of the following:

1. External beam and/or internal radiation therapy.

2. Surgery if the cancer comes back following treatment.

3. A clinical trial of chemotherapy before surgery or radiation therapy.

4. A clinical trial of chemotherapy following surgery with or without radiation therapy.

5. A clinical trial of chemotherapy combined with radiation therapy.

Recurrent

Treatment depends on the type of cancer, where the cancer is found, and the type of treatment the patient received before.

If cancer is in the maxillary sinus, treatment will probably be one of the following:

1. If surgery was done before, more extensive surgery followed by radiation therapy or radiation therapy alone.

2. If radiation therapy was given before, surgery.

3. Chemotherapy. Clinical trials are testing new chemotherapy drugs.

If cancer is in the ethmoid sinus, treatment may be one of the following:

1. If limited surgery was done before, more extensive surgery followed by radiation therapy or radiation therapy alone.

2. If radiation therapy was given before, surgery.

3. Chemotherapy. Clinical trials are testing new chemotherapy drugs.

If cancer is in the sphenoid sinus, treatment will probably be radiation therapy. Chemotherapy is given if radiation therapy does not work.

If cancer is in the nasal cavity, treatment may be one of the following:

1. If limited surgery was done before, radiation therapy alone or more extensive surgery followed by radiation therapy.

2. If radiation therapy was given before, surgery.

3. Chemotherapy. Clinical trials are testing new chemotherapy drugs.

If the cancer is an inverting papilloma, treatment will probably be surgery. If the cancer comes back after surgery, patients may receive more surgery or radiation therapy.

If the cancer is a melanoma or sarcoma, treatment may be surgery or chemotherapy.

If the cancer is a midline granuloma, treatment will probably be radiation therapy.

If the cancer is in the nose (nasal vestibule), treatment may be one of the following:

1. If radiation therapy was given before, surgery.

2. If surgery was done before, radiation therapy alone or more extensive surgery followed by radiation therapy.

3. Chemotherapy. Clinical trials are testing new chemotherapy drugs.

To Learn More

To learn more about cancer of the paranasal sinus and nasal cavity, call the National Cancer Institute's Cancer Information Service at 1-800-4-CANCER (1-800-422-6237); TTY at 1-800-332-8615. By dialing this toll-free number, trained information specialists can answer your questions.

The Cancer Information Service also has booklets about cancer that are available to the public and can be sent on request. The following general booklets on questions related to cancer may be helpful:

What You Need To Know About Cancer *

Taking Time: Support for People with Cancer and the People Who Care About Them

What Are Clinical Trials All About?

Chemotherapy and You: A Guide to Self-Help During Treatment *

Radiation Therapy and You: A Guide to Self-Help During Treatment *

Eating Hints for Cancer Patients *

Advanced Cancer: Living Each Day *

When Cancer Recurs: Meeting the Challenge Again *

* Reprinted in this volume — see Table of Contents

There are many other places where people can get material and information about cancer treatment and services. The social service office at a hospital can be checked for local and national agencies that help with getting information about finances, getting to and from treatment, getting care at home, and dealing with problems. For more information from the National Cancer Institute, please write to this address:

National Cancer Institute
Office of Cancer Communications
31 Center Drive, MSC 2580
Bethesda, MD 20892-2580

Chapter 8

Salivary Gland Cancer

What Is Cancer of the Salivary Gland?

Cancer of the salivary gland is a disease in which cancer (malignant) cells are found in the tissues of the salivary glands. The salivary glands make saliva, the fluid that is released into the mouth to keep it moist and to help dissolve food.

Major clusters of salivary glands are found below the tongue, on the sides of the face just in front of the ears, and under the jawbone. Smaller clusters of salivary glands are found in other parts of the upper digestive tract. The smaller glands are called the minor salivary glands.

Many growths in the salivary glands do not spread to other tissues and are not cancer. These tumors are called "benign" tumors and are not usually treated the same as cancer.

A doctor should be seen if there is a swelling under the chin or around the jawbone, the face becomes numb, muscles in the face cannot move, or if there is pain that does not go away in the face, chin, or neck.

If there are symptoms, a doctor will examine the throat and neck using a mirror and lights. The doctor may order a special x-ray called a CT scan, which uses a computer to make a picture of the inside of parts of the body. Another special scan that uses magnetic waves to make a picture of the head may also be done. If tissue that is not normal is found, the doctor will need to cut out a small piece and look at

PDQ Statement, National Cancer Institute, revised September 1998.

81

it under the microscope to see if there are any cancer cells. This is called a biopsy.

The chance of recovery (prognosis) depends on where the cancer is in the salivary glands, whether the cancer is just in the area where it started or has spread to other tissues (the stage), how the cancer cells look under a microscope (the grade), and the patient's general state of health.

Stages of Cancer of the Salivary Gland

Once cancer of the salivary gland is found, more tests will be done to find out if cancer cells have spread to other parts of the body. This is called staging. A doctor needs to know the stage of the disease to plan treatment. Salivary gland cancers are also classified by "grade", which tells how fast the cancer cells grow, based on how the cells look under a microscope. Low-grade cancers grow more slowly than high-grade cancers.

The following stages are used for cancer of the salivary gland:

Stage I

The cancer is no more than 4 centimeters (about 1½ inches) and has not spread into the tissue around it or to the lymph nodes in the area (lymph nodes are small bean-shaped structures that are found throughout the body; they produce and store infection-fighting cells).

Stage II

Either of the following may be true:

- The cancer is no more than 4 centimeters and has spread into the skin, soft tissue, bone, or nerve around the gland. The cancer has not spread to lymph nodes in the area.

- The cancer is between 4 and 6 centimeters (a little over 2 inches) and has not spread into the tissue around it or to lymph nodes in the area.

Stage III

Any of the following may be true:

- The cancer is between 4 and 6 centimeters and has spread into the skin, soft tissue, bone, or nerve around the gland. The cancer has not spread to lymph nodes in the area.

- The cancer is more than 6 centimeters but has not spread into the tissue around it or to lymph nodes in the area.

- The cancer is any size and has spread to only one lymph node on the same side of the neck as the cancer. If the cancer is more than 6 centimeters, it has not spread to tissues around the cancer. The lymph node that contains cancer measures no more than 3 centimeters (just over 1 inch).

Stage IV

Any of the following may be true:

- The cancer is more than 6 centimeters and has spread into the skin, soft tissue, bone, or nerve around the gland. The lymph nodes may or may not have cancer.

- The cancer is any size and has spread to more than one lymph node on the same side of the neck as the cancer, to lymph nodes on one or both sides of the neck, or to any lymph node that measures more than 6 centimeters.

- The cancer has spread to other parts of the body.

Recurrent

Recurrent disease means that the cancer has come back (recurred) after it has been treated. It may come back in the salivary gland or in another part of the body.

How Cancer of the Salivary Gland Is Treated

There are treatments for all patients with cancer of the salivary gland. Three kinds of treatment are used:

- surgery (taking out the cancer)

- radiation therapy (using high-dose x-rays or other high-energy rays to kill cancer cells)

- chemotherapy (using drugs to kill cancer cells)

Surgery is often used to remove cancers of the salivary gland. Depending on where the cancer is and how far it has spread, a doctor may need to cut out tissue around the cancer. If cancer has spread to lymph nodes in the neck, the lymph nodes may be removed (lymph node dissection).

Radiation therapy is also a common treatment of cancer of the salivary gland. Radiation therapy uses high-energy x-rays to kill cancer cells and shrink tumors. Radiation may come from a machine outside the body (external radiation therapy) or from putting materials that produce radiation (radioisotopes) through thin plastic tubes in the area where the cancer cells are found (internal radiation therapy). A special type of radiation therapy using tiny particles called neutrons has been shown to be effective in treating some salivary gland cancers. The use of drugs with the radiation therapy to make cancer cells more sensitive to radiation (radiosensitization) is being tested in clinical trials.

Chemotherapy uses drugs to kill cancer cells. Chemotherapy may be taken by pill, or it may be put into the body by a needle in a vein or muscle. Chemotherapy is called a systemic treatment because the drug enters the bloodstream, travels through the body, and can kill cancer cells throughout the body. Chemotherapy for cancer of the salivary gland is still being tested in clinical trials.

Because the salivary glands help digest food and are close to the jaw, a patient may need special help adjusting to the side effects of the cancer and its treatment. A doctor will consult with several kinds of doctors who can help determine the best treatment. Trained medical staff can also help in recovery from treatment. Plastic surgery may be needed if a large amount of tissue or bone around the salivary glands is taken out.

Treatment by Stage

Treatment of cancer of the salivary gland depends on where the cancer is, the stage of the disease, and the patient's age and overall health.

Standard treatment may be considered because of its effectiveness in patients in past studies, or participation in a clinical trial may be considered. Not all patients are cured with standard therapy and some standard treatments may have more side effects than are desired. For these reasons, clinical trials are designed to find better ways to treat cancer patients and are based on the most up-to-date information. Clinical trials are ongoing in some parts of the country for patients with cancer of the salivary gland. To learn more about clinical trials, call the Cancer Information Service at 1-800-4-CANCER (1-800-422-6237); TTY at 1-800-332-8615.

Stage I Salivary Gland Cancer

Treatment depends on whether the cancer is low grade (slow growing) or high grade (fast growing).

If the cancer is low grade, treatment will probably be surgery.
If the cancer is high grade, treatment may be one of the following:

1. Surgery.

2. Surgery followed by radiation therapy.

3. Clinical trials of new chemotherapy drugs.

Stage II Salivary Gland Cancer

Treatment depends on whether the cancer is low grade (slow growing) or high grade (fast growing).
If the cancer is low grade, treatment may be one of the following:

1. Surgery with or without radiation therapy.

2. Chemotherapy (if surgery or radiation is refused or if the cancer does not respond to surgery or radiation therapy).

If the cancer is high grade, treatment may be one of the following:

1. Surgery.

2. Surgery followed by radiation therapy.

3. Radiation therapy alone (if surgery is not possible). Neutron radiation is effective in treating this type of cancer. Clinical trials of drugs given with radiation to make the cancer cells more sensitive to radiation (radiosensitization).

4. Clinical trials of new chemotherapy drugs.

Stage III Salivary Gland Cancer

Treatment depends on whether the cancer is low grade (slow growing) or high grade (fast growing).
If the cancer is low grade, treatment may be one of the following:

1. Surgery with or without radiation therapy.

2. Clinical trials of neutron irradiation and chemotherapy drugs.

If the cancer is high grade, treatment may be one of the following:

1. Surgery.

2. Surgery followed by radiation therapy.

3. Radiation therapy if surgery is not possible. Neutron radiation is effective in treating this type of cancer.

4. Clinical trials of drugs given with radiation to make the cancer cells more sensitive to radiation (radiosensitization).

Stage IV Salivary Gland Cancer

Treatment may be one of the following:

1. Radiation therapy. Neutron radiation is effective in treating this type of cancer.

2. A clinical trial of chemotherapy.

Recurrent Salivary Gland Cancer

Treatment depends on the type of salivary gland cancer the patient has, where the cancer came back, the treatment the patient had before, and the patient's general health. Radiation therapy may be given, or a patient may choose to take part in a clinical trial of new treatments.

To Learn More

To learn more about cancer of the salivary gland, call the National Cancer Institute's Cancer Information Service at 1-800-4-CANCER (1-800-422-6237); TTY at 1-800-332-8615. By dialing this toll-free number, you can speak with a trained information specialist who can answer your questions.

The Cancer Information Service also has booklets about cancer that are available to the public and can be sent on request. The following booklet about oral cancer may be helpful:

What You Need To Know About Oral Cancer *

The following general booklets on questions related to cancer may be helpful:

What You Need To Know About Cancer *

Taking Time: Support for People with Cancer and the People Who Care About Them

What Are Clinical Trials All About?

Chemotherapy and You: A Guide to Self-Help During Treatment *

Radiation Therapy and You: A Guide to Self-Help During Treatment *

Eating Hints for Cancer Patients *

Advanced Cancer: Living Each Day *

When Cancer Recurs: Meeting the Challenge Again *

* Reprinted in this volume—see Table of Contents

There are many other places where people can get material and information about cancer treatment and services. The social service office at a hospital can be checked for local and national agencies that can help with getting information about finances, getting to and from treatment, getting care at home, and dealing with problems. For more information from the National Cancer Institute, please write to this address:

National Cancer Institute
Office of Cancer Communications
31 Center Drive, MSC 2580
Bethesda, MD 20892-2580

Chapter 9

Oral Cancer

Introduction

The National Cancer Institute (NCI) has written this information to help people with oral cancer and their families and friends better understand this disease. We hope others will also read it to learn more about oral cancer.

This chapter describes symptoms, diagnosis, and treatment. It also has information about rehabilitation and about sources of support to help patients cope with oral cancer.

Our knowledge about oral cancer keeps increasing. For up-to-date information or to order this publication, call the National Cancer Institute's Cancer Information Service (CIS). The toll-free number is 1-800-4-CANCER (1-800-422-6237).

The CIS uses a National Cancer Institute cancer information database called PDQ and other NCI resources to answer callers' questions. Cancer information specialists can also send information from PDQ and other NCI materials about cancer, its treatment, and living with the disease.

The Oral Cavity

This chapter deals with cancer of the oral cavity (mouth) and the oropharynx (the part of the throat at the back of the mouth). The oral

"What You Need To Know About Oral Cancer," National Cancer Institute (NCI) publication, updated September 1998.

cavity includes many parts: the lips; the lining inside the lips and cheeks, called the buccal mucosa; the teeth; the bottom (floor) of the mouth under the tongue; the front two-thirds of the tongue; the bony top of the mouth (hard palate); the gums; and the small area behind the wisdom teeth. The oropharynx includes the back one-third of the tongue, the soft palate, the tonsils, and the part of the throat behind the mouth. Salivary glands throughout the oral cavity make saliva, which keeps the mouth moist and helps digest food.

What Is Cancer?

Cancer is a group of diseases. It occurs when cells become abnormal and divide without control or order. More than 100 different types of cancer are known.

Like all organs of the body, the mouth and throat are made up of many kinds of cells. Cells normally divide in an orderly way to produce more cells only when the body needs them. This process helps keep the body healthy.

Cells that divide when new cells are not needed form too much tissue. The mass of extra tissue, call a tumor, can be benign or malignant.

- Benign tumors are not cancer. They can usually be removed, and in most cases, they don't grow back. Most important, the cells in benign tumors do not invade other tissues and do not spread to other parts of the body. Benign tumors usually are not a threat to life.

- Malignant tumors are cancer. They can invade and damage nearby tissues and organs. Also, cancer cells can break away from a malignant tumor and enter the bloodstream or the lymphatic system. This is how cancer spreads and forms secondary tumors in other parts of the body. The spread of cancer is called metastasis.

When oral cancer spreads, it usually travels through the lymphatic system. Cancer cells that enter the lymphatic system are carried along by lymph, an almost colorless, watery fluid containing cells that help the body fight infection and disease. Along the lymphatic channels are groups of small, bean-shaped organs called lymph nodes (sometimes called lymph glands). Oral cancer that spreads usually travels to the lymph nodes in the neck. It can also spread to other parts of the body. Cancer that spreads is the same disease and has the same name as the original (primary) cancer.

Early Detection

Regular checkups that include an examination of the entire mouth can detect precancerous conditions or the early stages of oral cancer. Your doctor and dentist should check the tissues in your mouth as part of your routine exams.

Symptoms

Oral cancer usually occurs in people over the age of 45 but can develop at any age. These are some symptoms to watch for:

- A sore on the lip or in the mouth that does not heal;
- A lump on the lip or in the mouth or throat;
- A white or red patch on the gums, tongue, or lining of the mouth;
- Unusual bleeding, pain, or numbness in the mouth;
- A sore throat that does not go away, or a feeling that something is caught in the throat;
- Difficulty or pain with chewing or swallowing;
- Swelling of the jaw that causes dentures to fit poorly or become uncomfortable;
- A change in the voice; and/or
- Pain in the ear.

These symptoms may be caused by cancer or by other, less serious problems. It is important to see a dentist or doctor about any symptoms like these, so that the problem can be diagnosed and treated as early as possible.

Diagnosis and Staging

If an abnormal area has been found in the oral cavity, a biopsy is the only way to know whether it is cancer. Usually, the patient is referred to an oral surgeon or an ear, nose, and throat surgeon, who removes part or all of the lump or abnormal-looking area. A pathologist examines the tissue under a microscope to check for cancer cells.

Almost all oral cancers are squamous cell carcinomas. Squamous cells line the oral cavity.

If the pathologist finds oral cancer, the patient's doctor needs to know the stage, or extent, of the disease in order to plan the best treatment. Staging tests and exams help the doctor find out whether the cancer has spread and what parts of the body are affected.

A patient who needs a biopsy may want to ask the doctor these questions:

- How much tissue will be removed for the biopsy?
- How long will the biopsy take? Will I be awake? Will it hurt?
- How should I care for the biopsy site afterward?
- How soon will I know the results?
- If I do have cancer, who will talk with me about treatment? When?

Staging generally includes dental x-rays and x-rays of the head and chest. The doctor may also want the patient to have a CT (or CAT) scan. A CT scan is a series of x-rays put together by a computer to form detailed pictures of areas inside the body. Ultrasonography is another way to produce pictures of areas in the body. High-frequency sound waves (ultrasound), which cannot be heard by humans, are bounced off organs and tissue. The pattern of echoes produced by these waves creates a picture called a sonogram. Sometimes the doctor asks for MRI (magnetic resonance imaging), a procedure in which pictures are created using a magnet linked to a computer. The doctor also feels the lymph nodes in the neck to check for swelling or other changes. In most cases, the patient will have a complete physical examination before treatment begins.

Treatment

After diagnosis and staging, the doctor develops a treatment plan to fit each patient's needs. Treatment for oral cancer depends on a number of factors. Among these are the location, size, type, and extent of the tumor and the stage of the disease. The doctor also considers the patient's age and general health. Treatment involves surgery, radiation therapy, or, in many cases, a combination of the two. Some patients receive chemotherapy, treatment with anticancer drugs.

For most patients, it is important to have a complete dental exam before cancer treatment begins. Because cancer treatment may make the mouth sensitive and more easily infected, doctors often advise patients to have any needed dental work done before treatment begins.

Most people with cancer want to learn all they can about their disease and their treatment choices so they can take an active part in decisions about their medical and dental care. The doctor is the best person to answer their questions. Also, the patient may want to talk with the doctor about taking part in a research study of new treatment methods. Such studies, called clinical trials, are designed to improve cancer treatment.

Many patients find it useful to make a list of questions before seeing the doctor. Taking notes can make it easier to remember what the doctor says. Some patients also find that it helps to have a family member or friend with them—to take part in the discussion, to take notes, or just to listen.

Before treatment begins, the patient may want to ask the doctor these questions:

- What are my treatment choices? Which do you recommend for me? Why?

- What are the risks and possible side effects of each treatment?

- What are the expected benefits of each kind of treatment?

- What can be done about side effects?

- Would a clinical trial be appropriate for me?

There is a lot to learn about cancer and its treatment. Patients do not need to ask all their questions or understand all the answers at once. They will have many chances to ask the doctor to explain things that are not clear and to ask for more information.

Planning Treatment

Treatment decisions can be complex. Before starting treatment, the patient may want to have another doctor review the diagnosis and treatment plan. A short delay will not reduce the chance that treatment will be successful. There are a number of ways to find a doctor for a second opinion:

- The patient's doctor or dentist may suggest a specialist who treats oral cancer.

- The Cancer Information Service, at 1-800-4-CANCER, can tell callers about cancer centers and other NCI-supported programs in their area.

- Patients can get the names of specialists from their local medical or dental society, a nearby hospital, or a medical or dental school.

- The *Directory of Medical Specialists* lists doctors' names along with their specialty and their background. This resource is available in most public libraries.

Methods of Treatment

Patients with oral cancer may be treated by a team of specialists. The medical team may include an oral surgeon; an ear, nose, and throat surgeon; a medical oncologist; a radiation oncologist; a prosthodontist; a general dentist; a plastic surgeon; a dietitian; a social worker; a nurse; and a speech therapist.

Surgery to remove the tumor in the mouth is the usual treatment for patients with oral cancer. If there is evidence that the cancer has spread, the surgeon may also remove lymph nodes in the neck. If the disease has spread to muscles and other tissues in the neck, the operation may be more extensive.

Before surgery, the patient may want to ask the doctor these questions:

- What kind of operation will it be?

- How will I feel after the operation? If I have pain, how will you help me?

- Will I have trouble eating?

- Where will the scars be? What will they look like?

- Do you expect that there will be long-term effects from the surgery?

- Will there be permanent changes in my appearance?

- Will I lose my teeth? Can they be replaced? How soon?

- If I need to have plastic surgery, when can that be done?

- Will I need to see a specialist for help with my speech?

- When can I get back to my normal activities?

Radiation therapy (also called radiotherapy) is the use of high-energy rays to damage cancer cells and stop them from growing. Like surgery, radiation therapy is local therapy; it affects only the cells in the treated area. The energy may come from a large machine (external radiation). It can also come from radioactive materials placed directly into or near the tumor (internal radiation). Radiation therapy is sometimes used instead of surgery for small tumors in the mouth. Patients with large tumors may need both surgery and radiation therapy.

Radiation therapy may be given before or after surgery. Before surgery, radiation can shrink the tumor so that it can be removed. Radiation after surgery is used to destroy cancer cells that may remain.

For external radiation therapy, the patient goes to the hospital or clinic each day for treatments. Usually, treatment is given 5 days a week for 5 to 6 weeks. This schedule helps protect healthy tissues by dividing the total amount of radiation into small doses.

Implant radiation therapy puts tiny "seeds" containing radioactive material directly into the tumor or in tissue near it. Generally, an implant is left in place for several days, and the patient will stay in the hospital in a private room. The length of time nurses and other caregivers, as well as visitors, can spend with the patient will be limited. The implant is removed before the patient goes home.

Before radiation therapy, a patient may want to ask the doctor these questions:

- When will the treatments begin? When will they end?
- How will I feel during therapy?
- What can I do to take care of myself during therapy?
- Can I continue my normal activities?
- How will my mouth and face look afterward?
- Will I need a special diet? For how long?
- If my mouth becomes dry, what can I do about it?

Chemotherapy is the use of drugs to kill cancer cells. Researchers are looking for effective drugs or drug combinations to treat oral cancer. They are also exploring ways to combine chemotherapy with other forms of cancer treatment to help destroy the tumor and prevent the disease from spreading.

Clinical Trials

Researchers are developing treatment methods that are more effective against oral cancer, and they are also finding ways to reduce side effects of treatment. When laboratory research shows that a new method has promise, doctors use it to treat cancer patients in clinical trials. These trials are designed to answer scientific questions about the new approach and to find out whether it is both safe and effective. Patients who take part in clinical trials make an important contribution to medical science and may have the first chance to benefit from improved treatment methods.

Clinical trials to study new treatments for oral cancer are under way in hospitals throughout the country. Some trials involve ways to shrink or destroy the primary tumor. In others, scientists are testing ways to prevent the cancer from coming back in the mouth or spreading to other parts of the body. Still others involve treatments to slow or stop cancer that has already spread.

Researchers are studying the timing of treatments and new ways to combine various types of treatment. For example, they are trying to increase the effectiveness of radiation therapy by giving treatments twice a day instead of once a day. They are also working with hyperthermia (heat) and with drugs called radiosensitizers to try to make cancer cells more sensitive to radiation. Researchers are also using drugs to help protect normal cells from radiation damage. In addition, they are exploring various new anticancer drugs and drug combinations.

People who have had oral cancer have an increased risk of getting a new cancer of the mouth or another part of the head or neck. Doctors are trying to find ways to prevent these new cancers. Some research has shown that a substance related to vitamin A may prevent a new cancer from developing in someone who has already been successfully treated for oral cancer.

Oral cancer patients who are interested in taking part in a trial should talk with their doctor. They may want to read *Taking Part in Clinical Trials: What Cancer Patients Need To Know*, a booklet that explains what treatment studies are and outlines some of their possible benefits and risks.

One way to learn about clinical trials is through PDQ, a computerized resource developed by the National Cancer Institute. PDQ contains information about cancer treatment and an up-to-date list of trials all over the country. The Cancer Information Service, at 1-800-4-CANCER, can provide PDQ information to patients and the public.

Side Effects of Treatment

It is hard to limit the effects of cancer treatment so that only cancer cells are removed or destroyed. Because healthy cells and tissues may also be damaged, treatment often causes side effects.

The side effects of cancer treatment vary. They depend mainly on the type and extent of the treatment and the specific area being treated. Also, each person reacts differently. Some side effects are temporary; others are permanent. Doctors try to plan the patient's therapy to keep side effects to a minimum. They also watch patients very carefully so they can help with any problems that occur.

Surgery to remove a small tumor in the mouth usually does not cause any lasting problems. For a larger tumor, however, the surgeon may need to remove part of the palate, tongue, or jaw. Such surgery is likely to change the patient's ability to chew, swallow, or talk. The patient may also look different.

After surgery, the patient's face may be swollen. This swelling usually goes away within a few weeks. However, removing lymph nodes can slow the flow of lymph, which may collect in the tissues; this swelling may last for a long time.

Before starting radiation therapy, a patient should see a dentist who is familiar with the changes this therapy can cause in the mouth. Radiation therapy can make the mouth sore. It can also cause changes in the saliva and may reduce the amount of saliva, making it hard to chew and swallow. Because saliva normally protects the teeth, mouth dryness can promote tooth decay. Good mouth care can help keep the teeth and gums healthy and can make the patient feel more comfortable. The health care team may suggest the use of a special kind of toothbrush or mouthwash. The dentist usually suggests a special fluoride program to keep the teeth healthy. To help relieve mouth dryness, the health care team may suggest the use of artificial saliva and other methods to keep the mouth moist. Mouth dryness from radiation therapy goes away in some patients, but it can be permanent.

Weight loss can be a serious problem for patients being treated for oral cancer because a sore mouth may make eating difficult. Your doctor may suggest ways to maintain a healthy diet. In many cases, it helps to have food and beverages in very small amounts. Many patients find that eating several small meals and snacks during the day works better than trying to have three large meals. Often, it is easier to eat soft, bland foods that have been moistened with sauces or gravies; thick soups, puddings, and high protein milkshakes are nourishing and easy to swallow. It may be helpful to prepare other foods in a blender. The doctor may also suggest special liquid dietary supplements for patients who have trouble chewing. Drinking lots of fluids helps keep the mouth moist and makes it easier to eat.

Some patients are able to wear their dentures during radiation therapy. Many, however, will not be able to wear dentures for up to a year after treatment. Because the tissues in the mouth that support the denture may change during or after treatment, dentures may no longer fit properly. After treatment is over, a patient may need to have dentures refitted or replaced.

Radiation therapy can also cause sores in the mouth and cracked and peeling lips. These usually heal in the weeks after treatment is completed. Often, good mouth care can help prevent these sores. Dentures should not be worn until the sores have healed.

During radiation therapy, patients may become very tired, especially in the later weeks of treatment. Resting is important, but doctors usually advise their patients to try to stay reasonably active. Patients should match their activities to their energy level. It's common for radiation to cause the skin in the treated area to become red and dry, tender, and itchy. Toward the end of treatment, the skin may become moist and "weepy." There may be permanent darkening or "bronzing" of the skin in the treated area. This area should be exposed to the air as much as possible but should also be protected from the sun. Good skin care is important at this time, but patients should not use any lotions or creams without the doctor's advice. Men may lose all or part of their beard, but facial hair generally grows back after treatment is done. Usually, men shave with an electric razor during treatment to prevent cuts that may lead to infection. Most effects of radiation therapy on the skin are temporary. The area will heal when the treatment is over.

The side effects of chemotherapy depend on the drugs that are given. In general, anticancer drugs affect rapidly growing cells, such as blood cells that fight infection, cells that line the mouth and the digestive tract, and cells in hair follicles. As a result, patients may have side effects such as lower resistance to infection, loss of appetite, nausea, vomiting, or mouth sores. They also may have less energy and may lose their hair.

The side effects of cancer treatment are different for each person, and they may even be different from one treatment to the next. Doctors, nurses, and dietitians can explain the side effects of cancer treatment and can suggest ways to deal with them. The booklets *Radiation Therapy and You* [reprinted in this volume as Chapter 66] and *Eating Hints for Cancer Patients* [reprinted in this volume as Chapter 77] contain helpful information about cancer treatment and coping with side effects. Patients receiving anticancer drugs will find useful information in *Chemotherapy and You* [reprinted in this volume as Chapter 63].

Rehabilitation

Rehabilitation is a very important part of treatment for patients with oral cancer. The goals of rehabilitation depend on the extent of the disease and the treatment a patient has received. The health care team makes every effort to help the patient return to normal activities as soon as possible. Rehabilitation may include dietary counseling, surgery, a dental prosthesis, speech therapy, and other services.

Sometimes, a patient needs reconstructive and plastic surgery to rebuild the bones or tissues of the mouth. If this is not possible, a prosthodontist may be able to make an artificial dental and/or facial part (prosthesis). Patients may need special training to use the device.

Speech therapy generally begins as soon as possible for a patient who has trouble speaking after treatment. Often, a speech therapist visits the patient in the hospital to plan therapy and teach speech exercises. Speech therapy usually continues after the patient returns home.

Followup Care

Regular followup exams are very important for anyone who has been treated for oral cancer. The physician and the dentist watch the patient closely to check the healing process and to look for signs that the cancer may have returned. Patients with mouth dryness from radiation therapy should have dental exams three times a year.

The patient may need to see a dietitian if weight loss or eating problems continue. Most doctors urge their oral cancer patients to stop using tobacco and alcohol to reduce the risk of developing a new cancer.

Support for Cancer Patients

Living with a serious disease isn't easy. Cancer patients and those who care about them face many problems and challenges. Finding the strength to cope with these difficulties is easier when people have helpful information and support services. Several useful booklets, including *Taking Time: Support for People With Cancer and the People Who Care About Them*, are available from the Cancer Information Service.

Cancer patients may worry about holding a job, caring for their family, or starting new relationships. Worries about tests, treatments, hospital stays, and medical bills are common. Doctors, nurses, and other members of the health care team can help calm fears and ease confusion about treatment, working, or daily activities. Also, meeting with a nurse, social worker, counselor, or member of the clergy can be helpful for patients who want to talk about their feelings or discuss their concerns.

Friends and relatives, especially those who have had personal experience with cancer, can be very supportive. Also, many patients find it helpful to discuss their concerns with others who are facing similar problems. Cancer patients often get together in support groups, where they can share what they have learned about cancer and its treatment and about coping with the disease. It is important to keep in mind, however, that each patient is different. Treatments and ways of dealing with cancer that work for one person may not be right for another—even if they both have the same kind of cancer. It is always a good idea to discuss the advice of friends and family members with the doctor.

Often, a social worker at the hospital or clinic can suggest groups that can help with rehabilitation, emotional support, financial aid, transportation, or home care.

What the Future Holds

Patients and their families are naturally concerned about what the future holds. Sometimes they use statistics to try to figure out whether the patient will be cured or how long he or she will live. It is important to remember, however, that statistics are averages based on large numbers of patients. They cannot be used to predict what will happen to a certain patient because no two cancer patients are alike. The doctor who takes care of the patient knows his or her medical history and is in the best position to discuss the person's outlook (prognosis).

People should feel free to ask the doctor about their chance of recovery, but not even the doctor knows for sure what will happen. When doctors talk about surviving cancer, they may use the term remission rather than cure. Even though many patients with oral cancer recover completely, doctors use this term because oral cancer can recur.

Causes and Prevention

Scientists at hospitals and medical centers all across the country are studying this disease to learn more about what causes it and how to prevent it. Doctors do know that no one can "catch" cancer from another person: it is not contagious. Two known causes of oral cancer are tobacco and alcohol use.

Tobacco use—smoking cigarettes, cigars, or pipes; chewing tobacco; or dipping snuff—accounts for 80 to 90 percent of oral cancers.

A number of studies have shown that cigar and pipe smokers have the same risk as cigarette smokers. Studies indicate that smokeless tobacco users are at particular risk of developing oral cancer. For long-time users, the risk is much greater, making the use of snuff or chewing tobacco among young people a special concern.

People who stop using tobacco—even after many years of use—can greatly reduce their risk of oral cancer. Special counseling or self-help groups may be useful for those who are trying to give up tobacco. Some hospitals have groups for people who want to quit. Also, the Cancer Information Service and the American Cancer Society may have information about groups in local areas to help people quit using tobacco.

Chronic and/or heavy use of alcohol also increases the risk of oral cancer, even for people who do not use tobacco. However, people who use both alcohol and tobacco have an especially high risk of oral cancer. Scientists believe that these substances increase each other's harmful effects.

Cancer of the lip can be caused by exposure to the sun. The risk can be avoided with the use of a lotion or lip balm containing a sunscreen. Wearing a hat with a brim can also block the sun's harmful rays. Pipe smokers are especially prone to cancer of the lip.

Some studies have shown that many people who develop oral cancer have a history of leukoplakia, a whitish patch inside the mouth. The causes of leukoplakia are not well understood, but it is commonly associated with heavy use of tobacco and alcohol. The condition often occurs in irritated areas, such as the gums and mouth lining of smokeless tobacco users and the lower lip of pipe smokers.

Another condition, erythroplakia, appears as a red patch in the mouth. Erythroplakia occurs most often in people 60 to 70 years of age. Early diagnosis and treatment of leukoplakia and erythroplakia are important because cancer may develop in these patches.

People who think they might be at risk for developing oral cancer should discuss this concern with their doctor or dentist, who may be able to suggest ways to reduce the risk and plan an appropriate schedule for checkups.

Resources

National Institute of Dental Research
Building 31, Room 2C35
9000 Rockville Pike
Bethesda, MD 20892

The National Institute of Dental Research, an agency of the Federal Government, is concerned with the causes, prevention, diagnosis, and treatment of oral and dental diseases. It can supply free printed material about oral health during and after cancer treatment.

Booklets

The NCI booklets listed below are available free of charge by calling the Cancer Information Service at 1-800-4-CANCER.

Booklets about Cancer Treatment

Radiation Therapy and You: A Guide to Self-Help During Treatment *

Chemotherapy and You: A Guide to Self-Help During Treatment *

Eating Hints for Cancer Patients *

Helping Yourself During Chemotherapy: 4 Steps for Cancer Patients

Taking Part in Clinical Trials: What Cancer Patients Need To Know *

Questions and Answers About Pain Control

Get Relief from Cancer Pain

Booklets about Living with Cancer

Taking Time: Support for People With Cancer and the People Who Care About Them

Facing Forward: A Guide for Cancer Survivors *

When Cancer Recurs: Meeting the Challenge Again *

Advanced Cancer: Living Each Day *

* Reprinted in this volume—see Table of Contents

National Cancer Institute Information Resources

You may want more information for yourself, your family, and your doctor. The following National Cancer Institute (NCI) services are available to help you.

Telephone

Cancer Information Service (CIS) Provides accurate, up-to-date information on cancer to patients and their families, health professionals, and the general public. Information specialists translate the latest scientific information into understandable language and respond in English, Spanish, or on TTY equipment.

Toll-free: 1-800-4-CANCER (1-800-422-6237)
TTY: 1-800-332-8615

Internet

These Web sites may be useful:

http://www.nci.nih.gov—NCI's primary Web site; contains information about the Institute and its programs.

http://cancertrials.nci.nih.gov—CancerTrials; NCI's comprehensive clinical trials information center for patients, health professionals, and the public. Includes information on understanding trials, deciding whether to participate in trials, finding specific trials, plus research news and other resources.

http://cancernet.nci.nih.gov—CancerNet; contains material for health professionals, patients, and the public, including information from PDQ about cancer treatment, screening, prevention, supportive care, and clinical trials, and CANCERLIT, a bibliographic database.

E-mail

CancerMail—Includes NCI information about cancer treatment, screening, prevention, and supportive care. To obtain a contents list, send e-mail to cancermail@icicc.nci.nih.gov with the word "help" in the body of the message.

Fax

CancerFax—Includes NCI information about cancer treatment, screening, prevention, and supportive care. To obtain a contents list, dial 301-402-5874 from a fax machine hand set and follow the recorded instructions.

Chapter 10

Cancer of the Esophagus

What You Need to Know about Cancer of the Esophagus

Each year, about 11,000 Americans find out they have cancer of the esophagus. The National Cancer Institute (NCI) has prepared this chapter to help patients and their families and friends better understand this type of cancer. We also hope it will encourage others to learn more about this disease.

This chapter has information on the symptoms, diagnosis, and treatment of cancer of the esophagus. Other NCI publications about cancer, its treatment, and living with the disease are listed in the section "For Further Information." However, materials like these cannot answer every question or take the place of talks with doctors, nurses, and other members of the health care team. We hope our booklets will help with those talks.

Researchers continue to look for better ways to diagnose and treat cancer of the esophagus. For up-to-date information, call the NCI-supported Cancer Information Service (CIS) toll free at 1-800-4-CANCER. The CIS is described below in the "Resources" section.

The Esophagus

The esophagus, part of the digestive tract, is a tube that connects the throat with the stomach. It lies between the trachea (windpipe) and the spine. In an adult, the esophagus is about 10 inches long.

"What You Need to Know about Cancer of the Esophagus," National Cancer Institute, updated September 1998.

Upper Digestive Tract

When a person swallows, the muscular walls of the esophagus contract to push food down into the stomach. Glands in the lining of the esophagus produce mucus, which keeps the passageway moist and makes swallowing easier.

The esophagus, like all other organs of the body, is made up of many types of cells. Normally, cells divide to produce more cells only when they are needed. This orderly process helps keep the body healthy.

What Is Cancer?

Cancer is a group of diseases with one thing in common: cells become abnormal, dividing too often and without any order.

When cells divide without control, they form too much tissue. The mass of extra tissue, called a tumor, can be benign or malignant.

- Benign tumors are not cancer. They do not spread to other parts of the body and are seldom a threat to life. Benign tumors can usually be removed by surgery, and they are not likely to return.

- Malignant tumors are cancer. They can invade and damage nearby healthy tissues and organs. Cancer cells can also break away from the tumor and enter the bloodstream or the lymphatic system. That is how cancer spreads and forms tumors in other parts of the body. The spread of cancer is called metastasis.

Cancer of the esophagus is also called esophageal cancer. It can develop in any part of the esophagus. If the cancer spreads outside the esophagus, it usually shows up in nearby lymph nodes (sometimes called lymph glands). In many cases, the cancer also spreads to the windpipe, the large blood vessels in the chest, and other nearby organs. Esophageal cancer can also spread to the lungs, liver, stomach, and other parts of the body.

Cancer that spreads is the same disease and has the same name as the original (primary) cancer. When cancer of the esophagus spreads, it is called metastatic esophageal cancer.

Symptoms

Very small tumors in the esophagus usually do not cause symptoms. As the tumor grows, the most common symptom is difficulty in swallowing. The person may have a feeling of fullness, pressure, or burning as food goes down the esophagus. Also, it may feel as if food gets stuck behind the breastbone. Problems with swallowing may come and go. At first, they may be noticed mainly when the person eats meat, bread, or coarse foods, such as raw vegetables. As the tumor grows larger and the pathway to the stomach becomes narrower, other foods—even liquids—may be hard to swallow, and swallowing may be painful. Cancer of the esophagus can also cause indigestion, heartburn, vomiting, and frequent choking on food. Because of these problems, weight loss is common.

Sometimes a tumor in the esophagus causes coughing and hoarseness. It can also cause pain behind the breastbone or in the throat.

Any of these symptoms may be caused by cancer or by other, less serious health problems. Only a doctor can tell for sure. People with symptoms like these often see a gastroenterologist, a doctor who specializes in diseases of the digestive tract.

Diagnosis

To find the cause of any of these symptoms, the doctor asks about the patient's personal and family medical history and does a complete physical exam. In addition to checking general signs of health, the doctor usually orders x-rays and other tests.

An esophagram (also called a barium swallow) is a series of x-rays of the esophagus. To prepare for this test, the patient drinks a barium solution. The barium, which shows up on x-rays, coats the inside of the esophagus. The esophagram shows changes in the shape of the esophagus. The doctor can also use a special x-ray machine called a fluoroscope to watch the barium move down the esophagus to the stomach as the patient swallows.

Most patients also have a test called esophagoscopy. For this procedure, the patient's throat is sprayed with a local anesthetic to reduce discomfort and gagging. The doctor then passes a thin, flexible, lighted instrument called an endoscope through the mouth and down the throat into the esophagus. The scope lets the doctor see the lining of the esophagus and the place where the esophagus joins the stomach. If an abnormal area is found, the doctor does a biopsy (removal of a small amount of tissue through the endoscope). Also, cells can be brushed or washed from the walls of the esophagus through the scope. A pathologist examines the samples under a microscope to see whether cancer is present.

If cancer is found, the pathologist can tell what type of cancer it is. Cancer that occurs in the middle or upper part of the esophagus is usually squamous cell carcinoma. When cancer develops at the lower end of the esophagus, near the stomach, it is usually adenocarcinoma. (Carcinoma is another name for cancer in the lining of tissues.)

If the pathologist finds esophageal cancer, the patient's doctor needs to know the stage, or extent, of the disease. Staging is a careful attempt to find out what parts of the body are affected by the cancer.

Treatment decisions depend on these findings. Staging usually involves a physical exam, with special attention to the neck and chest, blood tests, additional x-rays, and other tests. The results show whether the cancer is just in the esophagus or has spread.

The doctor usually orders CT scans (also called CAT scans) of the chest and upper abdomen. During a CT scan, many x-rays are taken and a computer combines them to create detailed pictures. Some patients also have an MRI scan , which produces pictures using a huge magnet linked to a computer.

The doctor uses special instruments to check the organs near the esophagus. For example, the doctor can look through a laryngoscope to see whether the cancer has spread to the larynx (voice box). A bronchoscope lets the doctor see into the trachea and bronchi (airways that lead into the lungs).

If lymph nodes near the esophagus are enlarged, the surgeon may do a biopsy to find out whether they contain cancer cells. Sometimes the surgeon also removes samples of other tissues in the area to see whether the cancer has spread.

Treatment

Treatment for esophageal cancer depends on a number of factors. Among these are the exact location, size, and extent of the tumor, and the type of cancer cells. The doctor also considers the person's age and general health to develop a treatment plan to fit each person's needs.

The patient's doctor may want to discuss the case with other doctors who treat cancer of the esophagus. Also, the patient may want to talk with the doctor about taking part in a research study of new treatment methods. Such studies, called clinical trials, are designed to improve cancer treatment. Treatment studies are discussed below in the section on "Treatment Studies."

Many patients want to learn all they can about their disease and their treatment choices so they can take an active part in decisions about their medical care. People with cancer have many questions and concerns about their health. The doctor is the best one to answer them.

Most patients want to know the extent of their cancer, how it will be treated, how successful the treatment is likely to be, and how much it will cost.

Here are some important questions to ask the doctor:

- What are my treatment choices?

- Would a clinical trial be appropriate for me?

- What are the expected benefits of treatment?

- What are the risks and possible side effects of treatment?

- What can be done about side effects?

- If I have pain, how will you help me?

- Can I keep working during or after treatment?

Many people find it helpful to make a list of questions before they see the doctor. Taking notes can make it easier to remember what the doctor says. Some patients also find that it helps to have a family member or friend with them when they talk to the doctor—either to take part in the discussion or just to listen.

There's a lot to learn about cancer and its treatment. Patients should not feel that they need to understand everything the first time they hear it. They will have many chances to ask the doctor to explain things that are not clear.

Planning Treatment

Treatment decisions are complex. Before starting treatment, the patient might want a second doctor to review the diagnosis and treatment plan. There are a number of ways to get a second opinion:

- The patient's doctor may be able to suggest a doctor who has a special interest in cancer of the esophagus.

- The Cancer Information Service, at 1-800-4-CANCER, can tell callers about cancer centers and other NCI-supported programs in their area.

- Patients can get the names of doctors from their local medical society, a nearby hospital, or a medical school.

- The *Directory of Medical Specialists* lists doctors' names and gives their background. It is in most public libraries.

Treatment Methods

Cancer of the esophagus usually cannot be cured unless it is found in the earliest stages, before it has begun to spread. Unfortunately, early esophageal cancer causes few symptoms, and the disease is usually advanced when the diagnosis is made. However, advanced esophageal cancer can be treated and symptoms can be relieved.

Esophageal cancer is usually treated with surgery or radiation therapy (also called radiotherapy). Doctors are studying chemotherapy to see whether anticancer drugs can be helpful in treating patients with this disease. The doctor may use just one treatment method or combine them, depending on the patient's needs.

In some cases, the patient is referred to doctors who specialize in different kinds of cancer treatment. Often, specialists work together as a team to plan and carry out the patient's care. The medical team may include a gastroenterologist, surgeon, oncologist (cancer specialist), radiation oncologist, nurse, dietitian, and social worker.

Surgery is often part of the treatment plan. Many patients with esophageal cancer have an operation called esophagectomy. Generally, the surgeon removes the tumor along with a portion of the esophagus, nearby lymph nodes, and other tissue in the area. Usually, it is possible to connect the stomach to the remaining part of the esophagus. In a few cases, the surgeon forms a new passageway from the throat to the stomach, using tissue from another part of the digestive tract (such as the colon) to replace the esophagus.

If a tumor blocks the esophagus but cannot be removed, the surgeon may be able to create a bypass, a new pathway to the stomach. In some cases, the surgeon can dilate (widen) the esophagus. This procedure may have to be repeated as the tumor grows. Sometimes, the doctor puts a tube into the esophagus to keep it open. Recently, some surgeons have used a laser to destroy cancerous tissue and relieve blockages.

Radiation therapy is the use of high-energy rays to damage cancer cells and stop them from growing. Like surgery, radiation therapy is local therapy; it affects cells only in the treated area. Radiation therapy can be used to shrink a tumor before surgery or to destroy cancer cells that may remain in the area after surgery. Radiation may also be used instead of surgery, especially if the size or location of the tumor would make an operation difficult. In some cases, radiation therapy is recommended for patients who cannot have surgery for other health reasons. Even if the tumor cannot be removed by surgery or destroyed entirely by radiation therapy, radiation therapy can still help relieve pain and make swallowing easier.

In radiation therapy for esophageal cancer, the energy usually comes from a machine outside the body (external radiation). Some patients also need treatment with radioactive materials placed in the tumor (implant radiation). Usually, patients receive external radiation therapy 5 days a week for several weeks. Most patients can stay at home and go to the hospital or clinic each day for this treatment. For implant radiation, patients must stay in the hospital for a short time. More information about radiation therapy can be found in the NCI booklet *Radiation Therapy and You* [reprinted in this volume as Chapter 66].

Chemotherapy is the use of drugs to kill cancer cells. The doctor may suggest one drug or a combination of drugs. Chemotherapy may be used alone or combined with radiation therapy to shrink a tumor before surgery or to destroy cancer cells that remain in the body after surgery. Chemotherapy may also be used if surgery is not possible and for patients whose cancer returns after surgery or radiation therapy.

Most anticancer drugs for esophageal cancer are given by injection into a vein or muscle. Some may be taken by mouth. Chemotherapy is systemic therapy, meaning that the drugs travel through the bloodstream and can reach cancer cells all over the body. Often the drugs are given in cycles: a treatment period followed by a rest period, then another treatment and rest period, and so on. Many patients have their chemotherapy as outpatients at the hospital, in the doctor's office, or at home. Depending on the drugs, the treatment plan, and the patient's general health, however, a hospital stay may be needed. The NCI booklet *Chemotherapy and You* [reprinted in this volume as Chapter 63] has helpful information about this type of treatment.

Treatment Studies

Because esophageal cancer is so hard to control, many researchers are looking for more effective treatments. They are also exploring ways to reduce side effects. When laboratory research shows that a new method has promise, it is used to treat cancer patients in clinical trials. These trials are designed to answer scientific questions and to find out whether the new approach is both safe and effective. Patients who take part in clinical trials make an important contribution to medical science and may have the first chance to benefit from improved treatment methods.

Many clinical trials of new treatments for esophageal cancer are under way. Doctors are studying the timing of treatments and new ways of combining various types of treatment. They are also trying new anticancer drugs and drug combinations, new forms of radiation therapy, and drugs that make cancer cells more sensitive to radiation. Another method under study is photodynamic therapy, the use of laser light and drugs that make the cancer cells sensitive to light so the laser can destroy them. Researchers are also exploring biological therapy, a new type of treatment intended to help the body's immune system fight cancer more effectively.

Esophageal cancer patients who are interested in taking part in a trial should discuss this option with their doctor. *What Are Clinical Trials All About?* is an NCI booklet that explains some of the benefits and risks of treatment studies.

One way to learn about clinical trials is through PDQ, a computerized resource of cancer treatment information. Developed by NCI, PDQ contains an up todate list of trials in progress all over the country. Doctors can use an office computer or the services of a medical library to get PDQ information. The Cancer Information Service, at 1-800-4-CANCER, is another source of PDQ information for doctors, patients, and the public.

Side Effects

The methods used to treat cancer are very powerful. It is hard to limit the effects of therapy so that only cancer cells are removed or destroyed. Because healthy cells also may be damaged, treatment often causes unpleasant side effects.

The side effects of cancer treatment vary. They depend mainly on the type and extent of the treatment. Also, each person reacts differently. Doctors try to plan the therapy to keep side effects to a minimum. They also monitor patients very carefully so they can help with any problems that occur.

Surgery for cancer of the esophagus is a major operation. Patients who have had trouble eating and drinking may need intravenous (IV) feedings and fluids for several days before and after the operation. They may need antibiotics to prevent or treat infections. Patients are taught special coughing and breathing exercises to keep their lungs clear. Discomfort or pain after surgery can be controlled with medicine. Patients should feel free to discuss pain relief with the doctor.

Patients receiving radiation therapy may become tired as treatment continues. Resting as much as possible is important. It is also common for the skin in the treated area to become red or dry. The skin should be exposed to the air but protected from the sun, and patients should avoid wearing clothes that rub the area. Good skin care is important at this time. The doctor may suggest certain kinds of soap, and patients should not use any lotion or cream on the skin without the doctor's advice. Radiation to the chest and neck can cause a dry, sore throat or a dry cough. Drinking extra liquids may be helpful, and doctors sometimes suggest cough medicine. If burning, tightness, or other pain makes it hard to swallow, the doctor may suggest a local anesthetic or soothing gargle for use before meals. Some patients find that antacids help relieve feelings of indigestion. A small number of patients feel short of breath during radiation therapy. The doctor may prescribe medicine to relieve this problem.

The side effects of chemotherapy depend on the drugs that are given. In general, anticancer drugs affect cells that divide rapidly. These include blood cells, which fight infection, cause the blood to clot, or carry oxygen to all parts of the body. When blood cells are affected by anticancer drugs, patients may have lower resistance to infection, may bruise or bleed easily, and may have less energy. Cells in hair follicles and cells that line the digestive tract also divide rapidly. So chemotherapy can cause hair loss and other problems such as poor appetite, mouth sores, nausea, and vomiting. These side effects usually go away gradually after treatment stops.

The patient's weight is checked regularly because weight loss can be a serious problem for patients with cancer of the esophagus. Swallowing food may be difficult, and patients may not feel hungry if they are uncomfortable or tired. Yet well-nourished patients generally feel better, have more energy, and are often better able to withstand the side effects of their treatment, so good nutrition is important. Patients with esophageal cancer are usually encouraged to have several small meals and snacks throughout the day, rather than try to eat three large meals. It often helps to sit up for a while after eating, and the doctor may prescribe medicine to control nausea and vomiting and to relieve discomfort.

When swallowing is difficult, many patients can still manage soft, bland foods moistened with sauces or gravies. It may be helpful to prepare other foods in a blender. In addition, puddings, ice cream, and soups are nourishing and easy to swallow. Doctors, nurses, and dietitians may have other suggestions to help patients and their families choose foods that supply enough calories to control weight loss and enough protein to keep up strength and rebuild normal tissues. For example, they may suggest liquid dietary supplements or milkshakes made with extra dry milk or protein powder for patients who cannot swallow solid foods.

The health care team can explain the effects of esophageal cancer and its treatment, and they can suggest ways to deal with them. In addition, the NCI booklets *Radiation Therapy and You*, *Chemotherapy and You*, and *Eating Hints* provide helpful information about cancer treatment and coping with side effects [these booklets are reprinted in this volume—see Table of Contents].

Living with Cancer

The diagnosis of esophageal cancer can change the lives of patients and the people who care about them. These changes can be hard to handle. It's common for patients and their families and friends to have many different and sometimes confusing emotions.

At times, patients and their loved ones may feel frightened, angry, or depressed. These are normal reactions when people face a serious health problem. Most people handle their problems better when they share their thoughts and feelings with those close to them. Sharing can help everyone feel more at ease and can open the way for people to show one another their concern and offer their support.

Worries about tests, treatments, hospital stays, and medical bills are common. Doctors, nurses, social workers, and other members of the health care team can help calm fears and ease confusion. They can also provide information and suggest resources.

Patients and their families are naturally concerned about what the future holds. Sometimes they use statistics to try to figure out whether the patient will be cured or how long he or she will live. It is important to remember, however, that statistics are averages based on large numbers of patients. They can't be used to predict what will happen to a certain patient because no two cancer patients are alike. The doctor who takes care of the patient and knows his or her medical history is in the best position to discuss the person's outlook (prognosis). Patients should feel free to ask the doctor about their prognosis, but they should keep in mind that not even the doctor knows for sure what will happen.

Support for Cancer Patients

Living with a serious disease isn't easy. Cancer patients and those who care about them face many problems and challenges. Finding the strength to cope with these difficulties is easier when people have helpful information and support services.

The doctor can explain the disease and give advice about treatment, working, or daily activities. If patients want to discuss concerns about the future, family relationships, and finances, it also may help to talk with a nurse, social worker, counselor, or member of the clergy.

Friends and relatives who have had personal experiences with cancer can be very supportive. Also, it helps many patients to meet and talk with others who are facing problems like theirs. Cancer patients often get together in self-help and support groups, where they can share what they have learned about cancer and its treatment and about coping with the disease. It's important to keep in mind, however, that each cancer patient is different. So treatments and ways of dealing with cancer that work for one person may not be right for another—even if they both have the same kind of cancer. It's always a good idea to discuss the advice of friends and family members with the doctor.

Often, a social worker at the hospital or clinic can suggest local and national groups that can help with emotional support, financial aid, transportation, or home care. The American Cancer Society is one such group. This nonprofit organization has many services for patients and their families. Local offices of the American Cancer Society are listed in the white pages of the telephone book. More information about this resource is in the "Resources" section below.

Information about other programs and services is available through the Cancer Information Service. The toll-free number is 1-800-4-CANCER.

The public library is a good place to find books and articles on living with cancer. Cancer patients and their families and friends also can find helpful suggestions in the booklet *Taking Time.*

Cause and Prevention

Cancer of the esophagus is fairly common in some parts of the world. But in the United States, this disease accounts for only about 1 percent of all cancers.

The exact causes of cancer of the esophagus are not known. Researchers are trying to solve this problem. The more they can find out about what causes this disease, the better the chance of finding ways to prevent it.

Studies in the United States show that esophageal cancer is found mainly in people over age 55. It affects men about twice as often as women, and it is more common in black people than in white people. But doctors still cannot explain why one person gets esophageal cancer and another doesn't.

So far, doctors know for sure that no one can "catch" esophageal cancer from another person. Cancer is not contagious.

Also, doctors know that certain risk factors increase a person's chance of getting esophageal cancer. In the United States, smoking and excessive use of alcohol are the major risk factors for this disease. Heavy users of both alcohol and tobacco are much more likely to get esophageal cancer than are people who do not drink or smoke.

Cutting down on the use of alcohol reduces the chance of getting esophageal cancer, as well as cancers of the mouth, throat, and larynx. By not smoking, people can lower their risk of cancers of the esophagus, lung, mouth, throat, larynx, bladder, and pancreas. Also, it's very important to know that people who develop cancer due to smoking are at risk of getting a second cancer. Most doctors urge esophageal cancer patients to stop smoking to cut down the risk of a new cancer and to reduce other problems, such as coughing.

The risk of cancer of the esophagus is also increased by long-term irritation of esophageal tissues. Tissue at the bottom of the esophagus can become irritated if the contents of the stomach frequently "back up" into the esophagus, a problem known as reflux. When cells in the irritated part of the esophagus change and begin to resemble the cells that line the stomach, doctors call this condition Barrett's esophagus. In some cases, Barrett's esophagus leads to esophageal cancer.

Other kinds of irritation or damage to the lining of the esophagus can also increase the risk of cancer. For example, people who have swallowed lye or other caustic substances have a higher-than-average risk because these substances damage esophageal tissue.

Poor nutrition is another factor that may increase a person's risk of esophageal cancer. Scientists are not sure exactly how diet changes the risk of developing this disease, but they think that it's important to have a well-balanced diet that includes generous amounts of fruits and vegetables.

Often, patients with esophageal cancer have no clear risk factors. In most cases, the disease is probably the result of several factors (known or unknown) acting together.

People who think they might be at increased risk for cancer of the esophagus should discuss this concern with their doctor. The doctor may be able to suggest ways to reduce the risk and can suggest an appropriate schedule of checkups.

Resources

General information about cancer is available from many sources. Two are listed below. You also may wish to check your local library or contact support groups in your community.

Cancer Information Service (CIS)
1-800-4-CANCER

The Cancer Information Service, a program of the National Cancer Institute, includes a telephone service for cancer patients and their families and friends, the public, and health care professionals. The staff can answer questions and send booklets about cancer. They also may know about local resources and services. One toll-free number, 1-800-4-CANCER, connects callers all over the country to the office that serves their area. Spanish-speaking staff members are available.

American Cancer Societ (ACS)
1599 Clifton Road, N.E.
Atlanta, GA 30329
1-800-ACS-2345

The American Cancer Society is a voluntary organization with a national office (at the above address) and local units all over the country. It supports research, conducts educational programs, and offers many services to patients and their families. To obtain information about services and activities in local areas, call the Society's tollfree number, 1-800-ACS-2345, or the number listed under "American Cancer Society" in the white pages of the telephone book.

For Further Information

Cancer patients, their families and friends, and others may find the following booklets useful. They are available free of charge by calling 1-800-4-CANCER or writing:

Office of Cancer Communications
National Cancer Institute
Building 31, Room 10A24
Bethesda, MD 20892

Booklets about Cancer Treatment

Radiation Therapy and You: A Guide to Self-Help During Treatment *

Chemotherapy and You: A Guide to Self-Help During Treatment *

Eating Hints: Recipes and Tips for Better Nutrition During Cancer Treatment *

Questions and Answers About Pain Control (also available from the American Cancer Society)

What Are Clinical Trials All About?

Booklets about Living with Cancer

Taking Time: Support for People With Cancer and the People Who Care About Them

When Cancer Recurs: Meeting the Challenge Again *

Advanced Cancer: Living Each Day *

* Reprinted in this volume—see Table of Contents

Chapter 11

Cancer of the Larynx

What You Need to Know about Cancer of the Larynx

Each year, more than 12,000 Americans find out they have cancer of the larynx. The National Cancer Institute (NCI) has prepared this chapter to help patients and their families and friends better understand this type of cancer. We also hope it will encourage all readers to learn more about this disease.

This chapter has information on the symptoms, diagnosis, and treatment of cancer of the larynx. Other NCI booklets about cancer, its treatment, and living with the disease are listed in the "For Further Information" section below. However, materials like these cannot answer every question or take the place of talks with doctors, nurses, and other members of the health care team. We hope our booklets will help with those talks.

Knowledge about cancer of the larynx is increasing. Research is leading to better ways to treat this disease. For up-to-date information about cancer of the larynx and its treatment, call the NCI-supported Cancer Information Service (CIS) at 1-800-4-CANCER. The CIS is described below in the "Resources" section.

The Larynx

The larynx, also called the voice box, is a 2-inch-long, tube-shaped organ in the neck. We use the larynx when we breathe, talk, or swallow.

"What You Need to Know about Cancer of the Larynx," National Cancer Institute, updated September 1998.

The larynx is at the top of the windpipe (trachea). Its walls are made of cartilage. The large cartilage that forms the front of the larynx is sometimes called the Adam's apple. The vocal cords, two bands of muscle, form a "V" inside the larynx.

Each time we inhale (breathe in), air goes into our nose or mouth, then through the larynx, down the trachea, and into our lungs. When we exhale (breathe out), the air goes the other way. When we breathe, the vocal cords are relaxed, and air moves through the space between them without making any sound.

When we talk, the vocal cords tighten up and move closer together. Air from the lungs is forced between them and makes them vibrate, producing the sound of our voice. The tongue, lips, and teeth form this sound into words.

The esophagus, a tube that carries food from the mouth to the stomach, is just behind the trachea and the larynx. The openings of the esophagus and the larynx are very close together in the throat. When we swallow, a flap called the epiglottis moves down over the larynx to keep food out of the windpipe.

What Is Cancer?

Cancer is a group of diseases that have one thing in common: cells become abnormal. These abnormal cells destroy body tissue and can spread to other parts of the body.

Cells make up all of the body's tissues. Healthy cells grow, divide, and replace themselves in an orderly way. This process keeps the body in good repair. If cells lose the ability to control their growth, they divide too often and without any order. They form too much tissue. The mass of extra tissue is called a tumor. Tumors can be benign or malignant.

- Benign tumors are not cancer. They do not spread to other parts of the body and are seldom a threat to life. Benign tumors can usually be removed, but certain types may return.

- Malignant tumors are cancer. They can invade and destroy nearby healthy tissues and organs. Cancer cells can also break away from the tumor and enter the bloodstream and the lymphatic system. That is how cancer spreads to other parts of the body. This spread is called metastasis.

Cancer of the larynx is also called laryngeal cancer. It can develop in any region of the larynx—the glottis (where the vocal cords are), the supraglottis (the area above the cords), or the subglottis (the area that connects the larynx to the trachea).

If the cancer spreads outside the larynx, it usually goes first to the lymph nodes (sometimes called lymph glands) in the neck. It can also spread to the back of the tongue, other parts of the throat and neck, the lungs, and sometimes other parts of the body.

Cancer that spreads is the same disease and has the same name as the original (primary) cancer. When cancer of the larynx spreads, it is called metastatic laryngeal cancer.

Symptoms

The symptoms of cancer of the larynx depend mainly on the size and location of the tumor. Most cancers of the larynx begin on the vocal cords. These tumors are seldom painful, but they almost always cause hoarseness or other changes in the voice. Tumors in the area above the vocal cords may cause a lump on the neck, a sore throat, or an earache. Tumors that begin in the area below the vocal cords are rare. They can make it hard to breathe, and breathing may be noisy.

A cough that doesn't go away or the feeling of a lump in the throat may also be warning signs of cancer of the larynx. As the tumor grows, it may cause pain, weight loss, bad breath, and frequent choking on food. In some cases, a tumor in the larynx can make it hard to swallow. Any of these symptoms may be caused by cancer or by other, less serious problems. Only a doctor can tell for sure. People with symptoms like these usually see an ear, nose, and throat specialist (otolaryngologist).

Diagnosis

To find the cause of any of these symptoms, the doctor asks about the patient's personal and family medical history and does a complete physical exam. In addition to checking general signs of health, the doctor carefully feels the neck to check for lumps, swelling, tenderness, or other changes. The doctor can also look inside the larynx in two ways:

- *Indirect laryngoscopy.* The doctor looks down the throat with a small, long-handled mirror to check for abnormal areas and to see whether the vocal cords move as they should. This test is painless, but a local anesthetic may be sprayed in the throat to prevent gagging. This exam is done in the doctor's office.

- *Direct laryngoscopy.* The doctor inserts a lighted tube (laryngoscope) through the patient's nose or mouth. As the tube goes down the throat, the doctor can look at areas that cannot be seen with a simple mirror. A local anesthetic eases discomfort and prevents gagging. Patients may also be given a mild sedative to help them relax. Sometimes the doctor uses a general anesthetic to put the person to sleep. This exam may be done in an outpatient clinic, a hospital, or a doctor's office.

If the doctor sees abnormal areas, the patient will need to have a biopsy. A biopsy is the only sure way to know whether cancer is present. For a biopsy, the patient is given a local or general anesthetic, and the doctor removes tissue samples through a laryngoscope. A pathologist then examines the tissue under a microscope to check for cancer cells. If cancer is found, the pathologist can tell what type it is. Almost all cancers of the larynx are squamous cell carcinomas. This type of cancer begins in the flat, scale-like cells that line the epiglottis, vocal cords, and other parts of the larynx.

If the pathologist finds cancer, the patient's doctor needs to know the stage (extent) of the disease to plan the best treatment. To find out the size of the tumor and whether the cancer has spread, the doctor usually orders more tests, such as x-rays, a CT (or CAT) scan, and/or an MRI scan. During a CT scan, many x-rays are taken. A computer then puts them together to create detailed pictures of areas inside the body. An MRI scan produces pictures using a huge magnet linked to a computer.

Treatment Options

Treatment for cancer depends on a number of factors. Among these are the exact location and size of the tumor and whether the cancer has spread. To develop a treatment plan to fit each patient's needs, the doctor also considers the person's age, general health, and feelings about the possible treatments.

The patient's doctor may want to discuss the case with other doctors who treat cancer of the larynx. Also, the patient may want to talk with the doctor about taking part in a research study of new treatment methods. Such studies, called clinical trials, are discussed below.

Many patients want to learn all they can about their disease and their treatment choices so they can take an active part in decisions about their medical care. The patient and the doctor should discuss the treatment choices very carefully because treatments for this disease may change the way a person looks and the way he or she breathes and talks. In many cases, the patient meets with both the doctor and a speech pathologist to talk about treatment options and possible changes in voice and appearance.

People with cancer of the larynx have many important questions. The doctor and other members of the health care team are the best ones to answer them. Most patients want to know the extent of their cancer, how it can be treated, how successful the treatment is expected to be, and how much it is likely to cost. These are some questions patients may want to ask the doctor:

- What are my treatment choices?

- Would a clinical trial be appropriate for me?

- What are the expected benefits of each kind of treatment?

- What are the risks and possible side effects of each treatment?

- How will I look?

- Will I need to change my normal activities? For how long?

- When will I be able to return to work?

- How often will I need to have checkups?

Many people find it helpful to make a list of their questions before they see the doctor. The doctor should be asked to explain anything that is not clear. Taking notes can make it easier to remember what the doctor says. Some patients also find it helps to have a family member or friend with them when they talk to the doctor—to take part in the discussion or just to listen.

Planning Treatment

Treatment decisions are complex. Before starting treatment, the patient might want a second doctor to review the diagnosis and treatment plan. A short delay will not reduce the chance that treatment will be successful. There are a number of ways to find a doctor for a second opinion:

- The patient's doctor may be able to suggest a doctor who has a special interest in cancer of the larynx.

- The Cancer Information Service, at 1-800-4-CANCER, can tell callers about cancer centers and other NCI-supported programs in their area.

- Patients can get the names of doctors from the local medical society, a nearby hospital, or a medical school.

- The *Directory of Medical Specialists* lists doctors' names and gives their background. It is in most public libraries.

Treatment Methods

Cancer of the larynx is usually treated with radiation therapy (also called radiotherapy) or surgery. These are types of local therapy; this means they affect cancer cells only in the treated area. Some patients may receive chemotherapy, which is called systemic therapy, meaning that drugs travel through the bloodstream. They can reach cancer cells all over the body. The doctor may use just one method or combine them, depending on the patient's needs.

In some cases, the patient is referred to doctors who specialize in different kinds of cancer treatment. Often several specialists work together as a team. The medical team may include a surgeon; ear, nose, and throat specialist; cancer specialist (oncologist); radiation oncologist; speech pathologist; nurse; and dietitian. A dentist may also be an important member of the team, especially for patients who will have radiation therapy (see below).

Radiation therapy uses high-energy rays to damage cancer cells and stop them from growing. The rays are aimed at the tumor and the area close to it. Whenever possible, doctors suggest this type of treatment because it can destroy the tumor and the patient does not lose his or her voice. Radiation therapy may be combined with surgery; it can be used to shrink a large tumor before surgery or to destroy cancer cells that may remain in the area after surgery. Also, radiation therapy may be used for tumors that can't be removed with surgery or for patients who cannot have surgery for other reasons. If a tumor grows back after surgery, it is generally treated with radiation.

Radiation therapy is usually given 5 days a week for 5 to 6 weeks. At the end of that time, the tumor site very often gets an extra "boost" of radiation.

Surgery or surgery combined with radiation is suggested for some newly diagnosed patients. Also, surgery is the usual treatment if a tumor does not respond to radiation therapy or grows back after radiation therapy. When patients need surgery, the type of operation depends mainly on the size and exact location of the tumor.

If a tumor on the vocal cord is very small, the surgeon may use a laser, a powerful beam of light. The beam can remove the tumor in much the same way that a scalpel does.

Surgery to remove part or all of the larynx is a partial or total laryngectomy. In either operation, the surgeon performs a tracheostomy, creating an opening called a stoma in the front of the neck. (The stoma may be temporary or permanent.) Air enters and leaves the trachea and lungs through this opening. A tracheostomy tube, also called a trach ("trake") tube, keeps the new airway open.

A partial laryngectomy preserves the voice. The surgeon removes only part of the voice box—just one vocal cord, part of a cord, or just the epiglottis—and the stoma is temporary. After a brief recovery period, the trach tube is removed, and the stoma closes up. The patient can then breathe and talk in the usual way. In some cases, however, the voice may be hoarse or weak.

In a total laryngectomy, the whole voice box is removed, and the stoma is permanent. The patient, called a laryngectomee, breathes through the stoma. A laryngectomee must learn to talk in a new way.

If the doctor thinks that the cancer may have started to spread, an operation called a neck dissection may be done. The surgeon removes the lymph nodes in the neck and some of the tissue around them because these nodes are often the first place to which laryngeal cancer spreads.

Chemotherapy is the use of drugs to kill cancer cells. The doctor may suggest one drug or a combination of drugs. In some cases, anticancer drugs are given to shrink a large tumor before the patient has radiation therapy or surgery. Also, chemotherapy may be used for cancers that have spread.

Anticancer drugs for cancer of the larynx are usually given by injection into the bloodstream. Often the drugs are given in cycles—a treatment period followed by a rest period, then another treatment and rest period, and so on. Some patients have their chemotherapy in the outpatient part of the hospital, at the doctor's office, or at home. However, depending on the drugs, the treatment plan, and the patient's general health, a hospital stay may be needed. The NCI publication *Chemotherapy and You* [reprinted in this volume as Chapter 63] has helpful information about this type of treatment and its possible side effects.

Treatment Studies

Researchers are looking for treatment methods that are more effective against cancer of the larynx and have fewer side effects. When laboratory research shows that a new method has promise, it is used to treat cancer patients in clinical trials. These trials are designed to answer scientific questions and to find out whether the new approach is both safe and effective. Patients who take part in clinical trials make an important contribution to medical science and may have the first chance to benefit from improved treatment methods.

Many clinical trials of new treatments for cancer of the larynx are under way. Doctors are studying new types and schedules of radiation therapy, new drugs, new drug combinations, and new ways of combining various types of treatment. Scientists are trying to increase the effectiveness of radiation therapy by giving treatments twice a day instead of once. Also, they are studying drugs called "radiosensitizers." These drugs make the cancer cells more sensitive to radiation.

People who have had cancer of the larynx have an increased risk of getting a new cancer in the larynx or in the lung, mouth, or throat. Doctors are looking for ways to prevent these new cancers. Some research has shown that a drug related to vitamin A may protect people from new cancers.

Patients interested in taking part in a trial should discuss this option with their doctor. *What Are Clinical Trials All About?* is an NCI booklet that explains some of the risks and possible benefits of treatment studies.

One way to learn about clinical trials is through PDQ, a computerized resource of cancer treatment information. Developed by NCI, PDQ contains an up todate list of trials in progress. Doctors can use a personal computer or the services of a medical library to get PDQ information. The Cancer Information Service, at 1-800-4-CANCER, is another source of PDQ information for doctors, patients, and the public.

Side Effects of Treatment

The methods used to treat cancer are very powerful. It is hard to limit the effects of therapy so that only cancer cells are removed or destroyed; healthy cells also may be damaged. That's why treatment often causes unpleasant side effects.

The side effects of cancer treatment vary. They depend mainly on the type and extent of the treatment. Also, each person reacts differently. Doctors try to plan the patient's therapy to keep problems to a minimum. Doctors, nurses, dietitians, and speech pathologists can explain the side effects of treatment and suggest ways to deal with them. It also may help to talk with another patient. In many cases, a social worker or another member of the medical team can arrange a visit with someone who has had the same treatment.

Radiation Therapy

During radiation therapy, healing after dental treatment may be a problem. That's why doctors want their patients to begin treatment with their teeth and gums as healthy as possible. They often recommend that patients have a complete dental exam and get any needed dental work done before the radiation therapy begins. It's also important to continue to see the dentist regularly because the mouth may be sensitive and easily irritated during cancer therapy.

In many cases, the mouth is tender during treatment, and some patients may get mouth sores. The doctor may suggest a special rinse to numb the mouth and reduce the discomfort.

Radiation to the larynx causes changes in the saliva and may reduce the amount of saliva. Because saliva normally protects the teeth, tooth decay can be a problem after treatment. Good mouth care can help keep the teeth and gums healthy and can make the patient feel more comfortable. Patients should do their best to keep their teeth clean. If it's hard to floss or brush the teeth in the usual way, patients can use gauze, a soft toothbrush, or a special toothbrush that has a spongy tip instead of bristles. A mouthwash made with diluted peroxide, salt water, and baking soda can keep the mouth fresh and help protect the teeth from decay. It also may be helpful to use a fluoride toothpaste and/or a fluoride rinse to reduce the risk of cavities. The dentist usually suggests a special fluoride program to keep the mouth healthy.

If reduced saliva makes the mouth uncomfortably dry, drinking plenty of liquids is helpful. Some patients use a special spray (artificial saliva) to relieve the dryness.

Patients who have radiation therapy instead of surgery do not have a stoma. They breathe and talk in the usual way, although the treatment can change the way their voice sounds. Also, the voice may be weak at the end of the day, and it is not unusual for the voice to be affected by changes in the weather. Voice changes and the feeling of a lump in the throat may come from swelling in the larynx caused by the radiation. The treatment can also cause a sore throat. The doctor may suggest medicine to reduce swelling or relieve pain.

During radiation therapy, patients may become very tired, especially in the later weeks. Resting as much as possible is important. It's also common for the skin in the treated area to become red or dry. The skin should be exposed to the air but protected from the sun, and patients should avoid wearing clothes that rub the area. During radiation therapy, hair usually does not grow in the treated area; if it

127

does, men should not shave. Good skin care is important at this time. Patients will be shown how to keep the area clean, and they should not put anything on the skin before their radiation treatments. Also, they should not use any lotion or cream at other times without the doctor's advice.

Some patients complain that radiation therapy makes their tongue sensitive. They may lose their sense of taste or smell or may have a bitter taste in their mouth. Drinking plenty of liquids may lessen the bitter taste. Often, the doctor or nurse can suggest other ways to ease these problems. And it helps to keep in mind that, although the side effects of radiation therapy may not go away completely, most of them gradually become less troublesome and patients feel better when the treatment is over.

Surgery

Keeping the patient comfortable is an important part of routine hospital care. If pain occurs, it can be relieved with medicine. Patients should feel free to discuss pain control with the doctor.

For a few days after surgery, the patient isn't able to eat or drink. At first, an intravenous (IV) tube supplies fluids. Within a day or two, the digestive tract is getting back to normal, but the patient still cannot swallow because the throat has not healed. Fluids and nutrition are given through a feeding tube (put in place during surgery) that goes through the nose and throat to the stomach. As the swelling in the throat goes away and the area begins to heal, the feeding tube is removed. Swallowing may be difficult at first, and the patient may need the guidance of a nurse or speech pathologist. Little by little, the patient returns to a regular diet.

After the operation, the lungs and windpipe produce a great deal of mucus. To remove it, the nurse applies gentle suction with a small plastic tube placed in the stoma. Soon, the patient learns to cough and to suction mucus through the stoma without the nurse's help. For a short time, it may also be necessary to suction saliva from the mouth because swelling in the throat prevents swallowing.

Normally, air is moistened by the tissues of the nose and throat before it reaches the windpipe. After surgery, air enters the trachea directly through the stoma and cannot be moistened in the same way. In the hospital, patients are kept comfortable with a special device that adds moisture to the air.

For several days after a partial laryngectomy, the patient breathes through the stoma. Soon the trach tube is removed; within the next few weeks, the stoma closes. The patient then breathes and speaks in the usual way, although the voice may not sound exactly the same as before.

After a complete laryngectomy, the stoma is permanent. The patient breathes, coughs, and "sneezes" through the stoma and has to learn to talk in a new way. The trach tube stays in place for at least several weeks (until the skin around the stoma heals), and some people continue to use the tube all or part of the time. If the tube is removed, it is usually replaced by a smaller tracheostomy button (also called a stoma button). After a while, some laryngectomees get along without either a tube or a button.

After a laryngectomy, parts of the neck and throat may be numb because nerves have been cut. Also, following a neck dissection, the shoulder and neck may be weak and stiff.

Chemotherapy

The side effects of chemotherapy depend on the drugs that are given. In general, anticancer drugs affect rapidly growing cells, such as blood cells that fight infection, cells that line the digestive tract, and cells in hair follicles. As a result, patients may have side effects such as lower resistance to infection, loss of appetite, nausea, vomiting, or mouth sores. They may also have less energy and may lose their hair.

Effects of Treatment on Eating

Loss of appetite can be a problem for patients treated for laryngeal cancer. People may not feel hungry when they are uncomfortable or tired.

Patients who have had a laryngectomy may lose their interest in food because the operation changes the way things smell and taste. Radiation therapy also tends to affect the sense of taste. The side effects of chemotherapy can also make it hard to eat. Yet patients who eat well may be better able to withstand the side effects of their treatment, so good nutrition is important. Eating well means getting enough calories and protein to prevent weight loss, regain strength, and rebuild normal tissues.

After surgery, learning to swallow again may take some practice with the help of a nurse or speech pathologist. Some patients find liquids easier to swallow; others do better with solid foods. If eating is difficult because the mouth is dry from radiation therapy, patients may want to try soft, bland foods moistened with sauces or gravies. Others enjoy thick soups, puddings, and high-protein milkshakes. The nurse and the dietitian will help the patient choose the right kinds of food. Also, many patients find that eating several small meals and snacks during the day works better than trying to have three large meals. The NCI booklets *Radiation Therapy and You*, *Chemotherapy and You*, and *Eating Hints* suggest a variety of other ways to deal with eating problems [These booklets are reprinted in this volume—see Table of Contents].

Rehabilitation

Learning to live with the changes brought about by cancer of the larynx is a special challenge. Rehabilitation is a very important part of the treatment plan. The medical team makes every effort to help patients return to their normal activities as soon as possible. Each laryngectomee must be able to care for the stoma. Before leaving the hospital, the patient learns to remove and clean the trach tube or stoma button, suction the trach, and care for the area around the stoma. The skin is less likely to become irritated if it is kept clean.

When shaving, men should keep in mind that the neck may be numb for several months after surgery. To avoid nicks and cuts, it may be best to use an electric shaver until normal feeling returns.

Most people continue to use a stoma cover after the area heals. Stoma covers—such as scarves, neckties, ascots, and special bibs—can be attractive as well as useful. They help keep moisture in and around the stoma. Also, laryngectomees may be sensitive to dust and smoke, and the cover filters the air that enters the stoma. The cover also catches any discharge from the windpipe when the person coughs or sneezes.

Whenever the air is too dry, as it may be in heated buildings in the winter, the tissues of the windpipe and lungs may react by producing extra mucus. Also, the skin around the stoma may get crusty and bleed. Using a humidifier at home or in the office can lessen these problems.

A person who has had a neck dissection may find that the neck is somewhat smaller. Also, the neck, shoulder, and arm may not be able to move as well as before. The doctor may advise physical therapy to help the person move more normally.

After surgery, laryngectomees work in almost every type of business and can do nearly all of the things they did before. However, they cannot hold their breath, so straining and heavy lifting may be difficult.

Also, laryngectomees have to give up swimming and water skiing unless they have special instruction and equipment because it would be very dangerous for water to get into the windpipe and lungs through the stoma. Wearing a special plastic stoma shield or holding a washcloth over the stoma keeps water out when showering or shaving.

Learning to Speak Again

It's natural to be fearful and upset if the voice box must be removed. Talking is part of nearly everything we do, and losing the ability to talk — even temporarily — can be frightening. Patients and their families and friends need one another's understanding and support during this very difficult time.

Until patients learn to talk again, it's important for them to be able to communicate in other ways. In the beginning, everyone who has had a laryngectomy has to communicate by writing, gesturing, or pointing to pictures, words, or letters. Some people like to use a "magic slate" for writing notes. Others use pads of paper and pens or pencils. It's handy to have a supply of pads that fit easily in a pocket or purse. In addition, some patients use a typewriter or computer. Others carry a small dictionary or a picture book (sometimes called a picture dictionary) and point to the words they need. Patients may want to select some of these items before the operation.

Within a week or so after a partial laryngectomy, most people can talk in the usual way. After a total laryngectomy, patients must learn to speak in a new way. A speech pathologist usually meets with the patient before surgery to explain the methods that can be used. In many cases, speech lessons can begin before the person leaves the hospital.

Patients may try out various new ways of talking. One way is to use air forced into the esophagus to produce the new voice (esophageal speech). Or the voice can come from some type of mechanical larynx. Some people rely on a mechanical larynx only until they learn esophageal speech, some decide to use this device instead of esophageal speech, and some use both.

Even though esophageal speech may sound low-pitched and gruff, many people want to use this method instead of a mechanical larynx because it sounds more like regular speech. Also, there's nothing to carry around, and the person's hands are free. In most cases, a speech pathologist teaches the laryngectomee how to force air into the top of the esophagus and then push it out again. The puff of air is like a burp. It vibrates the walls of the throat, producing sound for the new voice. The tongue, lips, and teeth form words as the sound passes through the mouth.

For some laryngectomees, air for esophageal speech comes through a tracheoesophageal puncture. The surgeon creates a small opening between the trachea and the esophagus. A plastic or silicone valve is inserted into this opening through the stoma. The valve keeps food out of the trachea.

When the stoma is covered, air from the lungs is forced into the esophagus through the valve. This air produces sound by making the walls of the throat vibrate. Words are formed in the mouth.

It takes practice and patience to learn esophageal speech, and not everyone is successful. How quickly a person learns, how natural the new voice sounds, and how understandable the speech is depend partly on the type and extent of the surgery. Other important factors are the patient's desire to learn and the help that's available. Patience and support from loved ones are important, too.

A mechanical larynx may be used until the person learns esophageal speech or if esophageal speech is too difficult. The device may be powered by batteries (electrolarynx) or by air (pneumatic larynx). The speech pathologist can help the patient choose a device and learn to use it.

One kind of electrolarynx looks like a small flashlight. It has a disk that makes a humming sound. The device is held against the neck, and the sound travels through the neck to the mouth. (This device may not be suitable for people who have had radiation therapy.) Another type of electrolarynx has a flexible plastic tube that carries sound to the person's mouth from a handheld device.

A pneumatic larynx is held over the stoma and uses air from the lungs instead of batteries to make it vibrate. The sound it makes travels to the mouth through a plastic tube.

Followup Care

Regular followup is very important after treatment for cancer of the larynx. The doctor will check closely to be sure that the cancer has not returned. Checkups include exams of the stoma, neck, and throat. From time to time, the doctor does a complete physical exam, blood and urine tests, and x-rays. People treated with radiation therapy or partial laryngectomy will have laryngoscopy.

People who have been treated for cancer of the larynx have a higher-than-average risk of developing a new cancer in the mouth, throat, or other areas of the head and neck. This is especially true for those who smoke. Most doctors strongly urge their patients to stop smoking to cut down the risk of a new cancer and to reduce other problems, such as coughing.

Living with Cancer

The diagnosis of cancer can change the lives of patients and the people who care about them. These changes can be hard to handle. It's natural for patients and their families and friends to have many different and sometimes confusing emotions. At times, patients and their loved ones may feel frightened, angry, or depressed. These are normal reactions when people face a serious health problem. Most people handle their problems better if they can share their thoughts and feelings with those close to them. Sharing can help everyone feel more at ease and can open the way for people to show one another their concern and offer their support.

Worries about tests, treatments, hospital stays, learning to talk again, and medical bills are common. Doctors, nurses, speech pathologists, social workers, and other members of the health care team can help calm fears and ease confusion. They also can provide information and suggest resources.

Patients and their families are naturally concerned about what the future holds. Sometimes they use statistics to try to figure out the chance of being cured. It is important to remember, however, that statistics are averages based on large numbers of patients. They can't be used to predict what will happen to a certain patient because no two cancer patients are alike. Only the doctor who takes care of the patient knows enough about that person to discuss his or her outlook (prognosis).

People should feel free to ask the doctor about their prognosis, but not even the doctor knows for sure what will happen. Doctors may talk about surviving cancer, or they may use the term remission rather than cure. Even though many people with cancer of the larynx recover completely, doctors use these terms because the disease can recur.

Support for Cancer Patients

Living with a serious disease isn't easy. Cancer patients and those who care about them face many problems and challenges. Finding the strength to cope with these difficulties is easier when people have helpful information and support services.

People who have cancer of the larynx may have concerns about the future, family and social relationships, and finances. Sometimes they worry that changes in how they look and talk will affect the way people feel about them. They may worry about holding a job, caring for their family, or starting new friendships.

The doctor can explain the disease and give advice about treatment, going back to work, or limiting daily activities. It also may help to talk with a nurse, social worker, counselor, or member of the clergy, especially about feelings or other very personal matters.

Many patients find that it's useful to get to know other people who are facing problems like theirs. They can meet other cancer patients through selfhelp and support groups. Often, a social worker at the hospital or clinic can suggest local and national groups that can help with emotional support, rehabilitation, financial aid, transportation, or home care.

The American Cancer Society is one such group. This nonprofit organization has many services for patients and their families. Local offices of the American Cancer Society are listed in the white pages of the telephone book. More information about the American Cancer Society is given in the "Resources" section below.

The International Association of Laryngectomees publishes educational materials and sponsors meetings and other activities for people who have lost their voice because of cancer. Many local laryngectomy clubs are members of this Association. For more information, patients may contact the national office, whose address and telephone number are in the "Resources" section. Information also is available from local American Cancer Society offices.

The public library is a good place to find books and articles on living with cancer. Cancer patients and their families can also find helpful suggestions in the NCI booklets *Taking Time* and *Facing Forward*.

Information about other programs and services is available through the Cancer Information Service. The toll-free number is 1-800-4-CANCER.

Cause and Prevention

Cancer of the larynx occurs most often in people over the age of 55. In the United States, it is four times more common in men than in women and is more common among black Americans than among whites. Scientists at hospitals and medical centers all across the country are studying this disease to learn more about what causes it and how to prevent it.

Doctors cannot explain why one person gets cancer of the larynx and another does not, but we are sure that no one can "catch" cancer from another person. Cancer is not contagious.

One known cause of cancer of the larynx is cigarette smoking. Smokers are far more likely than nonsmokers to develop this disease. The risk is even higher for smokers who drink alcohol heavily.

People who stop smoking can greatly reduce their risk of cancer of the larynx, as well as cancer of the lung, mouth, pancreas, bladder, and esophagus. Also, by quitting, those who have already had cancer of the larynx can cut down the risk of getting a second cancer of the larynx or a new cancer in another area. Special counseling or self-help groups are useful for some people who are trying to stop smoking. Some hospitals have groups for people who want to quit. Also, the Cancer Information Service and the American Cancer Society may have information about groups in local areas to help people quit smoking.

Working with asbestos can increase the risk of getting cancer of the larynx. Asbestos workers should follow work and safety rules to avoid inhaling asbestos fibers.

People who think they might be at risk for developing cancer of the larynx should discuss this concern with their doctor. The doctor may be able to suggest ways to reduce the risk and can suggest an appropriate schedule for checkups.

Resources

Information about cancer is available from many sources. Several are listed below. You also may wish to check your local library or contact support groups in your community.

Cancer Information Service (CIS)
1-800-4-CANCER

The Cancer Information Service, a program of the National Cancer Institute, includes a telephone service for cancer patients and their families and friends, the public, and health care professionals. The staff can answer questions and can send booklets about cancer. They also may know about local resources and services. One toll-free number, 1-800-4-CANCER, connects callers all over the country to the office that serves their area. Spanish-speaking staff members are available.

American Cancer Society (ACS)
1599 Clifton Road, N.E.
Atlanta, GA 30329
1-800-ACS-2345

The American Cancer Society is a voluntary organization with a national office (at the above address) and local units all over the country. It supports research, conducts educational programs, and offers many services to patients and their families. To obtain information about services and activities in local areas, including clubs for laryngectomees, call the Society's toll-free number, 1-800-ACS-2345, or the number listed under "American Cancer Society" in the white pages of the telephone book.

International Association of Laryngectomees (IAL)
1599 Clifton Road, N.E.
Atlanta, GA 30329
1-800-ACS-2345

The International Association of Laryngectomees is sponsored by the American Cancer Society. The Association supplies printed information and sponsors meetings and other activities. It publishes a directory of speech instructors and maintains a list of sources of supplies for laryngectomees. Most Lost Chord Clubs, New Voice Clubs, and other clubs for laryngectomees are members of this organization and are listed in its directory. Information about clubs is available from the American Cancer Society.

American Speech-Language-Hearing Association (ASHA)
Consumer Division
10801 Rockville Pike
Rockville, MD 20852
1-800-638-TALK
301-897-5700 (calls from Maryland)

The American Speech-Language-Hearing Association is a professional association. Its Consumer Division provides information on all types of communication problems and can refer patients to speech therapy programs.

The National Coalition for Cancer Survivorship (NCCS)
Suite 300
1010 Wayne Avenue
Silver Spring, MD 20910
301-585-2616

The National Coalition for Cancer Survivorship is a volunteer group concerned with issues faced by people with cancer and people who have recovered from cancer. It deals with legal, financial, emotional, and social matters. This group can advise people about their rights related to jobs and insurance. It has a speakers bureau and can supply printed information, including lists of cancer support groups in many areas.

For Further Information

Cancer patients, their families and friends, and others may find the following booklets useful. They are available free of charge by calling 1-800-4-CANCER or writing:

Office of Cancer Communications
National Cancer Institute
Building 31, Room 10A24
Bethesda, MD 20892

Booklets about Cancer Treatment

Radiation Therapy and You: A Guide to Self-Help During Treatment *

Chemotherapy and You: A Guide to Self-Help During Treatment *

Eating Hints: Recipes and Tips for Better Nutrition During Cancer Treatment *

Questions and Answers About Pain Control (also available from the American Cancer Society)

What Are Clinical Trials All About?

Booklets about Living with Cancer

Taking Time: Support for People With Cancer and the People Who Care About Them

When Cancer Recurs: Meeting the Challenge Again *

Advanced Cancer: Living Each Day *

* Reprinted in this volume—see Table of Contents

Chapter 12

Hypopharyngeal Cancer

What Is Cancer of the Hypopharynx?

Cancer of the hypopharynx is a disease in which cancer (malignant) cells are found in the tissues of the hypopharynx. The hypopharynx is the bottom part of the throat (also called the pharynx). The pharynx is a hollow tube about 5 inches long that starts behind the nose and goes down to the neck to become part of the esophagus, the tube that goes to the stomach. Air and food pass through the pharynx on the way to the windpipe (trachea) or the esophagus.

Cancer of the hypopharynx most commonly starts in the cells that line the hypopharynx, called squamous cells. If cancer has started in the lymph cells of the hypopharynx (a lymphoma), see the PDQ patient information summary on non-Hodgkin's lymphoma.

A doctor should be seen if a person has a sore throat that does not go away, trouble swallowing, a lump in the neck, a change in voice, or ear pain.

If there are symptoms, a doctor will examine the throat using a mirror and lights. A thin lighted tube called an endoscope may be put down the throat so the doctor can see if there is tissue that is not normal. The doctor will also feel the throat for lumps. If tissue that is not normal is found, the doctor will need to cut out a small piece and look at it under the microscope to see if there are any cancer cells. This is called a biopsy.

PDQ Statement, National Cancer Institute (NCI). Revised May 1998.

The chance of recovery (prognosis) depends on where the cancer is in the throat, whether the cancer is just in the throat or has spread to other tissues (the stage), and the patient's general state of health.

Stages of Cancer of the Hypopharynx

Once cancer of the hypopharynx is found, more tests will be done to find out if cancer cells have spread to other parts of the body. This is called staging. A doctor needs to know the stage of the disease to plan treatment. The following stages are used for cancer of the hypopharynx:

Stage I

The cancer is in only one part of the hypopharynx and has not spread to lymph nodes in the area (lymph nodes are small bean-shaped structures that are found throughout the body; they produce and store infection-fighting cells).

Stage II

The cancer is in more than one part of the hypopharynx or has spread to tissue next to the hypopharynx, but has not grown into the voice box (larynx). The cancer has not spread to lymph nodes in the area.

Stage III

Either of the following may be true:

- The cancer is in more than one part of the hypopharynx or has spread to tissue next to the hypopharynx. The cancer has grown into the larynx.

- The cancer is in the hypopharynx or has spread to the tissue around the hypopharynx. The cancer has spread to only one lymph node on the same side of the neck as the cancer. The lymph node that contains cancer measures no more than 3 centimeters (just over one inch).

Stage IV

Any of the following may be true:

- The cancer has spread to the connecting tissue or soft tissues of the neck. The lymph nodes in the area may or may not contain cancer.

- The cancer is in the hypopharynx or has spread to the tissues around the hypopharynx. The cancer has spread to more than one lymph node on the same side of the neck as the cancer, to lymph nodes on one or both sides of the neck, or to any lymph node that measures more than 6 centimeters (over 2 inches).

- The cancer has spread to other parts of the body.

Recurrent

Recurrent disease means that the cancer has come back (recurred) after it has been treated. It may come back in the hypopharynx or in another part of the body.

How Cancer of the Hypopharynx Is Treated

There are treatments for all patients with cancer of the hypopharynx. Two kinds of treatment are used:

- surgery (taking out the cancer)

- radiation therapy (using high-dose x-rays or other high-energy rays to kill cancer cells)

Chemotherapy (using drugs to kill cancer cells) is being tested in clinical trials.

Surgery is a common treatment of cancer of the hypopharynx. A doctor may remove the larynx and part of the throat in an operation called a laryngopharyngectomy. If the cancer is in the lymph nodes, the lymph nodes may be removed (lymph node dissection).

Radiation therapy uses high-energy x-rays to kill cancer cells and shrink tumors. Radiation may come from a machine outside the body (external radiation therapy) or from putting materials that produce radiation (radioisotopes) through thin plastic tubes in the area where the cancer cells are found (internal radiation therapy). Giving drugs with the radiation therapy to make the cancer cells more sensitive to radiation (radiosensitization) is being tested in clinical trials. If smoking is stopped before radiation therapy is started, a patient has a better chance of surviving longer. External radiation to the thyroid or the pituitary gland may change the way the thyroid gland works. The doctor may wish to test the thyroid gland before and after therapy to make sure it is working properly.

Chemotherapy uses drugs to kill cancer cells. Chemotherapy may be taken by pill, or it may be put into the body by a needle in the vein or muscle. Chemotherapy is called a systemic treatment because the drug enters the bloodstream, travels through the body, and can kill cancer cells throughout the body.

Because the hypopharynx helps people with breathing, eating, and talking, a patient may need special help adjusting to the side effects of the cancer and its treatment. The patient's doctor will consult with several kinds of doctors who can help determine the best treatment. Trained medical staff can also help the patient recover from treatment. The patient may need plastic surgery or help learning to eat and speak if all or part of the hypopharynx is taken out.

Treatment by Stage

Treatment of cancer of the hypopharynx depends on where the cancer is in the hypopharynx, the stage of the disease, and the patient's age and overall health.

Standard treatment may be considered because of its effectiveness in patients in past studies, or participation in a clinical trial may be considered. Not all patients are cured with standard therapy and some standard treatments may have more side effects than are desired. For these reasons, clinical trials are designed to find better ways to treat cancer patients and are based on the most up-to-date information. Clinical trials are ongoing in many parts of the country for patients with cancer of the hypopharynx. To learn more about clinical trials, call the Cancer Information Service at 1-800-4-CANCER (1-800-422-6237); TTY at 1-800-332-8615.

Stage I Hypopharyngeal Cancer

Treatment may be one of the following:

1. Surgery to remove the larynx and the pharynx (laryngopharyngectomy).

2. Surgery followed by radiation therapy.

3. Radiation therapy alone.

Stage II Hypopharyngeal Cancer

Treatment may be one of the following:

1. Surgery to remove the larynx and the pharynx (laryngopharyngectomy) and lymph nodes in the neck, followed by radiation therapy.

2. A clinical trial of chemotherapy followed by radiation therapy or surgery.

Stage III Hypopharyngeal Cancer

Treatment may be one of the following:

1. Surgery plus radiation therapy.
2. A clinical trial of chemotherapy followed by surgery or radiation therapy.
3. A clinical trial of chemotherapy combined with radiation therapy.

Stage IV Hypopharyngeal Cancer

If the cancer can be removed by surgery, treatment may be one of the following:

1. Surgery plus radiation therapy.
2. A clinical trial of chemotherapy followed by surgery or radiation therapy.
3. A clinical trial of chemotherapy combined with radiation therapy.
4. Radiation therapy with or without chemotherapy. Clinical trials are testing new ways of giving radiation therapy in smaller doses (hyperfractionated radiation therapy).

Recurrent Hypopharyngeal Cancer

Treatment may be one of the following:

1. Surgery to remove the cancer.
2. Radiation therapy.
3. A clinical trial of chemotherapy.

To Learn More

To learn more about cancer of the hypopharynx, call the National Cancer Institute's Cancer Information Service at 1-800-4-CANCER (1-800-422-6237); TTY at 1-800-332-8615. By dialing this toll-free number, trained information specialists can answer your questions.

The Cancer Information Service also has booklets about cancer that are available to the public and can be sent on request. The following general booklets on questions related to cancer may be helpful:

What You Need To Know About Cancer *

Taking Time: Support for People with Cancer and the People Who Care About Them

What Are Clinical Trials All About?

Chemotherapy and You: A Guide to Self-Help During Treatment *

Radiation Therapy and You: A Guide to Self-Help During Treatment *

Eating Hints for Cancer Patients *

Advanced Cancer: Living Each Day *

When Cancer Recurs: Meeting the Challenge Again *

* Reprinted in this volume—see Table of Contents

There are other places where people can get material and information about cancer treatment and services. The social service office at a hospital can be checked for local and national agencies that can help with getting information about finances, getting to and from treatment, getting care at home, and dealing with problems. For more information from the National Cancer Institute, please write to this address:

National Cancer Institute
Office of Cancer Communications
31 Center Drive, MSC 2580
Bethesda, MD 20892-2580

Chapter 13

Nasopharyngeal Cancer

What Is Cancer of the Nasopharynx?

Cancer of the nasopharynx is a disease in which cancer (malignant) cells are found in the tissues of the nasopharynx. The nasopharynx is behind the nose and is the upper part of the throat (also called the pharynx). The pharynx is a hollow tube about 5 inches long that starts behind the nose and goes down to the neck to become part of the esophagus (tube that goes to the stomach). Air and food pass through the pharynx on the way to the trachea (windpipe) or the esophagus. The nares, the holes in the nose through which people breathe, lead into the nasopharynx. Two openings on the side of the nasopharynx lead into the ear.

Cancer of the nasopharynx most commonly starts in the cells that line the oropharynx (the part of the throat behind the mouth). If a person has cancer that started in the lymph cells of the nasopharynx (a lymphoma), see the PDQ patient information summary on non-Hodgkin's lymphoma.

A doctor should be seen if a person has trouble breathing or speaking, frequent headaches, a lump in the nose or neck, pain or ringing in the ear, or trouble hearing.

If there are symptoms, the doctor will examine the throat using a mirror and lights. A special instrument (called a nasoscope) may be put into the nose to see into the nasopharynx. The doctor will also feel the neck for lumps. If tissue that is not normal is found, the doctor

PDQ Statement, National Cancer Institute (NCI). Revised February 1999.

will need to cut out a small piece and look at it under the microscope to see if there are any cancer cells. This is called a biopsy.

The chance of recovery (prognosis) depends on where the cancer is in the throat, whether the cancer is just in the throat or has spread to other tissues (the stage), and the patient's general state of health.

Stages of Cancer of the Nasopharynx

Once cancer of the nasopharynx is found, more tests will be done to find out if cancer cells have spread to other parts of the body. This is called staging. A doctor needs to know the stage of the disease to plan treatment. The following stages are used for cancer of the nasopharynx:

Stage I

The cancer is in only one part of the nasopharynx and has not spread to lymph nodes in the area (lymph nodes are small bean-shaped structures that are found throughout the body; they produce and store infection-fighting cells).

Stage II

The cancer is in more than one part of the nasopharynx and has not spread to lymph nodes in the area.

Stage III

Either of the following may be true:

- The cancer has spread into the nose or to the part of the throat behind the mouth (the oropharynx).

- The cancer is in the nasopharynx or has spread to the nose or the oropharynx. The cancer has spread to only one lymph node on the same side of the neck as the cancer. The lymph node that contains cancer measures no more than 3 centimeters (just over one inch).

Stage IV

Any of the following may be true:

- The cancer has spread to the bones or nerves in the head. The lymph nodes in the area may or may not contain cancer.

- The cancer is in the nasopharynx or has spread to the nose, the nasopharynx, or the bone or nerves in the head. The cancer has spread to more than one lymph node on the same side of the neck as the cancer, to lymph nodes on one or both sides of the neck, or to any lymph node that measures more than 6 centimeters (over 2 inches).

- The cancer has spread to other parts of the body.

Recurrent

Recurrent disease means that the cancer has come back (recurred) after it has been treated. It may come back in the nasopharynx or in another part of the body.

How Cancer of the Nasopharynx Is Treated

There are treatments for all patients with cancer of the nasopharynx. Three kinds of treatment are used:

- radiation therapy (using high-dose x-rays or other high-energy rays to kill cancer cells)

- surgery (taking out the cancer)

- chemotherapy (using drugs to kill cancer cells)

Biological therapy (using the body's immune system to fight cancer) is being tested in clinical trials.

Radiation therapy is the most common treatment for cancer of the nasopharynx. Radiation therapy uses high-energy x-rays to kill cancer cells and shrink tumors. Radiation may come from a machine outside the body (external radiation therapy) or from putting materials that produce radiation (radioisotopes) through thin plastic tubes in the area where the cancer cells are found (internal radiation therapy). External radiation to the thyroid or the pituitary gland may change the way the thyroid gland works. A doctor may wish to test the thyroid gland before and after therapy to make sure it is working properly.

Surgery is sometimes used for cancer of the nasopharynx that does not respond to radiation. If cancer has spread to lymph nodes, the lymph nodes may be removed (lymph node dissection).

Chemotherapy uses drugs to kill cancer cells. Chemotherapy may be taken by pill, or it may be put into the body by a needle in the vein or muscle. Chemotherapy is called a systemic treatment because the drug enters the bloodstream, travels through the body, and can kill cancer cells throughout the body.

Biological therapy tries to get the body to fight cancer. It uses materials made by the body or made in a laboratory to boost, direct, or restore the body's natural defenses against disease. Biological therapy is sometimes called biological response modifier (BRM) therapy or immunotherapy.

Because the nasopharynx helps in breathing and is close to the face, a patient may need special help adjusting to the side effects of the cancer and its treatment. A doctor will consult with several kinds of doctors who can help determine the best treatment. Trained medical staff can also help patients recover from treatment. Patients may need plastic surgery if a large part of the nasopharynx is taken out.

Treatment by Stage

Treatment for cancer of the nasopharynx depends on where the cancer is in the nasopharynx, the stage of the disease, and the patient's age and overall health.

Standard treatment may be considered because of its effectiveness in patients in past studies, or participation in a clinical trial may be considered. Not all patients are cured with standard therapy and some standard treatments may have more side effects than are desired. For these reasons, clinical trials are designed to find better ways to treat cancer patients and are based on the most up-to-date information. Clinical trials are ongoing in many parts of the country for patients with cancer of the nasopharynx. To learn more about clinical trials, call the Cancer Information Service at 1-800-4-CANCER (1-800-422-6237); TTY at 1-800-332-8615.

Stage I Nasopharyngeal Cancer

Treatment will probably be radiation therapy to the cancer and the lymph nodes in the neck.

Stage II Nasopharyngeal Cancer

Treatment will probably be radiation therapy to the cancer and the lymph nodes in the neck.

Stage III Nasopharyngeal Cancer

Treatment may be one of the following:

1. Radiation therapy to the cancer and the lymph nodes in the neck.

2. Radiation therapy followed by surgery to remove lymph nodes in the neck that remain large after radiation.

3. A clinical trial of chemotherapy followed by surgery or radiation therapy.

4. A clinical trial of radiation therapy followed by chemotherapy.

5. A clinical trial of surgery, radiation therapy, and chemotherapy.

6. A clinical trial of chemotherapy combined with radiation therapy.

Stage IV Nasopharyngeal Cancer

Treatment may be one of the following:

1. Radiation therapy to the cancer and the lymph nodes in the neck.

2. Radiation therapy followed by surgery to remove lymph nodes in the neck that remain large after radiation.

3. A clinical trial of chemotherapy followed by surgery or radiation therapy.

4. A clinical trial of surgery, radiation therapy, and chemotherapy.

5. A clinical trial of chemotherapy combined with radiation therapy.

Recurrent Nasopharyngeal Cancer

Treatment may be one of the following:

1. Radiation therapy.

2. Surgery to remove the cancer.

3. Chemotherapy.

4. A clinical trial of chemotherapy and/or biological therapy.

To Learn More

To learn more about cancer of the hypopharynx, call the National Cancer Institute's Cancer Information Service at 1-800-4-CANCER (1-800-422-6237); TTY at 1-800-332-8615. By dialing this toll-free number, trained information specialists can answer your questions.

The Cancer Information Service also has booklets about cancer that are available to the public and can be sent on request. The following general booklets on questions related to cancer may be helpful:

What You Need To Know About Cancer *

Taking Time: Support for People with Cancer and the People Who Care About Them

What Are Clinical Trials All About?

Chemotherapy and You: A Guide to Self-Help During Treatment *

Radiation Therapy and You: A Guide to Self-Help During Treatment *

Eating Hints for Cancer Patients *

Advanced Cancer: Living Each Day *

When Cancer Recurs: Meeting the Challenge Again *

* Reprinted in this volume—see Table of Contents

There are other places where people can get material and information about cancer treatment and services. The social service office at a hospital can be checked for local and national agencies that can help with getting information about finances, getting to and from treatment, getting care at home, and dealing with problems. For more information from the National Cancer Institute, please write to this address:

National Cancer Institute
Office of Cancer Communications
31 Center Drive, MSC 2580
Bethesda, MD 20892-2580

Chapter 14

Lung Cancer

Lung Cancer

Each year, more than 170,000 people in the United States learn that they have lung cancer. This chapter will give you some important information about this disease. It explains how lung cancer is diagnosed and treated, and it has information to help you deal with lung cancer if it affects you or someone you know.

Other NCI booklets are listed at the end of this chapter. Our materials cannot answer every question you may have about lung cancer. They cannot take the place of talks with doctors, nurses, and other members of the health care team. We hope our information will help with those talks.

Researchers continue to look for better ways to diagnose and treat lung cancer, and our knowledge is growing. For up-to-date information, call the NCI supported Cancer Information Service (CIS) toll free at 1-800-4-CANCER (1-800-422-6237).

The Lungs

The lungs, a pair of cone-shaped organs made up of spongy, pinkish-gray tissue, are part of the respiratory system. They take up most of the space in the chest and are separated from each other by the mediastinum, an area that contains the heart, trachea (windpipe),

"What You Need to Know About Lung Cancer," National Cancer Institute (NCI). NIH Publications No. 97-1553, September 1997.

esophagus, and many lymph nodes. The right lung has three sections, called lobes; it is a little larger than the left lung, which has two lobes.

When we breathe, air enters the body through the nose or the mouth. The air travels down the throat, through the larynx (voice box) and trachea, and into the lungs through tubes called main-stem bronchi. One main-stem bronchus leads to the right lung and one to the left lung. In the lungs, the main-stem bronchi divide into smaller bronchi and then into even smaller tubes called bronchioles. The bronchioles end in tiny air sacs called alveoli.

The lungs take in oxygen, which cells need to live and carry out their normal functions. The lungs also get rid of carbon dioxide, a waste product of the body's cells.

What Is Cancer?

Cancer is a group of more than 100 different diseases. Cancer occurs when cells become abnormal and keep dividing and forming more cells without control or order.

Like all the other organs of the body, the lungs are made up of many types of cells. Normally, cells divide to produce more cells only when the body needs them. This orderly process helps keep us healthy.

If cells divide when new cells are not needed, a mass of tissue forms. This mass of excess tissue, called a growth or tumor, can be benign or malignant.

- Benign tumors are not cancer. They can usually be removed and, in most cases, they do not come back. Most important, the cells in benign tumors do not invade other tissues and do not spread to other parts of the body. Benign tumors are rarely a threat to life.

- Malignant tumors are cancer. They can invade and damage nearby tissues and organs. Also, cancer cells can break away from a malignant tumor and enter the bloodstream or the lymphatic system. This is how cancer spreads from the original tumor and forms new tumors in other parts of the body. The spread of cancer is called metastasis.

Lung cancer often spreads to lymph nodes or other tissues in the chest (including the other lung). In many cases, lung cancer also spreads to other organs of the body, such as the bones, brain, or liver. Cancer that spreads is the same disease and has the same name as the original (primary) cancer. In other words, lung cancer that spreads to the brain (or another organ) is called metastatic lung cancer, even though the new tumor is in the brain (or another organ).

What Causes Lung Cancer?

Most lung cancer is caused by cigarette smoking. Tobacco smoke contains many carcinogens—harmful substances that damage cells. Over time, these cells can become cancerous. The more a person smokes, the higher the risk of getting cancer—not just lung cancer, but also cancers of the mouth, throat, esophagus, larynx, bladder, kidney, cervix, and pancreas.

It is clear that thousands of lives could be saved each year if people did not smoke. For this reason, NCI strongly encourages smokers to quit. The risk of lung cancer begins decreasing slowly as soon as a person quits smoking. The earlier the age at which a person quits, the closer a former smoker's risk of lung cancer will approach the risk for a person who never smoked.

Although quitting early is best, smokers should know that it is never too late to benefit from quitting—even if they have lung cancer. Lung cancer patients who stop smoking are less likely to get a second lung cancer than are patients who continue to smoke.

Many programs are available to help people stop smoking. The Cancer Information Service, the American Cancer Society, and the American Lung Association can offer advice about quitting and can give you information about programs in your area.

Although smoking is by far the major cause of lung cancer, it is not the only cause. Exposure to other people's tobacco smoke (environmental tobacco smoke) increases the risk of lung cancer among nonsmokers. Scientists have found that nonsmokers who live or work with smokers have a higher lung cancer risk than nonsmokers who do not face this type of exposure to environmental tobacco smoke.

Exposure to certain carcinogens in the workplace, such as asbestos, also increases the risk of lung cancer. (The risk is especially high for workers who smoke.) People should carefully follow work and safety rules to reduce their exposure to workplace carcinogens.

Workers (especially smokers) who are exposed to high levels of radon, a radioactive gas, have an increased risk of developing lung cancer. High levels of radon are found in some types of underground mines (for example, underground uranium mines). Radon also can build up in some homes, but the levels in homes are generally much lower than in mines. Researchers are studying whether exposure to radon in the home can increase lung cancer risk. The U.S. Environmental Protection

Agency can provide information about radon exposure and testing for radon in the home.

Types of Lung Cancer

Nearly all lung cancers are carcinomas. A carcinoma is a cancer that begins in the lining or covering tissues of an organ. Lung cancers are generally divided into two types: nonsmall cell lung cancer and small cell lung cancer. The tumor cells of each type of lung cancer grow and spread differently, and each type needs different treatment.

Nonsmall cell lung cancer is more common than small cell lung cancer. The three main kinds of nonsmall cell lung cancer are named for the type of cells in the tumor:

- Squamous cell carcinoma, also called epidermoid carcinoma, is the most common type of lung cancer in men. This disease often begins in the bronchi. It usually does not spread as quickly as other types of lung cancer.

- Adenocarcinoma usually begins along the outer edges of the lungs and under the lining of the bronchi. This is the most common type of lung cancer in women and in people who have never smoked.

- Large cell carcinomas are a group of cancers with large, abnormal-looking cells. These tumors usually begin along the outer edges of the lungs.

Small cell lung cancer is sometimes called oat cell cancer because the cancer cells may look like oats when viewed under a microscope. This type of lung cancer grows rapidly and quickly spreads to other organs.

Symptoms

Lung cancer usually does not cause symptoms when it first develops. Doctors sometimes discover lung cancer in a person with no symptoms after the individual has a chest x-ray for another medical reason. Usually, however, lung cancer is found after the growing tumor causes symptoms to appear.

A cough is the most common symptom of lung cancer. It is likely to occur when a tumor irritates the lining of the airways or blocks the passage of air. The person may have a "smoker's cough" that becomes worse. Another symptom is constant chest pain. Other symptoms may include shortness of breath, wheezing, repeated bouts of pneumonia or bronchitis, coughing up blood, or hoarseness. A tumor that presses on large blood vessels near the lung can cause swelling of the neck and face. If the tumor presses on certain nerves near the lung, it can cause pain and weakness in the shoulder, arm, or hand.

In addition, there may be symptoms that do not seem to be at all related to the lungs. Like all cancers, lung cancer can cause fatigue, loss of appetite, and loss of weight. If the cancer spreads to other parts of the body, it may cause headache, pain, or bone fractures.

Other symptoms can be caused by substances made by lung cancer cells. Doctors often refer to these symptoms as a paraneoplastic syndrome. For example, certain lung cancer cells produce a substance that causes a sharp drop in the level of salt (sodium) in the blood. A decrease in the sodium level can cause many symptoms, including confusion and sometimes even coma.

None of these symptoms is a sure sign of lung cancer. Only a doctor can tell whether a patient's symptoms are caused by cancer or by another problem.

Diagnosis

To find the cause of any of these symptoms, the doctor asks about the patient's personal and family medical background as well as smoking and work history. The doctor also does a physical exam and usually orders x-rays and other tests.

In addition to chest x-rays, the doctor may order other pictures of areas inside the body. For example, a CT scan (also called a CAT scan) is a series of x-ray images put together by a computer. These detailed pictures can reveal that a tumor is in the lung, but they cannot show whether the tumor is benign or malignant.

The only sure way to know whether cancer is present is to obtain cells from the lungs so that a pathologist can examine them under a microscope. Sometimes, cancer cells can be found in the sputum, a thick fluid that the patient coughs up from deep in the airways. Also, the doctor usually does a biopsy to remove a sample of cells from the lung. To do a biopsy, the doctor uses one of the procedures described below:

- An exam called bronchoscopy permits the doctor to look into the breathing passages through a bronchoscope (a thin, lighted tube). A local anesthetic reduces discomfort and gagging, and medicine helps the patient relax as the doctor inserts the tube through the nose or mouth. (A general anesthetic may be used instead to put the patient to sleep.) The doctor can brush or wash cells from the walls of bronchi or snip off small pieces of tissue for study under a microscope.

- Needle aspiration is a procedure to remove cells that are hard to reach with the bronchoscope. After the patient is given a local anesthetic, the doctor inserts a needle through the chest into the tumor to withdraw a small sample of tissue. Most often, the doctor uses fluoroscopy or CT scans to locate the tumor.

- Sometimes, examination of fluid from the pleura (the fluid-filled sac that surrounds the lungs) can reveal lung cancer. Using a needle, the doctor removes a sample of the fluid in the pleura and checks it for cancer cells. For this procedure, called thoracentesis, the patient receives a local anesthetic.

- For some patients, surgery is needed to diagnose lung cancer. Surgery to open the chest (for diagnosis or treatment) is called thoracotomy. This is major surgery and is done under a general anesthetic.

If the doctor can feel swollen lymph nodes or an enlarged liver, these areas may be biopsied to help with the diagnosis. The doctor also may biopsy other sites of the body where cancer is suspected. A patient who needs a biopsy may want to ask the doctor these questions:

- What type of biopsy will I have? Why?

- How long will it take? Will I be awake? Will it hurt?

- How soon will I know the results?

- If I do have cancer, who will talk with me about treatment? When?

Staging

If lung cancer is diagnosed, the patient's doctor needs to learn the stage, or extent, of the disease so that proper treatment can be given. Staging is a careful attempt to find out whether the cancer has spread and, if so, what parts of the body are affected.

To find out whether a patient's lung cancer has spread to the lymph nodes in the chest, the doctor removes a sample of tissue. In some patients, this can be done with a needle; in others, the doctor will need to perform surgery. Surgery to biopsy lymph nodes in the chest can often be done through a small incision near the breastbone. This procedure is called mediastinoscopy when the incision is above the breastbone and mediastinotomy when the incision is on one side of the breastbone. If a thoracotomy is planned, the doctor removes lymph nodes during the operation. Patients receive a general anesthetic for any of these operations.

Doctors may order CT scans to detect the spread of lung cancer to the lymph nodes and other parts of the body. Radionuclide scans of the bones, brain, or liver also may help doctors find out whether the cancer has spread. In these tests, a small amount of radioactive material is injected into a vein. A machine then scans the body to measure the radiation and reveal abnormal areas.

In another technique, called MRI (for magnetic resonance imaging), a strong magnet linked to a computer is used to produce images. Doctors may order MRI to see whether lung cancer has spread to the brain or spinal cord.

Treatment

The doctor develops a treatment plan to fit each patient's needs. This plan depends on many factors, including the type of lung cancer, the size and location of the tumor, and the stage of the disease. The doctor also considers the patient's age, medical history, and general health.

Most people with cancer want to learn all they can about their disease and their treatment choices so they can take an active part in decisions about their medical care. The doctor is the best person to answer questions about the extent of the cancer, how it can be treated, how successful the treatment is likely to be, and how much it is likely to cost. The patient also may want to talk with the doctor about taking part in a research study of new treatment methods. Such studies, called clinical trials, are designed to find ways to improve cancer treatment. More information about clinical trials appears below.

Many patients find it helps to make a list of questions before seeing the doctor. Taking notes during visits can make it easier to remember what the doctor says. Some patients also find that it helps to have a family member or friend with them—to take part in the discussion, to take notes, or just to listen.

A patient may want to ask the doctor these questions before treatment begins:

- What is my diagnosis?

- What is the stage of the disease?

- What are my treatment choices? Which do you recommend for me? Why ?

- Will I need to stay in the hospital, or will I be treated as an outpatient?

- Would a clinical trial be appropriate for me?

- What are the risks and possible side effects of each treatment?

- How long will treatment last?

- Will I need to change my normal activities?

- What is the treatment likely to cost?

There is a lot to learn about cancer and its treatment. Patients should not feel that they need to understand everything at once. They will have many chances to ask the doctor to explain things that are not clear and to ask for more information.

Getting a Second Opinion

Treatment decisions for lung cancer are complex. Before starting treatment, the patient might want another doctor to review the diagnosis and the treatment plan. There are a number of ways to find another doctor for a second opinion:

- The patient's doctor may be able to suggest a specialist. Specialists who treat lung cancer include thoracic surgeons, radiation oncologists, and medical oncologists.

- The Cancer Information Service, at 1 800-4-CANCER, can tell callers about cancer centers and other programs in their area supported by the National Cancer Institute.

- Patients can get the names of doctors from their local medical society, a nearby hospital, or a medical school.

Methods of Treatment

Surgery, radiation therapy, and chemotherapy are the usual treatments for lung cancer. Surgery is done when it is likely that all of the tumor can be removed. Radiation therapy (also called radiotherapy) is the use of high-energy rays to damage cancer cells and stop them from growing and dividing. Chemotherapy is the use of drugs to kill cancer cells. A patient may have just one form of treatment or a combination, depending on his or her needs. Several specialists may work together as a team to provide treatment.

Three main types of surgery are used in lung cancer treatment. The choice depends on the size and location of the tumor, the extent of the cancer, the general health of the patient, and other factors. An operation to remove only a small part of the lung is called a segmental or wedge resection. When the surgeon removes an entire lobe of the lung, the procedure is a lobectomy. Pneumonectomy is the removal of an entire lung.

A patient may want to ask the doctor these questions before surgery:

- What kind of operation will it be?
- How will I feel after the operation? If I have pain, how will you help me?
- How long must I stay in the hospital?
- Will I have to do special exercises?

Like surgery, radiation therapy is local treatment; it can affect cancer only in the treated area. The radiation, which comes from a large machine, is usually given 5 days a week for several weeks. The patient goes to the hospital or clinic each day to receive the treatments. A patient may want to ask the doctor these questions before radiation therapy:

- What will this treatment do?
- When will the treatments begin? When will they end?
- How will I feel during therapy?
- What can I do to take care of myself during therapy?

Chemotherapy is systemic treatment, meaning that the drugs flow through the bloodstream to nearly every part of the body. Most anticancer drugs are injected into a blood vessel or a muscle; some are given by mouth. Chemotherapy is most often given in cycles—a treatment period followed by a recovery period, then another treatment period, and so on.

Usually a patient has chemotherapy as an outpatient at the hospital, at the doctor's office, or at home. However, depending on which drugs the doctor orders and on the patient's health, the patient may need to stay in the hospital for a few days so that the drugs' side effects can be watched.

These are some questions a patient may want to ask the doctor before chemotherapy:

- What will this treatment do?

- What drugs will I be taking?

- Will there be side effects? What can I do about them'?

- How long will I need to take this treatment?

Treating Nonsmall Cell Lung Cancer

Patients with nonsmall cell lung cancer may be treated in several ways. The choice of treatment depends mainly on the extent of the disease.

Surgery is the usual treatment for patients whose cancer is in only one lung or in one lung and the closest lymph nodes. Patients who cannot have surgery because of other medical problems and patients with large tumors often receive radiation therapy. Radiation therapy also is the usual treatment for patients whose cancer has spread within the chest—to more distant lymph nodes or other tissues. Some patients have both surgery and radiation therapy.

Doctors may use radiation therapy and chemotherapy to treat patients whose cancer has spread from the lung to other parts of the body. Although it is very hard to control lung cancer that has spread, treatment can often shrink the tumors. This can help relieve pain and other symptoms.

Treating Small Cell Lung Cancer

Small cell lung cancer spreads quickly. In most cases, cancer cells have already spread to distant parts of the body when the disease is diagnosed. To be sure that treatment affects all cancer cells, doctors generally use chemotherapy, even when the disease appears to be limited to the lung and nearby lymph nodes. Usually, chemotherapy for small cell lung cancer includes a combination of two or more anticancer drugs.

In many cases treatment also includes radiation therapy—to shrink or destroy the primary tumor in the lung or tumors elsewhere in the body (such as in the brain). Some patients have radiation therapy to the brain even though no cancer is found there. This treatment, called prophylactic cranial irradiation or PCI, is given to prevent tumors from forming in the brain. Usually, PCI is reserved for patients whose lung tumor has responded well to treatment.

Surgery also can be part of the treatment plan for small cell lung cancer. This treatment is appropriate only for a small number of patients.

Side Effects of Treatment

It is hard to limit the effects of cancer therapy so that only cancer cells are removed or destroyed. Because treatment also damages healthy cells and tissues, it often causes unpleasant side effects.

The side effects of cancer treatment vary. They depend mainly on the type and extent of the treatment. Also, each person reacts differently to treatment.

Doctors try to plan the patient's therapy to keep side effects to a minimum.

Doctors and nurses can explain the side effects of cancer treatment and can suggest ways to deal with them. The National Cancer Institute booklets *Radiation Therapy and You* and *Chemotherapy and You* also have helpful information about cancer treatment and coping with side effects.

Surgery

Surgery for lung cancer is a major operation. It may take several weeks or months for patients to regain their energy and strength. This recovery time differs from patient to patient. The doctor and nurse will explain what will happen and what they and the patient can do to make recovery easier.

Doctors can prescribe medicine to control pain after surgery. The doctor or nurse also may suggest other ways to reduce discomfort. Patients should feel free to ask what can be done to relieve their pain or discomfort.

After lung surgery, air and fluid tend to collect in the chest. The air and fluid are drained out through flexible tubes put in place during surgery. Patients also are helped to turn, cough, and breathe deeply. All of these procedures are important for recovery because they help expand the remaining lung tissue and get rid of excess air and fluid.

Generally, patients who have had lung surgery receive respiratory therapy treatments and exercises to keep the lungs expanded and prevent fluid buildup. Patients may feel short of breath because they have less lung tissue to supply the body with oxygen. For this reason, they may have to limit their activities for some time. In most cases, the remaining lung tissue gradually expands somewhat, making it easier to breathe.

After surgery, the muscles of the chest and the arm on the affected side may become weak. Special exercises can help the patient regain strength in these muscles.

Radiation Therapy

Patients often become very tired during radiation therapy, especially in the later weeks of treatment. Resting is important, but doctors usually advise their patients to try to stay as active as they can.

It also is common for the skin in the treated area to become red, dry, tender, and itchy. There may be permanent darkening or "bronzing" in the treated area. The skin should be exposed to the air but protected from the sun, and patients should avoid wearing clothes that rub or irritate the treated area. Good skin care is important at this time, and patients will be shown how to keep the area clean. They should not use any lotion or cream on the skin without the doctor's advice.

During radiation therapy for lung cancer and for a short time afterward, patients may have a dry, sore throat, and it may be difficult to swallow. Many find it helpful to eat soft foods and drink extra liquids until these problems go away.

Radiation therapy to the lungs can cause certain permanent changes in lung tissues. These changes, called radiation fibrosis, tend to occur several months after the treatment is over. Fibrosis, which is similar to scarring, can interfere with the ability of the lung to supply the body with oxygen. Patients who have this problem may have to limit their activities.

Chemotherapy

The side effects of chemotherapy depend mainly on the drugs the patient is given. In addition, as with other types of treatment, side effects vary from person to person. Generally, anticancer drugs affect cells that divide rapidly. These include blood cells, which fight infection, help the blood to clot, or carry oxygen to all parts of the body. When blood cells are affected by anticancer drugs, patients are more likely to get infections, may bruise or bleed easily, and may have less energy. Cells in hair roots and cells that line the digestive tract also divide rapidly. When chemotherapy affects these cells, it can cause hair loss and other problems such as nausea and vomiting. Usually these side effects go away gradually during the recovery period or after treatment stops.

Nutrition for Cancer Patients

Some patients find it hard to eat well. They may lose their appetite. In addition, the common side effects of treatment, such as nausea, vomiting, or mouth sores, can make it hard to eat. For some patients, foods taste different. Also, people may not feel like eating when they are uncomfortable or tired.

Eating well means getting enough calories and protein to help prevent weight loss and regain strength. Patients who eat well during cancer treatment often feel better and have more energy. In addition, they may be better able to handle the side effects of treatment.

Doctors, nurses, and dietitians can offer advice for healthy eating during cancer treatment. Patients and their families also may want to read the National Cancer Institute booklet *Eating Hints for Cancer Patients*, which contains recipes and tips for better nutrition during cancer treatment.

Support for Cancer Patients

Living with a serious disease is not easy. Cancer patients and those who care about them face many problems and challenges. Coping with these difficulties is easier when people have helpful information and support services. Several useful booklets, including *Taking Time: Support for People With Cancer and the People Who Care About Them*, are available from the Cancer Information Service.

Cancer patients may worry about holding jobs, caring for their families, or keeping up with daily activities. Worries about tests, treatments, hospital stays, and medical bills also are common. Doctors, nurses, and other members of the health care team can answer questions and help calm fears about treatment, working, or other activities. Also, meeting with a social worker, counselor, or member of the clergy can be helpful to patients who want to talk about their feelings or discuss their concerns about the future or about personal relationships.

Friends and relatives, especially those who have had personal experience with cancer, can be very supportive. Also, many patients find it helps to discuss their concerns with others who are facing similar problems. Cancer patients often get together in support groups, where they can share what they have learned about coping with cancer and the effects of treatment. It is important to keep in mind, however, that each patient is different. Treatments and ways of dealing with cancer that work for one person may not be right for another even if they both have the same kind of cancer. It is always a good idea to discuss the advice of friends and family members with the doctor.

Often, a social worker at the hospital or clinic can suggest local and national groups that help with rehabilitation, emotional support, financial aid, transportation, or home care. The American Cancer Society is one such group. This nonprofit organization has many services for patients and their families. Local offices of the American Cancer Society are listed in the white pages of the telephone directory.

Information about other programs and services is available through the Cancer Information Service. The toll-free number is 1-800-4-CANCER.

The public library is a good place to find books and articles on living with cancer. Cancer patients and their families and friends also can find helpful suggestions in the booklets listed at the end of this file.

The Promise of Cancer Research

Researchers at hospitals and medical centers all across the country are studying lung cancer. They are trying to learn more about what causes this disease and how to prevent it. They also are looking for better ways to detect and treat it.

Cause and Prevention

Scientists are continuing to identify factors that may increase the risk for lung cancer. Recent research has shown that genetic factors play an important role in lung cancer risk. For example, certain genetic traits make some people very sensitive to carcinogens. Smokers with these traits may be more likely than other smokers to develop lung cancer.

Researchers also are studying ways to help people lower their risk of lung cancer. An important area of study is chemoprevention—the use of natural and laboratory-made substances to prevent or delay cancer. Vitamin A and substances like it may offer some protection against lung cancer. Other substances also are being studied. However, more research is needed, and some vitamins can be dangerous if taken in large doses. It is best to get a doctor's advice before taking vitamins or other nutrients.

Currently, we know that the best way to prevent lung cancer is not to smoke. The National Cancer Institute, the American Cancer Society, and other organizations have programs designed to reduce the number of smokers. If these efforts are successful, far fewer people will develop and die of lung cancer each year.

Detection

The earlier cancer is detected, the more successful treatment is likely to be. However, lung cancer is difficult to diagnose at an early stage. For this reason, scientists are studying ways of checking for lung cancer in people who have no symptoms of the disease. This is called screening. The goal of screening is to detect lung cancer before symptoms appear so that it can be treated as early as possible. Whether successful screening methods for this disease can be developed is not yet known.

Treatment

Because lung cancer is so hard to control, researchers are looking for more effective treatments. They also are exploring ways to reduce the side effects of treatment and improve the quality of patients' lives. When laboratory research shows that a new method has promise, cancer patients can receive the treatment in clinical trials. These trials are designed to find out whether the new approach is both safe and effective and to answer scientific questions. Some clinical trials compare a new treatment with a standard approach. Patients who take part in clinical trials make an important contribution to medical science and may have the first chance to benefit from improved treatment methods.

Trials are under way to study new treatments for patients with all stages of lung cancer. Some trials involve treatments to shrink or destroy the primary tumor. In others, scientists are testing ways to prevent lung cancer from coming back in the chest or spreading to other parts of the body after the primary tumor has been treated. Still others involve treatments to slow or stop the spread of lung cancer.

Researchers are studying the timing of treatments and new ways to combine various types of treatment. They also are trying new anticancer drugs and drug combinations, new forms of radiation therapy, and drugs that make cancer cells more sensitive to radiation. Another method under study is photodynamic therapy. In this treatment, cancer cells are destroyed with a combination of laser light and light-sensitive drugs. Other types of laser therapy are being studied as a way to open the airways in patients whose tumors block the bronchi. Some researchers also are working with biological therapy. This type of treatment includes efforts to help the body's immune system fight cancer more effectively or to protect the body from some of the side effects of treatment.

Patients with lung cancer may want to read a National Cancer Institute booklet called *What Are Clinical Trials All About?*, which explains some of the possible benefits and risks of treatment studies. Those who are interested in taking part in a trial should talk with their doctor.

One way to learn about clinical trials is through PDQ, a computerized resource developed by the National Cancer Institute. PDQ contains information about cancer treatment and about clinical trials in progress all over the country. The Cancer Information Service can provide PDQ information to doctors, patients, and the public.

Resources

Information about cancer is available from many sources, including the ones listed below. You also may wish to check for information at your local library or bookstore and from support groups in your community.

Cancer Information Service
1-800-4-CANCER

The Cancer Information Service, a program of the National Cancer Institute, is a nationwide telephone service for cancer patients and their families and friends, the public, and health care professionals. The staff can answer questions in English or Spanish and can send free National Cancer Institute booklets about cancer. They also know about local resources and services. One toll-free number, 1-800-4-CANCER (1-800-422-6237), connects callers all over the country with the office that serves their area.

American Cancer Society
1599 Clifton Road, N.E.
Atlanta, GA 30329
1 -800-ACS-2345

The American Cancer Society is a voluntary organization with a national office (at the above address) and local units all over the country. It supports research, conducts educational programs, sponsors support groups for cancer patients and for people who want to quit smoking, and offers many services to patients and their families. It provides free booklets on lung cancer and on caring for cancer patients at home. To request booklets or to obtain information about services and activities in local areas, call the Society's toll-free number, 1-800-ACS-2345 (1-800-227-2345), or the number listed under American Cancer Society in the white pages of the telephone book.

American Lung Association
1740 Broadway
New York, NY 10019
212-315-8700

The American Lung Association is a voluntary organization concerned with the prevention and treatment of lung diseases, including lung cancer. It supports many activities to make the public aware of the dangers of smoking. The Association offers free printed material on smoking and on lung cancer. It also sponsors programs to help people stop smoking. Local chapters are listed in the white pages of the telephone book.

U.S. Environmental Protection Agency
Public Information Center
401 M Street, S.W.
Washington, DC 20460
202-260-2080

The U.S. Environmental Protection Agency is the Federal agency responsible for keeping the environment safe. It supports research and sets regulations on air and water pollution, toxic substances, and radiation in the environment. It also provides free printed material on many topics, including radon, asbestos, and environmental tobacco smoke.

Other Booklets

The National Cancer Institute booklets listed below are available free of charge by calling 1-800-4-CANCER (1-800-422-6237).

Booklets about Cancer and Its Treatment

- *Research Report: Cancer of the Lung*
- *Chemotherapy and You: A Guide to Self-Help During Treatment* *

- *Radiation Therapy and You: A Guide to Self-Help During Treatment* *

- *Eating Hints: Recipes and Tips for Better Nutrition During Cancer Treatment*

- *What Are Clinical Trials All About?* *

- *Questions and Answers About Pain Control* (also available from the American Cancer Society)

Booklets about Living with Cancer

- *Facing Forward: A Guide for Cancer Survivors* *

- *Taking Time: Support for People With Cancer and the People Who Care About Them*

- *When Cancer Recurs: Meeting the Challenge Again* *

- *Advanced Cancer: Living Each Day* *

* Reprinted in this volume: see Table of Contents

Chapter 15

Non-Small Cell Lung Cancer

What Is Non-Small Cell Lung Cancer?

Lung cancers can be divided into two types: small cell lung cancer and non-small cell lung cancer. The cancer cells of each type grow and spread in different ways, and they are treated differently. Non-small cell lung cancer is usually associated with prior smoking, passive smoking, or radon exposure. (A separate patient information summary on small cell lung cancer is also available in PDQ).

The main kinds of non-small cell lung cancer are named for the type of cells found in the cancer: squamous cell carcinoma (also called epidermoid carcinoma), adenocarcinoma, large cell carcinoma, adeno-squamous carcinoma, and undifferentiated carcinoma.

Non-small cell lung cancer is a common disease. It is usually treated by surgery (taking out the cancer in an operation) or radiation therapy (using high-dose x-rays to kill cancer cells). However, chemotherapy may be used in some patients.

The prognosis (chance of recovery) and choice of treatment depend on the stage of the cancer (whether it is just in the lung or has spread to other places), tumor size, the type of lung cancer, whether there are symptoms, and the patient's general health.

National Cancer Institute (NCI) PDQ database, February 1999.

Stage Explanation

Stages of Non-Small Cell Lung Cancer

Once lung cancer has been found (diagnosis), more tests will be done to find out if the cancer has spread from the lung to other parts of the body (staging). A doctor needs to know the stage to plan treatment. The following stages are used for non-small cell lung cancer:

- *Occult stage*: Cancer cells are found in sputum, but no tumor can be found in the lung.

- *Stage 0*: Cancer is only found in a local area and only in a few layers of cells. It has not grown through the top lining of the lung. Another term for this type of lung cancer is carcinoma in situ.

- *Stage I*: The cancer is only in the lung, and normal tissue is around it.

- *Stage II*: Cancer has spread to nearby lymph nodes.

- *Stage III*: Cancer has spread to the chest wall or diaphragm near the lung; or the cancer has spread to the lymph nodes in the area that separates the two lungs (mediastinum); or to the lymph nodes on the other side of the chest or in the neck. Stage III is further divided into stage IIIA (usually can be operated on) and stage IIIB (usually cannot be operated on).

- *Stage IV*: Cancer has spread to other parts of the body.

- *Recurrent*: Cancer has come back (recurred) after previous treatment.

Treatment Option Overview

Chemotherapy uses drugs to kill cancer cells. Chemotherapy may be taken by pill, or it may be put into the body by a needle in the vein or muscle. Chemotherapy is called a systemic treatment because the drug enters the bloodstream, travels through the body, and can kill cancer cells outside the lungs.

Chemoprevention uses drugs to prevent a second cancer from occurring.

Radiation therapy uses high-energy x-rays to kill cancer cells and shrink tumors. Radiation may come from a machine outside the body (external radiation therapy) or from putting materials that produce radiation (radioisotopes) through thin plastic tubes in the area where the cancer cells are found (internal radiation therapy).

One new type of radiation therapy is called radiosurgery. In radiosurgery, radiation is directly focused on the tumor, and involves as little normal tissue as possible. Radiosurgery is usually used as treatment of tumors that involve the brain.

Cryosurgery freezes the tumor and kills it. Photodynamic therapy uses a certain type of light and a special chemical to kill cancer cells. Laser therapy uses a narrow beam of light to kill cancer cells. Cryosurgery and photodynamic therapy are usually used in clinical trials.

Surgery, radiation therapy, and chemotherapy are used to treat non-small cell lung cancer. However, these treatments often do not cure the disease.

If lung cancer is found, a patient may want to think about taking part in one of the many clinical trials being done to improve treatment. Clinical trials are ongoing in most parts of the country for all stages of non-small cell lung cancer. Treatment choices can be discussed with a doctor.

Patients with non-small cell lung cancer can be divided into three groups, depending on the stage of the cancer and the treatment that is planned. The first group (stages 0, I, and II) includes patients whose cancers can be taken out by surgery. The operation that takes out only a small part of the lung is called a wedge resection. When a whole section (lobe) of the lung is taken out, the operation is called a lobectomy. When one whole lung is taken out, it is called a pneumonectomy.

Radiation therapy may be used to treat patients in this group who cannot have surgery because they have other medical problems. Like surgery, radiation therapy is called local treatment because it works only on the cells in the area being treated.

The second group of patients has lung cancer that has spread to nearby tissue or to lymph nodes. These patients can be treated with radiation therapy alone or with surgery and radiation, chemotherapy and radiation, or chemotherapy alone.

The third group of patients has lung cancer that has spread to other parts of the body. Radiation therapy may be used to shrink the cancer and to relieve pain. Chemotherapy may be used to treat some patients in this group.

Treatment by Stage

Occult Non-Small Cell Lung Cancer

Tests are done to find the main tumor (cancer). Lung cancer that is found at this early stage can be cured by surgery.

Stage 0 Non-Small Cell Lung Cancer

Treatment may be one of the following:

1. Surgery to cure these very early cancers. However, these patients may get a second lung cancer that may not be able to be taken out by surgery.

2. Photodynamic therapy used internally.

Stage I Non-Small Cell Lung Cancer

Treatment may be one of the following:

1. Surgery.

2. Radiation therapy (for patients who cannot be operated on).

3. Clinical trials of chemotherapy following surgery.

4. Clinical trials of chemoprevention following other therapy.

5. Clinical trials of photodynamic therapy used internally.

Stage II Non-Small Cell Lung Cancer

Treatment may be one of the following:

1. Surgery to take out the tumor and lymph nodes.

2. Radiation therapy (for patients who cannot be operated on).

3. Surgery and/or radiation therapy with or without chemotherapy.

Stage III Non-Small Cell Lung Cancer

Stage IIIA Non-Small Cell Lung Cancer

Treatment may be one of the following:

1. Surgery alone.

2. Chemotherapy with other treatments.

3. Surgery and radiation therapy.

4. Radiation therapy alone.

5. Laser therapy and/or internal radiation therapy.

Stage IIIB Non-Small Cell Lung Cancer

Treatment may be one of the following:

1. Radiation therapy alone.

2. Chemotherapy plus radiation therapy.

3. Chemotherapy plus radiation therapy followed by surgery.

4. Chemotherapy alone.

5. Cryotherapy plus radiation therapy.

Stage IV Non-Small Cell Lung Cancer

Treatment may be one of the following:

1. Radiation therapy.

2. Chemotherapy.

3. Chemotherapy and radiation therapy.

4. Laser therapy and/or internal radiation therapy.

Recurrent Non-Small Cell Lung Cancer

Treatment may be one of the following:

1. Radiation therapy to control symptoms.

2. Chemotherapy.

3. Chemotherapy with radiation therapy.

4. For some patients who have a very small amount of tumor that has spread to the brain, surgery may be used to remove the tumor.

5. Laser therapy or internal radiation therapy.

6. Radiosurgery (for certain patients who cannot be operated on).

To Learn More

To learn more about lung cancer, call the National Cancer Institute's Cancer Information Service at 1-800-4-CANCER (1-800-422-6237); TTY at 1-800-332-8615. By dialing this toll-free number, trained information specialists can answer your questions.

The Cancer Information Service also has booklets about cancer that are available to the public and can be sent on request. The following booklets about lung cancer may be helpful:

Other Booklets

The National Cancer Institute booklets listed below are available free of charge by calling 1-800-4-CANCER (1-800-422-6237).

Booklets about Cancer and Its Treatment

- *Research Report: Cancer of the Lung*

- *Chemotherapy and You: A Guide to Self-Help During Treatment* *

- *Radiation Therapy and You: A Guide to Self-Help During Treatment* *

- *Eating Hints: Recipes and Tips for Better Nutrition During Cancer Treatment*

- *What Are Clinical Trials All About?* *

- *Questions and Answers About Pain Control* (also available from the American Cancer Society)

Booklets about Living with Cancer

- *Facing Forward: A Guide for Cancer Survivors* *

- *Taking Time: Support for People With Cancer and the People Who Care About Them*

- *When Cancer Recurs: Meeting the Challenge Again* *

- *Advanced Cancer: Living Each Day* *

* Reprinted in this volume: see Table of Contents

There are many other places where people can get material and information about cancer treatment and services. The social service office at a hospital can be checked for local and national agencies that help with getting information about finances, getting to and from treatment, getting care at home, and dealing with problems.

For more information from the National Cancer Institute, please write to this address:

National Cancer Institute
Office of Cancer Communications
31 Center Drive, MSC 2580
Bethesda, MD 20892-2580

Chapter 16

Small Cell Lung Cancer

What Is Small Cell Lung Cancer?

Small cell lung cancer is a disease in which cancer (malignant) cells are found in the tissues of the lungs. The lungs are a pair of cone-shaped organs that take up much of the room inside the chest. The lungs bring oxygen into the body and take out carbon dioxide, which is a waste product of the body's cells. Tubes called bronchi make up the inside of the lungs.

There are two kinds of lung cancer based on how the cells look under a microscope: small cell and non-small cell. If a patient has non-small cell lung cancer, see the PDQ patient information summary on non-small cell lung cancer.

Small cell lung cancer is usually found in people who smoke or who used to smoke cigarettes. A doctor should be seen if there are any of the following symptoms: a cough or chest pain that doesn't go away, a wheezing sound when breathing, shortness of breath, coughing up blood, hoarseness, or swelling in the face and neck.

If there are symptoms, a doctor may want to look into the bronchi through a special instrument, called a bronchoscope, that slides down the throat and into the bronchi. This test, called bronchoscopy, is usually done in the hospital. Before the test, the patient will be given a local anesthetic (a drug that causes a loss of feeling for a short period of time) in the back of the throat. Some pressure may be felt,

National Cancer Institute (NCI) PDQ database. July 1998.

usually with no pain. The doctor can take cells from the walls of the bronchi tubes or cut small pieces of tissue to look at under the microscope to see if there are any cancer cells. This is called a biopsy.

The doctor may also use a needle to remove tissue from a place in the lung that may be hard to reach with the bronchoscope. A cut will be made in the skin and the needle will be put in between the ribs. This is called a needle aspiration biopsy. The doctor will look at the tissue under the microscope to see if there are any cancer cells. Before the test, a local anesthetic will be given to keep the patient from feeling pain.

The chance of recovery (prognosis) and choice of treatment depend on the stage of the cancer (whether it is just in the lung or has spread to other places), and the patient's gender and general state of health.

Stage Explanation

Stages of Small Cell Lung Cancer

Once small cell lung cancer has been found, more tests will be done to find out if cancer cells have spread from one or both lungs to other parts of the body (staging). A doctor needs to know the stage of the disease to plan treatment. The following stages are used for small cell lung cancer:

- *Limited stage*: Cancer is found only in one lung and in nearby lymph nodes. (Lymph nodes are small, bean-shaped structures that are found throughout the body. They produce and store infection-fighting cells.)

- *Extensive stage*: Cancer has spread outside of the lung where it began to other tissues in the chest or to other parts of the body.

- *Recurrent stage*: Recurrent disease means that the cancer has come back (recurred) after it has been treated. It may come back in the lungs or in another part of the body.

Treatment Option Overview

How Small Cell Lung Cancer Is Treated

There are treatments for all patients with small cell lung cancer. Three kinds of treatment are used:

- surgery (taking out the cancer)

- radiation therapy (using high-dose x-rays or other high-energy rays to kill cancer cells)

- chemotherapy (using drugs to kill cancer cells)

Additionally, clinical trials are testing the effect of new therapies on the treatment of small cell lung cancer.

Surgery may be used if the cancer is found only in one lung and in nearby lymph nodes. Because this type of lung cancer is usually not found in only one lung, surgery alone is not often used. Occasionally, surgery may be used to help determine exactly which type of lung cancer the patient has. If a patient does have surgery, the doctor may take out the cancer in one of the following operations:

- Wedge resection removes only a small part of the lung.

- Lobectomy removes an entire section (lobe) of the lung.

- Pneumonectomy removes the entire lung.

During surgery, the doctor will also take out lymph nodes to see if they contain cancer.

Radiation therapy uses x-rays or other high-energy rays to kill cancer cells and shrink tumors. Radiation therapy for small cell lung cancer usually comes from a machine outside the body (external beam radiation therapy). It may be used to kill cancer cells in the lungs or in other parts of the body where the cancer has spread. Radiation therapy may also be used to prevent the cancer from growing in the brain. This is called prophylactic cranial irradiation (PCI). Because PCI may affect brain function, the doctor will help the patient decide whether to have this kind of radiation therapy. Radiation therapy can be used alone or in addition to surgery and/or chemotherapy.

Chemotherapy is the most common treatment of all stages of small cell lung cancer. Chemotherapy may be taken by pill, or it may be put into the body by a needle in the vein or muscle. Chemotherapy is called a systemic treatment because the drug enters the bloodstream, travels through the body, and can kill cancer cells outside the lungs, including cancer cells that have spread to the brain.

Treatment by Stage

Treatment of small cell lung cancer depends on the stage of the disease, and the patient's age and overall condition.

Standard treatment may be considered because of its effectiveness in patients in past studies, or participation in a clinical trial may be considered. Most patients are not cured with standard therapy and some standard treatments may have more side effects than are desired. For these reasons, clinical trials are designed to find better ways to treat cancer patients and are based on the most up-to-date information. Clinical trials are ongoing in most parts of the country for most stages of small cell lung cancer. To learn more about clinical trials, call the Cancer Information Service at 1-800-4-CANCER (1-800-422-6237); TTY at 1-800-332-8615.

Limited State Small Cell Lung Cancer

Treatment may be one of the following:

1. Chemotherapy and radiation therapy to the chest with or without radiation therapy to the brain to prevent spread of the cancer (prophylactic cranial irradiation).

2. Chemotherapy with or without prophylactic cranial irradiation.

3. Surgery followed by chemotherapy with or without prophylactic cranial irradiation.

Clinical trials are testing new drugs and new ways of giving all of the above treatments.

Extensive Stage Small Cell Lung Cancer

Treatment may be one of the following:

1. Chemotherapy with or without radiation therapy to the brain to prevent spread of the cancer (prophylactic cranial irradiation).

2. Radiation therapy to places in the body where the cancer has spread, such as the brain, bone, or spine to relieve symptoms.

Clinical trials are testing new drugs and new ways of giving all of the above treatments.

Recurrent Stage Small Cell Lung Cancer

Treatment may be one of the following:

1. Radiation therapy to reduce discomfort.

2. Chemotherapy to reduce discomfort.

3. Laser therapy, radiation therapy, and/or surgical implantation of devices to keep the airways open to relieve discomfort.

4. A clinical trial testing new drugs.

To Learn More

To learn more about lung cancer, call the National Cancer Institute's Cancer Information Service at 1-800-4-CANCER (1-800-422-6237); TTY at 1-800-332-8615. By dialing this toll-free number, trained information specialists can answer your questions.

The Cancer Information Service also has booklets about cancer that are available to the public and can be sent on request. The following booklets about lung cancer may be helpful:

Other Booklets

The National Cancer Institute booklets listed below are available free of charge by calling 1-800-4-CANCER (1-800-422-6237).

Booklets about Cancer and Its Treatment

- *Research Report: Cancer of the Lung*

- *Chemotherapy and You: A Guide to Self-Help During Treatment* *

- *Radiation Therapy and You: A Guide to Self-Help During Treatment* *

- *Eating Hints: Recipes and Tips for Better Nutrition During Cancer Treatment*

- *What Are Clinical Trials All About?* *

- *Questions and Answers About Pain Control* (also available from the American Cancer Society)

Booklets about Living with Cancer

- *Facing Forward: A Guide for Cancer Survivors* *

- *Taking Time: Support for People With Cancer and the People Who Care About Them*

- *When Cancer Recurs: Meeting the Challenge Again* *

- *Advanced Cancer: Living Each Day* *

* Reprinted in this volume: see Table of Contents

There are many other places where people can get material and information about cancer treatment and services. The social service office at a hospital can be checked for local and national agencies that help with getting information about finances, getting to and from treatment, getting care at home, and dealing with problems.

For more information from the National Cancer Institute, please write to this address:

National Cancer Institute
Office of Cancer Communications
31 Center Drive, MSC 2580
Bethesda, MD 20892-2580

Chapter 17

Cancer of the Pancreas

Introduction

Each year, more than 26,000 people in the United States learn that they have cancer of the pancreas. The National Cancer Institute (NCI) has written this chapter to help people with cancer of the pancreas and their families and friends. We hope others will read it as well to learn about this disease.

This chapter discusses symptoms, diagnosis, and treatment. It also has information about resources and sources of support to help patients cope with cancer of the pancreas.

Researchers continue to look for better ways to diagnose and treat cancer of the pancreas. For up-to-date information or to order this publication, call the National Cancer Institute's Cancer Information Service (CIS). The toll-free number is 1-800-4-CANCER (1-800-422-6237).

The CIS staff uses a National Cancer Institute cancer information database called PDQ and other NCI resources to answer callers' questions. The staff can mail information from PDQ and other NCI materials about cancer, its treatment, and living with the disease (see Other Booklets).

The Pancreas

The pancreas is located in the abdomen. It is surrounded by the stomach, intestines, and other organs. The pancreas is about 6 inches

"What You Need To Know About Cancer of the Pancreas," National Cancer Institute (NCI), updated September 1998

long and is shaped like a long, flattened pear—wide at one end and narrow at the other. The wide part of the pancreas is called the head, the narrow end is the tail, and the middle section is called the body of the pancreas.

The pancreas is a gland that has two main functions. It makes pancreatic juices, and it produces several hormones, including insulin.

Pancreatic juices contain proteins called enzymes that help digest food. The pancreas releases these juices, as they are needed, into a system of ducts. The main pancreatic duct joins the common bile duct from the liver and gallbladder. (The common bile duct carries bile, a fluid that helps digest fat.) Together these ducts form a short tube that empties into the duodenum, the first section of the small intestine.

Pancreatic hormones help the body use or store the energy that comes from food. For example, insulin helps control the amount of sugar (a source of energy) in the blood. The pancreas releases insulin and other hormones when they are needed. The hormones enter the bloodstream and travel throughout the body.

What Is Cancer?

Cancer is a group of many different diseases. Cancer occurs when cells divide without order and invade and destroy the tissue around them. To understand cancer, it is helpful to know about normal cells and about what happens when cells become cancerous.

The body is made up of many types of cells. Normally, cells grow and divide to produce more cells only when the body needs them. This orderly process helps keep the body healthy.

Sometimes cells keep dividing when new cells are not needed, forming a mass of extra tissue called a growth or tumor. Tumors can be benign or malignant.

- Benign tumors are not cancer. They often can be removed, and they usually do not come back. Cells in benign tumors do not spread to other parts of the body. Most important, benign tumors are rarely a threat to life.

- Malignant tumors are cancer. Cells in malignant tumors are abnormal and divide without control or order. These cancer cells can invade and destroy the tissue around them. Also, cancer cells can break away from malignant tumor and enter the bloodstream or the lymphatic system. This process is the way cancer spreads from the original (primary) tumor to form new tumors in other parts of the body. The spread of cancer is called metastasis.

More than 100 different types of cancer are known—and several types of cancer can develop in the pancreas. Cancer of the pancreas is also called pancreatic cancer or carcinoma of the pancreas. Most pancreatic cancers begin in the ducts that carry pancreatic juices. A rare type of pancreatic cancer begins in the cells that produce insulin and other hormones. These cells are called islet cells, or the islets of Langerhans. Cancers that begin in these cells are called islet cell cancers.

As pancreatic cancer grows, the tumor may invade organs that surround the pancreas, such as the stomach or small intestine. Pancreatic cancer cells also may break away from the tumor and spread to other parts of the body. When pancreatic cancer cells spread, they often form new tumors in lymph nodes and the liver, and sometimes in the lungs or bones. The new tumors have the same kind of abnormal cells and the same name as the primary (original) tumor in the pancreas. For example, if pancreatic cancer spreads to the liver, the cancer cells in the liver are pancreatic cancer cells. The disease is metastatic pancreatic cancer; it is not liver cancer.

Symptoms

Pancreatic cancer has been called a "silent" disease because it usually does not cause symptoms early on. The cancer may grow for some time before it causes pressure in the abdomen, pain, or other problems. When symptoms do appear, they may be so vague that they are ignored at first. For these reasons, pancreatic cancer is hard to find early. In many cases, the cancer has spread outside the pancreas by the time it is found.

When symptoms appear, they depend on the location and size of the tumor. If the tumor blocks the common bile duct so that bile cannot pass into the intestines, the skin and whites of the eyes may become yellow, and the urine may become dark. This condition is called jaundice.

As the cancer grows and spreads, pain often develops in the upper abdomen and sometimes spreads to the back. The pain may become worse after the person eats or lies down. Cancer of the pancreas can also cause nausea, loss of appetite, weight loss, and weakness.

Islet cell cancer can cause the pancreas to make too much insulin or other hormones. When this happens, the person may feel weak or dizzy and may have chills, muscle spasms, or diarrhea.

These symptoms may be caused by cancer or by other, less serious problems. Only a doctor can tell for sure.

Diagnosis and Staging

To find the cause of a person's symptoms, the doctor performs a physical exam and asks about the person's medical history. In addition to checking general signs of health, the doctor may perform blood, urine, and stool tests.

The doctor usually orders procedures that produce pictures of the pancreas and the area around it. Pictures can help the doctor diagnose cancer of the pancreas. They also can help the doctor determine the stage, or extent, of the disease by showing whether the cancer affects nearby organs. Pictures that show the location and extent of the cancer help the doctor decide how to treat it. Procedures to produce pictures of the pancreas and nearby organs may include:

- An upper GI series, sometimes called a barium swallow. A series of x-rays of the upper digestive system is taken after the patient drinks a barium solution. The barium shows an outline of the digestive organs on the x-rays.

- CT (computerized tomography) scanning, the use of an x-ray machine linked with a computer. The x-ray machine is shaped like a doughnut with a large hole. The patient lies on a bed that passes through the hole, and the machine moves along the patient's body, taking many x-rays. The computer puts the x-rays together to produce detailed pictures.

- MRI (magnetic resonance imaging), the use of a powerful magnet linked to a computer. The MRI machine is very large, with space for the patient to lie in a tunnel inside the magnet. The machine measures the body's response to the magnetic field, and the computer uses this information to make detailed pictures of areas inside the body.

- Ultrasonography, the use of high-frequency sound waves that cannot be heard by humans. An instrument sends sound waves into the patient's abdomen. The echoes that the sound waves produce as they bounce off internal organs create a picture called a sonogram. Healthy tissues and tumors produce different echoes.

- ERCP (endoscopic retrograde cholangiopancreatograpy), a method for taking x-rays of the common bile duct and pancreatic ducts. The doctor passes a long, flexible tube (endoscope) down the throat, through the stomach, and into the small intestine. The doctor then injects dye into the ducts and takes x-rays.

- PTC (percutaneous transhepatic cholangiography), in which a thin needle is put into the liver through the skin on the right side of the abdomen. Dye is injected into the bile ducts in the liver so that blockages in the ducts can be seen on x-rays.

- Angiography, x-rays of blood vessels taken after the injection of dye that makes the blood vessels show up on the x-rays.

The doctor can explain what is involved in each of these exams and what will be done to keep the patient comfortable.

Pictures of the pancreas and nearby organs provide important clues as to whether a person has cancer. However, doing a biopsy is the only sure way for the doctor to learn whether pancreatic cancer is present. In a biopsy, the doctor removes a tissue sample. A pathologist looks at the tissue under a microscope to check for cancer cells.

There are several ways to do a biopsy to diagnose pancreatic cancer, and some people may need to have more than one type of biopsy. One way to remove tissue is called a needle biopsy. The doctor inserts a long needle through the skin of the abdomen into the pancreas. Ultrasonography or x-rays guide the placement of the needle. Another type of biopsy is a brush biopsy. This is done at the same time as ERCP. The doctor inserts a very small brush through the endoscope into the opening from the bile duct and main pancreatic duct to rub off cells to examine under a microscope.

Sometimes, the biopsy to diagnose pancreatic cancer is done during surgery. In one type of surgery, called laparoscopy, the doctor inserts a lighted instrument shaped like a thin tube into the abdomen through a small incision. In addition to removing tissue samples to be examined under the microscope, the doctor can see inside the abdomen to determine the location and extent of the disease. During the laparoscopy, the doctor can decide whether a larger operation called a laparotomy is needed to remove the tumor or to relieve symptoms caused by the cancer.

In some cases, a laparotomy is necessary to make a diagnosis. In this operation, the doctor makes a larger incision and directly examines the organs in the abdomen. If cancer is found, the doctor can go ahead with further surgery. (The types of surgery done to treat pancreatic cancer are described in the Treatment Methods section.)

A person who needs a biopsy may want to ask the doctor some of the following questions:

- What type of biopsy do I need? Why?

- How long will it take? Will I be awake? Will it hurt?

- How soon will I know the results?

- If I do have cancer, who will talk with me about treatment? When?

Treatment

Cancer of the pancreas is very hard to control. This disease can be cured only when it is found at an early stage, before it has spread. However, treatment can improve the quality of a person's life by controlling the symptoms and complications of this disease.

People with pancreatic cancer are often treated by a team of specialists, which may include surgeons, medical oncologists, radiation oncologists, and endocrinologists. The choice of treatment depends on the type of cancer, the location and size of the tumor, the extent (stage) of the disease, the person's age and general health, and other factors. Cancer that begins in the pancreatic ducts may be treated with surgery, radiation therapy, or chemotherapy. Doctors sometimes use combinations of these treatments. Researchers are also studying biological therapy to see whether it can help when pancreatic cancer has spread to other parts of the body or has recurred. Islet cell cancer is usually treated with surgery or chemotherapy. Doctors may decide to use one method or a combination of treatment methods.

Some people take part in a clinical trial (research study) using new treatment methods. Such studies are designed to improve cancer treatment.

Getting a Second Opinion

Before starting treatment, the patient may want a second pathologist to confirm the diagnosis and another specialist to review the treatment plan. Some insurance companies require a second opinion; many others will cover a second opinion if the patient requests it. There are a number of ways to find a doctor who can give a second opinion:

- A patient's doctor may be able to suggest pathologists and specialists to consult.

- The Cancer Information Service, at 1-800-4-CANCER, can tell callers about treatment facilities, including cancer centers and other programs supported by the National Cancer Institute.

- Local medical societies, nearby hospitals, or medical schools can supply the names of doctors.

- The *Directory of Medical Specialists* lists doctors' names along with their specialty and their background. It is in most public libraries.

Preparing for Treatment

Many people with cancer want to learn all they can about their disease and their treatment choices so they can take an active part in decisions about their medical care. When a person is diagnosed with cancer, shock and stress are natural reactions. These feelings may make if difficult for people to think of everything they want to ask the doctor. Often, it helps to make a list of questions. To help remember what the doctor says, people may take notes or ask whether they may use a tape recorder. Some patients also want to have a family member or friend with them when they talk to the doctor—to take part in the discussion, to take notes, or just to listen.

Patients do not need to ask all their questions or remember all of the answers at one time. They will have other chances to ask the doctor to explain things and to get more information.

These are some questions a patient may want to ask the doctor before treatment begins:

- What is my diagnosis?

- What is the stage of the disease?

- What are my treatment choices? What does each treatment involve? Which do you recommend? Why?

- What are the risks and possible side effects of each treatment?

- What are the chances that the treatment will be successful?

- What new treatments are being studied in clinical trials? Would a clinical trial be appropriate for me?

- Will treatment affect my normal activities?

- What is the treatment likely to cost?

Treatment Methods

Surgery may be done to remove all or part of the pancreas and other nearby tissue. The type of surgery depends on the type of pancreatic cancer, the location of the tumor in the pancreas, the person's symptoms, whether the cancer involves other organs, and whether the cancer can be completely removed. In the Whipple procedure, the surgeon removes the head of the pancreas, the duodenum, part of the stomach, and other nearby tissue. A total pancreatectomy is surgery to remove the entire pancreas as well as the duodenum, common bile duct, gallbladder, spleen, and nearby lymph nodes.

Sometimes, the cancer cannot be completely removed. However, surgery can help to relieve symptoms that occur if the duodenum or bile duct is blocked. To relieve such symptoms, the surgeon creates a bypass around the blockage.

See the discussion about the side effects of surgery.

These are some questions a patient may want to ask the doctor before having surgery:

- What kind of operation will it be?

- Will further treatment be necessary? What kind?

- How will I feel after the operation?

- If I have pain, how will you help?

- How long will I be in the hospital?

- When will I be able to resume my normal activities?

Radiation therapy (also called radiotherapy) is the use of high-energy rays to damage cancer cells and stop them from growing and dividing. Like surgery, radiation therapy is local therapy; the radiation can affect cancer cells only in the treated area. The radiation to treat pancreatic cancer comes from a machine that aims the rays from radioactive material at a specific area of the body.

These are some questions a patient may want to ask the doctor before having radiation therapy:

- What is the goal of this treatment?

- How will the radiation be given?

- When will the treatments begin? When will they end?

- How will I feel during therapy? What are the possible side effects?

- What can I do to take care of myself during treatment?

- Will I be able to continue my normal activities during treatment?

Chemotherapy is the use of drugs to kill cancer cells. It may be given alone or along with radiation therapy to relieve symptoms of the disease if the cancer cannot be removed. When the cancer can be removed, doctors sometimes give chemotherapy after surgery to help control the growth of cancer cells that may remain in the body. The doctor may use one drug or a combination of drugs.

Chemotherapy is usually given in cycles: a treatment period followed by a recovery period, then another treatment period, and so on. Most anticancer drugs are given by injection into a vein (IV); some are given by mouth. Chemotherapy is a systemic therapy, meaning that the drugs flow through the body in the bloodstream.

Usually a person has chemotherapy as an outpatient (at the hospital, at the doctor's office, or at home). However, depending on which drugs are given and the person's general health, a short hospital stay may be needed. Read about the side effects of chemotherapy.

These are some questions patients may want to ask the doctor before starting chemotherapy:

- What is the goal of this treatment?

- What drugs will I be taking? How will they be given? Will I need to stay in the hospital?

- Will the drugs cause side effects? What can I do about them?

- How long will I need to take this treatment?

- What can I do to take care of myself during treatment?

Biological therapy (also called immunotherapy) is a form of treatment that uses the body's natural ability (immune system) to fight disease or to protect the body from treatment side effects. Researchers are testing several types of biological therapy, alone or in combination with chemotherapy. These treatments may be used when pancreatic cancer has spread to other organs or when it has recurred. People receiving biological therapy may need to stay in the hospital so that the side effects of their treatment can be watched. Read about the side effects of biological therapy.

These are some questions patients may want to ask the doctor before starting biological therapy:

- What kind of treatment will be used?

- What side effects can I expect? How long do the side effects last? What can be done to manage them?

- How will we know whether the treatment is working?

Clinical Trials

Many people with pancreatic cancer take part in clinical trials. Doctors conduct clinical trials to learn about the effectiveness and side effects of new treatments. In some clinical trials, all patients receive the new treatment. In other trials, doctors compare different therapies by giving the new treatment to one group of patients and the standard therapy to another group.

People who take part in these studies have the first chance to benefit from treatments that have shown promise in earlier research. They also make an important contribution to medical science.

In clinical trials for pancreatic cancer, doctors are studying different ways of giving radiation therapy, aiming the rays at the cancer during surgery or implanting radioactive material in the abdomen. They also are exploring new ways of giving chemotherapy, new drugs and drug combinations, biological therapy, and new ways of combining various types of treatment. Some trials are designed to study ways to reduce the side effects of treatment and to improve quality of life.

People interested in taking part in a trial should talk with their doctor. They may want to read the National Cancer Institute booklet *Taking Part in Clinical Trials: What Cancer Patients Need To Know*, which explains the possible benefits and risks of treatment studies.

One way to learn about clinical trials is through PDQ, a computerized resource developed by the National Cancer Institute. PDQ contains information about cancer treatment and about clinical trials in progress all over the country. The Cancer Information Service can provide PDQ information to patients and the public.

Side Effects of Treatment

It is hard to limit the effects of therapy so that only cancer cells are removed or destroyed. Because treatment also damages healthy cells and tissues, it often causes unpleasant side effects.

The side effects of cancer treatment depend mainly on the type and extent of the treatment. Also, they may not be the same for each person, and they may even change from one treatment to the next. Doctors monitor patients closely so they can help with any problems that occur. Doctors and nurses can explain the possible side effects of treatment and suggest ways to help relieve symptoms that may occur during and after treatment.

Surgery

Surgery for cancer of the pancreas is a major operation. The side effects of surgery depend on the extent of the operation, the person's general health, and other factors. Although patients often have pain during the first few days after surgery, their pain can be controlled with medicine. People should feel free to discuss pain relief with the doctor or nurse. See more information about pain control.

It is also common for patients to feel tired or weak for a while. The length of time it takes to recover from an operation varies for each person.

During recovery from surgery, a patient's diet and weight are checked carefully. At first, patients may be fed only liquids and may be given extra nourishment by IV. Foods are added gradually.

When the entire pancreas is removed, and even sometimes when only part of the pancreas is removed, people with pancreatic cancer may not have enough pancreatic juices or hormones. When a patient does not have enough pancreatic juices, problems with digestion may occur. The doctor can suggest an appropriate diet and prescribe medicine to help relieve diarrhea or other problems such as pain, feelings of fullness, or cramping. See more information about nutrition for people with cancer. Patients who do not have enough pancreatic hormones may develop other problems. For example, those who do not have enough insulin may develop diabetes. The doctor can treat this problem by giving patients hormones to replace those no longer produced by the pancreas.

Radiation Therapy

With radiation therapy, the side effects depend on the treatment dose and the part of the body that is treated. During radiation therapy people are likely to become very tired, especially in the later weeks of treatment. Getting plenty of rest is important.

It is common to lose hair in the treated area and for the skin to become red, tender, and itchy. There may be permanent darkening or "bronzing" of the skin in the treated areas. This area should be exposed to the air as much as possible but protected from the sun, and it is important to avoid wearing clothes that rub. Patients will be shown how to take care of the treated area. Lotion or cream should not be used on the treated skin without the doctor's advice.

Radiation therapy to the pancreas and nearby tissues and organs may cause nausea, vomiting, diarrhea, or problems with digestion.

Usually, the doctor can suggest certain diet changes or medicine to treat or control these problems. In most cases, side effects go away when treatment is over. The National Cancer Institute booklet *Radiation Therapy and You* [reprinted in this volume as Chapter 66] has helpful information about radiation therapy and coping with its side effects.

Chemotherapy

The side effects of chemotherapy depend mainly on the specific drugs and the doses received. As with other types of treatment, side effects also vary from person to person. Generally, anticancer drugs affect cells that divide rapidly. These include blood cells, which fight infection, help the blood to clot, or carry oxygen to all parts of the body. When blood cells are affected, people are more likely to get infections, may bruise or bleed easily, and may have less energy. Cells in hair roots and cells that line the digestive tract also divide rapidly. As a result, people may lose their hair and may have other side effects such as poor appetite, nausea and vomiting, diarrhea, or mouth sores. Usually these side effects go away gradually during the recovery periods between treatments or after treatment is over. The National Cancer Institute booklets *Chemotherapy and You* [reprinted in this volume as Chapter 63] and *Helping Yourself During Chemotherapy* have useful information about this form of treatment and about managing the side effects it can cause.

Biological Therapy

The side effects caused by biological therapy vary with the type of treatment. These treatments may cause flu-like symptoms such as chills, fever, muscle aches, weakness, loss of appetite, nausea, vomiting, and diarrhea. Patients also may bleed or bruise easily, get a rash, or have swelling. These problems can be severe, but they usually go away after the treatment stops.

Pain Control

Pain is a common problem for people with pancreatic cancer, especially when the cancer grows outside the pancreas and presses against nerves and other organs. However, the doctor can usually relieve or reduce pain. It is important for patients to report their pain so the doctor can take steps to help relieve it.

There are several ways to control pain caused by pancreatic cancer. In most cases, the doctor prescribes medicine to control the pain. Sometimes a combination of pain medicines is needed. Medicines that relieve pain may make people drowsy and constipated, but resting and taking laxatives can help. In some cases, pain medicine is not enough. The doctor may use other treatments that affect nerves in the abdomen. For example, the doctor may inject alcohol into the area around certain nerves to block the feeling of pain. The injection can be done during surgery or by using a long needle inserted through the skin into the abdomen. This procedure rarely causes problems and usually provides pain relief. Sometimes, the doctor cuts nerves in the abdomen during surgery to block the feeling of pain. In addition, radiation therapy can help relieve pain by shrinking the tumor.

The Cancer Information Service can supply booklets called *Questions and Answers About Pain Control* and *Get Relief From Cancer Pain*. People with pancreatic cancer and their families may find these booklets helpful.

Nutrition for Cancer Patients

Eating well during cancer treatment means getting enough calories and protein to help prevent weight loss and maintain strength. Eating well often helps people feel better and have more energy.

Some people with cancer find it hard to eat well. They may lose their appetite. In addition, common side effects of treatment, such as nausea, vomiting, or mouth sores, can make eating difficult. Often, foods taste different. Also, people being treated for cancer may not feel like eating when they are uncomfortable or tired.

Cancer of the pancreas and its treatment may interfere with production of pancreatic enzymes and insulin. As a result, patients may have problems digesting food and maintaining the proper blood sugar level. They may need to take medicines to replace the enzymes and hormones normally produced by the pancreas. These medicines must be given in just the right amount for each patient. The doctor will watch the patient closely and adjust the doses or suggest diet changes when needed. Careful planning and checkups are important to help avoid nutrition problems leading to weight loss, weakness, and lack of energy.

Doctors, nurses, and dietitians can offer advice on how to eat well during cancer treatment. Patients and their families also may want to read the National Cancer Institute booklet *Eating Hints for Cancer Patients* [reprinted in this volume as Chapter 77], which contains many useful suggestions.

Followup Care

Regular followup exams are very important after treatment for pancreatic cancer. The doctor will continue to check the person closely so that, if the cancer returns or progresses, it can be treated. Checkups may include a physical exam; blood, urine, and stool tests; chest x-rays; and CT scans.

People taking medicine to replace pancreatic hormones or digestive juices need to see their doctor regularly so that the dose can be adjusted if necessary. Also, it is important for the patient to let the doctor know about pain or any changes or problems that occur.

Support for Cancer Patients

Living with a serious disease is not easy. People with cancer and those who care about them face many problems and challenges. Coping with these problems is often easier when people have helpful information and support services. Several useful booklets, including *Taking Time*, are available from the Cancer Information Service.

Worries about tests, treatments, hospital stays, and medical bills are common. Doctors, nurses, and other members of the health care team can talk with patients and their families about treatment, managing daily activities, and other concerns. Meeting with a social worker, counselor, or member of the clergy also can be helpful to those who want to talk about their feelings or discuss their concerns.

Cancer patients and their families may want to know what the future holds. Sometimes they use statistics to try to predict what may happen. It is important to remember, however, that statistics are averages based on large numbers of patients. They cannot be used to predict what will happen to a particular patient because no two patients are alike; treatments and responses vary greatly. The doctor who takes care of the patient is in the best position to talk about the person's outlook (prognosis).

Friends and relatives can be very supportive. Also, many people find it helpful to discuss their concerns with others who have cancer. People with cancer often get together in support groups, where they can share what they have learned about coping with cancer and the effects of treatment. It is important to keep in mind, however, that each patient is different. Treatment and ways of dealing with cancer that work for one person may not be right for another—even if they both have the same kind of cancer. It is always a good idea to discuss the advice of friends and family members with the doctor.

Often, a social worker at the hospital or clinic can suggest groups that provide emotional support or that help with rehabilitation, financial aid, transportation, or home care. For example, the American Cancer Society has many services for patients and their families. Local offices of the American Cancer Society are listed in the white pages of the telephone directory.

The Cancer Information Service also can supply information about pancreatic cancer and about programs and services for patients and their families.

Possible Causes and Prevention

Scientists across the country are studying pancreatic cancer and trying to learn what causes this disease. The more they can find out about the cause of this disease, the better the chance of finding ways to prevent it.

At this time, scientists do not know exactly what causes cancer of the pancreas, and they can seldom explain why one person gets this disease and another does not. However, it is clear that pancreatic cancer is not contagious; no one can "catch" this disease from another person.

Scientists have learned that some things increase a person's chance of getting this disease. As with most other types of cancer, studies show that the risk of pancreatic cancer increases with age. This disease rarely occurs before age 40; the average age at diagnosis is about 70.

Research also shows that smoking is a risk factor for several types of cancer, including cancer of the pancreas. Cigarette smokers develop this disease two to three times more often than nonsmokers. Quitting smoking reduces the risk of pancreatic, lung, and certain other cancers, as well as a number of other diseases.

Having diabetes is another risk factor for pancreatic cancer. People who have diabetes develop pancreatic cancer about twice as often as people who do not have diabetes.

Research suggests that a person's diet may affect the chances of getting some types of cancer. In several studies, the risk of pancreatic cancer was higher among people whose diet was high in fat and low in fruits and vegetables. Although the possible link between diet and cancer of the pancreas is still under study, some scientists believe that choosing a low-fat diet and eating well-balanced meals with plenty of fruits and vegetables may lower a person's risk.

Some studies suggest that occupational exposure to petroleum and certain chemicals may increase the risk of pancreatic cancer. These possible links have not been proven, but workers should follow safety rules provided by their employers.

People who think they may be at risk for pancreatic cancer should discuss this concern with their doctor. The doctor may be able to suggest ways to reduce the risk and can suggest an appropriate schedule of checkups.

Other Booklets

The National Cancer Institute booklets listed below and others are available from the Cancer Information Service by calling 1-800-4-CANCER.

Booklets about Cancer Treatment

- *Chemotherapy and You: A Guide to Self-Help During Treatment* *

- *Radiation Therapy and You: A Guide to Self-Help During Treatment* *

- *Eating Hints for Cancer Patients* *

- *Taking Part in Clinical Trials: What Cancer Patients Need To Know*

- *Questions and Answers About Pain Control*

- *Get Relief From Cancer Pain*

Booklets about Living with Cancer

- *Taking Time: Support for People With Cancer and the People Who Care About Them*

- *When Cancer Recurs: Meeting the Challenge Again* *

- *Advanced Cancer: Living Each Day* *

* Reprinted in this volume—see Table of Contents

National Cancer Institute Information Resources

You may want more information for yourself, your family, and your doctor. The following National Cancer Institute (NCI) services are available to help you.

Telephone: Cancer Information Service (CIS) Provides accurate, up-to-date information on cancer to patients and their families, health professionals, and the general public. Information specialists translate the latest scientific information into understandable language and respond in English, Spanish, or on TTY equipment. Toll-free: 1-800-4-CANCER (1-800-422-6237) TTY: 1-800-332-8615

Internet: These Web sites may be useful:

- http://www.nci.nih.gov—NCI's primary Web site; contains information about the Institute and its programs.

- http://cancernet.nci.nih.gov—CancerNet contains material for health professionals, patients, and the public, including information from PDQ about cancer treatment, screening, prevention, supportive care, and clinical trials, and CANCERLIT, a bibliographic database.

- http://cancertrials.nci.nih.gov—CancerTrials, NCI's comprehensive clinical trials information center for patients, health professionals, and the public. Includes information on understanding trials, deciding whether to participate in trials, finding specific trials, plus research news and other resources.

CancerMail: Includes NCI information about cancer treatment, screening, prevention, and supportive care. To obtain a contents list, send e-mail to cancermail@icicc.nci.nih.gov with the word "help" in the body of the message.

CancerFax: Includes NCI information about cancer treatment, screening, prevention, and supportive care. To obtain a contents list, dial 301-402-5874 from a fax machine hand set and follow the recorded instructions.

Chapter 18

Islet Cell Pancreatic Cancer

What Is Islet Cell Cancer?

Islet cell cancer, a rare cancer, is a disease in which cancer (malignant) cells are found in certain tissues of the pancreas. The pancreas is about 6 inches long and is shaped like a thin pear, wider at one end and narrower at the other. The pancreas lies behind the stomach, inside a loop formed by part of the small intestine. The broader right end of the pancreas is called the head, the middle section is called the body, and the narrow left end is the tail.

The pancreas has two basic jobs in the body. It produces digestive juices that help break down (digest) food, and hormones (such as insulin) that regulate how the body stores and uses food. The area of the pancreas that produces digestive juices is called the exocrine pancreas. About 95% of pancreatic cancers begin in the exocrine pancreas. The hormone-producing area of the pancreas has special cells called islet cells and is called the endocrine pancreas. Only about 5% of pancreatic cancers start here. This summary has information on cancer of the endocrine pancreas (islet cell cancer). For more information on cancer of the exocrine pancreas, see the PDQ patient information summary on cancer of the pancreas.

The islet cells in the pancreas make many hormones, including insulin, which help the body store and use sugars. When islet cells in the pancreas become cancerous, they may make too many hormones.

PDQ Statement, National Cancer Institute (NCI), updated February 1998.

201

Islet cell cancers that make too many hormones are called functioning tumors. Other islet cell cancers may not make extra hormones and are called nonfunctioning tumors. Tumors that do not spread to other parts of the body can also be found in the islet cells. These are called benign tumors and are not cancer. A doctor will need to determine whether the tumor is cancer or a benign tumor.

A doctor should be seen if there is pain in the abdomen, diarrhea, stomach pain, a tired feeling all the time, fainting, or weight gain without eating too much.

If there are symptoms, the doctor will order blood and urine tests to see whether the amounts of hormones in the body are normal. Other tests, including x-rays and special scans, may also be done.

The chance of recovery (prognosis) depends on the type of islet cell cancer the patient has, how far the cancer has spread, and the patient's overall health.

Stages of Islet Cell Cancer

Once islet cell cancer is found, more tests will be done to find out if cancer cells have spread to other parts of the body. This is called staging. The staging system for islet cell cancer is still being developed. These tumors are most often divided into one of three groups:

- islet cell cancers occurring in one site within the pancreas
- islet cell cancers occurring in several sites within the pancreas
- islet cell cancers that have spread to lymph nodes near the pancreas or to distant sites

A doctor also needs to know the type of islet cell tumor to plan treatment. The following types of islet cell tumors are found:

Gastrinoma

The tumor makes large amounts of a hormone called gastrin, which causes too much acid to be made in the stomach. Ulcers may develop as a result of too much stomach acid.

Insulinoma

The tumor makes too much of the hormone insulin and causes the body to store sugar instead of burning the sugar for energy. This causes too little sugar in the blood, a condition called hypoglycemia.

Miscellaneous

Other types of islet cell cancer can affect the pancreas and/or small intestine. Each type of tumor may affect different hormones in the body and cause different symptoms.

Recurrent

Recurrent disease means that the cancer has come back (recurred) after it has been treated. It may come back in the pancreas or in another part of the body.

How Islet Cell Cancer Is Treated

There are treatments for all patients with islet cell cancer. Three types of treatment are used:

- surgery (taking out the cancer)
- chemotherapy (using drugs to kill cancer cells)
- hormone therapy (using hormones to stop cancer cells from growing)

Surgery is the most common treatment of islet cell cancer. The doctor may take out the cancer and most or part of the pancreas. Sometimes the stomach is taken out (gastrectomy) because of ulcers. Lymph nodes in the area may also be removed and looked at under a microscope to see if they contain cancer.

Chemotherapy uses drugs to kill cancer cells. Chemotherapy may be taken by pill, or it may be put into the body by a needle in the vein or muscle. Chemotherapy is called a systemic treatment because the drug enters the bloodstream, travels through the body, and can kill cancer cells throughout the body.

Hormone therapy uses hormones to stop the cancer cells from growing or to relieve symptoms caused by the tumor.

Hepatic arterial occlusion or embolization uses drugs or other agents to reduce or block the flow of blood to the liver in order to kill cancer cells growing in the liver.

Treatment by Type

Treatment of islet cell cancer depends on the type of tumor, the stage, and the patient's overall health.

Standard treatment may be considered because of its effectiveness in patients in past studies, or participation in a clinical trial may be considered. Not all patients are cured with standard therapy and some standard treatments may have more side effects than are desired. For these reasons, clinical trials are designed to find better ways to treat cancer patients and are based on the most up-to-date information. Clinical trials are ongoing in many parts of the country for patients with islet cell cancer. To learn more about clinical trials, call the Cancer Information Service at 1-800-4-CANCER (1-800-422-6237); TTY at 1-800-332-8615.

Gastrinoma

Treatment may be one of the following:

1. Surgery to remove the cancer.

2. Surgery to remove the stomach (gastrectomy).

3. Surgery to cut the nerve that stimulates the pancreas.

4. Chemotherapy.

5. Hormone therapy.

6. Hepatic arterial occlusion or embolization to kill cancer cells growing in the liver.

Insulinoma

Treatment may be one of the following:

1. Surgery to remove the cancer.

2. Chemotherapy.

3. Hormone therapy.

4. Drugs to relieve symptoms.

5. Hepatic arterial occlusion or embolization to kill cancer cells growing in the liver.

Miscellaneous Islet Cell Cancer

Treatment may be one of the following:

1. Surgery to remove the cancer.

2. Chemotherapy.

3. Hormone therapy.

4. Hepatic arterial occlusion or embolization to kill cancer cells growing in the liver.

Recurrent Islet Cell Carcinoma

Treatment depends on many factors, including what treatment the patient had before and where the cancer has come back. Treatment may be chemotherapy, or patients may want to consider taking part in a clinical trial.

To Learn More

To learn more about islet cell cancer, call the National Cancer Institute's Cancer Information Service at 1-800-4-CANCER (1-800-422-6237); TTY at 1-800-332-8615. By dialing this toll-free number, trained information specialists can answer your questions.

The Cancer Information Service also has booklets about cancer that are available to the public and can be sent on request. The following booklets about pancreatic cancer may be helpful:

What You Need To Know About Cancer of the Pancreas *

Research Report: Cancer of the Pancreas

Booklets about Cancer Treatment

Radiation Therapy and You: A Guide to Self-Help During Treatment *

Chemotherapy and You: A Guide to Self-Help During Treatment *

Eating Hints: Recipes and Tips for Better Nutrition During Cancer Treatment *

Questions and Answers About Pain Control

What Are Clinical Trials All About?

Booklets about Living with Cancer

What You Need To Know About Cancer *

Taking Time: Support for People With Cancer and the People Who Care About Them

When Cancer Recurs: Meeting the Challenge Again *

Advanced Cancer: Living Each Day *

* Reprinted in this volume—see Table of Contents

Chapter 19

Liver Cancer

What Is Adult Primary Liver Cancer?

Adult primary liver cancer is a disease in which cancer (malignant) cells start to grow in the tissues of the liver. The liver is one of the largest organs in the body, filling the upper right side of the abdomen and protected by the rib cage. The liver has many functions. It has an important role in making food into energy and also filters and stores blood.

People who have hepatitis B or C (viral infections of the liver) or a disease of the liver called cirrhosis are more likely than other people to get adult primary liver cancer. Primary liver cancer is different from cancer that has spread from another place in the body to the liver. (A separate PDQ summary is available for childhood liver cancer).

A doctor should be seen if the following symptoms appear: a hard lump just below the rib cage on the right side where the liver has swollen, discomfort in the upper abdomen on the right side, pain around the right shoulder blade, or yellowing of the skin (jaundice). If there are symptoms, a doctor may order special x-rays, such as a computed tomographic scan or a liver scan. If a lump is seen on an x-ray, a doctor may use a needle inserted into the abdomen to remove a small amount of tissue from the liver. This procedure is called a needle biopsy, and a doctor usually will use an x-ray for guidance. The doctor will have the tissue looked

This Chapter is comprised of two documents: PDQ Statement on Adult Primary Liver Cancer, revised June 1998; and Questions and Answers about Liver Cancer, revised June 1997. Both documents are from the National Cancer Institute (NCI).

at under a microscope to see if there are any cancer cells. Before the test, a patient will be given a local anesthetic (a drug that causes loss of feeling for a short period of time) in the area so that no pain is felt.

A doctor may also want to look at the liver with an instrument called a laparoscope, which is a small tube-shaped instrument with a light on the end. For this test, a small cut is made in the abdomen so that the laparoscope can be inserted. The doctor may also take a small piece of tissue (biopsy specimen) during the laparoscopy and look at it under the microscope to see if there are any cancer cells. An anesthetic will be given so no pain is felt.

A doctor may also order an examination called an angiography. During this examination, a tube (catheter) is inserted into the main blood vessel that takes blood to the liver. Dye is then injected through the tube so that the blood vessels in the liver can be seen on an x-ray. Angiography can help a doctor tell whether the cancer is primary liver cancer or cancer that has spread from another part of the body. This test is usually done in the hospital.

Certain blood tests (such as alpha-fetoprotein, or AFP) may also help a doctor diagnose primary liver cancer.

The chance of recovery (prognosis) and choice of treatment depend on the stage of the cancer (whether it is just in the liver or has spread to other places) and the patient's general state of health.

Stages of Adult Primary Liver Cancer

Once adult primary liver cancer is found, more tests will be done to find out if the cancer cells have spread to other parts of the body (staging). The following stages are used for adult primary liver cancer:

Localized Resectable

Cancer is found in one place in the liver and can be totally removed in an operation.

Localized Unresectable

Cancer is found only in one part of the liver, but the cancer cannot be totally removed.

Advanced

Cancer has spread through much of the liver or to other parts of the body.

Recurrent

Recurrent disease means that the cancer has come back (recurred) after it has been treated. It may come back in the liver or in another part of the body.

How Adult Primary Liver Cancer Is Treated

There are treatments for all patients with adult primary liver cancer. Three kinds of treatment are used:

- surgery (taking out the cancer in an operation)
- radiation therapy (using high-dose x-rays to kill cancer cells)
- chemotherapy (using drugs to kill cancer cells)

Surgery may be used to take out the cancer or to replace the liver.

- Resection of the liver takes out the part of the liver where the cancer is found.
- A liver transplant is the removal of the entire liver and replacement with a healthy liver donated from someone else. Only a very few patients with liver cancer are eligible for this procedure.
- Cryosurgery is a type of surgery that kills cancer by freezing it.

Radiation therapy is the use of x-rays or other high-energy rays to kill cancer cells and shrink tumors. Radiation may come from a machine outside the body (external-beam radiation therapy) or from putting materials that contain radiation through thin plastic tubes (internal radiation therapy) in the area where the cancer cells are found. Drugs may be given with the radiation therapy to make the cancer cells more sensitive to radiation (radiosensitization).

Radiation may also be given by attaching radioactive substances to antibodies (radiolabeled antibodies) that search out certain cells in the liver. Antibodies are made by the body to fight germs and other harmful things; each antibody fights specific cells.

Chemotherapy is the use of drugs to kill cancer cells. Chemotherapy for liver cancer is usually put into the body by inserting a needle into a vein or artery. This type of chemotherapy is called a systemic treatment because the drug enters the bloodstream, travels through the body, and can kill cancer cells outside the liver. In another type of chemotherapy called regional chemotherapy, a small pump containing drugs is placed in the body. The pump puts drugs directly into the blood vessels that go to the tumor.

If a doctor removes all the cancer that can be seen at the time of the operation, the patient may be given chemotherapy after surgery to kill any remaining cells. Chemotherapy that is given after surgery to remove the cancer is called adjuvant chemotherapy.

Hyperthermia (warming the body to kill cancer cells) and biological therapy (using the body's immune system to fight cancer) are being tested in clinical trials.

Hyperthermia therapy is the use of a special machine to heat the body for a certain period of time to kill cancer cells. Because cancer cells are often more sensitive to heat than normal cells, the cancer cells die and the tumor shrinks.

Biological therapy is the use of methods to get the body to fight cancer. Materials made by the body or made in a laboratory are used to boost, direct, or restore the body's natural defenses against disease. Biological therapy is sometimes called biological response modifier therapy or immunotherapy.

Treatment by Stage

Treatments for adult primary liver cancer depend on the stage of the disease the condition of the liver, and the patient's age and general health. Standard treatment may be considered, based on its effectiveness in patients in past studies, or participation into a clinical trial. Many patients are not cured with standard therapy, and some standard treatments may have more side effects than are desired. For these reasons, clinical trials are designed to find better ways to treat cancer patients and are based on the most up-to-date information. Clinical trials are ongoing in most parts of the country for most stages of adult liver cancer. For more information, call the Cancer Information Service at 1-800-4-CANCER (1-800-422-6237); TTY at 1-800-332-8615.

Localized Resectable Adult Primary Liver Cancer

Treatment is usually surgery (resection). Liver transplantation may be done in certain patients. Clinical trials are testing adjuvant systemic or regional chemotherapy following surgery.

Localized Unresectable Adult Primary Liver Cancer

Treatment may be one of the following:

1. Cryosurgery (in patients whose tumors can not be surgically removed).

2. Liver transplantation (in certain patients).

3. Regional chemotherapy, including local infusion of chemotherapy.

4. Systemic chemotherapy.

5. Surgery or cryosurgery followed by chemotherapy. Hyperthermia or radiation therapy with or without drugs to make the cancer cells more sensitive to radiation may be given in addition to chemotherapy.

6. Local injection of pure alcohol for small tumors.

7. Radiation therapy.

Advanced Adult Primary Liver Cancer

Treatment may be one of the following:

1. A clinical trial of biological therapy.

2. A clinical trial of chemotherapy.

3. A clinical trial of chemotherapy, radiation therapy, and drugs to make the cancer cells more sensitive to radiation (radiosensitizers).

4. A clinical trial of external radiation therapy plus chemotherapy followed by radiolabeled antibodies.

Recurrent Adult Primary Liver Cancer

Treatment of recurrent adult primary liver cancer depends on what treatment a patient has already received, the part of the body where the cancer has come back, whether the liver has cirrhosis, and other factors. Patients may wish to consider taking part in a clinical trial.

To Learn More

To learn more about adult primary liver cancer, call the National Cancer Institute's Cancer Information Service at 1-800-4-CANCER (1-800-422-6237); TTY at 1-800-332-8615. By dialing this toll-free number, trained information specialists can help answer your questions.

The Cancer Information Service also has booklets about cancer that are available to the public and can be sent on request. The following booklet about liver cancer may also be helpful: *In Answer to Your Questions About Liver Cancer.*

For Further Information

Cancer patients, their families and friends, and others may find the following booklets useful. They are available free of charge by calling 1-800-4-CANCER or writing:

Office of Cancer Communications
National Cancer Institute
Building 31, Room 10A24
Bethesda, MD 20892

Booklets about Cancer Treatment

Radiation Therapy and You: A Guide to Self-Help During Treatment *

Chemotherapy and You: A Guide to Self-Help During Treatment *

Eating Hints: Recipes and Tips for Better Nutrition During Cancer Treatment *

Questions and Answers About Pain Control

What Are Clinical Trials All About?

Booklets about Living with Cancer

Taking Time: Support for People With Cancer and the People Who Care About Them

When Cancer Recurs: Meeting the Challenge Again *

Advanced Cancer: Living Each Day *

* Reprinted in this volume—see Table of Contents

If you want to know more about cancer and how it is treated, or if you wish to know about clinical trials for your type of cancer, you can call the NCI's Cancer Information Service at 1-800-422-6237, toll free. A trained information specialist can talk with you and answer your questions.

Questions and Answers about Liver Cancer

1. Where is the liver and what is its function?

The liver is a large organ located on the tight side of the abdomen and is protected by the rib cage. The liver has many functions. It plays a role in converting food into energy. It also filters and stores blood.

2. What is liver cancer?

Liver cancer is a disease in which liver cells become abnormal grow out of control, and form a cancerous tumor. This type of cancer is called primary liver cancer. Primary liver cancer is also called malignant hepatoma or hepatocellular carcinoma. Very young children may develop another form of liver cancer known as hepatoblastoma. Cancer that spreads to the liver from another part of the body (metastatic cancer) is not the same as primary liver cancer. This fact sheet deals with primary liver cancer in adults. For information on hepatoblastoma or cancer that has spread to the liver from another site, contact the National Cancer Institute's Cancer Information Service.

3. What are the risk factors for liver cancer?

The development of liver cancer is believed to be related to infection with the hepatitis-B virus (HBV) and hepatitis-C virus (HCV). Scientists estimate that 10 to 20 percent of people infected with HBV will develop cancer of the liver. Evidence of HBV infection is found in nearly one-fourth of Americans with liver cancer. The exact relationship between HCV and cancer of the liver is being studied.

Researchers have found that people with certain other liver diseases have a higher-than-average chance of developing primary liver cancer. For example, 5 to 10 percent of people with cirrhosis of the liver (a progressive disorder that leads to scarring of the liver) will eventually develop liver cancer. Some research suggests that lifestyle factors, such as alcohol consumption and malnutrition, cause both cirrhosis and liver cancer.

Aflatoxins—a group of chemicals produced by a mold that can contaminate certain foods, such as peanuts, com, grains, and seeds—are carcinogens (cancer-causing agents) for liver cancer.

4. What are the symptoms of liver cancer?

Primary liver cancer is difficult to detect at an early stage because its first symptoms are usually vague. As with other types of cancer, this disease can cause a general feeling of poor health. Cancer of the liver can lead to loss of appetite, weight loss, fever, fatigue, and weakness.

As the cancer grows, pain may develop in the upper abdomen on the right side and may extend into the back and shoulder. Some people can feel a mass in the upper abdomen. Liver cancer can also lead to abdominal swelling and a feeling of fullness or bloating. Some people have episodes of fever and nausea, or develop jaundice, a condition in which the skin and the whites of the eyes become yellow and the urine becomes dark. It is important to note that these symptoms can be caused by primary or metastatic cancer in the liver, by a benign (noncancerous) liver tumor, or by other, less serious conditions. Only a doctor can tell for sure.

5. How is liver cancer diagnosed?

To make a diagnosis of liver cancer, the doctor takes a medical history, does a careful physical examination, and orders certain tests.

Certain blood tests are used to see how well the liver is functioning. Blood tests can also be used to check for tumor markers, substances often found in abnormal amounts in patients with liver cancer. The tumor marker alpha-fetoprotein (AFP) can be useful to help diagnose liver cancer. About 50 to 70 percent of people who have primary liver cancer have elevated levels of AFP. However, other cancers such as germ cell cancer and, in some cases, pancreatic and gastric cancer, also cause elevated AFP levels. X-rays of the chest and abdomen, angiograms (x-rays of blood vessels), CT scans (x-rays put together by computer), and MRI's (images created by using a magnetic field) may all be part of the diagnostic process. Liver scans using radioactive materials can help identify abnormal areas in the liver.

The presence of liver cancer is confirmed with a biopsy. Tissue from the liver (biopsy specimen) is removed (through a needle or during an operation) and checked under a microscope for the presence of cancer cells. The doctor may also look at the liver with an instrument called a laparoscope, which is a small tube-shaped instrument with a light on one end. For this procedure, a small is made in the abdomen so that the laparoscope can be inserted. doctor may take a small piece of tissue during the laparoscopy. A pathologist then examines the tissue under the microscope to see if cancer cells are present.

6. How is liver cancer treated?

Liver cancer is difficult to control unless the cancer is found when it is very small. However, treatment can relieve symptoms and improve the patient's quality of life. Treatment depends on the stage (extent) of disease, the condition of liver, and the patient's age and general health. The doctor may recommend surgery, chemotherapy (treatment with anticancer drugs), radiation therapy (treatment with high-energy rays), biological therapy (treatment using substances that help the body fight the cancer), or a combination of these treatment methods.

7. Are treatment studies (clinical trials) available for patients with liver cancer?

Treatment studies (clinical trials) are research studies designed to find more effective treatments and better ways to use current treatments. Participation in treatment studies is an option for many patients with liver cancer. In some studies, all patients receive the new treatment. In others, doctors compare different therapies by giving the new treatment to one group of patients and standard therapy to another group. In this way, doctors can compare different therapies. In treatment studies for cancer of the liver, doctors are studying new anticancer drugs and drug combinations. They are also studying new ways to give chemotherapy, such as putting the drugs directly into the liver. Other research approaches include cryotherapy (surgery that uses extreme cold to destroy cancer cells) and combinations of several standard treatments.

Chapter 20

Extrahepatic Bile Duct Cancer

What Is Extrahepatic Bile Duct Cancer?

Extrahepatic bile duct cancer, a rare cancer, is a disease in which cancer (malignant) cells are found in the tissues of the extrahepatic bile duct. The bile duct is a tube that connects the liver and the gallbladder to the small intestine. The part of the bile duct that is outside the liver is called the extrahepatic bile duct. A fluid called bile, which is made by the liver and breaks down fats during digestion, is stored in the gallbladder. When food is being broken down in the intestines, bile is released from the gallbladder through the bile duct to the first part of the small intestine.

A doctor should be seen if there are any of the following symptoms: yellowing of the skin (jaundice), pain in the abdomen, fever, or itching.

If there are symptoms, a doctor will perform an examination and order tests to see if there is cancer. A patient may have an ultrasound, a test that uses sound waves to find tumors. A patient may also have a CT (computed tomographic) scan, which is a special type of x-ray that uses a computer to make a picture of the inside of the abdomen. Another special scan called magnetic resonance imaging (MRI), which uses magnetic waves to make a picture of the inside of the abdomen, may be done as well.

A doctor may perform a test called an ERCP (endoscopic retrograde cholangiopancreatography). During this test, a flexible tube is put

PDQ Statement, National Cancer Institute (NCI), updated December 1997.

down the throat, through the stomach, and into the small intestine. The doctor can see through the tube and inject dye into the drainage tube (duct) of the pancreas so that the area can be seen more clearly on an x-ray.

PTC (percutaneous transhepatic cholangiography) is another test that can help find cancer of the extrahepatic bile duct. During this test, a thin needle is put into the liver through the right side of the patient. Dye is injected through the needle into the bile duct in the liver so that blockages can be seen on x-rays.

If tissue that is not normal is found, the doctor may remove a small amount of fluid or tissue from the bile duct and look at it under the microscope to see if there are any cancer cells. This procedure is called a biopsy and is usually done during the PTC or ERCP.

Because it is sometimes hard to tell whether a patient has cancer or another disease, surgery may be needed to see if there is cancer of the bile duct. If this is the case, the doctor will cut into the abdomen and look at the bile duct and the tissues around it for cancer. If there is cancer and if it looks like it has not spread to other tissues, the doctor may remove the cancer or relieve blockages caused by the tumor.

The chance of recovery (prognosis) and choice of treatment depends on the location of the cancer in the bile duct, the stage of the cancer (whether it is only in the bile duct or has spread to other places), and the patient's general health.

Stages of Extrahepatic Bile Duct Cancer

Once extrahepatic bile duct cancer is found (diagnosed), more tests will be done to find out if cancer cells have spread to other parts of the body. This is called staging. To plan treatment, a doctor needs to know the stage of the cancer. The following stages are used for extrahepatic bile duct cancer:

Localized

The cancer is only in the area where it began and can be removed in an operation.

Unresectable

All of the cancer cannot be removed in an operation. The cancer may have spread to nearby organs and lymph nodes or to other parts of the body. (Lymph nodes are small bean-shaped structures that are found throughout the body. They produce and store infection-fighting cells.)

Recurrent

Recurrent disease means that the cancer has come back (recurred) after it has been treated. It may come back in the bile duct or in another part of the body.

How Extrahepatic Bile Duct Cancer Is Treated

There are treatments for all patients with extrahepatic bile duct cancer. Two kinds of treatment are used:

- surgery (taking out the cancer or taking steps to relieve symptoms caused by the cancer)
- radiation therapy (using high-dose x-rays to kill cancer cells)

Other treatments for extrahepatic bile duct cancer are being studied in clinical trials. These include:

- chemotherapy (using drugs to kill cancer cells)
- biological therapy (using the body's immune system to fight cancer)

Surgery is a common treatment of extrahepatic bile duct cancer. If the cancer is small and is only in the bile duct, a doctor may remove the whole bile duct and make a new duct by connecting the duct openings in the liver to the intestine. The doctor will also remove lymph nodes and look at them under the microscope to see if they contain cancer. If the cancer has spread outside the bile duct, a surgeon may remove the bile duct and the tissues around it.

If the cancer has spread and it cannot be removed, the doctor may do surgery to relieve symptoms. If the cancer is blocking the small intestine and bile builds up in the gallbladder, the doctor may do surgery to go around (bypass) all or part of the small intestine. During this operation, the doctor will cut the gallbladder or bile duct and sew it to the small intestine. This is called biliary bypass. Surgery or x-ray procedures may also be done to put in a tube (catheter) to drain bile that has built up in the area. During these procedures, the doctor may make the catheter drain through a tube to the outside of the body or the catheter may go around the blocked area and drain the bile to the small intestine. In addition, if the cancer is blocking the flow of food from the stomach, the stomach may be sewn directly to the small intestine so the patient can continue to eat normally.

Radiation therapy is the use of high-energy x-rays to kill cancer cells and shrink tumors. Radiation may come from a machine outside the body (external- beam radiation therapy) or from putting materials that produce radiation (radioisotopes) through thin plastic tubes into the area where the cancer cells are found (internal radiation therapy).

Chemotherapy is the use of drugs to kill cancer cells. Chemotherapy may be taken by pill, or it may be put into the body by inserting a needle into a vein or muscle. Chemotherapy is called a systemic treatment because the drug enters the bloodstream, travels through the body, and can kill cancer cells outside the bile duct.

Biological therapy tries to get the body to fight cancer. It uses materials made by the body or made in a laboratory to boost, direct, or restore the body's natural defenses against disease. Biological therapy is sometimes called biological response modifier (BRM) therapy or immunotherapy. This treatment is currently only being given in clinical trials.

Treatment by Stage

Treatment depends on the stage of the disease, and the patient's age and overall health.

Standard treatment may be considered because of its effectiveness in patients in past studies, or participation in a clinical trial may be considered. Not all patients are cured with standard therapy and some standard treatments may have more side effects than are desired. For these reasons, clinical trials are designed to find better ways to treat cancer patients and are based on the most up-to-date information. Clinical trials are ongoing in some parts of the country for patients with extrahepatic bile duct cancer. To learn more about clinical trials, call the Cancer Information Service at 1-800-4-CANCER (1-800-422-6237); TTY at 1-800-332-8615.

Localized Extrahepatic Bile Duct Cancer

Treatment may be one of the following:

1. Surgery to remove the cancer.

2. Surgery to remove the cancer followed by external-beam radiation therapy.

Unresectable Extrahepatic Bile Duct Cancer

Treatment may be one of the following:

1. Surgery or other procedures to bypass blockage in the bile duct.

2. Surgery or other procedures to bypass blockage in the bile duct followed by external-beam radiation therapy or internal radiation therapy.

3. Clinical trials of radiation therapy with drugs to make the cancer cells more sensitive to radiation (radiosensitizers).

4. Clinical trials of chemotherapy or biological therapy.

Recurrent Extrahepatic Bile Duct Cancer

Treatment depends on many factors, including where the cancer came back and what treatment the patient received before. Clinical trials are testing new treatments.

To Learn More

To learn more about extrahepatic bile duct cancer, call the National Cancer Institute's Cancer Information Service at 1-800-4-CANCER (1-800-422-6237); TTY at 1-800-332-8615. By dialing this toll-free number, trained information specialists can answer your questions.

Cancer patients, their families and friends, and others may find the following booklets useful. They are available free of charge by calling 1-800-4-CANCER or writing:

Office of Cancer Communications
National Cancer Institute
Building 31, Room 10A24
Bethesda, MD 20892

Booklets about Cancer Treatment

Radiation Therapy and You: A Guide to Self-Help During Treatment *

Chemotherapy and You: A Guide to Self-Help During Treatment *

Eating Hints: Recipes and Tips for Better Nutrition During Cancer Treatment *

Questions and Answers About Pain Control

What Are Clinical Trials All About?

Booklets about Living with Cancer

Taking Time: Support for People With Cancer and the People Who Care About Them

When Cancer Recurs: Meeting the Challenge Again *

Advanced Cancer: Living Each Day *

* Reprinted in this volume—see Table of Contents

Chapter 21

Kidney Cancer

Introduction

Each year, more than 28,000 people in the United States learn that they have kidney cancer. The National Cancer Institute (NCI) has written this chapter to help people with kidney cancer and their families and friends better understand this disease. We hope others will read it as well to learn more about kidney cancer.

This chapter discusses symptoms, diagnosis, treatment, and followup care. It also has information to help patients cope with kidney cancer.

Our knowledge about kidney cancer keeps increasing. For up-to-date information or to order this publication, call the NCI-supported Cancer Information Service (CIS) toll free at 1-800-4-CANCER (1-800-422-6237).

The CIS staff uses a National Cancer Institute cancer information database called PDQ and other NCI resources to answer callers' questions. Cancer information specialists can send callers information from PDQ and other NCI materials about cancer, its treatment, and living with the disease.

The Kidneys

The kidneys are two reddish-brown, bean-shaped organs located just above the waist, one on each side of the spine. They are part of the urinary system. Their main function is to filter blood and produce

"What You Need To Know About Kidney Cancer," National Cancer Institute (NCI), updated September 1998.

urine to rid the body of waste. As blood flows through the kidneys, they remove waste products and unneeded water. The resulting liquid, urine, collects in the middle of each kidney in an area called the renal pelvis. Urine drains from each kidney through a long tube, the ureter, into the bladder, where it is stored. Urine leaves the body through another tube, called the urethra.

The kidneys also produce substances that help control blood pressure and regulate the formation of red blood cells.

What Is Cancer?

Cancer is a group of many different diseases that have some important things in common. They all affect cells, the body's basic unit of life. To understand cancer, it is helpful to know about normal cells and about what happens when cells become cancerous.

The body is made up of many types of cells. Normally, cells grow and divide to produce more cells only when the body needs them. This orderly process helps keep the body healthy. Sometimes cells keep dividing when new cells are not needed. A mass of extra tissue forms, and this mass is called a growth or tumor. Tumors can be benign or malignant.

- Benign tumors are not cancer. They often can be removed and, in most cases, they do not come back. Cells in benign tumors do not spread to other parts of the body. Most important, benign tumors are rarely a threat to life.

- Malignant tumors are cancer. Cells in malignant tumors are abnormal and divide without control or order. These cancer cells can invade and destroy the tissue around them. Also, cancer cells can break away from a malignant tumor and enter the bloodstream or lymphatic system. This process is how cancer spreads from the original (primary) tumor to form new tumors in other parts of the body. The spread of cancer is called metastasis.

Kidney Cancer

Several types of cancer can develop in the kidney. This chapter discusses kidney cancer in adults. Transitional cell cancer (carcinoma), which affects the renal pelvis, is a less common form of kidney cancer. It is similar to cancer that occurs in the bladder and is often treated like bladder cancer. Wilms' tumor, the most common type of childhood kidney cancer, is different from kidney cancer in adults. The

Cancer Information Service can provide information about transitional cell cancer and Wilms' tumor.

As kidney cancer grows, it may invade organs near the kidney, such as the liver, colon, or pancreas. Kidney cancer cells may also break away from the original tumor and spread (metastasize) to other parts of the body. When kidney cancer spreads, cancer cells may appear in the lymph nodes. For this reason, lymph nodes near the kidney may be removed during surgery. If the pathologist finds cancer cells in the lymph nodes, it may mean that the disease has spread to other parts of the body. Kidney cancer may spread and form new tumors, most often in the bones or lungs. The new tumors have the same kind of abnormal cells and the same name as the original (primary) tumor in the kidney. For example, if kidney cancer spreads to the lungs, the cancer cells in the lungs are kidney cancer cells. The disease is metastatic kidney cancer; it is not lung cancer.

Symptoms

In its early stages, kidney cancer usually causes no obvious signs or troublesome symptoms. However, as a kidney tumor grows, symptoms may occur. These may include:

- Blood in the urine. Blood may be present one day and not the next. In some cases, a person can actually see the blood, or traces of it may be found in urinalysis, a lab test often performed as part of a regular medical checkup.

- A lump or mass in the kidney area.

Other less common symptoms may include:

- Fatigue;

- Loss of appetite;

- Weight loss;

- Recurrent fevers;

- A pain in the side that doesn't go away; and/or

- A general feeling of poor health.

High blood pressure or a lower than normal number of red cells in the blood (anemia) may also signal a kidney tumor; however, these symptoms occur less often.

These symptoms may be caused by cancer or by other, less serious problems such as an infection or a cyst. Only a doctor can make a diagnosis. People with any of these symptoms may see their family doctor or a urologist, a doctor who specializes in diseases of the urinary system. Usually, early cancer does not cause pain; it is important not to wait to feel pain before seeing a doctor.

In most cases, the earlier cancer is diagnosed and treated, the better a person's chance for a full recovery.

Diagnosis

To find the cause of symptoms, the doctor asks about the patient's medical history and does a physical exam. In addition to checking for general signs of health, the doctor may perform blood and urine tests. The doctor may also carefully feel the abdomen for lumps or irregular masses.

The doctor usually orders tests that produce pictures of the kidneys and nearby organs. These pictures can often show changes in the kidney and surrounding tissue. For example, an IVP (intravenous pyelogram) is a series of x-rays of the kidneys, ureters, and bladder after the injection of a dye. The dye may be placed in the body through a needle or a narrow tube called a catheter. The pictures produced can show changes in the shape of these organs and nearby lymph nodes.

Another test, arteriography, is a series of x-rays of the blood vessels. Dye is injected into a large blood vessel through a catheter. X-rays show the dye as it moves through the network of smaller blood vessels in and around the kidney.

Other imaging tests may include CT scan, MRI, and ultrasonography, which can show the difference between diseased and healthy tissues.

If test results suggest that kidney cancer may be present, a biopsy may be performed; it is the only sure way to diagnose cancer. During a biopsy for kidney cancer, a thin needle is inserted into the tumor and a sample of tissue is withdrawn. A pathologist then examines the tissue under a microscope to check for cancer cells.

Once kidney cancer is diagnosed, the doctor will want to learn the stage, or extent, of the disease. Staging is a careful attempt to find out whether the cancer has spread and, if so, what parts of the body are affected. This information is needed to plan a patient's treatment.

To stage kidney cancer, the doctor may use additional MRI and x-ray studies of the tissues and blood vessels in and around the kidney.

The doctor can check for swollen lymph nodes in the chest and abdomen through CT scans. Chest x-rays can often show whether cancer has spread to the lungs. Bone scans reveal changes that may be a sign that the cancer has spread to the bones.

A person who needs a biopsy may want to ask the doctor some of the following questions:

- How long will it take? Will I be awake? Will it hurt?
- How soon will I know the results?
- If I do have cancer, who will talk with me about treatment? When?

Treatment

Treatment for kidney cancer depends on the stage of the disease, the patient's general health and age, and other factors. The doctor develops a treatment plan to fit each patient's needs.

People with kidney cancer are often treated by a team of specialists, which may include a urologist, an oncologist, and a radiation oncologist. Kidney cancer is usually treated with surgery, radiation therapy, biological therapy, chemotherapy, or hormone therapy. Sometimes a special treatment called arterial embolization is used. The doctors may decide to use one treatment method or a combination of methods.

Some people take part in a clinical trial (research study) using new treatment methods. Such studies are designed to improve cancer treatment.

Getting a Second Opinion

Before starting treatment, the patient may want a second pathologist to review the diagnosis and another specialist to review the treatment plan. A short delay will not reduce the chance that treatment will be successful. Some insurance companies require a second opinion; many others will cover a second opinion if the patient requests it.

There are a number of ways a person can find a doctor who can give a second opinion:

- The person's doctor may be able to suggest pathologists and specialists to consult.
- The Cancer Information Service, at 1-800-4-CANCER, can tell callers about treatment facilities, including cancer centers and other programs supported by the National Cancer Institute.

- People can get the names of doctors from a local medical society, a nearby hospital, or a medical school.

- The *Directory of Medical Specialists* lists doctors' names along with their specialty and their background. This book is in most public libraries.

Preparing for Treatment

Many people with cancer want to learn all they can about their disease and their treatment choices so they can take an active part in decisions about their medical care. When a person is diagnosed with cancer, shock and stress are natural reactions. These feelings may make it difficult for patients to think of everything they want to ask the doctor. Often, it helps to make a list of questions. To help remember what the doctor says, people may take notes or ask whether they may use a tape recorder. Some patients also want to have a family member or friend with them when they talk to the doctor—to take part in the discussion, to take notes, or just to listen.

These are some questions a patient may want to ask the doctor before treatment begins:

- What type of kidney cancer do I have?

- What is the stage of the disease?

- What are the treatment choices? Which do you recommend? Why?

- What are the risks and possible side effects of each treatment?

- What are the chances that the treatment will be successful?

- What new treatments are being studied in clinical trials? Would a clinical trial be appropriate?

- How long will treatment last?

- Will I have to stay in the hospital?

- Will treatment affect my normal activities? If so, for how long?

- What is the treatment likely to cost?

People do not need to ask all their questions or remember all the answers at one time. Questions may arise throughout the treatment process. Patients may wish to ask doctors, nurses, or other members of the health care team to explain things further or to provide more information.

Methods of Treatment

Surgery is the most common treatment for kidney cancer. An operation to remove the kidney is called a nephrectomy. Most often, the surgeon removes the whole kidney along with the adrenal gland and the tissue around the kidney. Some lymph nodes in the area may also be removed. This procedure is called a radical nephrectomy. In some cases, the surgeon removes only the kidney (simple nephrectomy). The remaining kidney generally is able to perform the work of both kidneys. In another procedure, partial nephrectomy, the surgeon removes just the part of the kidney that contains the tumor.

Arterial embolization is sometimes used before an operation to make surgery easier. It also may be used to provide relief from pain or bleeding when removal of the tumor is not possible. Small pieces of a special gelatin sponge or other material are injected through a catheter to clog the main renal blood vessel. This procedure shrinks the tumor by depriving it of the oxygen-carrying blood and other substances it needs to grow.

These are some questions a patient may want to ask the doctor before surgery:

- What kind of operation will it be?

- Will further treatment be necessary? What kind?

- How will I feel after the operation?

- If I have pain, how will you help?

- When will I be able to resume my normal activities?

Radiation therapy (also called radiotherapy) uses high-energy rays to kill cancer cells. Doctors sometimes use radiation therapy to relieve pain (palliative therapy) when kidney cancer has spread to the bone.

Radiation therapy for kidney cancer involves external radiation, which comes from radioactive material outside the body. A machine aims the rays at a specific area of the body. Most often, treatment is given on an outpatient basis in a hospital or clinic 5 days a week for several weeks. This schedule helps protect normal tissue by spreading out the total dose of radiation. The patient does not need to stay in the hospital for radiation therapy, and patients are not radioactive during or after treatment.

These are some questions a patient may want to ask the doctor before having radiation therapy:

- What is the goal of this treatment?
- When will the treatments begin? When will they end?
- How will I feel during therapy? What are the possible side effects?
- What can I do to take care of myself during therapy?
- How will I know if the radiation therapy is working?
- Will I be able to continue my normal activities during treatment?

Surgery and arterial embolization are local therapy; they affect cancer cells only in the treated area. Biological therapy, chemotherapy, and hormone therapy, explained below, are systemic treatments because they travel through the bloodstream and can reach cells throughout the body.

Biological therapy (also called immunotherapy) is a form of treatment that uses the body's natural ability (immune system) to fight cancer. Interleukin-2 and interferon are types of biological therapy used to treat advanced kidney cancer. Clinical trials continue to examine better ways to use biological therapy while reducing the side effects patients may experience. Many people having biological therapy stay in the hospital during treatment so that these side effects can be monitored.

These are some questions patients may want to ask the doctor before starting biological therapy:

- What is the goal of the treatment?
- What drugs will be used?
- Will the treatment cause side effects? If so, what can be done about them?
- Will I have to be in the hospital to receive treatment?
- When will I be able to resume my normal activities?

Chemotherapy is the use of drugs to kill cancer cells. Although useful in the treatment of many other cancers, chemotherapy has shown only limited effectiveness against kidney cancer. However, researchers continue to study new drugs and new drug combinations that may prove to be more useful.

Hormone therapy is used in a small number of patients with advanced kidney cancer. Some kidney cancers may be treated with hormones to try to control the growth of cancer cells. More often, it is used as palliative therapy.

These are some questions a patient may want to ask the doctor before having chemotherapy or hormone therapy:

- What is the goal of this treatment?
- What drugs will I be taking?
- Will I have side effects? What can I do about them?
- How long will I be on the treatment?

Clinical Trials

Many people with kidney cancer take part in clinical trials (treatment studies). Doctors conduct clinical trials to learn about the effectiveness and side effects of new treatments. In some clinical trials, all patients receive the new treatment. In other trials, doctors compare different therapies by giving the new treatment to one group of patients and the standard therapy to another group.

People who take part in these studies have the first chance to benefit from treatments that have shown promise in early research. They also make an important contribution to medical science.

In clinical trials for kidney cancer, doctors are studying new ways of giving radiation therapy and chemotherapy, new drugs and drug combinations, biological therapies, and new ways of combining various types of treatment. Some trials are designed to study ways to reduce the side effects of treatment and to improve quality of life.

Patients who are interested in taking part in a trial should talk with their doctor. They may want to read the National Cancer Institute booklet *Taking Part in Clinical Trials: What Cancer Patients Need To Know*, which explains the possible benefits and risks of treatment studies.

One way to learn about clinical trials is through PDQ, a computerized resource developed by the National Cancer Institute. PDQ contains information about cancer treatment and about clinical trials in progress throughout the country. The Cancer Information Service can provide PDQ information to patients and the public.

Side Effects of Treatment

It is hard to limit the effects of therapy so that only cancer cells are removed or destroyed. Because treatment also damages healthy cells and tissues, it often causes unwanted side effects.

The side effects of cancer therapy depend mainly on the type and extent of the treatment. Also, side effects may not be the same for each person, and they may even change from one treatment to the next. Doctors and nurses can explain the possible side effects of therapy, and they can help relieve problems that may occur during and after treatment. Patients should notify a doctor of the side effects they are having, as some may require immediate medical attention.

Surgery

The side effects of kidney surgery depend on the type of operation, the patient's general health, and other factors. Nephrectomy is major surgery, and after the operation most people have pain and discomfort. Patients may find it difficult to breathe deeply due to discomfort from surgery; they may have to do special coughing and breathing exercises to help keep their lungs clear. It is also common for patients who have had surgery to feel tired or weak for a while.

In addition, patients may need intravenous (IV) feeding and fluids for several days before and after the operation. When a kidney is removed, the one remaining kidney takes over the work of both. Nurses will monitor the amount of fluid a person takes in and the amount of urine produced. The length of time it takes to recover from an operation varies for each person.

Arterial Embolization

Arterial embolization can cause pain, fever, nausea, or vomiting. Often, people need IV fluids as the body recovers from this procedure.

Radiation Therapy

With radiation therapy, the side effects depend on the treatment dose and the part of the body that is treated. Patients are likely to become very tired, especially in the later weeks of treatment. Resting is important, but doctors usually advise patients to try to stay as active as they can.

It is common for the skin in the treated area to become red, dry, tender, and itchy. There may be permanent darkening or "bronzing" of the skin in the treated area. Radiation to the kidney and nearby areas may cause nausea, vomiting, diarrhea, or urinary discomfort. It may also cause a decrease in the number of white blood cells, cells that help protect the body against infection. The National Cancer Institute booklet *Radiation Therapy and You* [reprinted in this volume as

Chapter 66] has helpful information about radiation therapy and managing its side effects.

Biological Therapy

The side effects caused by biological therapy vary with the type of treatment. These treatments may cause flu-like symptoms such as chills, fever, muscle aches, weakness, loss of appetite, nausea, vomiting, and diarrhea. Patients often feel very tired after treatment, and they may bleed or bruise easily. Some people also get a skin rash. In addition, interleukin therapy can cause swelling and can interfere with normal liver or kidney function. These problems can be severe, but they go away after the treatment stops.

Chemotherapy

The side effects of chemotherapy depend on the drugs that are given. In general, anticancer drugs affect rapidly growing cells, such as blood cells that fight infection, cells that line the digestive tract, and cells in the hair follicles. As a result, patients may have side effects such as lower resistance to infection, loss of appetite, nausea, vomiting, or mouth sores. They may also have less energy and may lose their hair.

Hormone Therapy

The side effects of hormone therapy are usually mild. Progesterone is the hormone most often used to treat kidney cancer. Drugs containing progesterone may cause changes in appetite and weight. They may also cause swelling or fluid retention. These side effects generally go away after treatment.

Nutrition for Cancer Patients

Eating well during cancer treatment means getting enough calories and protein to help prevent weight loss and regain strength. Patients who eat well often feel better and have more energy.

Some people find it hard to eat well during treatment for kidney cancer. They may lose their appetite. In addition to loss of appetite, common side effects of treatment, such as nausea, vomiting, or mouth sores, can make eating difficult. For some people, food tastes different. Also, people may not feel like eating when they are uncomfortable or tired.

Doctors, nurses, and dietitians can offer advice for healthy eating during cancer treatment. Patients and their families also may want to read the National Cancer Institute booklet, *Eating Hints for Cancer Patients* [reprinted in this volume as Chapter 77], which contains many useful suggestions.

Followup Care

Regular followup by the doctor is important after treatment for kidney cancer. The doctor will suggest appropriate followup that may include a physical exam, chest x-rays, and laboratory tests. The doctor sometimes orders scans and other tests. Patients should continue to have followup visits. They should also report any problem as soon as it appears.

Support for Cancer Patients

Living with a serious illness is not easy. People with cancer and those who care about them face many problems and challenges. Coping with these problems is often easier when people have helpful information and support services. Several useful booklets, including *Taking Time*, are available from the Cancer Information Service.

Friends and relatives can be very supportive. Also, it helps many people to discuss their concerns with others who have or have had cancer. Cancer patients often get together in support groups, where they can share what they have learned about coping with cancer and the effects of treatment. It is important to keep in mind, however, that each person is different. Treatments and ways of dealing with cancer that work for one person may not be right for another—even if they both have the same kind of cancer. It is always a good idea to discuss the advice of friends and family members with the doctor.

People living with cancer may worry about the future. They may worry about holding their job, caring for their family, or keeping up with daily activities. Concerns about tests, treatments, hospital stays, and medical bills are also common. Doctors, nurses, and other members of the health care team can answer questions about treatment, working, or other activities. They can also discuss outlook (prognosis) and the activity level people may be able to manage. Meeting with a social worker, counselor, or member of the clergy also can be helpful to people who want to talk about their feelings or discuss their concerns. Often, a social worker at the hospital or clinic can suggest groups that can help with rehabilitation, emotional support, financial aid, transportation, or home care. For example, the American Cancer Society has many services for patients and their families. Local offices of the American Cancer Society are listed in the white pages of the telephone directory.

What the Future Holds

People with kidney cancer and their families are naturally concerned about what the future holds. Sometimes they use statistics to try to figure out the chances of being cured. It is important to remember, however, that statistics are averages based on large numbers of people. They cannot be used to predict what will happen to a particular person because no two people are alike; treatments and responses vary greatly. The doctor who takes care of the patient is in the best position to talk with the patient about the chance of recovery.

The outlook for people with early stage kidney cancer is positive. Kidney cancer is often cured if it is found and treated before it has spread. Many researchers are trying to find better ways to detect kidney cancer at an early stage. They are also continuing to look for new and better ways to treat advanced kidney cancer.

When doctors talk about surviving cancer, they may use the term remission rather than cure. Although many kidney cancer patients are cured, doctors use this term because the disease can return. (The return of cancer after treatment is called a recurrence.)

Possible Causes and Prevention

Scientists at hospitals and medical centers all across the country are studying kidney cancer. They are trying to learn what causes this disease and how to prevent it. At this time, scientists do not know exactly what causes kidney cancer, and they can seldom explain why one person gets this disease and another does not. However, it is clear that this disease is not contagious; no one can "catch" kidney cancer from another person.

Researchers study patterns of cancer in the population to look for factors that are more common in people who get kidney cancer than in people who don't get this disease. These studies help researchers find possible risk factors for kidney cancer. It is important to know that most people with these risk factors do not get cancer, and people who do get kidney cancer may have none of these factors.

As with most other types of cancer, studies show that the risk of kidney cancer increases with age. It occurs most often between the ages of 50 and 70. It affects almost twice as many men as women. In addition, kidney cancer is somewhat more common among African American men than White men. Other risk factors for kidney cancer include:

- *Tobacco use:* Research shows that smokers are twice as likely to develop kidney cancer as nonsmokers. In addition, the longer a person smokes, the higher the risk. However, the risk of kidney cancer decreases for those who quit smoking.

- *Obesity:* Obesity may increase the risk of developing kidney cancer. In several studies, obesity has been associated with increased risk in women. One report suggests that being overweight may be a risk factor for men, too. The reasons for this possible link are not clear.

- *Occupational exposure:* A number of studies have examined occupational exposures to see whether they increase workers' chances of developing kidney cancer. Studies suggest, for example, that coke oven workers in steel plants have above-average rates of kidney cancer. In addition, there is some evidence that asbestos in the workplace, which has been linked to cancers of the lung and mesothelium (a membrane that surrounds internal organs of the body), also increases the risk of some kidney cancers.

- *Radiation:* Women who have been treated with radiation therapy for disorders of the uterus may have a slightly increased risk of developing kidney cancer. Also, people who were exposed to thorotrast (thorium dioxide), a radioactive substance used in the 1920s with certain diagnostic x-rays, have an increased rate of kidney cancer. However, this substance is no longer in use, and scientists think that radiation accounts for an extremely small percentage of the total number of kidney cancers.

- *Phenacetin:* Some people have developed kidney cancer after heavy, long-term use of this drug. This painkilling drug is no longer sold in the United States.

- *Dialysis:* Patients on long-term use of dialysis to treat chronic kidney failure have an increased risk of developing renal cysts and renal cancer. Further study is needed to learn more about the long-term effects of dialysis on patients with kidney failure.

- *Von Hippel-Lindau (VHL) disease:* Researchers have found that people who have this inherited disorder are at greater risk of developing renal cell carcinoma, as well as tumors in other organs. Researchers have found the gene responsible for VHL, and they believe that the isolation of this gene may lead to improved methods of diagnosis, treatment, and even prevention of some kidney cancers.

People who think they may be at risk for developing kidney cancer should discuss this concern with their doctor. The doctor may suggest ways to reduce the risk and help plan an appropriate schedule for checkups.

For Further Information

National Kidney and Urologic Disease Information Clearinghouse. This clearinghouse is a service of the Federal Government's National Institute of Diabetes and Digestive and Kidney Diseases. It can supply free information about noncancerous kidney conditions and other urinary tract problems. The address is NKUDIC, Three Information Way, Bethesda, MD 20892-3580; the telephone number is 301-654-4415.

Cancer patients, their families and friends, and others may find the following booklets useful. They are available free of charge by calling 1-800-4-CANCER or writing:

Office of Cancer Communications
National Cancer Institute
Building 31, Room 10A24
Bethesda, MD 20892

Booklets about Cancer Treatment

Radiation Therapy and You: A Guide to Self-Help During Treatment *

Chemotherapy and You: A Guide to Self-Help During Treatment *

Eating Hints: Recipes and Tips for Better Nutrition During Cancer Treatment *

Questions and Answers About Pain Control

What Are Clinical Trials All About?

Booklets about Living with Cancer

Taking Time: Support for People With Cancer and the People Who Care About Them

When Cancer Recurs: Meeting the Challenge Again *

Advanced Cancer: Living Each Day *

* Reprinted in this volume—see Table of Contents

Chapter 22

Renal Cell Cancer

What Is Renal Cell Cancer?

Renal cell cancer (also called cancer of the kidney or renal adeno-carcinoma) is a disease in which cancer (malignant) cells are found in certain tissues of the kidney. Renal cell cancer is one of the less common kinds of cancer. It occurs more often in men than in women.

The kidneys are a "matched" pair of organs found on either side of the backbone. The kidneys of an adult are about 5 inches long and 3 inches wide and are shaped like a kidney bean. Inside each kidney are tiny tubules that filter and clean the blood, taking out waste products, and making urine. The urine made by the kidneys passes through a tube called a ureter into the bladder where it is held until it is passed from the body. Renal cell cancer is a cancer of the lining of the tubules in the kidney. If cancer is found in the part of the kidney that collects urine and drains it to the ureters (the renal pelvis), or is found in the ureters, refer to the PDQ patient information summary on transitional cell cancer of the renal pelvis and ureter.

A doctor should be seen if one or more of the following symptoms appear: blood in the urine, a lump (mass) in the abdomen, or a pain in the side that doesn't go away. Tiredness, loss of appetite, weight loss without dieting, and anemia (too few red blood cells) may also be symptoms.

PDQ Statement, National Cancer Institute (NCI), updated June 1998.

If there are signs of cancer, a doctor will usually feel the abdomen for lumps. A doctor may order a special x-ray called an intravenous pyelogram (IVP). During this test, a dye containing iodine is injected into the bloodstream. This allows the doctor to see the kidney more clearly on the x-ray. The doctor may also do an ultrasound, which uses sound waves to find tumors, or a special x-ray called a CT scan to look for lumps in the kidney. A special scan called magnetic resonance imaging (MRI), which uses magnetic waves to find tumors, may also be done.

The chance of recovery (prognosis) and choice of treatment depend on the stage of the cancer (whether it is just in the kidney or has spread to other places in the body) and the patient's general state of health.

Stages of Renal Cell Cancer

Once renal cell cancer has been found, more tests will be done to find out if cancer cells have spread to other parts of the body. This is called staging. A doctor needs to know the stage of the disease to plan treatment. The following stages are used for renal cell cancer:

Stage I

Cancer is found only in the kidney.

Stage II

Cancer has spread to the fat around the kidney, but the cancer has not spread beyond this to the capsule that contains the kidney.

Stage III

Cancer has spread to the main blood vessel that carries clean blood from the kidney (renal vein), to the blood vessel that carries blood from the lower part of the body to the heart (inferior vena cava), or to lymph nodes around the kidney. (Lymph nodes are small, bean-shaped structures that are found throughout the body; they produce and store infection-fighting cells.)

Stage IV

Cancer has spread to nearby organs such as the bowel or pancreas or has spread to other places in the body such as the lungs.

Recurrent

Recurrent disease means that the cancer has come back (recurred) after it has been treated. It may come back in the original area or in another part of the body.

How Renal Cell Cancer Is Treated

There are treatments for most patients with renal cell cancer. Five kinds of treatment are used:

- surgery (taking out the cancer in an operation)
- chemotherapy (using drugs to kill cancer cells)
- radiation therapy (using high-dose x-rays or other high-energy rays to kill cancer cells)
- hormone therapy (using hormones to stop cancer cells from growing)
- biological therapy (using the body's immune system to fight cancer)

Surgery is a common treatment of renal cell cancer. A doctor may take out the cancer using one of the following:

- Partial nephrectomy removes the cancer and part of the kidney around the cancer. This is usually done only in special cases, such as when the other kidney is damaged or has already been removed.
- Simple nephrectomy removes the whole kidney. The kidney on the other side of the body can take over filtering the blood.
- Radical nephrectomy removes the kidney with the tissues around it. Some lymph nodes in the area may also be removed.

Chemotherapy uses drugs to kill cancer cells. Chemotherapy may be taken by pill, or it may be put into the body by a needle in a vein or muscle. Chemotherapy is called a systemic treatment because the drugs enter the bloodstream, travel through the body, and can kill cancer cells throughout the body.

Radiation therapy uses x-rays or other high-energy rays to kill cancer cells and shrink tumors. Radiation may come from a machine outside the body (external radiation therapy) or from putting materials that contain radiation through thin plastic tubes (internal radiation therapy) in the area where the cancer cells are found. Radiation can be used alone or before or after surgery and/or chemotherapy.

Hormone therapy uses hormones (taken by pill or injected with a needle) to stop cancer cells from growing.

Biological therapy tries to get the body to fight cancer. It uses materials made by the body or made in a laboratory to boost, direct, or restore the body's natural defenses against disease. Biological therapy is sometimes called biological response modifier (BRM) therapy or immunotherapy.

Sometimes a special treatment called arterial embolization is used to treat renal cell cancer. A narrow tube (catheter) is used to inject small pieces of a special gelatin sponge into the main blood vessel that flows into the kidney to block the blood cells that feed the tumor. This prevents the cancer cells from getting oxygen or other substances they need to grow.

Treatment by Stage

Treatment of renal cell cancer depends on the type and stage of the disease, and the patient's age and general health.

Standard treatment may be considered because of its effectiveness in patients in past studies, or participation in a clinical trial may be considered. Not all patients are cured with standard therapy and some standard treatments may have more side effects than are desired. For these reasons, clinical trials are designed to find better ways to treat cancer patients and are based on the most up-to-date information. Clinical trials are ongoing in most parts of the country for most stages of renal cell cancer. To learn more about clinical trials, call the Cancer Information Service at 1-800-4-CANCER (1-800-422-6237); TTY at 1-800-332-8615.

Stage I Renal Cell Cancer

Treatment may be one of the following:

1. Surgery to remove the kidney and the tissues around it (radical nephrectomy). Lymph nodes in the area may also be removed.

2. Surgery to remove only the kidney (simple nephrectomy).

3. Surgery to remove the part of the kidney where the cancer is found (partial nephrectomy).

4. External beam radiation therapy to relieve symptoms in patients who cannot have surgery.

5. Injection of small pieces of a special gelatin sponge into the main artery that flows to the kidney to block blood flow to the cancer cells (arterial embolization). This is usually done only in patients who cannot have surgery.

6. Clinical trials.

Stage II Renal Cell Cancer

Treatment may be one of the following:

1. Surgery to remove the kidney and the tissues around it (radical nephrectomy). Lymph nodes in the area may also be removed.

2. External beam radiation therapy before or after radical nephrectomy.

3. Surgery to remove the part of the kidney where the cancer is found (partial nephrectomy).

4. External beam radiation therapy to relieve symptoms in patients who cannot have surgery.

5. Injection of small pieces of a special gelatin sponge into the main artery that flows to the kidney to block blood flow to the cancer cells (arterial embolization). This is usually done only in patients who cannot have surgery.

6. Clinical trials.

Stage III Renal Cell Cancer

Treatment may be one of the following:

1. Surgery to remove the kidney and the tissues around it (radical nephrectomy). Lymph nodes in the area may also be removed. If the cancer has spread to the main blood vessels that carry blood to and from the kidney (the renal vein or vena cava), part of the blood vessel may also be removed.

2. Injection of small pieces of a special gelatin sponge into the main artery that flows to the kidney to block blood flow to the cancer cells (arterial embolization) followed by radical nephrectomy.

3. External beam radiation therapy to relieve symptoms.

4. Arterial embolization to relieve symptoms.

5. Surgery to remove the kidney (simple or radical nephrectomy) to relieve symptoms.

6. External beam radiation therapy before or after radical nephrectomy.

7. Clinical trials of biological therapy in addition to other therapy.

Stage IV Renal Cell Cancer

Treatment may be one of the following:

1. Biological therapy.

2. External radiation therapy to relieve symptoms.

3. Surgery to remove the kidney (nephrectomy) to relieve symptoms.

4. If cancer has spread only to the area around the kidney, surgery to remove the kidney and the tissue around it (radical nephrectomy). If the cancer has spread to a limited area, surgery to remove the cancer where it has spread (metastasized) in addition to radical nephrectomy.

5. Clinical trials.

Recurrent Renal Cell Cancer

Treatment may be one of the following:

1. Biological therapy.

2. External radiation therapy to relieve symptoms.

3. Chemotherapy.

To Learn More

To learn more about renal cell cancer, call the National Cancer Institute's Cancer Information Service at 1-800-4-CANCER (1-800-422-6237); TTY at 1-800-332-8615. By dialing this toll-free number, trained information specialists can answer your questions.

The Cancer Information Service also has booklets about cancer that are available to the public and can be sent on request. The following booklet about renal cell cancer may be helpful: *What You Need To Know About Kidney Cancer* *

Booklets about Cancer Treatment

Radiation Therapy and You: A Guide to Self-Help During Treatment *

Chemotherapy and You: A Guide to Self-Help During Treatment *

Eating Hints: Recipes and Tips for Better Nutrition During Cancer Treatment *

Questions and Answers About Pain Control

What Are Clinical Trials All About?

Booklets about Living with Cancer

Taking Time: Support for People With Cancer and the People Who Care About Them

When Cancer Recurs: Meeting the Challenge Again *

Advanced Cancer: Living Each Day *

* Reprinted in this volume—see Table of Contents

Chapter 23

Renal Pelvis and Ureter Cancer

What Is Transitional Cell Cancer of the Renal Pelvis and Ureter?

Transitional cell cancer (TCC) of the renal pelvis and ureter is a disease in which cancer (malignant) cells are found in the tissues in the kidneys that collect urine (the renal pelvis) and/or in the tube that connects the kidney to the bladder (ureter).

The kidneys are a "matched" pair of organs found on either side of your backbone. The kidneys of an adult are about 5 inches long and 3 inches wide and are shaped like a kidney bean. Inside each kidney are tiny tubules that clean your blood, taking out waste products and making urine. The urine made by the kidneys passes through the ureter into the bladder where it is held until it is passed from your body. The renal pelvis is the part of the kidney that collects urine and drains it to the ureters. The cells that line the renal pelvis and ureters are called transitional cells, and it is these cells that are affected in TCC. If you have a more common type of kidney cancer called renal cell cancer, see the patient information statement on renal cell cancer.

Like most cancers, TCC of the renal pelvis and ureter is best treated when it is found (diagnosed) early. In the early stages of TCC you may not have any symptoms. The symptoms of TCC and other types of kidney cancer are similar to other types of kidney disease.

PDQ Statement, National Cancer Institute (NCI), updated September 1997.

You should see your doctor if you have blood in your urine or pain in your back.

If you have symptoms, your doctor will usually feel your abdomen for lumps. A narrow lighted tube called a ureteroscope may be inserted through the bladder into the ureter so that your doctor can look inside the ureter and renal pelvis for signs of cancer. If cancer cells are found, your doctor may take out a small piece of the tissue to look at under the microscope. This is called a biopsy. Your doctor may also do a special x-ray called a CT scan or a scan that uses magnetic waves (MRI) to look for lumps.

Your chance of recovery (prognosis) and choice of treatment depend on the stage of your cancer (whether it is just in the tissue lining the inside of the ureter or renal pelvis or has spread to other places) and your general state of health.

Stages of Transitional Cell Cancer of the Renal Pelvis and Ureter

Once transitional cell cancer is found, more tests will be done to find out if cancer cells have spread to other parts of the body (staging). Your doctor needs to know the stage to plan treatment. The following stages are used for TCC of the renal pelvis and ureter:

Localized

The cancer is only in the area where it started and has not spread outside the kidney or ureter.

Regional

The cancer has spread to the tissue around the kidney or to lymph nodes in the pelvis. (Lymph nodes are bean-shaped structures that are found throughout the body. They produce infection-fighting cells.)

Metastatic

The cancer has spread to other parts of the body.

Recurrent

Recurrent disease means that the cancer has come back (recurred) after it has been treated. It may come back in the original area or in another part of the body.

How Transitional Cell Cancer of the Renal Pelvis and Ureter Is Treated

There are treatments for all patients with transitional cell cancer of the renal pelvis and ureter. The primary treatment is surgery (taking out the cancer in an operation). Radiation therapy (using high-dose x-rays to kill cancer cells), biological therapy (using your body's immune system to fight cancer), and chemotherapy (using drugs to kill cancer cells) are being tested in clinical trials.

Surgery is the most common treatment of transitional cell cancer of the renal pelvis and ureter. Your doctor may remove the tumor using one of the following operations:

- The kidney, ureter, and top part of the bladder may be removed in an operation called a nephroureterectomy.

- Segmental resection removes only part of the ureter or kidney.

- Electrosurgery uses an electric current to remove the cancer. The tumor and the area around it are burned away and then removed with a sharp tool.

- Laser therapy uses a narrow beam of intense light to remove cancer cells.

Electrosurgery and laser therapy are used only for cancers that are on the surface of the renal pelvis or ureter.

Chemotherapy uses drugs to kill cancer cells. Chemotherapy may be taken by pill, or it may be put into the body by a needle in the vein or muscle. Chemotherapy is called a systemic treatment because the drug enters the bloodstream, travels through the body, and can kill cancer cells throughout the body. Chemotherapy may also be put directly into the ureter or pelvis (intraureteral or intrapelvic chemotherapy).

Biological therapy tries to get your own body to fight cancer. It uses materials made by your own body or made in a laboratory to boost, direct, or restore your body's natural defenses against disease. Biological therapy is sometimes called biological response modifier (BRM) therapy or immunotherapy.

Radiation therapy uses high-energy x-rays to kill cancer cells and shrink tumors. Radiation may come from a machine outside the body (external beam radiation therapy) or from putting materials that produce radiation (radioisotopes) through thin plastic tubes (internal radiation therapy) in the area where the cancer cells are found.

249

Treatment by Stage

Your choice of treatment depends on how far the cancer has spread and your general health.

You may receive treatment that is considered standard based on its effectiveness in a number of patients in past studies, or you may choose to go into a clinical trial. Not all patients are cured with standard therapy and some standard treatments may have more side effects than are desired. For these reasons, clinical trials are designed to find better ways to treat cancer patients and are based on the most up-to-date information. Clinical trials are going on in most parts of the country for most stages of transitional cell cancer of the renal pelvis and ureter. If you want more information, call the Cancer Information Service at 1-800-4-CANCER (1-800-422-6237); TTY at 1-800-332-8615.

Localized Transitional Cell Cancer of the Renal Pelvis and Ureter

Your treatment may be one of the following:

1. Surgery to remove the kidney, ureter, and the top part of the bladder (nephroureterectomy).

2. Surgery to remove part of the ureter or kidney (segmental resection).

3. A clinical trial of electrosurgery or laser therapy.

4. A clinical trial of intrapelvic or intraureteral chemotherapy or biological therapy.

Regional Transitional Cell Cancer of the Renal Pelvis and Ureter

Your treatment will probably be a clinical trial of radiation therapy and/or chemotherapy.

Metastatic Transitional Cell Cancer of the Renal Pelvis and Ureter

Your treatment will probably be a clinical trial of chemotherapy.

Recurrent Transitional Cell Cancer of the Renal Pelvis and Ureter

Your treatment will probably be a clinical trial of new treatments.

To Learn More

To learn more about renal cell cancer, call the National Cancer Institute's Cancer Information Service at 1-800-4-CANCER (1-800-422-6237); TTY at 1-800-332-8615. By dialing this toll-free number, trained information specialists can answer your questions.

The Cancer Information Service also has booklets about cancer that are available to the public and can be sent on request. The following booklet about renal cell cancer may be helpful: *What You Need To Know About Kidney Cancer* *

Booklets about Cancer Treatment

Radiation Therapy and You: A Guide to Self-Help During Treatment *

Chemotherapy and You: A Guide to Self-Help During Treatment *

Eating Hints: Recipes and Tips for Better Nutrition During Cancer Treatment *

Questions and Answers About Pain Control

What Are Clinical Trials All About?

Booklets about Living with Cancer

Taking Time: Support for People With Cancer and the People Who Care About Them

When Cancer Recurs: Meeting the Challenge Again *

Advanced Cancer: Living Each Day *

* Reprinted in this volume—see Table of Contents

Chapter 24

Stomach Cancer

Introduction

Each year, about 24,000 people in the United States learn that they have cancer of the stomach. This chapter from the National Cancer Institute (NCI) will give you important information about the symptoms, diagnosis, and treatment of stomach cancer. This chapter also has information to help you deal with this disease if it affects you or someone you know.

Other NCI publications are listed in the Other Booklets section. Our materials cannot answer every question you may have about stomach cancer. They cannot take the place of talks with doctors, nurses, and other members of the health care team. We hope our information will help with those talks.

Researchers continue to look for better ways to diagnose and treat cancer of the stomach, and our knowledge is growing. For up-to-date information or to order this publication, call the NCI-supported Cancer Information Service (CIS) toll free at 1-800-4-CANCER (1-800-422-6237).

The Stomach

The stomach is part of the digestive system. It is located in the upper abdomen, under the ribs. The upper part of the stomach connects to the esophagus, and the lower part leads into the small intestine.

"What You Need To Know About Stomach Cancer," National Cancer Institute (NCI), updated September 1998.

When food enters the stomach, muscles in the stomach wall create a rippling motion that mixes and mashes the food. At the same time, juices made by glands in the lining of the stomach help digest the food. After about 3 hours, the food becomes a liquid and moves into the small intestine, where digestion continues.

What Is Cancer?

Cancer is a group of more than 100 different diseases. They affect the body's basic unit, the cell. Cancer occurs when cells become abnormal and divide without control or order.

Like all other organs of the body, the stomach is made up of many types of cells. Normally, cells divide to produce more cells only when the body needs them. This orderly process helps keep us healthy.

If cells keep dividing when new cells are not needed, a mass of tissue forms. This mass of extra tissue, called a growth or tumor, can be benign or malignant.

- Benign tumors are not cancer. They can usually be removed and, in most cases, they do not come back. Most important, cells from benign tumors do not spread to other parts of the body. Benign tumors are rarely a threat to life.

- Malignant tumors are cancer. Cancer cells can invade and damage tissues and organs near the tumor. Also, cancer cells can break away from a malignant tumor and enter the bloodstream or lymphatic system. This is how cancer spreads from the original (primary) tumor to form new tumors in other parts of the body. The spread of cancer is called metastasis.

Stomach cancer (also called gastric cancer) can develop in any part of the stomach and may spread throughout the stomach and to other organs. It may grow along the stomach wall into the esophagus or small intestine.

It also may extend through the stomach wall and spread to nearby lymph nodes and to organs such as the liver, pancreas, and colon. Stomach cancer also may spread to distant organs, such as the lungs, the lymph nodes above the collar bone, and the ovaries.

When cancer spreads to another part of the body, the new tumor has the same kind of abnormal cells and the same name as the primary tumor. For example, if stomach cancer spreads to the liver, the cancer cells in the liver are stomach cancer cells. The disease is metastatic stomach cancer (it is not liver cancer). However, when stomach cancer spreads to an ovary, the tumor in the ovary is called a Krukenberg tumor. (This tumor, named for a doctor, is not a different disease; it is metastatic stomach cancer. The cancer cells in a Krukenberg tumor are stomach cancer cells, the same as the cancer cells in the primary tumor.)

Symptoms

Stomach cancer can be hard to find early. Often there are no symptoms in the early stages and, in many cases, the cancer has spread before it is found. When symptoms do occur, they are often so vague that the person ignores them. Stomach cancer can cause the following:

- Indigestion or a burning sensation (heartburn);
- Discomfort or pain in the abdomen;
- Nausea and vomiting;
- Diarrhea or constipation;
- Bloating of the stomach after meals;
- Loss of appetite;
- Weakness and fatigue; and
- Bleeding (vomiting blood or having blood in the stool).

Any of these symptoms may be caused by cancer or by other, less serious health problems, such as a stomach virus or an ulcer. Only a doctor can tell the cause. People who have any of these symptoms should see their doctor. They may be referred to a gastroenterologist, a doctor who specializes in diagnosing and treating digestive problems. These doctors are sometimes called gastrointestinal (or GI) specialists.

Diagnosis

To find the cause of symptoms, the doctor asks about the patient's medical history, does a physical exam, and may order laboratory studies. The patient may also have one or all of the following exams:

Fecal occult blood test—a check for hidden (occult) blood in the stool. This test is done by placing a small amount of stool on a plastic slide or on special paper. It may be tested in the doctor's office or sent to a laboratory. This test is done because stomach cancer sometimes causes bleeding that cannot be seen. However, noncancerous conditions also may cause bleeding, so having blood in the stool does not necessarily mean that a person has cancer.

Upper GI series—x-rays of the esophagus and stomach (the upper gastrointestinal, or GI, tract. The x-rays are taken after the patient drinks a barium solution, a thick, chalky liquid. (This test is sometimes called a barium swallow.) The barium outlines the stomach on the x-rays, helping the doctor find tumors or other abnormal areas. During the test, the doctor may pump air into the stomach to make small tumors easier to see.

Endoscopy—an exam of the esophagus and stomach using a thin, lighted tube called a gastroscope, which is passed through the mouth and esophagus to the stomach. The patient's throat is sprayed with a local anesthetic to reduce discomfort and gagging. Patients also may receive medicine to relax them. Through the gastroscope, the doctor can look directly at the inside of the stomach. If an abnormal area is found, the doctor can remove some tissue through the gastroscope. Another doctor, a pathologist, examines the tissue under a microscope to check for cancer cells. This procedure—removing tissue and examining it under a microscope—is called a biopsy. A biopsy is the only sure way to know whether cancer cells are present.

A patient who needs a biopsy may want to ask the doctor some of these questions:

- How long will the procedure take? Will I be awake? Will it hurt?

- How soon will I know the results?

- If I do have cancer, who will talk with me about treatment? When?

Staging

If the pathologist finds cancer cells in the tissue sample, the patient's doctor needs to know the stage, or extent, of the disease. Staging exams and tests help the doctor find out whether the cancer has spread and, if so, what parts of the body are affected. Because stomach cancer can spread to the liver, the pancreas, and other organs near the stomach as well as to the lungs, the doctor may order a CT (or CAT) scan, an ultrasound exam, or other tests to check these areas.

Staging may not be complete until after surgery. The surgeon removes nearby lymph nodes and may take samples of tissue from other areas in the abdomen. All of these samples are examined by a pathologist to check for cancer cells. Decisions about treatment after surgery depend on these findings.

Treatment

The doctor develops a treatment plan to fit each patient's needs. Treatment for stomach cancer depends on the size, location, and extent of the tumor; the stage of the disease; the patient's general health; and other factors.

Many people who have cancer want to learn all they can about the disease and their treatment choices so they can take an active part in decisions about their medical care. The doctor is the best person to answer questions about their diagnosis and treatment plan.

When a person is diagnosed with cancer, shock and stress are natural reactions. These feelings may make it difficult for people to think of everything they want to ask the doctor. Often, it helps to make a list of questions. Also, to help remember what the doctor says, patients may take notes or ask whether they may use a tape recorder. Some people also want to have a family member or friend with them when they talk to the doctor—to take part in the discussion, to take notes, or just to listen. Patients should not feel the need to ask all their questions or remember all the answers at one time. They will have other chances to ask the doctor to explain things and to get more information.

When talking about treatment choices, the patient may want to ask about taking part in a research study. Such studies, called clinical trials, are designed to improve cancer treatment. More information about clinical trials is in the Clinical Trials section.

These are some questions a patient may want to ask the doctor before treatment begins:

- What is the stage of the disease?

- What are my treatment options? Which do you suggest for me? Why?

- Would a clinical trial be appropriate for me?

- What are the expected benefits of the treatment?

- What are the risks and possible side effects of the treatment?

- What can be done about side effects?

- What can I do to take care of myself during therapy?

- How long will my treatment last?

Patients and their loved ones are naturally concerned about the effectiveness of the treatment. Sometimes they use statistics to try to figure out whether the patient will be cured, or how long he or she will live. It is important to remember, however, that statistics are averages based on large numbers of patients. They cannot be used to predict what will happen to a particular person because no two cancer patients are alike; treatments and responses vary greatly. Patients may want to talk with the doctor about the chance of recovery (prognosis). When doctors talk about surviving cancer, they may use the term remission rather than cure. Even though many patients recover completely, doctors use this term because the disease can return. (The return of cancer is called a recurrence.)

Getting a Second Opinion

Treatment decisions are complex. Sometimes it is helpful for patients to have a second opinion about the diagnosis and the treatment plan. (Some insurance companies require a second opinion; others may pay for a second opinion if the patient requests it.) There are several ways to find another doctor to consult:

- The patient's doctor may be able to suggest a specialist. Specialists who treat this disease include gastroenterologists, surgeons, medical oncologists and radiation oncologists.

- The Cancer Information Service, at 1-800-4-CANCER, can tell callers about treatment facilities, including cancer centers and other programs supported by the National Cancer Institute.

- Patients can get the names of doctors from their local medical society, a nearby hospital, or a medical school.

Methods of Treatment

Cancer of the stomach is difficult to cure unless it is found in an early stage (before it has begun to spread). Unfortunately, because early stomach cancer causes few symptoms, the disease is usually advanced when the diagnosis is made. However, advanced stomach cancer can be treated and the symptoms can be relieved. Treatment for stomach cancer may include surgery, chemotherapy, and/or radiation therapy. New treatment approaches such as biological therapy and improved ways of using current methods are being studied in clinical trials. A patient may have one form of treatment or a combination of treatments.

Surgery is the most common treatment for stomach cancer. The operation is called gastrectomy. The surgeon removes part (subtotal or partial gastrectomy) or all (total gastrectomy) of the stomach, as well as some of the tissue around the stomach. After a subtotal gastrectomy, the doctor connects the remaining part of the stomach to the esophagus or the small intestine. After a total gastrectomy, the doctor connects the esophagus directly to the small intestine. Because cancer can spread through the lymphatic system, lymph nodes near the tumor are often removed during surgery so that the pathologist can check them for cancer cells. If cancer cells are in the lymph nodes, the disease may have spread to other parts of the body.

These are some questions a patient may want to ask the doctor before surgery:

- What kind of operation will I have?

- What are the risks of this operation?

- How will I feel afterwards? If I have pain, how will you help me?

- Will I need a special diet? Who will teach me about my diet?

Chemotherapy is the use of drugs to kill cancer cells. This type of treatment is called systemic therapy because the drugs enter the bloodstream and travel through the body.

Clinical trials are in progress to find the best ways to use chemotherapy to treat stomach cancer. Scientists are exploring the benefits of giving chemotherapy before surgery to shrink the tumor, or as adjuvant therapy after surgery to destroy remaining cancer cells. Combination treatment with chemotherapy and radiation therapy is also under study. Doctors are testing a treatment in which anticancer drugs are put directly into the abdomen (intraperitoneal chemotherapy). Chemotherapy also is being studied as a treatment for cancer that has spread, and as a way to relieve symptoms of the disease.

Most anticancer drugs are given by injection; some are taken by mouth. The doctor may use one drug or a combination of drugs. Chemotherapy is given in cycles: a treatment period followed by a recovery period, then another treatment, and so on. Usually a person receives chemother apy as an outpatient (at the hospital, at the doctor's office, or at home). However, depending on which drugs are given and the patient's general health, a short hospital stay may be needed.

These are some questions patients may want to ask about chemotherapy:

- What is the goal of this treatment?

- What drugs will I be taking?

- Will the drugs cause side effects? What can I do about them?

- How long will I need to take this treatment?

- How will we know if the treatment is working?

Radiation therapy (also called radiotherapy) is the use of high-energy rays to damage cancer cells and stop them from growing. Like surgery, it is local therapy; the radiation can affect cancer cells only in the treated area. Radiation therapy is sometimes given after surgery to destroy cancer cells that may remain in the area. Researchers are conducting clinical trials to find out whether it is helpful to give radiation therapy during surgery (intraoperative radiation therapy). Radiation therapy may also be used to relieve pain or blockage.

The patient goes to the hospital or clinic each day for radiation therapy. Usually treatments are given 5 days a week for 5 to 6 weeks.

These are some questions a patient may want ask the doctor before receiving radiation therapy:

- What is the goal of this treatment?

- How will the radiation be given?

- When will the treatment begin? When will it end?

- Will I have side effects? What can I do about them?

- How will we know if the radiation therapy is working?

Biological therapy (also called immunotherapy) is a form of treatment that helps the body's immune system attack and destroy cancer cells; it may also help the body recover from some of the side effects of treatment. In clinical trials, doctors are studying biological therapy in combination with other treatments to try to prevent a recurrence of stomach cancer. In another use of biological therapy, patients who have low blood cell counts during or after chemotherapy may receive colony-stimulating factors to help restore the blood cell levels. Patients may need to stay in the hospital while receiving some types of biological therapy.

Clinical Trials

Many patients with stomach cancer are treated in clinical trials (treatment studies). Doctors conduct clinical trials to find out whether a new approach is both safe and effective and to answer scientific questions. Patients who take part in these studies are often the first to receive treatments that have shown promise in laboratory research. In clinical trials, some patients may receive the new treatment while others receive the standard approach. In this way, doctors can compare different therapies. Patients who take part in a trial make an important contribution to medical science and may have the first chance to benefit from improved treatment methods. Researchers also use clinical trials to look for ways to reduce the side effects of treatment and to improve the quality of patients' lives.

Many clinical trials for people with stomach cancer are under way. Patients who are interested in taking part in a trial should talk with their doctor. The booklet *Taking Part in Clinical Trials: What Cancer Patients Need To Know* explains the possible benefits and risks of treatment studies.

One way to learn about clinical trials is through PDQ, a computer database developed by the National Cancer Institute. PDQ contains information about cancer treatment and about clinical trials. The Cancer Information Service can provide PDQ information to doctors, patients, and the public.

Side Effects of Treatment

It is hard to limit the effects of therapy so that only cancer cells are removed or destroyed. Because healthy cells and tissues also may be damaged, treatment can cause unpleasant side effects.

The side effects of cancer treatment are different for each person, and they may even be different from one treatment to the next. Doctors try to plan treatment in ways that keep side effects to a minimum; they can help with any problems that occur. For this reason, it is very important to let the doctor know about any problems during or after treatment.

The National Cancer Institute booklets *Radiation Therapy and You* [reprinted in this volume as Chapter 66] and *Chemotherapy and You* [reprinted in this volume as Chapter 63] have helpful information about cancer treatment and coping with side effects.

Surgery

Gastrectomy is major surgery. For a period of time after the surgery, the person's activities are limited to allow healing to take place. For the first few days after surgery, the patient is fed intravenously (through a vein). Within several days, most patients are ready for liquids, followed by soft, then solid, foods. Those who have had their

261

entire stomach removed cannot absorb vitamin B12, which is necessary for healthy blood and nerves, so they need regular injections of this vitamin. Patients may have temporary or permanent difficulty digesting certain foods, and they may need to change their diet. Some gastrectomy patients will need to follow a special diet for a few weeks or months, while others will need to do so permanently. The doctor or a dietitian (a nutrition specialist) will explain any necessary dietary changes.

Some gastrectomy patients have cramps, nausea, diarrhea, and dizziness shortly after eating because food and liquid enter the small intestine too quickly. This group of symptoms is called the dumping syndrome. Foods containing high amounts of sugar often make the symptoms worse. The dumping syndrome can be treated by changing the patient's diet. Doctors often advise patients to eat several small meals throughout the day, to avoid foods that contain sugar, and to eat foods high in protein. To reduce the amount of fluid that enters the small intestine, patients are usually encouraged not to drink at mealtimes. Medicine also can help control the dumping syndrome. The symptoms usually disappear in 3 to 12 months, but they may be permanent.

Following gastrectomy, bile in the small intestine may back up into the remaining part of the stomach or into the esophagus, causing the symptoms of an upset stomach. The patient's doctor may prescribe medicine or suggest over-the-counter products to control such symptoms.

Chemotherapy

The side effects of chemotherapy depend mainly on the drugs the patient receives. As with any other type of treatment, side effects also vary from person to person. In general, anticancer drugs affect cells that divide rapidly. These include blood cells, which fight infection, help the blood to clot, or carry oxygen to all parts of the body. When blood cells are affected by anticancer drugs, patients are more likely to get infections, may bruise or bleed easily, and may have less energy. Cells in hair roots and cells that line the digestive tract also divide rapidly. As a result of chemotherapy, patients may have side effects such as loss of appetite, nausea, vomiting, hair loss, or mouth sores. For some patients, the doctor may prescribe medicine to help with side effects, especially with nausea and vomiting. These effects usually go away gradually during the recovery period between treatments or after the treatments stop.

Radiation Therapy

Patients who receive radiation to the abdomen may have nausea, vomiting, and diarrhea. The doctor can prescribe medicine or suggest dietary changes to relieve these problems. The skin in the treated area may become red, dry, tender, and itchy. Patients should avoid wearing clothes that rub; loose-fitting cotton clothes are usually best. It is important for patients to take good care of their skin during treatment, but they should not use lotions or creams without the doctor's advice.

Patients are likely to become very tired during radiation therapy, especially in the later weeks of treatment. Resting is important, but doctors usually advise patients to try to stay as active as they can.

Biological Therapy

The side effects of biological therapy vary with the type of treatment. Some cause flu-like symptoms, such as chills, fever, weakness, nausea, vomiting, and diarrhea. Patients sometimes get a rash, and they may bruise or bleed easily. These problems may be severe, and patients may need to stay in the hospital during treatment.

Nutrition for Cancer Patients

It is sometimes difficult for patients who have been treated for stomach cancer to eat well. Cancer often causes loss of appetite, and people may not feel like eating when they are uncomfortable or tired. It is hard for patients to eat when they have nausea, vomiting, mouth sores, or the dumping syndrome. Patients who have had stomach surgery are likely to feel full after eating only a small amount of food. For some patients, the taste of food changes. Still, good nutrition is important. Eating well means getting enough calories and protein to help prevent weight loss, regain strength, and rebuild normal tissues.

Doctors, nurses, and dietitians can offer advice for healthy eating during and after cancer treatment. Patients and their families also may want to read the National Cancer Institute booklet *Eating Hints for Cancer Patients* [reprinted in this volume as Chapter 77], which contains many useful suggestions.

Support for Cancer Patients

Living with a serious disease is not easy. Cancer patients and those who care about them face many problems and challenges. Coping with these problems is often easier when people have helpful information and support services. Several useful booklets, including *Taking Time*, are available from the Cancer Information Service.

Cancer patients may worry about holding their job, caring for their family, or keeping up with their daily activities. Concerns about tests, treatments, hospital stays, and medical bills are common. Doctors, nurses, and other members of the health care team can answer questions about treatment, working, or other activities. Meeting with a social worker, counselor, or member of the clergy also can be helpful for patients who want to talk about their feelings or discuss their concerns about the future or about personal relationships.

Friends and relatives can be very supportive. Also, it helps many patients to discuss their concerns with others who have cancer. Cancer patients often get together in support groups, where they can share what they have learned about coping with cancer and the effects of treatment. It is important to keep in mind, however, that each patient is different. Treatments and ways of dealing with cancer that work for one person may not be right for another—even if they both have the same kind of cancer. It is always a good idea to discuss the advice of friends and family members with the doctor.

Often, a social worker at the hospital or clinic can suggest groups that can help with rehabilitation, emotional support, financial aid, transportation, or home care. For example, the American Cancer Society has many services for cancer patients and their families. Local offices of the American Cancer Society are listed in the white pages of the telephone directory. The Cancer Information Service also has information on local resources.

Causes of Stomach Cancer

The stomach cancer rate in the United States and the number of deaths from this disease have gone down dramatically over the past 60 years. Still, stomach cancer is a serious disease, and scientists all over the world are trying to learn more about what causes this disease and how to prevent it. At this time, doctors cannot explain why one person gets stomach cancer and another does not. They do know, however, that stomach cancer is not contagious; no one can "catch" cancer from another person.

Researchers have learned that some people are more likely than others to develop stomach cancer. The disease is found most often in people over age 55. It affects men twice as often as women, and is more common in black people than in white people. Also, stomach cancer is more common in some parts of the world—such as Japan, Korea, parts of Eastern Europe, and Latin America—than in the United States. People in these areas eat many foods that are preserved by drying, smoking, salting, or pickling. Scientists believe that eating foods preserved in these ways may play a role in the development of stomach cancer. On the other hand, fresh foods (especially fresh fruits and vegetables and properly frozen or refrigerated fresh foods) may protect against this disease.

Stomach ulcers do not appear to increase a person's risk (chance) of getting stomach cancer. However, some studies suggest that a type of bacteria, *Helicobacter pylori*, which may cause stomach inflammation and ulcers, may be an important risk factor for this disease. Also, research shows that people who have had stomach surgery or have pernicious anemia, achlorhydria, or gastric atrophy (which generally result in lower than normal amounts of digestive juices) have an increased risk of stomach cancer.

Exposure to certain dusts and fumes in the workplace has been linked to a higher than average risk of stomach cancer. Also, some scientists believe smoking may increase stomach cancer risk.

People who think they might be at risk for stomach cancer should discuss this concern with their doctor. The doctor can suggest an appropriate schedule of checkups so that, if cancer appears, it can be detected as early as possible.

Other Booklets

Cancer patients, their families and friends, and others may find the following booklets useful. They are available free of charge by calling 1-800-4-CANCER or writing:

Office of Cancer Communications
National Cancer Institute
Building 31, Room 10A24
Bethesda, MD 20892

Booklets about Cancer Treatment

Radiation Therapy and You: A Guide to Self-Help During Treatment *

Chemotherapy and You: A Guide to Self-Help During Treatment *

Eating Hints: Recipes and Tips for Better Nutrition During Cancer Treatment *

Questions and Answers About Pain Control

What Are Clinical Trials All About?

Booklets about Living with Cancer

Taking Time: Support for People With Cancer and the People Who Care About Them

When Cancer Recurs: Meeting the Challenge Again *

Advanced Cancer: Living Each Day *

* Reprinted in this volume—see Table of Contents

Chapter 25

Gallbladder Cancer

What Is Cancer of the Gallbladder?

Cancer of the gallbladder, an uncommon cancer, is a disease in which cancer (malignant) cells are found in the tissues of the gallbladder. The gallbladder is a pear-shaped organ that lies just under the liver in the upper abdomen. Bile, a fluid made by the liver, is stored in the gallbladder. When food is being broken down (digested) in the stomach and the intestines, bile is released from the gallbladder through a tube called the bile duct that connects the gallbladder and liver to the first part of the small intestine. The bile helps to digest fat.

Cancer of the gallbladder is more common in women than in men. It is also more common in people who have hard clusters of material in their gallbladder (gallstones).

Cancer of the gallbladder is hard to find (diagnose) because the gallbladder is hidden behind other organs in the abdomen. Cancer of the gallbladder is sometimes found after the gallbladder is removed for other reasons. The symptoms of cancer of the gallbladder may be like other diseases of the gallbladder, such as gallstones or infection, and there may be no symptoms in the early stages. A doctor should be seen if the following symptoms persist: pain above the stomach, loss of weight without trying, fever, or yellowing of the skin (jaundice).

If there are symptoms, a doctor may order x-rays and other tests to see what is wrong. However, usually the cancer cannot be found

PDQ Statement, National Cancer Institute (NCI), updated January 1998.

unless the patient has surgery. During surgery, a cut is made in the abdomen so that the gallbladder and other nearby organs and tissues can be examined.

The chance of recovery (prognosis) and choice of treatment depend on the stage of cancer (whether it is just in the gallbladder or has spread to other places) and on the patient's general health.

Stages of Cancer of the Gallbladder

Once cancer of the gallbladder is found, more tests will be done to find out if cancer cells have spread to other parts of the body. A doctor needs to know the stage to plan treatment. The following stages are used for cancer of the gallbladder:

Localized

Cancer is found only in the tissues that make up the wall of the gallbladder, and it can be removed completely in an operation.

Unresectable

All of the cancer cannot be removed in an operation. Cancer has spread to the tissues around the gallbladder, such as the liver, stomach, pancreas, or intestine and/or to lymph nodes in the area. (Lymph nodes are small, bean-shaped structures that are found throughout the body. They produce and store infection-fighting cells.)

Recurrent

Recurrent disease means that the cancer has come back (recurred) after it has been treated. It may come back in the gallbladder or in another part of the body.

How Cancer of the Gallbladder Is Treated

There are treatments for all patients with cancer of the gallbladder. Three treatments are used:

- surgery (taking out the cancer or relieving symptoms of the cancer in an operation)
- radiation therapy (using high-dose x-rays to kill cancer cells)
- chemotherapy (using drugs to kill cancer)

Surgery is a common treatment of cancer of the gallbladder if it has not spread to surrounding tissues. The doctor may take out the gallbladder in an operation called a cholecystectomy. Part of the liver around the gallbladder and lymph nodes in the abdomen may also be removed.

If the cancer has spread and cannot be removed, the doctor may do surgery to relieve symptoms. If the cancer is blocking the bile ducts and bile builds up in the gallbladder, the doctor may do surgery to go around (bypass) the cancer. During this operation, the doctor will cut the gallbladder or bile duct and sew it to the small intestine. This is called biliary bypass. Surgery or other procedures may also be done to put in a tube (catheter) to drain bile that has built up in the area. During these procedures, the doctor may place the catheter so that it drains through a tube to the outside of the body or so that it goes around the blocked area and drains the bile into the small intestine.

Radiation therapy is the use of high-energy x-rays to kill cancer cells and shrink tumors. Radiation for gallbladder cancer usually comes from a machine outside the body (external-beam radiation therapy). Radiation may be used alone or in addition to surgery.

Chemotherapy is the use of drugs to kill cancer cells. Chemotherapy for cancer of the gallbladder is usually put into the body by a needle inserted into a vein. Chemotherapy is called a systemic treatment because the drug enters the bloodstream, travels through the body, and can kill cancer cells outside the gallbladder. Chemotherapy or other drugs may be given with radiation therapy to make cancer cells more sensitive to radiation (radiosensitizers).

Treatment by Stage

Treatments for cancer of the gallbladder depend on the stage of the disease and the patient's general health.

Standard treatment may be considered because of its effectiveness in past studies, or participation in a clinical trial may be considered. Most patients with gallbladder cancer are not cured with standard therapy and some standard treatments may have more side effects than are desired. For these reasons, clinical trials are designed to find better ways to treat cancer patients and are based on the most up-to-date information. Clinical trials are ongoing in many parts of the country for patients with cancer of the gallbladder. To learn more about clinical trials, call the Cancer Information Service at 1-800-4-CANCER (1-800-422-6237); TTY at 1-800-332-8615.

Localized Gallbladder Cancer

Treatment may be one of the following:

1. Surgery to remove the gallbladder and some of the tissues around it (cholecystectomy).

2. External-beam radiation therapy.

3. Surgery followed by external-beam radiation therapy.

4. Clinical trials of radiation therapy plus chemotherapy or drugs to make the cancer cells more sensitive to radiation (radiosensitizers).

Unresectable Gallbladder Cancer

Treatment may be one of the following:

1. Surgery or other procedures to relieve symptoms.

2. External-beam radiation therapy with or without surgery or other procedures to relieve symptoms.

3. Chemotherapy to relieve symptoms. Clinical trials are testing new chemotherapy drugs.

4. Clinical trials of radiation therapy plus chemotherapy or drugs to make the cancer cells more sensitive to radiation (radiosensitizers).

Recurrent Gallbladder Cancer

Treatment for recurrent cancer of the gallbladder depends on the type of treatment the patient received before, the place where the cancer has recurred and other facts about the cancer, and the patient's general health. The patient may wish to consider taking part in a clinical trial.

To Learn More

To learn more about cancer of the gallbladder, call the National Cancer Institute's Cancer Information Service at 1-800-4-CANCER (1-800-422-6237); TTY at 1-800-332-8615. By dialing this toll-free number, trained information specialists can answer your questions.

The Cancer Information Service also has booklets about cancer that are available to the public and can be sent on request. The following general booklets on questions related to cancer may be helpful:

Booklets about Cancer Treatment

Radiation Therapy and You: A Guide to Self-Help During Treatment *

Chemotherapy and You: A Guide to Self-Help During Treatment *

Eating Hints: Recipes and Tips for Better Nutrition During Cancer Treatment *

Questions and Answers About Pain Control

What Are Clinical Trials All About?

Booklets about Living with Cancer

Taking Time: Support for People With Cancer and the People Who Care About Them

When Cancer Recurs: Meeting the Challenge Again *

Advanced Cancer: Living Each Day *

* Reprinted in this volume—see Table of Contents

Chapter 26

Bladder Cancer

Introduction

Each year, nearly 55,000 people in the United States learn that they have bladder cancer. The National Cancer Institute (NCI) has written this chapter to help patients with bladder cancer and their families and friends better understand this disease. We hope others will read it as well to learn more about bladder cancer.

This chapter discusses symptoms, diagnosis, treatment, and rehabilitation. It also has information to help patients cope with bladder cancer.

Our knowledge about bladder cancer keeps increasing. For up-to-date information or to order this publication, call the NCI-supported Cancer Information Service (CIS) toll free at 1-800-4-CANCER (1-800-422-6237).

The CIS staff uses a National Cancer Institute cancer information database called PDQ and other NCI resources to answer callers' questions. Cancer information specialists can send callers information from PDQ and other NCI materials about cancer, its treatment, and living with the disease (see Other Booklets section).

The Bladder

The bladder is a hollow organ in the lower abdomen. It stores urine, the waste that is produced when the kidneys filter the blood. The bladder has a muscular wall that allows it to get larger and smaller as

What You Need To Know About Bladder Cancer, National Cancer Institute, NIH Publication 97-1559, updated 28 September 1998.

urine is stored or emptied. The wall of the bladder is lined with several layers of transitional cells.

Urine passes from the two kidneys into the bladder through two tubes called ureters. Urine leaves the bladder through another tube, the urethra.

What Is Cancer?

Cancer is a group of many different diseases that have some important things in common. They all affect cells, the body's basic unit of life. To understand different types of cancer, such as bladder cancer, it is helpful to know about normal cells and what happens when they become cancerous.

The body is made up of many types of cells. Normally, cells grow and divide to produce more cells only when the body needs them. This orderly process helps keep the body healthy. Sometimes cells keep dividing when new cells are not needed. These cells form a mass of extra tissue, called a growth or tumor. Tumors can be benign or malignant.

- Benign tumors are not cancer. They often can be removed and, in most cases, they do not come back. Cells in benign tumors do not spread to other parts of the body. Most important, benign tumors are rarely a threat to life.

- Malignant tumors are cancer. Cells in malignant tumors are abnormal and divide without control or order. These cancer cells can invade and destroy the tissues around them. Also, cancer cells can break away from a malignant tumor and enter the bloodstream or the lymphatic system. This process is the way cancer spreads from the original (primary) tumor to form new tumors in other parts of the body. The spread of cancer is called metastasis.

Bladder Cancer

Most cancers are named for the part of the body or type of cells in which they begin. About 90 percent of bladder cancers are transitional cell carcinomas, cancers that begin in the cells lining the bladder. Cancer that is confined to the lining of the bladder is called superficial bladder cancer. After treatment, superficial bladder cancer can recur; if this happens, most often it recurs as another superficial cancer.

274

In some cases, cancer that begins in the transitional cells spreads through the lining of the bladder and invades the muscular wall of the bladder. This is known as invasive bladder cancer. Invasive cancer may grow through the bladder wall and spread to nearby organs.

Bladder cancer cells may also be found in the lymph nodes surrounding the bladder. If the cancer has reached these nodes, it may mean that cancer cells have spread to other lymph nodes and to distant organs, such as the lungs. The cancer cells in the new tumor are still bladder cancer cells. The new tumor is called metastatic bladder cancer rather than lung cancer because it has the same kind of abnormal cells that were found in the bladder.

Symptoms

Some common symptoms of bladder cancer include:

- Blood in the urine (slightly rusty to deep red in color).
- Pain during urination.
- Frequent urination, or feeling the need to urinate without results.

When symptoms occur, they are not sure signs of bladder cancer. They may also be caused by infections, benign tumors, bladder stones, or other problems. Only a doctor can make a diagnosis. (People with symptoms like these generally see their family doctor or a urologist, a doctor who specializes in diseases of the urinary system.) It is important to see a doctor so that any illness can be diagnosed and treated as early as possible.

Diagnosis and Staging

To find the cause of symptoms, the doctor asks about the patient's medical history and does a physical exam. The physical will include a rectal or vaginal exam that allows the doctor to check for tumors that can be felt. In addition, urine samples are sent to the laboratory for testing to check for blood and cancer cells.

The doctor may use an instrument to look directly into the bladder, a procedure called cystoscopy. This procedure may be done with local or general anesthesia. The doctor inserts a thin, lighted tube (called a cystoscope) into the bladder through the urethra to examine the lining of the bladder. The doctor can remove samples of tissues through this tube. The sample is then examined under a microscope by a pathologist. The removal of tissue to look for cancer cells is called a biopsy. In many cases, performing a biopsy is the only sure way to tell whether cancer is present. If the entire cancer is removed during the biopsy, bladder cancer can be diagnosed and treated in a single procedure.

A patient who needs a biopsy may want to ask the doctor some of the following questions:

- Why do I need to have a biopsy?

- How long will it take? Will I be awake? Will it hurt?

- What side effects can I expect?

- How soon will I know the results?

- If I do have cancer, who will talk with me about treatment? When?

Once bladder cancer is diagnosed, the doctor will want to learn the grade of the cancer and the stage, or extent, of the disease. Grade is important because it tells how closely the cancer resembles normal tissue and suggests how fast the cancer is likely to grow. Low-grade cancers more closely resemble normal tissue and are likely to grow and spread more slowly than high-grade cancers.

Staging is a careful attempt to find out whether the cancer has spread and, if so, what parts of the body are affected. The stage of bladder cancer may be determined at the time of diagnosis, or it may be necessary to perform additional tests. Such tests may include imaging tests—CT scan, MRI, sonogram, IVP, bone scan, or chest x-ray.

Treatment

Treatment for bladder cancer depends on the stage of the disease (particularly if, or how deeply, the cancer has invaded the bladder wall), the grade of the cancer, the patient's general health, and other factors. People with bladder cancer are often treated by a team of specialists, which may include a urologist, oncologist, and radiation oncologist. The doctors develop a treatment plan to fit each patient's needs. Depending on its stage and grade, bladder cancer may be treated with surgery, radiation therapy, chemotherapy, or biological therapy. Doctors may recommend one treatment method or a combination of methods. It is important for patients to discuss the treatment plan with their doctors.

Some patients take part in a clinical trial (research study) using new treatment methods. Such studies are designed to improve cancer treatment.

Getting a Second Opinion

Before starting treatment, the patient may want a second specialist to review the diagnosis and the treatment plan. It may take a week or two to arrange for a second opinion. A short delay will not reduce the chance that treatment will be successful. Some insurance companies require a second opinion; others may cover a second opinion if the patient requests it.

There are a number of ways to find a doctor who can give a second opinion:

- The patient's doctor may be able to suggest specialists to consult.

- The Cancer Information Service, at 1-800-4-CANCER, can tell callers about treatment facilities, including cancer centers and other programs supported by the National Cancer Institute.

- Patients can get the names of doctors from their local medical society, a nearby hospital, or a medical school.

- The *Directory of Medical Specialists* lists doctors' names along with their specialty and their background. This resource is in most public libraries.

Preparing for Treatment

Many people with cancer want to learn all they can about the disease and their treatment choices so they can take an active part in decisions about their medical care. When a person is diagnosed with cancer, shock and stress are natural reactions. These feelings may make it difficult to think of everything to ask the doctor. Often, it helps to make a list of questions. To help remember what the doctor says, patients may take notes or ask whether they may use a tape recorder. Some people also want to have a family member or friend with them when they talk to the doctor—to take part in the discussion, to take notes, or just to listen.

People do not need to ask all of their questions or remember all of the answers at one time. Questions may arise throughout the treatment process. Patients may ask doctors, nurses, or other members of the health care team to explain things further or to provide more information.

These are some questions a patient may want to ask the doctor before treatment begins:

- What is the diagnosis?
- What is the stage of the disease?
- What is the grade of the disease?
- What are the treatment choices? Which do you recommend? Why?
- What are the risks and possible side effects of each treatment?
- What are the chances that the treatment will be successful?
- What new treatments are being studied in clinical trials? Would a clinical trial be appropriate?
- How long will treatment last?
- Will treatment affect my normal activities? If so, for how long?
- What is the treatment likely to cost?

Methods of Treatment

Surgery is a common form of treatment for bladder cancer. Early (superficial) bladder cancer may be treated at the time of diagnosis through a procedure called transurethral resection (TUR). During TUR, the doctor inserts a cystoscope into the bladder through the urethra. The doctor then uses a tool with a small wire loop on the end to remove the cancer or to burn away cancer cells with an electric current (fulguration). TUR requires anesthesia and may be done in the hospital.

Surgery to remove part or all of the bladder is called cystectomy. The most common form of surgery for invasive bladder cancer is radical cystectomy. This surgery may be done when the bladder cancer invades the muscle wall, or when superficial cancer involves a large part of the bladder.

Radical cystectomy removes the entire bladder, nearby lymph nodes, and any surrounding organs that contain cancerous cells. In men, the nearby organs that are removed are the prostate and the seminal vesicles. In women, the uterus, the ovaries, and part of the vagina are removed. Sometimes, when the cancer has spread outside the bladder and cannot be completely removed, surgery to remove only the bladder may be done to relieve urinary symptoms caused by the cancer. When the bladder must be removed, the doctor creates another way for urine to leave the body. (See the Side Effects of Treatment and Rehabilitation sections).

In some cases, patients may have part of the bladder removed in an operation called segmental cystectomy. This type of surgery may be done when a patient has a low-grade cancer that has invaded the wall of the bladder but is limited to one area of the organ. Because most of the bladder remains intact, a patient urinates normally after recovering from this surgery.

These are some questions a patient may want to ask the doctor before surgery:

- What kind of operation will it be?

- Will I need more treatment after surgery? What kind?

- How will I feel after the operation?

- If I have pain, how will you help?

- Will I urinate in a normal way?

- How will surgery affect my normal activities?

In radiation therapy (also called radiotherapy), high-energy rays are used to kill cancer cells. Like surgery, radiation therapy is local therapy; it affects cancer cells only in the treated area. Sometimes, radiation is given before or after surgery or along with anticancer drugs. When bladder cancer has spread to other organs, radiation therapy may be used to relieve symptoms caused by the cancer.

Radiation may come from a machine outside the body (external radiation) or from a small container of radioactive material, called a radiation implant, placed directly into the bladder (internal radiation). Some patients have both kinds of radiation therapy.

External radiation therapy is usually given on an outpatient basis in a hospital or clinic 5 days a week for 5 to 7 weeks. Treatment may be shorter when external radiation is given along with radiation implants.

These are some questions a patient may want to ask the doctor before having radiation therapy:

- What is the goal of this treatment?

- How will the radiation be given?

- What type of treatment schedule will I follow?

- How will I feel during therapy?
- What can I do to take care of myself during therapy?
- How will we know if the radiation is working?
- When will I be able to resume my normal activities?

For internal radiation, radiation implants are placed in the bladder either through the urethra or during surgery. The patient stays in the hospital for several days while the implant is in place. To protect others from exposure to radiation, patients may not be able to have visitors or may have visitors for only a short time. Once an implant is removed, there is no radioactivity in the body.

Chemotherapy is the use of drugs to kill cancer cells. The doctor may use one drug or a combination of drugs. Chemotherapy may be used alone or after TUR with fulguration to treat superficial bladder cancer. In a treatment called intravesical chemotherapy, anticancer drugs are placed in the bladder through a tube called a catheter, which is inserted through the urethra. When given in this way, the anticancer drugs, which remain in the bladder for several hours, affect mainly the cells of the bladder. The treatment is usually done once a week for several weeks. Sometimes, the treatments continue once or several times a month for up to a year.

Chemotherapy also may be used to help control the disease when cancer cells have deeply invaded the bladder or spread to lymph nodes or other organs. In this case, the anticancer drugs are usually given by injection into a vein (IV); some may be given by mouth. This form of chemotherapy is systemic therapy, meaning that the drugs flow through the bloodstream to nearly every part of the body. The drugs are usually given in cycles: a treatment period followed by a recovery period, then another treatment period, and so on. Chemotherapy may be used alone or in combination with surgery or radiation therapy.

These are some questions patients may want to ask the doctor before starting chemotherapy:

- What is the goal of this treatment?
- What drugs will I be taking?
- Will the drugs cause side effects? What can I do about them?
- How long will I need to take this treatment?
- What can I do to take care of myself during treatment?
- How will I know if the drugs are working?

Usually a patient has chemotherapy as an outpatient (at the hospital, at the doctor's office, or at home). However, depending on which drugs are given and the patient's general health, a short hospital stay may be needed.

Biological therapy (also called immunotherapy) is a form of treatment that uses the body's natural ability (immune system) to fight cancer. Biological therapy for bladder cancer is most often used when the disease is superficial. Like chemotherapy, biological therapy may be used alone to treat bladder cancer or after TUR with fulguration to help prevent the cancer from recurring. This form of treatment involves placing a solution of BCG, a substance that stimulates the immune system, into the bladder. The medicine stays in the bladder for about 2 hours before the patient is allowed to empty the bladder by urinating. This treatment is usually done once a week for 6 weeks and may need to be prolonged or repeated. Doctors are also studying the use of other forms of biological therapy for other stages of bladder cancer.

These are some questions patients may want to ask the doctor before starting biological therapy:

- What is the goal of this treatment?
- What drugs will be used?
- What type of treatment schedule will I follow?
- Will the treatment cause side effects? If so, what can I do about them?
- Will I have to be in the hospital to receive treatment?
- How long will I be on treatment?
- Will I be able to continue my normal activities?

Clinical Trials

Another treatment option for people with bladder cancer is to take part in clinical trials (treatment studies). Doctors conduct clinical trials to learn the effectiveness and side effects of new treatments. In some clinical trials, all patients receive the new treatment. In other trials, doctors compare different therapies by giving the new treatment to one group of patients and the standard therapy to another group.

People who take part in these studies have the first chance to benefit from treatments that have shown promise in earlier research. They also make an important contribution to medical science.

Doctors are studying new ways of treating bladder cancer with radiation therapy, chemotherapy, biological therapies, and ways of combining various types of treatment. In addition, some trials are designed to study ways to reduce the side effects of treatment and to improve the quality of life.

Patients who are interested in taking part in a trial should talk with their doctor. They may want to read the National Cancer Institute booklet *Taking Part in Clinical Trials: What Cancer Patients Need To Know* [reprinted in this volume—see Table of Contents] which explains the possible benefits and risks of clinical trials.

One way to learn about clinical trials is through PDQ, a cancer information database developed by the National Cancer Institute. PDQ contains information about cancer treatment and about clinical trials in progress all over the country. The Cancer Information Service can provide PDQ information to doctors, patients, and the public.

Side Effects of Treatment

It is hard to limit the effects of cancer therapy so that only cancer cells, not healthy cells, are removed or destroyed. Because treatment can damage healthy cells and tissues, it often causes side effects.

These side effects depend mainly on the type and extent of the cancer treatment. Also, the effects may not be the same for each person, and they may even change from one treatment to the next. Doctors and nurses can explain the possible side effects of treatment, and they can help relieve symptoms that may occur during and after treatment.

Surgery

TUR causes few problems. Patients may have some blood in their urine and difficulty or pain when urinating for a few days afterward.

After any bladder surgery, particularly radical cystectomy, patients are often uncomfortable during the first few days. However, this pain can be controlled with medicine. Patients should feel free to discuss pain relief with the doctor or nurse. It is also common for patients to feel tired or weak for a while. The length of time it takes to recover from an operation varies for each patient.

After segmental cystectomy, patients may not be able to hold as much urine in their bladder. In most cases, this problem is temporary, but some patients may have long-lasting changes in bladder capacity.

When the bladder is removed, the patient needs a new way to store and pass urine. Various methods are used. In one common method, the surgeon uses a piece of the person's small intestine to form a new tube through which urine can pass. The ureters are attached to one end, and the other end is brought out through an opening in the wall of the abdomen. This new opening is called a stoma. A flat bag fits over the stoma to collect urine, and special adhesive holds it in place. The patient will be taught how to care for the stoma. The surgical procedure to create a stoma is called a urostomy or an ostomy. (See Rehabilitation section).

A newer method uses part of the small intestine to make a new storage pouch (called a continent reservoir) inside the body. Urine collects there instead of emptying into a bag. The pouch is connected either to a stoma or to the urethra. The patient learns to use a catheter to drain the urine through the stoma or the urethra.

Women who have had a radical cystectomy are not able to have children because their uterus has been removed. In addition, the vagina may be narrower or shallower, which may make sexual intercourse difficult.

In the past, nearly all men were impotent after radical cystectomy, but improvements in surgery have made it possible to prevent this side effect in some cases. However, men who have had their prostate and seminal vesicles removed no longer produce semen, so they do not ejaculate when they have an orgasm and are not able to father children.

Radiation Therapy

With radiation therapy, the side effects depend mainly on the treatment dose and the part of the body that is treated. Patients are likely to become very tired during radiation therapy, especially in the later weeks of treatment. Resting is important, but doctors usually advise patients to try to stay as active as they can.

With external radiation, there may be permanent darkening or "bronzing" of the skin in the treated area. In addition, it is common to lose hair in the treated area and for the skin to become red, dry, tender, and itchy. These problems are temporary, and the doctor may be able to suggest ways to relieve them.

Radiation therapy to the abdomen may cause nausea, vomiting, diarrhea, or urinary discomfort. Radiation therapy also may cause a decrease in the number of white blood cells, cells that help protect the body against infection. Usually, the doctor can suggest certain diet changes or medicine to ease these problems. For both men and women, radiation treatment for bladder cancer can affect sexuality. Women may experience vaginal dryness, and men may have difficulty with erections.

Although the side effects of radiation therapy can be distressing, the doctor can usually treat or control them. It also helps to know that, in most cases, side effects are not permanent. The National Cancer Institute booklet *Radiation Therapy and You* [reprinted in this volume as Chapter 66] has helpful information about radiation therapy and managing its side effects.

Chemotherapy

The side effects of chemotherapy depend mainly on the drugs and the doses the patient receives as well as how the drugs are given. In addition, as with other types of treatment, side effects vary from person to person.

Anticancer drugs that are placed in the bladder may irritate the bladder for a few days after treatment, causing some discomfort or bleeding. Some drugs, if they come into contact with the skin or genitals, may cause a rash.

Systemic chemotherapy affects rapidly dividing cells throughout the body. These cells include blood cells, which fight infection, help the blood to clot, or carry oxygen to all parts of the body. When blood cells are affected by anticancer drugs, patients are more likely to get infections, may bruise or bleed easily, and may have less energy. Cells in hair roots and cells that line the digestive tract also divide rapidly. As a result, patients may lose their hair and may have other side effects such as poor appetite, nausea and vomiting, or mouth sores. Usually, these side effects go away gradually during the recovery periods between treatments or after treatment is over. Certain drugs used in the treatment of bladder cancer also may cause kidney damage. Patients are given large amounts of fluid while taking these drugs. Anticancer drugs can also cause tingling in the fingers, ringing in the ears, or hearing loss. These problems may not clear up after treatment stops. The National Cancer Institute booklet *Chemotherapy and You* [reprinted in this volume as Chapter 63] has helpful information about chemotherapy and coping with side effects.

Biological Therapy

Treatment with BCG can irritate the bladder for a few days after treatment. This may cause pain, especially while urinating, and the feeling of an urgent need to urinate. Patients also may have some blood in their urine, have a low fever, or feel tired or nauseated.

Other types of biological therapy may cause flu-like symptoms such as chills, fever, muscle aches, weakness, loss of appetite, nausea, vomiting, and diarrhea. Patients also may bleed or bruise easily, get a rash, or have swelling. These problems can be severe, but they go away after the treatment stops.

Nutrition for Cancer Patients

Eating well during cancer treatment means getting enough calories and protein to help prevent weight loss and regain strength. Eating well often helps people feel better and have more energy.

Some people with cancer find it hard to eat well. They may lose their appetite. In addition to loss of appetite, common side effects of treatment, such as nausea, vomiting, or mouth sores, can make eating difficult. Often, foods taste different. Also, people being treated for cancer may not feel like eating when they are uncomfortable or tired.

Doctors, nurses, and dietitians can offer advice for healthy eating during cancer treatment. Patients and their families also may want to read the National Cancer Institute booklet *Eating Hints for Cancer Patients* [reprinted in this volume as Chapter 77], which contains many useful suggestions.

Rehabilitation

Rehabilitation after cancer is an important part of the overall treatment process. The goal of rehabilitation is to improve a person's quality of life after cancer treatment. The medical team, which may include doctors, nurses, a physical therapist, or a social worker, develops a rehabilitation plan to meet the patient's physical and emotional needs, helping the patient to return to normal activities as soon as possible. People who have had cancer and their families may discuss any concerns about rehabilitation with the medical team.

Bladder cancer patients who have a urostomy need special instructions for care. Enterostomal therapists teach them to care for themselves and their stomas after surgery. They often visit patients before surgery to discuss what to expect and talk about lifestyle issues including emotional, physical, and sexual concerns. Enterostomal therapists can also provide information about resources and support groups for people who have a urostomy.

Recovery and Outlook

People with bladder cancer and their families are naturally concerned about recovery from cancer and their outlook for the future. Sometimes people use statistics to try to figure out their chances of being cured. It is important to remember, however, that statistics are averages based on large numbers of patients. They cannot be used to predict what will happen to a particular patient because no two patients are alike; treatments and responses vary greatly. The patient's doctor is in the best position to discuss the issue of prognosis, or chance of recovery.

When doctors talk about surviving cancer, they may use the term remission rather than cure. Although many cancer patients are cured, doctors use this term because cancer can return. (The return of cancer is called a recurrence.) Superficial bladder cancer tends to recur as an another superficial cancer in the bladder. The disease can also recur in the bladder muscle or elsewhere in the body. Therefore, people who have had bladder cancer may wish to discuss the possibility of recurrence with the doctor.

Followup Care

It is important for people who have had cancer to have regular followup examinations after their treatment is over. For people with bladder cancer who have not had their bladder removed, the doctor will check the bladder with a cystoscope and remove any superficial tumors that may have recurred. Patients also may have urine tests to check for cancer cells. Followup care may also include blood tests, a CT scan, a chest x-ray, or other tests.

Followup care is an important part of the overall treatment process, and people with cancer should not hesitate to discuss it with the doctor. Regular followup care ensures that changes in health are noted so that recurrent cancer or other problems can be treated as soon as possible. Between checkups, people who have had bladder cancer should report any health problems as soon as they appear.

Support for People with Cancer

Living with a serious disease is not easy. People with cancer and those who care about them face many problems and challenges. Coping with these problems is often easier when people have helpful information and support services. Several useful booklets, including *Taking Time*, are available from the Cancer Information Service.

Friends and relatives can be very supportive. Also, it helps many patients to discuss their concerns with others who have cancer. Cancer patients often get together in support groups, where they can share what they have learned about coping with cancer and the effects of treatment. It is important to keep in mind, however, that each person is different. Treatments and ways of dealing with cancer that work for one person may not be right for another—even if they both have the same kind of cancer. It is always a good idea to discuss the advice of friends and family members with the doctor.

People living with cancer may worry about what the future holds. They may worry about caring for their family, holding their job, or continuing daily activities. Concerns about tests, treatments, hospital stays, and medical bills are also common. Doctors, nurses, and other members of the health care team can answer questions about treatment, working, or other activities. Meeting with a social worker, counselor, or member of the clergy can be helpful to people who want to talk about their feelings or discuss their concerns.

Often, a social worker can suggest groups that can help with rehabilitation, emotional support, financial aid, transportation, or home care.

The Cancer Information Service can supply information about bladder cancer and about programs and services for patients and their families.

Possible Causes and Prevention

Researchers at hospitals and medical centers all across the country are studying bladder cancer. They are trying to learn what causes the disease and how to prevent it.

At this time, the causes of bladder cancer are not fully understood. It is clear, however, that this disease is not contagious; no one can "catch" cancer from another person.

Some researchers study patterns of cancer in the population. They look for factors that are more common in people who get bladder cancer than in people who don't get this disease. Studying such patterns helps researchers identify risk factors for bladder cancer. However, most people with these risk factors do not get cancer, and many people who do get bladder cancer have none of the known risk factors.

Researchers have found that white people in the United States get bladder cancer twice as often as African-Americans, and men are affected about three times as often as women. People with family members who have bladder cancer may be more likely to get the disease as well. Most bladder cancers occur after the age of 55, but the disease can also develop in younger people.

Known and possible risk factors for bladder cancer include:

- *Smoking:* This is a major risk factor. Cigarette smokers develop bladder cancer two to three times more often than do nonsmokers. Quitting smoking reduces the risk of bladder cancer, lung cancer, and several other types of cancer, as well as a number of other diseases.

- *Occupational risk:* Workers in some occupations are at higher risk of getting bladder cancer because of exposure to carcinogens in the workplace. Increased risk is seen in people in the rubber, chemical, and leather industries, as well as in hairdressers, machinists, metal workers, printers, painters, textile workers, and truck drivers.

People who think they may be at risk for developing bladder cancer should discuss this concern with their doctor. The doctor may suggest ways to reduce the risk and can plan an appropriate schedule for checkups.

The Promise of Cancer Research

Research advances in detection, treatment, rehabilitation, and pain control have improved the outlook and quality of life for people with bladder cancer. By using a combination of therapies, doctors can treat some bladder cancers without removing the patient's bladder. However, when cystectomy is necessary, new surgical techniques allow doctors to create new ways of storing and passing urine, which improve patients' recovery and long-term comfort. Researchers are also conducting studies to learn more about what causes the development of bladder cancer. Although there is still much more work to be done, there are many reasons to be optimistic about the future.

Other Booklets

The National Cancer Institute booklets listed below and others are available from the Cancer Information Service by calling 1-800-4-CANCER.

Booklets about Cancer Treatment

Chemotherapy and You: A Guide to Self-Help During Treatment *

Helping Yourself During Chemotherapy: 4 Steps for Patients

Radiation Therapy and You: A Guide to Self-Help During Treatment *

Eating Hints for Cancer Patients *

Taking Part in Clinical Trials: What Cancer Patients Need To Know

Questions and Answers About Pain Control

Get Relief from Cancer Pain

Booklets about Living with Cancer

Taking Time: Support for People With Cancer and the People Who Care About Them

Facing Forward: A Guide for Cancer Survivors *

When Someone in Your Family Has Cancer

When Cancer Recurs: Meeting the Challenge Again *

Advanced Cancer: Living Each Day *

* Reprinted in this volume—see Table of Contents.

National Cancer Institute Information Resources

You may want more information for yourself, your family, and your doctor. The following National Cancer Institute (NCI) services are available to help you.

Telephone

Cancer Information Service (CIS): Provides accurate, up-to-date information on cancer to patients and their families, health professionals, and the general public. Information specialists translate the latest scientific information into understandable language and respond in English, Spanish, or on TTY equipment.
Toll-free: 1-800-4-CANCER (1-800-422-6237)
TTY: 1-800-332-8615

Internet

These Web sites may be useful:

http://www.nci.nih.gov: NCI's primary Web site; contains information about the Institute and its programs.

http://cancertrials.nci.nih.gov: Cancer Trials; NCI's comprehensive clinical trials information center for patients, health professionals, and the public. Includes information on understanding trials, deciding whether to participate in trials, finding specific trials, plus research news and other resources.

http://cancernet.nci.nih.gov: CancerNet; contains material for health professionals, patients, and the public, including information from PDQ about cancer treatment, screening, prevention, supportive care, and clinical trials, and CANCERLIT, a bibliographic database.

E-mail

CancerMail includes NCI information about cancer treatment, screening, prevention, and supportive care. To obtain a contents list, send e-mail to cancermail@icicc.nci.nih.gov with the word "help" in the body of the message.

Fax

CancerFax includes NCI information about cancer treatment, screening, prevention, and supportive care. To obtain a contents list, dial 301-402-5874 from a fax machine hand set and follow the recorded instructions.

Chapter 27

Small Intestine Cancer

What Is Cancer of the Small Intestine?

Cancer of the small intestine, a rare cancer, is a disease in which cancer (malignant) cells are found in the tissues of the small intestine. The small intestine is a long tube that folds many times to fit inside the abdomen. It connects the stomach to the large intestine (bowel). In the small intestine, food is broken down to remove vitamins, minerals, proteins, carbohydrates, and fats.

A doctor should be seen if there are any of the following: pain or cramps in the middle of the abdomen, weight loss without dieting, a lump in the abdomen, or blood in the stool.

If there are symptoms, a doctor will usually order an upper gastrointestinal x-ray (also called an upper GI series). For this examination, a patient drinks a liquid containing barium, which makes the stomach and intestine easier to see in the x-ray. This test is usually performed in a doctor's office or in a hospital radiology department.

The doctor may also do a CT scan, a special x-ray that uses a computer to make a picture of the inside of the abdomen. An ultrasound, which uses sound waves to find tumors, or an MRI scan, which uses magnetic waves to make a picture of the abdomen, may also be done.

PDQ Statement, National Cancer Institute (NCI), updated July 1998.

The doctor may put a thin lighted tube called an endoscope down the throat, through the stomach, and into the first part of the small intestine. The doctor may cut out a small piece of tissue during the endoscopy. This is called a biopsy. The tissue is then looked at under a microscope to see if it contains cancer cells.

The chance of recovery (prognosis) depends on the type of cancer, whether it is just in the small intestine or has spread to other tissues, and the patient's overall health.

Stages of Cancer of the Small Intestine

Once small intestine cancer is found, more tests will be done to find out if cancer cells have spread to other parts of the body. Although there is a staging system for cancer of the small intestine, for treatment purposes this cancer is grouped based on what kind of cells are found. Four types of cancer are found in the small intestine: adenocarcinoma, lymphoma, sarcoma, and carcinoid tumors. If a tumor called a carcinoid tumor is found, see the PDQ patient information summary on gastrointestinal carcinoid tumor. If a patient has lymphoma, more information can be obtained from the PDQ patient information summary on adult or childhood non-Hodgkin's lymphoma. If a tumor called a sarcoma is found, see the patient information summary on adult soft tissue sarcoma for more information than is given here.

Adenocarcinoma

Adenocarcinoma starts in the lining of the small intestine and is the most common type of cancer of the small intestine. These tumors occur most often in the part of the small intestine nearest the stomach. These cancers often grow and block the bowel.

Lymphoma

A lymphoma starts from lymph tissue in the small intestine. Lymph tissue is part of the body's immune system, which helps the body fight infections. Most of these tumors are a type of lymphoma called non-Hodgkin's lymphomas.

Leiomyosarcoma

Leiomyosarcomas are cancers that start growing in the smooth muscle lining of the small intestine.

Recurrent

Recurrent disease means that the cancer has come back (recurred) after it has been treated. It may come back in the small intestine or in another part of the body.

How Cancer of the Small Intestine Is Treated

There are treatments for all patients with cancer of the small intestine. Three kinds of treatment are used:

* surgery (taking out the cancer)

* radiation therapy (using high-dose x-rays to kill cancer cells)

* chemotherapy (using drugs to kill cancer cells)

Surgery to remove the cancer is the most common treatment. Lymph nodes in the area may also be removed and looked at under a microscope to see if they contain cancer. If the tumor is large, a doctor may cut out a section of the small intestine containing the cancer and reconnect the intestine.

Radiation therapy uses high-energy x-rays to kill cancer cells and shrink tumors. Radiation may come from a machine outside the body (external radiation therapy) or from putting materials that produce radiation (radioisotopes) through thin plastic tubes in the area where the cancer cells are found (internal radiation therapy). Drugs that make the cancer cells more sensitive to radiation (radiosensitizers) are sometimes given along with radiation. Radiation can be used alone or in addition to surgery and/or chemotherapy.

Chemotherapy uses drugs to kill cancer cells. Chemotherapy may be taken by pill, or it may be put in the body through a needle in a vein or muscle. Chemotherapy is called a systemic treatment because the drug enters the bloodstream, travels through the body, and can kill cancer cells outside the intestine.

If the doctor removes all the cancer that can be seen at the time of the operation, the patient may be given chemotherapy after surgery to kill any cancer cells that are left. Chemotherapy given after an operation is called adjuvant chemotherapy.

Biological therapy (using the body's immune system to fight cancer) is being studied in clinical trials. Biological therapy tries to get the body to fight cancer. It uses materials made by the body or made in a laboratory to boost, direct, or restore the body's natural defenses against disease. Biological therapy is sometimes called biological response modifier (BRM) therapy or immunotherapy.

Treatment by Stage

Treatments for cancer of the small intestine depend on the type of cancer, how far it has spread, and the patient's general health and age.

Standard treatment may be considered because of its effectiveness in patients in past studies, or participation in a clinical trial may be considered. Not all patients are cured with standard therapy and some standard treatments may have more side effects than are desired. For these reasons, clinical trials are designed to find better ways to treat cancer patients and are based on the most up-to-date information. Clinical trials are ongoing in some parts of the country for patients with cancer of the small intestine. To learn more about clinical trials, call the Cancer Information Service at 1-800-4-CANCER (1-800-422-6237); TTY at 1-800-332-8615.

Small Intestine Adenocarcinoma

Treatment may be one of the following:

1. Surgery to cut out the tumor.

2. Surgery to allow food in the small intestine to go around the cancer (bypass) if the cancer cannot be removed.

3. Radiation therapy to relieve symptoms.

4. A clinical trial of radiation plus drugs to make cancer cells more sensitive to radiation (radiosensitizers), with or without chemotherapy.

5. A clinical trial of chemotherapy or biological therapy.

Small Intestine Lymphoma

Treatment may be one of the following:

1. Surgery to remove the cancer and nearby lymph nodes.

2. Surgery followed by adjuvant chemotherapy or radiation therapy.

3. Chemotherapy with or without radiation therapy.

See the PDQ patient information summary on adult or childhood non-Hodgkin's lymphoma for more information.

Small Intestine Leiomyosarcoma

Treatment may be one of the following:

1. Surgery to remove the cancer.

2. Surgery to allow food in the small intestine to go around the cancer (bypass) if the cancer cannot be removed.

3. Radiation therapy.

4. Surgery, chemotherapy, or radiation therapy to relieve symptoms.

5. A clinical trial of chemotherapy or biological therapy.

See the PDQ patient information summary on adult or childhood soft tissue sarcoma for more information.

Recurrent Small Intesine Cancer

If the cancer comes back in another part of the body, treatment will probably be a clinical trial of chemotherapy or biological therapy.

If the cancer has come back only in one area, treatment may be one of the following:

1. Surgery to remove the cancer.

2. Radiation therapy or chemotherapy to relieve symptoms.

3. A clinical trial of radiation with drugs to make the cancer cells more sensitive to radiation (radiosensitizers), with or without chemotherapy.

See the PDQ patient information summary on adult or childhood non-Hodgkin's lymphoma for treatment of recurrent small intestine lymphoma or the summary on adult or childhood soft tissue sarcoma for treatment of recurrent small intestine sarcoma.

To Learn More

Cancer patients, their families and friends, and others may find the following booklets useful. They are available free of charge by calling 1-800-4-CANCER or writing:

Office of Cancer Communications
National Cancer Institute
Building 31, Room 10A24
Bethesda, MD 20892

Booklets about Cancer Treatment

Radiation Therapy and You: A Guide to Self-Help During Treatment *

Chemotherapy and You: A Guide to Self-Help During Treatment *

Eating Hints: Recipes and Tips for Better Nutrition During Cancer Treatment *

Questions and Answers About Pain Control

What Are Clinical Trials All About?

Booklets about Living with Cancer

Taking Time: Support for People With Cancer and the People Who Care About Them

When Cancer Recurs: Meeting the Challenge Again *

Advanced Cancer: Living Each Day *

* Reprinted in this volume—see Table of Contents

Chapter 28

Gastrointestinal Carcinoid Tumor

What Is Gastrointestinal Carcinoid Tumor?

Gastrointestinal carcinoid tumors are cancers in which cancer (malignant) cells are found in certain hormone-making cells of the digestive, or gastrointestinal, system. The digestive system absorbs vitamins, minerals, carbohydrates, fats, proteins, and water from the food that is eaten and stores waste until the body eliminates it. The digestive system is made up of the stomach and the small and large intestines. The last six feet of intestine is called the colon. The last 10 inches of the colon is the rectum. The appendix is an organ attached to the large intestine.

There are often no signs of a gastrointestinal carcinoid tumor in its early stages. Often the cancer will make too much of some of the hormones, which can cause symptoms. A doctor should be seen if the following symptoms persist: pain in the abdomen, flushing and swelling of the skin of the face and neck, wheezing, diarrhea, and symptoms of heart failure, including breathlessness.

If there are symptoms, a doctor may order blood and urine tests to look for signs of cancer. Other tests may also be done. If there is a carcinoid tumor, the patient has a greater chance of getting other cancers in the digestive system, either at the same time or at a later time.

PDQ Statement, National Cancer Institute (NCI), updated January 1998.

The chance of recovery (prognosis) and choice of treatment depend on whether the cancer is just in the gastrointestinal system or has spread to other places, and on the patient's general state of health.

Stages of Gastrointestinal Carcinoid Tumors

Once gastrointestinal carcinoid tumor is found, more tests will be done to find out if cancer cells have spread to other parts of the body. This is called staging. A doctor needs to know the stage of the disease to plan treatment. The following stages are used for gastrointestinal carcinoid tumor:

Localized

The cancer is found in the appendix, the colon or rectum, the small intestine, or stomach, but it has not spread to other parts of the body.

Regional

Cancer has spread from the appendix, colon or rectum, stomach, or small intestine to nearby tissues or lymph nodes. (Lymph nodes are small, bean-shaped structures that are found throughout the body. They produce and store infection-fighting cells.)

Metastatic

Cancer has spread to other parts of the body.

Recurrent

Recurrent disease means that the cancer has come back (recurred) after it has been treated. It may come back in the first place it was found or in another part of the body.

How Gastrointestinal Carcinoid Tumors Are Treated

There are treatments for all patients with gastrointestinal carcinoid tumors. Four kinds of treatment are used:

- surgery (taking out the cancer)
- radiation therapy (using high-dose x-rays to kill cancer cells)
- biological response modifier therapy (using the body's natural immune system to fight cancer)

- chemotherapy (using drugs to kill cancer cells)

Depending on where the cancer started, the doctor may take out the cancer using one of the following operations:

- A simple appendectomy removes the appendix. If part of the colon is also taken out, the operation is called a hemicolectomy. The doctor may also remove lymph nodes and look at them under a microscope to see if they contain cancer.

- Local excision uses a special instrument inserted into the colon or rectum through the anus to cut the tumor out. This operation can be used for very small tumors.

- Fulguration uses a special tool inserted into the colon or rectum through the anus. An electric current is then used to burn the tumor away.

- Bowel resection takes out the cancer and a small amount of healthy tissue on either side. The healthy parts of the bowel are then sewn together. The doctor will also remove lymph nodes and have them looked at under a microscope to see if they contain cancer.

- Cryosurgery kills the cancer by freezing it.

- Hepatic artery ligation cuts and ties off the main blood vessel that brings blood into the liver (the hepatic artery).

- Hepatic artery embolization uses drugs or other agents to reduce or block the flow of blood to the liver in order to kill cancer cells growing in the liver.

Radiation therapy uses high-energy x-rays to kill cancer cells and shrink tumors. Radiation may come from a machine outside the body (external radiation therapy) or from putting materials that produce radiation (radioisotopes) through thin plastic tubes in the area where the cancer cells are found (internal radiation therapy).

Chemotherapy uses drugs to kill cancer cells. Chemotherapy may be taken by pill, or it may be put into the body by a needle in the vein or muscle. Chemotherapy is called a systemic treatment because the drug enters the bloodstream, travels through the body, and can kill cancer cells outside the digestive system.

Biological therapy tries to get the patient's body to fight the cancer. It uses materials made by the body or made in a laboratory to boost, direct, or restore the body's natural defenses against disease. Biological therapy is sometimes called biological response modifier (BRM) therapy or immunotherapy.

Treatment by Type

Treatment of gastrointestinal carcinoid tumor depends on the type of tumor, the stage, and the patient's overall health.

Standard treatment may be considered because of its effectiveness in patients in past studies, or participation in a clinical trial may be considered. Not all patients are cured with standard therapy and some standard treatments may have more side effects than are desired. For these reasons, clinical trials are designed to find better ways to treat cancer patients and are based on the most up-to-date information. Clinical trials are ongoing in most parts of the country for most stages of gastrointestinal carcinoid tumor. To learn more about clinical trials, call the Cancer Information Service at 1-800-4-CANCER (1-800-422-6237); TTY at 1-800-332-8615.

Localized Gastrointestinal Carcinoid Tumor

If the cancer started in the appendix, the treatment will probably be surgery to remove the appendix (appendectomy) with or without removal of part of the colon (hemicolectomy).

If the cancer started in the rectum, treatment may be one of the following:

1. Local excision.

2. Simple fulguration.

3. Surgery to remove part of the bowel (bowel resection).

If the cancer started in the small intestine, the treatment will probably be surgery to remove part of the bowel (bowel resection). Lymph nodes may also be taken out and looked at under the microscope to see if they contain cancer.

If the cancer started in the stomach, pancreas, or colon, the treatment will probably be surgery to remove part of the gastrointestinal tract.

Regional Gastrointestinal Carcinoid Tumor

The treatment will probably be surgery to remove the cancer.

Metastatic Gastrointestinal Carcinoid Tumor

Treatment may be one of the following:

1. Surgery to remove the cancer. If the cancer has spread to the liver, treatment may include cryosurgery.

2. Chemotherapy.

3. Hepatic arterial embolization to kill cancer cells growing in the liver.

4. Radiation therapy to relieve pain and discomfort.

Carcinoid Syndrome

Treatment may be one of the following:

1. Surgery to remove the cancer.

2. Surgery to cut and tie the main artery that goes to the liver (hepatic artery ligation).

3. Hepatic arterial embolization to kill cancer cells growing in the liver.

4. Drugs to relieve symptoms such as diarrhea.

5. Biological therapy to relieve symptoms.

6. Chemotherapy.

7. A clinical trial of chemotherapy to relieve symptoms.

Recurrent Gastrointestinal Carcinoid Tumor

The treatment depends on many factors, including where the cancer came back and what treatment the patient received before. Clinical trials are studying new treatments.

To Learn More

To learn more about gastrointestinal carcinoid tumors, call the National Cancer Institute's Cancer Information Service at 1-800-4-CANCER (1-800-422-6237); TTY at 1-800-332-8615. By dialing this toll-free number, trained information specialists can answer your questions.

Booklets about Cancer Treatment

Radiation Therapy and You: A Guide to Self-Help During Treatment *

Chemotherapy and You: A Guide to Self-Help During Treatment *

Eating Hints: Recipes and Tips for Better Nutrition During Cancer Treatment *

Questions and Answers About Pain Control

What Are Clinical Trials All About?

Booklets about Living with Cancer

Taking Time: Support for People With Cancer and the People Who Care About Them

When Cancer Recurs: Meeting the Challenge Again *

Advanced Cancer: Living Each Day *

* Reprinted in this volume—see Table of Contents

Chapter 29

Cancer of the Colon and Rectum

Introduction

The diagnosis of cancer raises many questions and a need for clear, understandable answers. We hope this chapter from the National Cancer Institute (NCI) will help. It provides information about some of the possible causes and prevention of colorectal cancer and describes the symptoms, detection and diagnosis, and treatment of this disease. Having this important information can make it easier for patients and their families to handle the challenges they face.

Colorectal cancer is one of the most common cancers in the United States. It occurs in both men and women and is most often found among people who are over the age of 50.

Cancer research has led to real progress against colorectal cancer— a lower chance of death and an improved quality of life. And our knowledge is increasing. The NCI resources listed in the National Cancer Institute Resources section can provide the latest, most accurate information on colorectal cancer. To order this publication, call the Cancer Information Service (CIS) toll free at 1-800-4-CANCER (1-800-422-6237).

Understanding the Cancer Process

Cancer affects our cells, the body's basic unit of life. To understand cancer, it is helpful to know how normal cells become cancerous.

"What You Need To Know About Cancer of the Colon and Rectum," National Cancer Institute (NCI), updated September 1998.

The body is made up of many types of cells. Normally, cells grow, divide, and produce more cells to keep the body healthy and functioning properly. Sometimes, however, the process goes astray—cells keep dividing when new cells are not needed. The mass of extra cells forms a growth or tumor. Tumors can be benign or malignant.

- Benign tumors are not cancer. They often can be removed and, in most cases, they do not come back. Cells in benign tumors do not spread to other parts of the body. Most important, benign tumors are rarely a threat to life.

- Malignant tumors are cancer. Cells in malignant tumors are abnormal and divide without control or order. These cancer cells can invade and destroy the tissue around them. Cancer cells can also break away from a malignant tumor and enter the bloodstream or lymphatic system (the tissues and organs that produce and store cells which fight infection and disease). This process, called metastasis, is how cancer spreads from the original tumor to form new tumors in other parts of the body.

The Colon and Rectum

The colon and rectum are parts of the body's digestive system, which removes nutrients from food and stores waste until it passes out of the body. Together, the colon and rectum form a long, muscular tube called the large intestine (also called the large bowel). The colon is the first 6 feet of the large intestine and the rectum is the last 8 to 10 inches.

Understanding Colorectal Cancer

Cancer that begins in the colon is called colon cancer, and cancer that begins in the rectum is called rectal cancer. Cancers affecting either of these organs may also be called colorectal cancer.

Colorectal Cancer: Who's at Risk?

The exact causes of colorectal cancer are not known. However, studies show that the following factors increase a person's likelihood of developing colorectal cancer:

- *Age:* Colorectal cancer is more likely to occur as people get older. Most people who develop colorectal cancer are over the age of 50. However, the disease can occur at any age.

- *Diet:* The development of colorectal cancer seems to be associated with a diet that is high in fat and calories and low in foods with fiber, such as whole grains, fruits, and vegetables. Researchers are exploring how these and other dietary components play a role in the development of colorectal cancer.

- *Polyps:* Polyps are benign growths on the inner wall of the colon and rectum. They are relatively common in people over age 50. Because most colorectal cancers develop in polyps, detecting and removing these growths may be a way to prevent colorectal cancer. Familial polyposis is a rare, inherited condition in which hundreds of polyps develop in the colon and rectum. Unless this condition is treated, a person who has it is extremely likely to develop colorectal cancer at some point in his or her lifetime.

- *Personal history:* A person who has already had colorectal cancer may develop colorectal cancer a second time. Research studies also show that women with a history of ovarian, uterine, or breast cancer have a somewhat increased chance of developing colorectal cancer.

- *Family history:* First-degree relatives (parents, siblings, children) of a person who has had colorectal cancer are somewhat more likely to develop this type of cancer themselves, especially if the relative developed the cancer at a young age. If many family members have had colorectal cancer, the chances increase even more.

- *Ulcerative colitis:* Ulcerative colitis is a condition in which the lining of the colon becomes inflamed. People who have ulcerative colitis are more likely to develop colorectal cancer.

Having one or more of these factors does not guarantee a person will develop colorectal cancer. It just increases the chances. People who are concerned about their health may want to talk with a doctor. The doctor may be able to suggest ways to reduce the chance of developing colorectal cancer and can plan an appropriate schedule for checkups.

Cancer Prevention

The National Cancer Institute is supporting and conducting research on the causes and prevention of colorectal cancer. Researchers are evaluating the benefits of lifestyle changes, including smoking cessation, use of dietary supplements, use of aspirin or similar products, decreased alcohol consumption, and increased physical activity, in preventing colorectal cancer. They have also discovered that changes in certain genes (basic units of heredity) are responsible for inherited colorectal cancer. Individuals in families with many cases of colorectal cancer may have a special blood test to see if they have the genetic change that increases the chance of developing this disease. Although having such a genetic change does not mean that a person is sure to develop colorectal cancer, those who have the change may want to discuss prevention and early detection options with their doctor.

Detecting Cancer Early

People who have any of the risk factors described above should ask their doctor when to begin screening for colorectal cancer, what tests to have, and how often to schedule appointments. Doctors may suggest one or more of the tests listed below as a part of regular checkups. These tests are used to detect polyps, cancer, or other abnormalities, even when a person does not have symptoms.

- A fecal occult blood test (FOBT), a test used to check for hidden blood in the stool, has been proved to reduce the death rate of colorectal cancer.

- A sigmoidoscopy is an examination of the rectum and lower colon with a lighted instrument.

- A colonoscopy is an examination of the rectum and entire colon with a lighted instrument.

- A double contrast barium enema is a series of x-rays of the large intestine. The x-rays are taken after the patient is given an enema with a white, chalky solution that contains barium to outline the colon on the x-rays.

- A digital rectal exam (DRE) is a test in which the doctor inserts a lubricated, gloved finger into the rectum to feel for abnormal areas.

Recognizing Symptoms

Common signs and symptoms of colorectal cancer include:

- A change in bowel habits

- Diarrhea, constipation, or feeling that the bowel does not empty completely

- Blood in the stool (either bright red or very dark in color)

- Stools that are narrower than usual

- General abdominal discomfort (frequent gas pains, bloating, fullness, and/or cramps)

- Weight loss with no known reason

- Constant tiredness

- Vomiting

These symptoms are often caused by other conditions. It is important to check with a doctor.

Diagnosing Colorectal Cancer

To help find the cause of symptoms, the doctor evaluates a person's medical history. The doctor also performs a physical exam and may order one or more diagnostic tests.

- X-rays of the gastrointestinal tract are sometimes taken.

- A sigmoidoscopy is a procedure in which the doctor looks inside the rectum and the lower part of the colon (sigmoid colon) through a lighted instrument. The doctor may remove polyps and other abnormal tissue for examination.

- A colonoscopy is a procedure in which the doctor examines the rectum and the entire colon with a lighted instrument. It can be used to remove polyps or other abnormal tissue.

- A biopsy is the removal of tissue for examination by a pathologist under a microscope to determine if a person has cancer.

- A CEA (carcinoembryonic antigen) assay is a blood test used to measure a protein called carcinoembryonic antigen that is sometimes higher in patients with colorectal cancer.

If the diagnosis is cancer, the doctor will want to learn the stage (or extent) of disease. Staging is a careful attempt to find out whether the cancer has spread and, if so, to what parts of the body. Knowing the stage of the disease helps the doctor plan treatment. Additional laboratory or imaging tests may also be performed to help determine the stage.

Treatment for Colorectal Cancer

Treatment depends on a number of factors, including the general health of the patient and the size, location, and extent of the tumor. Patients are often treated by a team of specialists, which may include a gastroenterologist, surgeon, medical oncologist, and radiation oncologist. Many different treatments and combinations of treatments are used to treat colorectal cancer.

Surgery to remove cancer is the most common treatment for colorectal cancer. The type of surgery that a doctor performs depends on where the cancer is found. If colon cancer is found in a polyp, the polyp is often removed using a colonoscope in an operation called a polypectomy. If a larger area is affected, the doctor may need to perform abdominal surgery to remove the tumor along with part of the healthy colon or rectum and nearby lymph nodes.

In most cases, the doctor is able to reconnect the remaining healthy portions of the colon or rectum. When the surgeon cannot reconnect the healthy portions, a temporary or permanent colostomy may be necessary. A colostomy is a surgical opening (stoma) through the wall of the abdomen into the colon that provides a new path for waste material to leave the body. If a colostomy is needed, the patient will need to wear a special bag to collect body wastes. Some patients need a temporary colostomy to help the lower colon or rectum heal after surgery. About 15 percent of colorectal cancer patients require a permanent colostomy.

Chemotherapy is the use of anticancer drugs to kill cancer cells throughout the body. Chemotherapy may be given to destroy any cancerous cells that may remain in the body after surgery, control tumor growth, or relieve symptoms of the disease. Most anticancer drugs are given by injection into a vein (IV); some are given in the form of a pill. Another way to get IV chemotherapy is by means of a catheter, a thin tube that is placed into a large vein and remains there as long as it is needed.

Radiation therapy, also called radiotherapy, involves the use of high-energy x-rays to kill cancer cells. Radiation therapy is a local treatment and affects the cancer cells only in the treated area. Most often it is used in patients whose cancer is in the rectum. Doctors may use radiation therapy before surgery to shrink a tumor so that it is easier to remove or after surgery to destroy any cancer cells that remain in the treated area. Radiation therapy is also used to relieve symptoms. The radiation may come from a machine (external radiation) or from an implant (a small container of radioactive material) placed directly into or near the tumor (internal radiation). Some patients have both kinds of radiation therapy.

Biological therapy, also called immunotherapy, uses the body's immune system, either directly or indirectly, to fight cancer. The immune system recognizes cancer cells in the body and works to eliminate them. Biological therapies are designed to repair, stimulate, or enhance the immune system's natural anticancer function. Biological therapy may be given after surgery, either alone or in combination with chemotherapy or radiation treatment. Most biological treatments are given by injection into a vein (IV).

Clinical trials (treatment studies) to evaluate new ways to treat cancer are an appropriate treatment option for many cancer patients with colorectal cancer. In some studies, all cancer patients receive the new treatment. In others, doctors compare different therapies by giving the promising new treatment to one group of patients and the usual (standard) therapy to another group. Research has led to significant advances in the treatment of colorectal cancer. Through research, doctors learn new ways to treat cancer that may be more effective than the standard therapy. The NCI publication *Taking Part in Clinical Trials: What Cancer Patients Need To Know* provides information about how these studies work. Detailed information about ongoing studies for colorectal cancer can be found in PDQ, NCI's cancer information database.

PDQ, NCI's cancer information database, contains current information on cancer prevention, screening, treatment, and supportive care. PDQ also describes active research studies. The Cancer Information Service can provide information from PDQ for patients and their families and health professionals. PDQ is also easily accessible through the resources listed in the Resources section.

Side Effects

The side effects of cancer treatment depend on the type of treatment and may be different for each person. Most often the side effects are temporary. Doctors and nurses can explain the possible side effects of treatment. Patients should report troublesome or severe side effects to their doctor. Doctors can suggest ways to help relieve symptoms that may occur during and after treatment.

Surgery causes short-term pain and tenderness in the area of the operation. Occasionally, the wound may become infected. Surgery for colorectal cancer may also cause temporary constipation or diarrhea. Patients who have a colostomy may have irritation on the skin around the stoma. The doctor, nurse, or enterostomal therapist can teach the patient how to clean the area and prevent irritation and infection.

Chemotherapy affects normal as well as cancerous cells. Side effects depend largely on the specific drugs and the dose (amount of drug administered). Common side effects of chemotherapy include nausea and vomiting, hair loss, mouth sores, diarrhea, and fatigue. Less often, serious side effects may occur, such as infection or bleeding.

Radiation therapy, like chemotherapy, affects normal as well as cancerous cells. Side effects of radiation therapy depend mainly on the treatment dose. Common side effects of radiation therapy are fatigue, skin changes at the site where the treatment is given, a loss of appetite, nausea, and diarrhea. Sometimes, radiation therapy can cause bleeding through the rectum (bloody stools).

Biological therapy may cause side effects that vary with the specific type of treatment. Often, treatments cause flu-like symptoms, such as chills, fever, weakness, and nausea.

Several useful NCI booklets, including *Chemotherapy and You* [reprinted in this volume as Chapter 63], *Radiation Therapy and You* [Chapter 66] and *Eating Hints for Cancer Patients* [Chapter 77], suggest ways for patients to cope with the side effects they experience during cancer treatment.

Doctors and nurses can explain the possible side effects of treatment. Patients should report troublesome or severe side effects to their doctor. Doctors can suggest ways to help relieve symptoms that may occur during and after treatment.

The Importance of Followup Care

Followup care after treatment for colorectal cancer is important. Regular checkups may include a physical exam, a fecal occult blood test, a colonoscopy, chest x-rays, and blood tests. The doctor may also perform additional tests. In addition to having followup exams to check for the return of colorectal cancer, patients may also want to ask their doctor about checking them for other types of cancer. Persons who have had colorectal cancer are somewhat more likely to develop certain other cancers during their lifetime.

Providing Emotional Support

Living with a serious disease, such as cancer, is challenging. Apart from having to cope with the physical and medical challenges, people with cancer face many worries, feelings, and concerns that can make life difficult. They may find they need help coping with the emotional as well as the practical aspects of their disease. In fact, attention to the emotional burden of having cancer is often a part of a patient's treatment plan. The support of the health care team (doctors, nurses, social workers), support groups, and patient-to-patient networks can help people feel less isolated and distressed, and improve the quality of their lives. Cancer support groups provide a safe environment where cancer patients can talk about living with cancer with others who may be having similar experiences. Patients may want to speak to a member of their health care team about finding a support group. Many also find useful information in NCI fact sheets and booklets, including *Taking Time* and *Facing Forward.*

Questions for Your Doctor

This chapter is designed to help you get information you need from your doctor, so that you can make informed decisions about your health care. In addition, asking your doctor the following questions will help you further understand your condition. To help you remember what the doctor says, you may takes notes or ask whether you may use a tape recorder. Some people also want to have a family member or friend with them when they talk to the doctor—to take part in the discussion, to take notes, or just to listen.

Diagnosis

- What tests can diagnose colorectal cancer? Are they painful?
- How soon after the tests will I learn the results?

Treatment

- What is the stage of my cancer?
- What treatments are recommended for me?
- What clinical trials are appropriate for my type of cancer?
- Will I need a colostomy? When is a permanent colostomy necessary?
- What will happen if I don't have the suggested treatment?
- Will I need to be in the hospital to receive my treatment? For how long?
- How might my normal activities change during my treatment?

- After treatment, how often do I need to be checked? What type of followup care should I have?

Side Effects

- What side effects should I expect? How long will side effects last?

- Who should I call if I am concerned about the type or length of time a side effect lasts?

The Health Care Team

- Who will be involved with my treatment an rehabilitation? What role does each member of the health care team play in my care?

- What has been your experience in caring for patients with colorectal cancer?

Resources

- Are there support groups in the area with people I can talk to?

- Are there organizations where I can get more information about cancer, specifically colorectal cancer?

National Cancer Institute Information Resources

You may want more information for yourself, your family, and your doctor. The following National Cancer Institute (NCI) services are available to help you.

Telephone

Cancer Information Service (CIS) Provides accurate, up-to-date information on cancer to patients and their families, health professionals, and the general public. Information specialists translate the latest scientific information into understandable language and respond in English, Spanish, or on TTY equipment.
Toll-free: 1-800-4-CANCER (1-800-422-6237)
TTY: 1-800-332-8615

Internet

These Web sites may be useful:

http://www.nci.nih.gov—NCI's primary Web site; contains information about the Institute and its programs.

http://cancertrials.nci.nih.gov—CancerTrials; NCI's comprehensive clinical trials information center for patients, health professionals, and the public. Includes information on understanding trials, deciding whether to participate in trials, finding specific trials, plus research news and other resources.

http://cancernet.nci.nih.gov—CancerNet; contains material for health professionals, patients, and the public, including information from PDQ about cancer treatment, screening, prevention, supportive care, and clinical trials, and CANCERLIT, a bibliographic database.

E-mail

CancerMail—Includes NCI information about cancer treatment, screening, prevention, and supportive care. To obtain a contents list, send e-mail to cancermail@icicc.nci.nih.gov with the word "help" in the body of the message.

Fax

CancerFax—Includes NCI information about cancer treatment, screening, prevention, and supportive care. To obtain a contents list, dial 301-402-5874 from a fax machine hand set and follow the recorded instructions.

Chapter 30

Anal Cancer

What Is Anal Cancer?

Anal cancer, an uncommon cancer, is a disease in which cancer (malignant) cells are found in the anus. The anus is the opening at the end of the rectum (the end part of the large intestine) through which body waste passes. Cancer in the outer part of the anus is more likely to occur in men; cancer of the inner part of the rectum (anal canal) is more likely to occur in women. If the anus is often red, swollen, and sore, there is a greater chance of getting anal cancer. Tumors found in the area of skin with hair on it just outside the anus are skin tumors, not anal cancer.

A doctor should be seen if one or more of the following symptoms appear: bleeding from the rectum (even a small amount), pain or pressure in the area around the anus, itching or discharge from the anus, or a lump near the anus.

If there are signs of cancer, a doctor will usually examine the outside part of the anus and give a patient a rectal examination. In a rectal examination, a doctor, wearing thin gloves, puts a greased finger into the rectum and gently feels for lumps. The doctor may also check any material on the glove to see if there is blood in it. The doctor may give the patient general anesthesia, medicine that puts patients to sleep, to continue the examination if pain is felt during it. The doctor may cut out a small piece of tissue and look at it under a microscope to see if there are any cancer cells. This procedure is called a biopsy.

PDQ Statement, National Cancer Institute (NCI), updated January 1999.

The prognosis (chance of recovery) and choice of treatment depend on the stage of the cancer (whether it is just in the anus or has spread to other places in the body) and the patient's general health.

Stages of Anal Cancer

Once anal cancer is found (diagnosed), more tests will be done to find out if cancer cells have spread to other parts of the body. This testing is called staging. To plan treatment, a doctor needs to know the stage of the disease. The following stages are used for anal cancer.

Stage 0 or Carcinoma in Situ

Stage 0 anal cancer is very early cancer. The cancer is found only in the top layer of anal tissue.

Stage I

The cancer has spread beyond the top layer of anal tissue and is smaller than 2 centimeters (less than 1 inch).

Stage II

Cancer has spread beyond the top layer of anal tissue and is larger than 2 centimeters (about 1 inch), but it has not spread to nearby organs or lymph nodes. (Lymph nodes are small, bean-shaped structures found throughout the body. They produce and store infection-fighting cells.)

Stage IIIA

Cancer has spread to the lymph nodes around the rectum or to nearby organs such as the vagina or bladder.

Stage IIIB

Cancer has spread to the lymph nodes in the middle of the abdomen or in the groin, or the cancer has spread to both nearby organs and the lymph nodes around the rectum.

Stage IV

Cancer has spread to distant lymph nodes within the abdomen or to organs in other parts of the body.

Recurrent

Recurrent disease means that the cancer has come back (recurred) after it has been treated. It may come back in the anus or in another part of the body.

How Anal Cancer Is Treated

There are treatments for all patients with anal cancer. Three kinds of treatment are used:

- surgery (taking out the cancer in an operation)
- radiation therapy (using high-dose x-rays or other high-energy rays to kill cancer cells)
- chemotherapy (using drugs to kill cancer cells)

Surgery is a common way to diagnose and treat anal cancer. A doctor may take out the cancer using one of the following methods:

- Local resection is an operation that takes out only the cancer. Often the ring of muscle around the anus that opens and closes it (the sphincter muscle) can be saved during surgery so that you will be able to pass the body wastes as before.

- Abdominoperineal resection is an operation in which the doctor removes the anus and the lower part of the rectum by cutting into the abdomen and the perineum, which is the space between the anus and the scrotum (in men) or the anus and the vulva (in women). A doctor will then make an opening (stoma) on the outside of the body for waste to pass out of the body. This opening is called a colostomy. Although this operation was once commonly used for anal cancer, it is not used as much today because radiation therapy with or without chemotherapy is an equally effective treatment option but does not require a colostomy. If a patient has a colostomy, a special bag will need to be worn to collect body wastes. This bag, which sticks to the skin around the stoma with a special glue, can be thrown away after it is used. This bag does not show under clothing, and most people take care of these bags themselves. Lymph nodes may also be taken out at the same time or in a separate operation (lymph node dissection).

Radiation therapy uses x-rays or other high-energy rays to kill cancer cells and shrink tumors. Radiation may come from a machine outside the body (external radiation therapy) or from putting materials that produce radiation (radioisotopes) through thin plastic tubes in the area where the cancer cells are found (internal radiation therapy). Radiation can be used alone or in addition to other treatments.

Chemotherapy uses drugs to kill cancer cells. Chemotherapy may be taken by pill, or it may be put into the body by a needle in a vein or muscle. Chemotherapy is called a systemic treatment because the drugs enter the bloodstream, travel through the body, and can kill cancer cells throughout the body. Some chemotherapy drugs can also make cancer cells more sensitive to radiation therapy. Radiation therapy and chemotherapy can be used together to shrink tumors and make an abdominoperineal resection unnecessary. When only limited surgery is required, the sphincter muscle can often be saved.

Treatment by Stage

Treatments for anal cancer depend on the type of disease, stage of disease, and the patient's age and general health.

Standard treatment may be considered, based on its effectiveness in patients in past studies, or participation in a clinical trial. Not all patients are cured with standard therapy, and some standard treatments may have more side effects than are desired. For these reasons, clinical trials are designed to find better ways to treat cancer patients and are based on the most up-to-date information. Clinical trials are ongoing in most parts of the country for most stages of anal cancer. For more information about clinical trials, call the Cancer Information Service at 1-800-4-CANCER (1-800-422-6237); TTY at 1-800-332-8615.

Stage O Anal Cancer

Treatment will probably be local resection.

Stage I Anal Cancer

Treatment may be one of the following:

1. Local resection (for some small tumors).

2. External radiation therapy with or without chemotherapy. Some patients may also receive internal radiation therapy.

3. If cancer cells remain following therapy, surgery may be needed to remove cancer in the anal canal.

4. If cancer cells remain following therapy, additional chemotherapy and radiation therapy may be needed.

5. External radiation therapy followed by internal radiation therapy.

Stage II Anal Cancer

Treatment may be one of the following:

1. Local resection (for small tumors).

2. External radiation therapy with chemotherapy. Some patients may also receive internal radiation therapy.

3. If cancer cells remain following therapy, surgery may be needed to remove cancer in the anal canal.

4. If cancer cells remain following therapy, additional chemotherapy and radiation therapy may be needed.

Stage IIIA Anal Cancer

Treatment may be one of the following:

1. Radiation therapy with chemotherapy.

2. Depending on how much cancer remains following the initial radiation therapy and chemotherapy, additional radiation therapy and chemotherapy may be given. Some patients may also receive internal radiation therapy.

3. Surgery. Depending on how much cancer remains following chemotherapy and radiation, local resection or surgery may be done to remove cancer in the anal canal.

4. Surgery (resection) followed by radiation therapy.

Stage IIIB Anal Cancer

Treatment will probably be radiation therapy and chemotherapy followed by surgery. Depending on how much cancer remains following chemotherapy and radiation, local resection or surgery to remove the anus and the lower part of the rectum (abdominoperineal resection) may be done. During surgery, the lymph nodes in the groin may be removed (lymph node dissection).

Stage IV Anal Cancer

Treatment may be one of the following:

1. Surgery to relieve symptoms.

2. Radiation therapy to relieve symptoms.

3. Chemotherapy and radiation therapy to relieve symptoms.

4. Clinical trials.

Recurrent Anal Cancer

The choice of treatment will be based on what treatment the patient received when the cancer was first treated. If the patient was treated with surgery, radiation therapy may be given if the cancer recurs. If the patient were treated with radiation, surgery may be used if the cancer recurs. Clinical trials are studying new chemotherapy drugs with or without radiation therapy. The patient may also receive additional chemotherapy and radiation therapy.

To Learn More

To learn more about anal cancer, call the National Cancer Institute's Cancer Information Service at 1-800-4-CANCER (1-800-422-6237); TTY at 1-800-332-8615. By dialing this toll-free number, you can speak with a trained information specialist who can answer your questions.

Cancer patients, their families and friends, and others may find the following booklets useful. They are available free of charge by calling 1-800-4-CANCER or writing:

Office of Cancer Communications
National Cancer Institute
Building 31, Room 10A24
Bethesda, MD 20892

Booklets about Cancer Treatment

Radiation Therapy and You: A Guide to Self-Help During Treatment *

Chemotherapy and You: A Guide to Self-Help During Treatment *

Eating Hints: Recipes and Tips for Better Nutrition During Cancer Treatment *

Questions and Answers About Pain Control

What Are Clinical Trials All About?

Booklets about Living with Cancer

Taking Time: Support for People With Cancer and the People Who Care About Them

When Cancer Recurs: Meeting the Challenge Again *

Advanced Cancer: Living Each Day *

* Reprinted in this volume—see Table of Contents

Chapter 31

Urethral Cancer

What Is Cancer of the Urethra?

Cancer of the urethra, a rare type of cancer, is a disease in which cancer (malignant) cells are found in the urethra. The urethra is the tube that empties urine from the bladder, the hollow organ in the lower abdomen that stores urine. In women, the urethra is about 1½ inches long and opens to the outside of the body above the vagina. In men, the urethra is about 8 inches long and goes through the prostate gland and then through the penis to the outside of the body. Cancer of the urethra affects women more often then men.

There may be no symptoms of early cancer of the urethra. A doctor should be seen if there is a lump or growth on the urethra, or pain, bleeding, or other difficulty during urination.

If there are symptoms, a doctor will examine the patient and feel for lumps in the urethra. In men, a thin lighted tube called a cystoscope may be inserted into the penis so the doctor can see inside the urethra. If the doctor finds cells or other signs that are not normal, a small piece of tissue (called a biopsy) may be cut out and looked at under a microscope for cancer cells.

The chance of recovery (prognosis) and choice of treatment depend on the stage of the cancer (whether it is just in one area or has spread to other places) and the patient's general state of health.

PDQ Statement, National Cancer Institute (NCI), updated July 1998.

Stages of Cancer of the Urethra

Once cancer of the urethra is found, more tests will be done to find out if cancer cells have spread to other parts of the body (staging). A doctor needs to know the stage of the disease to plan treatment. For cancer of the urethra, patients are grouped into stages depending on where the tumor is and whether it has spread to other places. The following stage groupings are used for cancer of the urethra:

Anterior Urethral Cancer

The part of the urethra that is closest to the outside of the body is called the anterior urethra, and cancers that start here are called anterior urethral cancers.

Posterior Urethral Cancer

The part of the urethra that connects to the bladder is called the posterior urethra, and cancers that start here are called posterior urethral cancers. Because the posterior urethra is closer to the bladder and other tissues, cancers that start here are more likely to grow through the inner lining of the urethra and affect nearby tissues.

Urethral Cancer Associated with Invasive Bladder Cancer

Occasionally, patients who have bladder cancer also have cancer of the urethra. This is called urethral cancer associated with invasive bladder cancer.

Recurrent Urethral Cancer

Recurrent cancer means that the cancer has come back (recurred) after it has been treated. It may come back in the same place, or in another part of the body.

How Cancer of the Urethra Is Treated

There are treatments for all patients with cancer of the urethra. Three kinds of treatment are used:

- Surgery (taking out the cancer in an operation)
- Radiation therapy (using high-dose x-rays or other high-energy rays to kill cancer cells)
- Chemotherapy (using drugs to kill cancer cells)

Surgery is the most common treatment of cancer of the urethra. A doctor may take out the cancer using one of the following operations:

- Electrofulguration uses an electric current to remove the cancer. The tumor and the area around it are burned away and then removed with a sharp tool.

- Laser therapy uses a narrow beam of intense light to kill cancer cells.

- Cystourethrectomy removes the bladder and the urethra.

In men, the part of the penis containing the urethra that has cancer may be removed in an operation called a partial penectomy. Sometimes the entire penis is removed (penectomy). A patient may need plastic surgery to make a new penis if all or part of the penis is removed. The bladder and prostate may also be removed in an operation called cystoprostatectomy. Lymph nodes in the pelvis may also be removed (lymph node dissection). Lymph nodes are small bean-shaped structures that are found throughout the body. They produce and store infection-fighting cells.

In women, surgery to remove the urethra, the bladder, and the vagina (anterior exenteration) may also be done. Lymph nodes in the pelvis may be removed (lymph node dissection). Plastic surgery may be needed to make a new vagina after this operation.

If the urethra is removed, the doctor will need to make a new way for the urine to pass from the body. This is called urinary diversion.

If the bladder is removed, the doctor will need to make a new way for the patient to store and pass urine. There are several ways to do this. Sometimes the doctor will use part of the small intestine to make a tube through which urine can pass out of the body through an opening (stoma) on the outside of the body. This is sometimes called an ostomy or urostomy. If a patient has an ostomy, a special bag will need to be worn to collect urine. This special bag, which sticks to the skin around the stoma with a special glue, can be thrown away after it is used. This bag does not show under clothing, and most people take care of these bags themselves. The doctor may also use part of the small intestine to make a new storage pouch (a continent reservoir) inside the body where the urine can collect. The patient would then need to use a tube (catheter) to drain the urine through a stoma.

Radiation therapy uses x-rays or other high-energy rays to kill cancer cells and shrink tumors. Radiation may come from a machine outside the body (external radiation therapy) or from putting materials that produce radiation (radioisotopes) through thin plastic tubes (internal radiation therapy) in the area where cancer cells are found. Radiation may be used alone or with surgery and/or chemotherapy.

Chemotherapy uses drugs to kill cancer cells. Chemotherapy may be taken by mouth, or it may be put in the body through a needle in a vein or muscle. Chemotherapy is called a systemic treatment because the drug enters the bloodstream, travels through the body and can kill cancer cells outside the urethra.

Treatment by Stage

Treatment depends on where the cancer is found, whether it has spread to other areas in the body, and the patient's sex, age, and overall health.

Standard treatment may be considered because of its effectiveness in patients in past studies, or participation in a clinical trial may be considered. Not all patients are cured with standard therapy and some standard treatments may have more side effects than are desired. For these reasons, clinical trials are designed to find better ways to treat cancer patients and are based on the most up-to-date information. Clinical trials are going on in many parts of the country for patients with cancer of the urethra. To learn more about clinical trials, call the Cancer Information Service at 1-800-4-CANCER (1-800-422-6237); TTY at 1-800-332-8615.

Anterior Urethral Cancer

Treatment is different for men and women.

For women, treatment may be one of the following:

1. Electrofulguration.

2. Laser therapy.

3. External and/or internal radiation therapy.

4. Radiation therapy followed by surgery or surgery alone to remove the urethra and the organs in the lower pelvis (anterior exenteration), or the tumor only, if it is small. A new way is made for urine to pass out of the body (urinary diversion).

For men, treatment may be one of the following:

1. Electrofulguration.

2. Laser therapy.

3. Surgery to remove a part of the penis (partial penectomy).

4. Radiation therapy.

Posterior Urethral Cancer

Treatment is different for men and women.

For women, treatment will probably be radiation therapy followed by surgery or surgery alone to remove the urethra, the organs in the lower pelvis (anterior exenteration), or the tumor only, if it is small. Lymph nodes in the pelvis are usually removed (lymph node dissection), and lymph nodes in the upper thigh may or may not be removed. A new way is made for urine to pass out of the body (urinary diversion).

For men, treatment will probably be radiation therapy followed by surgery or surgery alone to remove the bladder and prostate (cysto-prostatectomy) and the penis and urethra (penectomy). Lymph nodes in the pelvis are usually removed (lymph node dissection), and lymph nodes in the upper thigh may or may not be removed. A new way is made for urine to pass out of the body (urinary diversion).

Urethral Cancer Associated with Invasive Bladder Cancer

Because people with bladder cancer sometimes also have cancer of the urethra, the urethra may be removed at the same time the bladder is taken out (cystourethrectomy). If the urethra is not removed during surgery for bladder cancer, the doctor may follow the patient closely so treatment can be started if cancer of the urethra develops.

Recurrent Urethral Cancer

Treatment depends on what treatment the patient received before. If the patient had surgery, treatment may be radiation therapy and surgery to remove the cancer. If the patient had radiation therapy, treatment may be surgery to remove the cancer. Clinical trials are testing chemotherapy for cancer of the urethra that has spread to other parts of the body.

To Learn More

To learn more about cancer of the urethra, call the National Cancer Institute's Cancer Information Service at 1-800-4-CANCER (1-800-422-6237); TTY at 1-800-332-8615. By dialing this toll-free number, you can speak with a trained information specialist who can answer your questions.

Cancer patients, their families and friends, and others may find the following booklets useful. They are available free of charge by calling 1-800-4-CANCER or writing:

Office of Cancer Communications
National Cancer Institute
Building 31, Room 10A24
Bethesda, MD 20892

Booklets about Cancer Treatment

Radiation Therapy and You: A Guide to Self-Help During Treatment *

Chemotherapy and You: A Guide to Self-Help During Treatment *

Eating Hints: Recipes and Tips for Better Nutrition During Cancer Treatment *

Questions and Answers About Pain Control

What Are Clinical Trials All About?

Booklets about Living with Cancer

Taking Time: Support for People With Cancer and the People Who Care About Them

When Cancer Recurs: Meeting the Challenge Again *

Advanced Cancer: Living Each Day *

* Reprinted in this volume—see Table of Contents

Chapter 32

Testicular Cancer

The Testicles

The testicles (also called testes or gonads) are the male sex glands. They are located behind the penis in a pouch of skin called the scrotum. The testicles produce and store sperm, and they are also the body's main source of male hormones. These hormones control the development of the reproductive organs and other male characteristics, such as body and facial hair, low voice, and wide shoulders.

What Is Cancer?

Cancer is a group of more than 100 diseases. Although each kind differs from the others in many ways, every type of cancer is a disease of some of the body's cells.

Healthy cells that make up the body's tissues grow, divide, and replace themselves in an orderly way. This process keeps the body in good repair. Sometimes, however, some cells lose the ability to limit and direct their growth. They grow too rapidly and without any order. Too much tissue is produced, and tumors are formed. Tumors can be either benign or malignant.

- Benign tumors are not cancer. They do not spread to other parts of the body and are seldom a threat to life. Benign tumors

Excerpted from "What You Need To Know About Testicular Cancer," National Cancer Institute, August 3, 1999; and "Testicular Self-Examination," NIH publication 94-2636.

can often be removed by surgery, and they are not likely to return.

- Malignant tumors are cancer. They can invade and destroy nearby healthy tissues and organs. Also, cancer cells can spread, or metastasize, to other parts of the body and form new tumors.

Cancer that develops in a testicle is called testicular cancer. When testicular cancer spreads, the cancer cells are carried by blood or by lymph, an almost colorless fluid produced by tissues all over the body. The fluid passes through lymph nodes, which filter out bacteria and other abnormal substances such as cancer cells. Surgeons often remove the lymph nodes deep in the abdomen to learn whether testicular cancer cells have spread.

Symptoms

Testicular cancer is one of the most common cancers in young men between the ages of 15 and 34. But the disease also occurs in other age groups, so all men should be aware of its symptoms.

Most testicular cancers are found by men themselves. The testicles are smooth, oval-shaped, and rather firm. Anything unusual should be reported to a doctor.

Testicular cancer can cause a number of symptoms. Listed below are warning signs that men should watch for:

- A lump in either testicle;

- Any enlargement of a testicle;

- A feeling of heaviness in the scrotum;

- A dull ache in the lower abdomen or the groin;

- A sudden collection of fluid in the scrotum;

- Pain or discomfort in a testicle or in the scrotum;

- Enlargement or tenderness of the breasts.

These symptoms are not sure signs of cancer. They can also be caused by other conditions. However, any illness should be diagnosed and treated as soon as possible. Early diagnosis of testicular cancer is important because the sooner cancer is found and treated, the better a man's chance for complete recovery.

Diagnosing Testicular Cancer

When a man's symptoms suggest that there might be cancer in a testicle, the doctor will ask about his personal and family history and do a complete physical exam. In addition to checking for general signs of health (temperature, pulse, blood pressure, and so on), the doctor will carefully examine the scrotum. Also, the patient will usually have a chest x-ray and blood and urine tests. If the physical exam and lab tests do not show an infection or another disorder, the doctor is likely to suspect cancer because most tumors in the testicles are cancer.

The only sure way to know whether cancer is present is for a pathologist to examine a sample of tissue under a microscope. To obtain the tissue, the affected testicle is removed through the groin. This operation is called inguinal orchiectomy. The surgeon does not cut through the scrotum and does not remove just a part of the testicle because, if the problem is cancer, cutting through the outer layer of the testicle might cause local spread of the disease.

The most common types of testicular cancer are seminoma and nonseminoma.

- Seminomas make up about 40 percent of all cases.

- Nonseminomas are actually a group of cancers. They include choriocarcinoma, embryonal carcinoma, teratoma, and yolk sac tumors.

Each of these two major types of testicular cancer grows and spreads differently—and they are treated differently.

Treating the Disease

Testicular cancer is almost always curable if it is found early. This disease responds well to treatment, even if it has spread to other parts of the body.

Staging

If a man has testicular cancer, it is important to find out the extent, or stage, of the disease (whether it has spread from the testicle to other parts of the body). Staging procedures include a thorough physical exam, blood tests, x-rays and scans, and, in some cases, additional surgery.

Most patients have computed tomography, also call CT or CAT scan, which is a series of x-rays of various sections of the body. Some have intravenous pyelography (IVP), x-rays used with a special dye to outline the urinary system. Some doctors recommend lymphangiography, x-rays taken with a special dye that outlines the lymph system in the abdomen. Ultrasonography, which creates a picture from the echoes of high-frequency sound waves bounced off internal organs, also may be useful.

Special lab tests can reveal certain substances in the blood. These substances are called tumor markers because they often are found in abnormal amounts in patients with some types of cancer. The levels of specific tumor markers in the blood can help the doctor determine what type of testicular cancer the patient has.

Surgery may be recommended to remove the lymph nodes deep in the abdomen. A pathologist then examines the nodes to see whether they contain cancer cells. For patients with nonseminoma, removing the nodes helps stop the spread of their disease. Seminoma patients do not need this surgery because cancer cells in their lymph nodes can be destroyed with radiation therapy.

Planning Treatment

Decisions about treatment for testicular cancer are complex. Sometimes it is helpful to have more than one doctor's advice. Before starting treatment, the patient might want a second opinion about the diagnosis and treatment plan. It may take a week or two to arrange to see another doctor. This short delay will not make treatment less effective. There are a number of ways to find a doctor for a second opinion:

The patient's doctor may be able to suggest a doctor who has a special interest in testicular cancer.

The Cancer Information Service, at 1-800-4-CANCER, can tell callers about cancer centers and other NCI-supported programs in their area.

Patients can get the names of doctors from their local medical society, a nearby hospital, or a medical school.

Methods of Treating Testicular Cancer

Testicular cancer can be treated with surgery, radiation therapy, and chemotherapy. The doctor may use just one method or a combination. Often, the patient is referred to medical centers that specialize in testicular cancer treatment.

Surgery. In most cases, surgery is done to remove the testicle. Sometimes it also is necessary to remove lymph nodes in the abdomen. In addition, tumors that have spread to other parts of the body may be partly or entirely removed by surgery.

Radiation therapy. In radiation therapy (also called x-ray therapy, radiotherapy, cobalt treatment, or irradiation), high-energy rays are used to damage cancer cells and stop their growth. Like surgery, radiation therapy is a local therapy; it affects only the cells in the treated area. The patient usually receives radiation therapy as an outpatient.

Seminomas are highly sensitive to radiation. Following surgery, men with seminomas generally have radiation therapy to their abdominal lymph nodes.

Nonseminomas are somewhat less sensitive to radiation. Patients with this type of cancer usually have other types of treatment.

Chemotherapy. The use of drugs to treat cancer is called chemotherapy. Anticancer drugs are recommended when there are signs that the cancer has spread.

Also, chemotherapy is sometimes used when the doctor suspects that undetected cancer cells remain in the body after surgery or irradiation. The use of anticancer drugs following surgery for early stage cancer is known as adjuvant therapy.

Chemotherapy may be given by mouth or by injection into a muscle or a blood vessel. Chemotherapy is a systemic treatment—the drugs enter the bloodstream and reach cells all over the body. Depending on the specific drugs and the patient's general condition, chemotherapy may be taken as an outpatient—at the hospital, at the doctor's office, or at home. Sometimes, however, the person must be hospitalized for a time, so the effects of the treatment can be watched.

Side Effects of Treatment

The treatments used against cancer must be very powerful. That's why patients may have some unpleasant side effects.

Many men worry that losing one testicle will affect their ability to have sexual intercourse or make them sterile. But a man with one healthy testicle can still have a normal erection and produce sperm. Therefore, an operation to remove just one testicle does not make a patient impotent and seldom interferes with fertility. Men can also have an artificial testicle, called a prosthesis, placed in the scrotum. The implant has the weight and feel of a normal testicle.

Surgery to remove the lymph nodes does not change a man's ability to have an erection or an orgasm, but the operation can cause sterility because it interferes with ejaculation. Some men recover the ability to ejaculate without treatment; others may be helped by medication. Patients should talk with the doctor about the possibility of removing the lymph nodes using a special surgical technique that may protect the ability to ejaculate.

Radiation therapy affects both normal and cancerous cells, but normal cells are able to recover. Having treatments 5 days a week for several weeks spreads out the total dose of radiation and gives the patient weekend rest breaks. Nevertheless, the body must work very hard during radiation therapy to repair the tissues injured by the treatment. Patients may feel unusually tired, and they should try to rest as much as possible. Radiation therapy does not change the ability to have sex. Radiation therapy does, however, interfere with sperm production. Usually the effect is temporary, and most patients regain their fertility within a matter of months.

Other unpleasant effects of radiation therapy include diarrhea, nausea, and vomiting. These problems can usually be controlled with medication. Also, there may be skin reactions in the area being treated, and it is important to treat the skin gently. Lotions and creams should not be used on these areas without the doctor's advice.

Chemotherapy causes side effects because it damages not only cancer cells, but other rapidly growing cells as well. Often anticancer drugs are given in cycles; treatment periods alternate with rest periods. The side effects of chemotherapy depend on the specific drugs that are given and the response of the individual patient. These drugs commonly affect hair cells, blood-forming cells, and cells that line the digestive tract. As a result, they may cause various problems, including hair loss, lowered resistance to infection, loss of appetite, nausea and vomiting, and mouth sores. Most men who receive chemotherapy for testicular cancer can continue to function sexually, although some anticancer drugs interfere with sperm production. Although this effect is permanent for some patients, many recover their fertility later on.

Loss of appetite can be a serious problem for patients receiving radiation therapy or chemotherapy. Researchers are learning that patients who eat well are better able to withstand the side effects of their treatment. Therefore, good nutrition is important. Eating well means getting enough calories to prevent weight loss and having enough protein to build and repair skin, hair, muscles, and organs. Many patients find that having several small meals and snacks throughout the day is easier than trying to eat three large meals.

The side effects of cancer therapy vary from person to person and may even be different from one treatment to the next. Patients may find that they are less interested in sexual activity if they are tired or feel ill. Doctors try to plan treatment to keep problems to a minimum, and fortunately, most side effects are temporary. Doctors, nurses, and dietitians can explain the side effects of cancer treatment and suggest ways to deal with them. Helpful information about cancer treatment and coping with side effects is given in the NCI publications *Radiation Therapy and You*, *Chemotherapy and You*, and *Eating Hints for Cancer Patients*.

Followup Care

Regular followup exams are very important for anyone treated for testicular cancer. The doctor will continue to watch the patient closely for several years to be sure the cancer is completely gone. If the cancer does recur, it is very important for the doctor to detect it right away and start additional treatment.

Followup care may vary for different types and stages of testicular cancer. Generally, patients are checked and have blood tests to measure tumor marker levels every month for the first 2 years after treatment. They also have regular x-rays and scans. After that, checkups may be needed just once or twice a year. Testicular cancer seldom recurs after a patient has been free of the disease for 3 years.

Patients who have been treated for cancer in one testicle have about a 1 percent chance of developing cancer in the remaining one. If cancer does arise in the second testicle, it is nearly always a new disease rather than a metastasis from the first tumor. Patients should be checked regularly by their doctor. Between checkups, they should report any unusual symptoms to the doctor without delay.

Adjusting to the Disease

When people have cancer, life can change—for them and for the people who care about them. These changes in daily life can be difficult to handle. When a man learns that he has testicular cancer, it's natural to have many different and sometimes confusing emotions.

At times, patients and family members may be frightened, angry, or depressed. Their feelings may vary from hope to despair or from courage to fear. Patients are usually better able to handle these feelings if they talk about their illness and share their feelings with family members and friends.

Concerns about the future—as well as about medical tests and treatments, hospital stays, medical bills, and sexuality—are common.

Talking with doctors, nurses, or other members of the health care team may help ease fear and confusion. Patients should ask questions about their disease and its treatment and take an active part in decisions about their medical care. Patients and family members often find it helpful to write down questions as they think of them to prepare for the next visit to the doctor. Taking notes during talks with the doctor can be a useful aid to memory. Patients should ask the doctor to repeat or explain anything that is not clear.

Most people want to know what kind of cancer they have, how it can be treated, and how successful the treatment is likely to be. The following are some other questions patients might want to ask the doctor:

- What are the expected benefits of treatment?

- What are the risks and side effects of treatment?

- Will my sex life change?

- Will I be able to father children?

- Is it possible to keep working during treatment?

- Will changes in my normal daily activities be required?

- How often are checkups needed?

The patient's doctor is the best person to answer questions and give advice about working or other activities. If it is hard to talk with the doctor about feelings and other very personal matters, patients may find it helpful to talk with others facing similar problems. This kind of help is available through support groups, such as those described in the next section. If the patient or his family finds that emotional problems become too hard to handle, a mental health counselor may be able to help.

The public library is a good source of books and articles on living with cancer. Also, cancer patients and their families and friends can find helpful suggestions in the NCI booklets in the Other Booklets section.

Support for Cancer Patients

Adapting to the changes that are brought about by having cancer is easier for patients and those who care about them when they have helpful information and support services. Often, the social service office at the hospital or clinic can suggest local and national agencies that will help with emotional support, financial aid, transportation, home care, or rehabilitation.

The American Cancer Society (ACS), for example, is a nonprofit organization that offers a variety of services to patients and their families. Local ACS offices are listed in the telephone directory.

Information about other programs and services for cancer patients and their families is available through the Cancer Information Service (CIS), whose toll-free number is 1-800-4-CANCER.

What the Future Holds

More than 8 million Americans living today have had some type of cancer. The outlook for men with testicular cancer is excellent. Because researchers have found better ways to diagnose and treat this disease, the chance of recovery has improved dramatically. Today, a large majority of testicular cancer patients are cured by their initial treatment, and many of those who have a recurrence can be cured too.

The Promise of Cancer Research

Scientists at hospitals and medical centers throughout the United States are studying testicular cancer. They are working toward a better understanding of its causes, prevention, diagnosis, and treatment.

Cause and Prevention

Researchers study patterns of cancer in the population to discover whether some people are more likely than others to get certain cancers. If they can learn what causes the disease, they may be able to suggest ways to prevent it.

Although any man can get testicular cancer, the disease is rare. It accounts for only about 1 percent of all cancers in American men. Although most other cancers affect mostly older people, testicular cancer usually occurs in young men. It is more common in white men than in black.

We know that testicular cancer is not contagious. No one can "catch" it from another person. However, doctors do not know exactly what causes this disease. They can seldom explain why one person gets it while another doesn't, but research does show that some men are more likely to develop testicular cancer. For example, the risk is higher than average for boys born with their testicles in the lower abdomen rather than in the scrotum. The cancer risk for boys with this condition (called undescended testicles or cryptorchidism) is increased if the problem is not corrected in early childhood. Research has also shown that testicular cancer is sometimes linked to certain other rare conditions in which the testicles do not develop normally.

Some men whose mothers took a hormone called DES (diethylstilbestrol) during pregnancy to prevent miscarriage have testicular abnormalities. But scientists do not know whether prenatal exposure to DES (or any other female hormone) increases the risk of testicular cancer.

Some patients with testicular cancer have a history of injury to the scrotum. But no one knows whether such an injury can actually cause cancer. Many doctors think such an injury simply calls attention to a tumor that was already growing.

Detection and Diagnosis

Every man can help himself by seeing a doctor promptly if he notices any symptoms of testicular disease. [See the section at the end of this chapter on testicular self-examination.]

Researchers are looking for additional tumor markers that may be present in abnormal amounts in the blood or urine of a person with very early testicular cancer. If such markers are found, it might be possible to detect testicular cancer even before any symptoms are noticed. Several such markers have been studied, and research is continuing.

Treatment

Researchers are looking for treatment methods that are more effective and easier for patients to tolerate. They are studying new drugs and drug combinations, varied doses, and different treatment schedules.

When research shows that a new treatment method has promise, the method is used to treat cancer patients in clinical trials. These trials are designed to answer scientific questions and find out whether a new approach is both safe and effective. Patients who take part in research make an important contribution to medical science and may have the first chance to benefit from improved treatment methods.

Patients with testicular cancer are encouraged to consider participating in a trial and should discuss this option with their doctor. The NCI booklet *Taking Part in Clinical Trials: What Cancer Patients Need To Know* is for patients who may be interested in taking part in clinical research.

One way to learn about clinical trials is through PDQ, a computerized resource of cancer treatment information. Developed by NCI, PDQ contains an up-to-date list of trials all over the country. Doctors can obtain an access code and use a personal computer to get PDQ information, or they can use the services of a medical library. Also, the Cancer Information Service, at 1-800-4-CANCER, can provide PDQ information to doctors, patients, and the public.

There is much yet to learn about what causes testicular cancer and how it might be prevented. Our understanding is growing, and as new knowledge is gained, we hope that fewer men will develop the disease. At the same time, better methods of detection and treatment already have contributed to greatly increased survival rates for men with testicular cancer. The remarkable improvements in dealing with this disease may, in fact, lead the way in other types of cancer.

Other Booklets

The booklets listed below may be helpful to testicular cancer patients and their families. They are available free of charge from the National Cancer Institute. You may request them by calling 1-800-4-CANCER or writing:

Office of Cancer Communications
National Cancer Institute
Building 31, Room 10A24
Bethesda, MD 20892

Booklets about Cancer Treatment

Chemotherapy and You: A Guide to Self-Help During Treatment *

Radiation Therapy and You: A Guide to Self-Help During Treatment *

Eating Hints for Cancer Patients *

Questions and Answers About Pain Control

Taking Part in Clinical Trials: What Cancer Patients Need To Know

Booklets about Living with Cancer

Taking Time: Support for People With Cancer and the People Who Care About Them

Facing Forward: A Guide for Cancer Survivors *

When Cancer Recurs: Meeting the Challenge Again *

Advanced Cancer: Living Each Day *

* Reprinted in this volume—see Table of Contents

Testicular Self-Examination

Testicular cancer is the most common type of cancer in men ages 20 to 35. Yet, because it accounts for only about 1 percent of all cancers in men, many people have never heard of this type of cancer.

Testicular cancer is of special concern to young men. It can occur anytime after age 15. It is less common in middle-aged and older men. White men are four times more likely to develop testicular cancer than black men. The rate among Hispanic men lies between those of blacks and whites.

Two groups of men have a greater risk of developing testicular cancer—those whose testicles have not descended into the scrotum and those whose testicles descended after age 6. Testicular cancer is 3 to 17 times more likely to develop in these men.

Testicles are male reproductive organs. They produce and store sperm, They also produce testosterone, a hormone that causes such male traits as facial hair and lower voice pitch. Testicles are smooth, oval-shaped, and somewhat firm to the touch. They are below the penis in a sac of skin called the scrotum.

The testicles normally descend into the scrotum before birth. Parents should have their infant sons examined by a doctor to be sure that the testicles have properly descended. If they have not, this can be easily corrected with surgery.

Fifteen years ago, testicular cancer was often fatal because it spread quickly to vital organs such as the lungs. Today, due to advances in treatment, testicular cancer is one of the most curable cancers, especially if detected and treated promptly.

The most common symptom of testicular cancer is a small, painless lump in a testicle or a slightly enlarged testicle. It is important for men to become familiar with the size and feeling of their own testicles, so that they can detect changes if they occur.

Other possible symptoms include a feeling of heaviness in the scrotum, a dull ache in the lower stomach or groin, a change in the way a testicle feels, or a sudden accumulation of blood or fluid in the scrotum. These symptoms can also be caused by infections or other conditions that are not cancer. A doctor can tell you if you have cancer and what the proper treatment should be.

How to Do TSE

A simple procedure called testicular self-exam (TSE) can increase the chances of finding a tumor early.

Men should perform TSE once a month after a warm bath or shower. The heat causes the scrotal skin to relax, making it easier to find anything unusual. TSE is simple and only takes a few minutes.

Examine each testicle gently with both hands. The index and middle fingers should be placed underneath the testicle while the thumbs are placed on the top. Roll the testicle gently between the thumbs and fingers, One testicle may be larger than the other. This is normnal.

- The epididymis is a cord-like structure on the top and back of the testicle that stores and transports the sperm. Do not confuse the epididymis with an abnormal lump.

- Feel for any abnormal lumps—about the size of a pea—on the front or the side of the testicle. These lumps are usually painless.

If you do find a lump, you should contact your doctor right away. The lump may be due to an infection, and a doctor can decide the proper treatment. If the lump is not an infection, it is likely to be cancer. Remember that testicular cancer is highly curable, especially when detected and treated early. Testicular cancer almost always occurs in only one testicle, and the other testicle is all that is needed for full sexual function.

Routine testicular self-exams are important, but they cannot substitute for a doctor's examination. Your doctor should examine your testicles when you have a physical exam. You also can ask your doctor to check the way you do TSE.

Chapter 33

Prostate Cancer

Introduction

Prostate cancer is the most common type of cancer in men in the United States (other than skin cancer). The National Cancer Institute (NCI) has written this chapter to help patients with prostate cancer and their families and friends better understand this disease. We hope others will read it as well to learn more about prostate cancer. This chapter discusses symptoms, diagnosis, and treatment. It also has information to help patients cope with prostate cancer.

Our knowledge about prostate cancer keeps increasing. For up-to-date information, call the National Cancer Institute's Cancer Information Service (CIS). The toll-free number is 1-800-4-CANCER (1-800-422-6237).

The CIS staff use a National Cancer Institute cancer information database called PDQ and other NCI resources to answer callers' questions. Cancer Information Specialists can send callers information from PDQ and other NCI materials about cancer, its treatment, and living with the disease.

The Prostate

The prostate is a male sex gland. It produces a thick fluid that forms part of the semen. The prostate is about the size of a walnut.

"What You Need To Know About Prostate Cancer," National Cancer Institute (NCI), updated September 1998.

It is located below the bladder and in front of the rectum. The prostate surrounds the upper part of the urethra, the tube that empties urine from the bladder.

The prostate needs male hormones to function. The main male hormone is testosterone, which is made mainly by the testicles. Some male hormones are produced in small amounts by the adrenal glands.

What Is Cancer?

Cancer is a group of many different diseases that have some important things in common. They all affect cells, the body's basic unit of life. To understand cancer, it is helpful to know about normal cells and what happens when cells become cancerous.

The body is made up of many types of cells. Normally, cells grow and divide to produce more cells only when the body needs them. This orderly process helps keep the body healthy.

If the cells keep dividing when new cells are not needed, they form too much tissue. Excess tissue can form a mass, called a tumor. Excess tissue can be benign or malignant.

- Benign tissue is not cancer. The cells do not invade nearby tissue or spread to other parts of the body.

- Malignant tissue is cancer. The cancer cells divide out of control. They can invade and destroy nearby healthy tissue. Also, cancer cells can break away from the tumor they form and enter the bloodstream and lymphatic system, This is how cancer spreads from the original (primary) tumor to form new tumors in other parts of the body. The spread of cancer is called metastasis.

Benign prostatic hyperplasia (BPH) is the abnormal growth of benign prostate cells. In BPH, the prostate grows larger and pushes against the urethra and bladder, blocking the normal flow of urine. More than half of the men in the United States between the ages of 60 and 70 and as many as 90 percent between the ages of 70 and 90 have symptoms of BPH. Although this condition is seldom a threat to life, it may require treatment to relieve symptoms.

Most cancers are named for the type of cell or organ in which they begin. Cancer that begins in the prostate is called primary prostate cancer (or prostatic cancer). Prostate cancer may remain in the prostate gland, or it may spread to nearby lymph nodes. Prostate cancer may also spread to the bones, bladder, rectum, and other organs.

When cancer spreads to other parts of the body, the new tumor has the same malignant cells and the same name as the primary tumor. For example, if prostate cancer spreads to the bones, the cancer cells in the new tumor are prostate cancer cells. The disease is metastatic prostate cancer; it is not bone cancer.

Symptoms

Early prostate cancer often does not cause symptoms. When symptoms of prostate cancer do occur, they may include some of the following problems:

- A need to urinate frequently, especially at night;
- Difficulty starting urination or holding back urine;
- Inability to urinate;
- Weak or interrupted flow of urine;
- Painful or burning urination;
- Painful ejaculation;
- Blood in urine or semen; and/or
- Frequent pain or stiffness in the lower back, hips, or upper thighs.

Any of these symptoms may be caused by cancer or by other, less serious health problems, such as BPH or an infection. Only a doctor can tell the cause. A man who has symptoms like these should see his family doctor or a urologist (a doctor who specializes in treating diseases of the genitourinary system). Do not wait to feel pain; early prostate cancer does not cause pain.

Diagnosis

If symptoms occur, the doctor asks about the patient's medical history, performs a physical exam, and may order laboratory tests. The exams and tests may include the following:

- Digital rectal exam—the doctor inserts a gloved, lubricated finger into the rectum and feels the prostate through the rectal wall to check for hard or lumpy areas.
- Blood tests—a lab measures the levels of prostate-specific antigen (PSA) and prostatic acid phosphatase (PAP) in the blood.

345

The level of PSA in the blood may rise in men who have prostate cancer, BPH, or an infection in the prostate. The level of PAP rises above normal in many prostate cancer patients, especially if the cancer has spread beyond the prostate. The doctor cannot diagnose prostate cancer with these tests alone because elevated PSA or PAP levels may also indicate other, noncancerous problems. However, the doctor will take the results of these tests into account in deciding whether to check the patient further for signs of cancer.

• Urine test—a lab checks the urine for blood or infection.

The doctor may order other tests to learn more about the cause of the symptoms and to help determine whether conditions of the prostate are benign or malignant, such as:

• Transrectal ultrasonography—sound waves that cannot be heard by humans (ultrasound) are sent out by a probe inserted into the rectum. The waves bounce off the prostate, and a computer uses the echoes to create a picture called a sonogram.

• Intravenous pyelogram—a series of x-rays of the organs of the urinary tract.

• Cystoscopy—a procedure in which a doctor looks into the urethra and bladder through a thin, lighted tube.

If test results suggest that cancer may be present, the patient will need to have a biopsy. A biopsy is the only sure way to know whether a problem is cancer. During a biopsy, the doctor removes a small amount of prostate tissue, usually with a needle. A pathologist looks at the tissue under a microscope to check for cancer cells. If cancer is present, the pathologist usually reports the grade of the tumor. The grade tells how closely the tumor resembles normal prostate tissue and suggests how fast the tumor is likely to grow. One way of grading prostate cancer, called the Gleason system, uses scores of 2 to 10. Another system uses G1 through G4. Tumors with lower scores are less likely to grow or spread than tumors with higher scores.

A man who needs a biopsy may want to ask the doctor some of the following questions:

• How long will the procedure take? Will I be awake? Will it hurt?

• How soon will I know the results?

• If I do have cancer, who will talk to me about treatment? When?

If the physical exam and test results do not suggest cancer, the doctor may recommend medicine to reduce the symptoms caused by an enlarged prostate. Surgery is another way to relieve these symptoms. The surgery used in such cases is transurethral resection of the prostate (TURP or TUR). In TURP, an instrument is inserted through the penis to remove prostate tissue that is pressing against the upper part of the urethra.

Staging

If cancer is found in the prostate, the doctor needs to know the stage, or extent, of the disease. Staging is a careful attempt to find out whether the cancer has spread and, if so, what parts of the body are affected. The doctor may use various blood and imaging tests to learn the stage of the disease. Treatment decisions depend on these findings.

The results of staging tests help the doctor decide which stage best describes a patient's disease:

Stage I (A)

The cancer cannot be detected by rectal exam and causes no symptoms. The cancer is usually found during surgery to relieve problems with urination. Stage I tumors may be in more than one area of the prostate, but there is no evidence of spread outside the prostate.

Stage II (B)

The tumor is felt in a rectal exam or detected by a blood test, but there is no evidence that the cancer has spread outside the prostate.

Stage III (C)

The cancer has spread outside the prostate to nearby tissues.

Stage IV (D)

Cancer cells have spread to lymph nodes or to other parts of the body.

Treating Prostate Cancer

Getting a Second Opinion

Decisions about prostate cancer treatment are complex. It may be helpful to have the opinion of more than one doctor. Before starting treatment, men may want to have a second doctor review their diagnosis and treatment options. A short delay will not reduce the chance that treatment will be successful. Some health insurance companies require a second opinion; many others will cover a second opinion if the patient requests it. There are a number of ways to find a doctor who can give a second opinion:

- The doctor may be able to recommend a specialist. Doctors who specialize in treating prostate cancer are urologists, radiation oncologists, and medical oncologists.

- The Cancer Information Service, at 1-800-4-CANCER, can tell callers about treatment facilities, including cancer centers and other programs supported by the National Cancer Institute.

- People can get the names of doctors from their local medical society, a nearby hospital, or a medical school.

- The *Directory of Medical Specialists* lists doctors by state and specialty and gives information about their background. This resource is in most public libraries.

Preparing for Treatment

The doctor develops a treatment plan to fit each patient's needs. Treatment for prostate cancer depends on the stage of the disease and the grade of the tumor (how fast the cells are likely to grow or spread to other organs). Other important factors in planning treatment are the man's age and general health and his feelings about the treatments and their possible side effects.

Many people with cancer want to learn all they can about their disease, their treatment choices, and possible side effects of treatment, so they can take an active part in decisions about their medical care. There are a number of available treatments for men with prostate cancer (surgery, radiation therapy, and hormone therapy). Not all men require treatment. The patient and his doctor may want to consider both the benefits and possible side effects of each option, especially the effects on sexual activity and urination, and other concerns about quality of life. Patients may find helpful information in Methods of Treatment, Side Effects of Treatment, and Support for Cancer Patients. Also, the patient may want to talk with his doctor about taking part in a research study to help determine the best approach or to study new kinds of treatment. To find more information about such studies, see the Clinical Trials section.

When a person is diagnosed with cancer, shock and stress are natural reactions. These feelings may make it difficult for patients to think of everything they want to ask the doctor. Often it helps to make a list of questions. Also, to help remember what the doctor says, patients may take notes or ask the doctor whether they may use a tape recorder. Some patients also may want to have a family member or friend with them when they talk to the doctor—to take part in the discussion, to take notes, or just to listen.

Questions may arise throughout the treatment process. From time to time, patients may wish to ask members of their health care team to explain things further.

These are some questions a patient may want to ask the doctor before treatment begins:

- What is the stage of the disease?

- What is the grade of the disease?

- Do I need to be treated? What are the treatment choices? What do you recommend for me?

- What are the expected benefits of each kind of treatment?

- What are the risks and possible side effects of each treatment?

- Is treatment likely to affect my sex life?

- Am I likely to have urinary problems?

- Are new treatments being studied in clinical trials? Would a trial be appropriate for me?

Methods of Treatment

Many men whose prostate cancer is slow growing and found at an early stage may not need treatment. Also, treatment may not be advised for older men or men with other serious medical problems. For these men, the possible side effects and the risks of treatment may outweigh the possible benefits of treatment; instead, the doctor may suggest "watchful waiting"—following the patient closely and treating the patient later for symptoms that may arise. Researchers are studying men with early stage prostate cancer to determine when and in whom treatment may be necessary and effective.

Treatment for prostate cancer may involve surgery, radiation therapy, or hormone therapy. Sometimes, patients receive a combination of these treatments. In addition, doctors are studying other methods of treatment to find out whether they are effective against this disease.

Surgery is a common treatment for the early stages of prostate cancer. Surgery to remove the entire prostate is called radical prostatectomy. It is done in one of two ways. In retropubic prostatectomy, the prostate and nearby lymph nodes are removed through an incision in the abdomen. In perineal prostatectomy, the prostate is removed through an incision between the scrotum and the anus. Nearby lymph nodes are sometimes removed through a separate incision in the abdomen. If the pathologist finds cancer cells in the lymph nodes, it may mean that the disease has spread to other parts of the body.

These are some questions a patient may want to ask the doctor before having surgery:

- What kind of operation will it be?

- How will I feel after the operation?

- If I have pain, how will you help?

- Will I have any lasting side effects?

Radiation therapy is another way to treat prostate cancer. In radiation therapy (also called radiotherapy), high-energy rays are used to damage cancer cells and stop them from growing and dividing. Like surgery, radiation therapy is local therapy; it can affect cancer cells only in the treated area. In early stage prostate cancer, radiation can be used instead of surgery, or it may be used after surgery to destroy any cancer cells that may remain in the area. In advanced stages, it may be given to relieve pain or other problems.

Radiation may be directed at the body by a machine (external radiation), or it may come from a small container of radioactive material placed directly into or near the tumor (internal radiation). Some patients receive both kinds of radiation therapy.

For external radiation therapy for prostate cancer, the patient is treated in an outpatient department of a hospital or clinic. Treatment generally is given 5 days a week for about 6 weeks. This schedule helps protect healthy tissues by spreading out the total dose of radiation. The rays are aimed at the pelvic area. At the end of treatment, an extra "boost" of radiation is often directed at a smaller area, where the tumor developed.

For internal (or implant) radiation therapy, a brief stay in the hospital may be needed when the radioactive material is implanted. The implant may be temporary or permanent. When a temporary implant is removed, there is no radioactivity in the body. The amount of radiation in a permanent implant is not generally dangerous to other people, but patients may be advised to avoid prolonged close contact with others for a period of time.

These are some questions a patient may want to ask the doctor before having radiation therapy:

- What is the goal of this treatment?
- How will the radiation be given?
- When will the treatment begin? When will it end?
- How will I feel during therapy?
- What can I do to take care of myself during therapy?
- How will we know if the radiation therapy is working?
- Will I be able to continue my normal activities during treatment?

Hormone therapy prevents the prostate cancer cells from getting the male hormones they need to grow. When a man undergoes hormone therapy, the level of male hormones is decreased. This drop in hormone level can affect all prostate cancer cells, even if they have spread to other parts of the body. For this reason, hormone therapy is called systemic therapy.

There are several forms of hormone therapy. One is surgery to remove the testicles. This operation, called orchiectomy, eliminates the main source of male hormones.

The use of luteinizing hormone-releasing hormone (LHRH) agonist is another type of hormone therapy. LHRH agonists prevent the testicles from producing testosterone.

In another form of hormone therapy, patients take the female hormone estrogen to stop the testicles from producing testosterone.

After orchiectomy or treatment with an LHRH agonist or estrogen, the body no longer gets testosterone from the testicles. However, the adrenal glands still produce small amounts of male hormones. Sometimes, the patient is also given an antiandrogen, a drug that blocks the effect of any remaining male hormones. This combination of treatment is known as a total androgen blockade.

Prostate cancer that has spread to other parts of the body usually can be controlled with hormone therapy for a period of time, often several years. Eventually, however, most prostate cancers are able to grow with very little or no male hormones. When this happens, hormone therapy is no longer effective, and the doctor may suggest other forms of treatment that are under study.

Clinical Trials

Many men with prostate cancer take part in clinical trials (treatment studies). Doctors conduct clinical trials to learn about the effectiveness and side effects of new treatments. In some clinical trials, all patients receive the new treatment. In the trials, doctors compare different therapies by giving the new treatment to one group of patients and the standard therapy to another group; or they may compare one standard treatment to another.

People who take part in these studies have the first chance to benefit from treatments that have shown promise in earlier research. They also make an important contribution to medical science.

Many clinical trials of treatments for prostate cancer are under way. For example, researchers are comparing treatment against careful observation of men with early stage prostate cancer. The results of this work will help doctors to know whether to treat early stage prostate cancer immediately or only later on, if symptoms occur.

Doctors are studying new ways of using radiation therapy and hormone therapy. Some doctors also are exploring the use of cryosurgery, which uses extreme cold to destroy cancer cells, as an alternative to surgery and radiation therapy. In cryosurgery, an instrument called a cryoprobe is placed in direct contact with the tumor to freeze it, sparing nearby healthy tissue.

Researchers also are testing the effectiveness of chemotherapy and biological therapy for patients whose cancer does not respond or stops responding to hormone therapy. In addition, scientists are looking for new ways of combining various types of treatment.

Men with prostate cancer who are interested in taking part in a clinical trial should discuss this option with their doctor. *Taking Part in Clinical Trials: What Cancer Patients Need To Know* is a National Cancer Institute booklet that explains the possible benefits and the risks of participating in treatment studies.

One way to learn about clinical trials is through PDQ, a computerized resource developed by the National Cancer Institute. This resource contains information about cancer treatment and about clinical trials in progress all over the country. The Cancer Information Service can provide PDQ information to patients and the public.

Side Effects of Treatment

Although doctors plan treatment very carefully, it is hard to limit the effects of treatment so that only cancer cells are removed or destroyed. Because treatment also damages healthy cells and tissues, it often causes unwanted, and sometimes serious, side effects.

The side effects of cancer treatment depend mainly on the type and extent of the treatment. Also, each patient reacts differently. Doctors and nurses can explain the possible side effects of treatment, and they can often suggest ways to help relieve symptoms that may occur during and after treatment. It is important to let the doctor know if any side effects occur.

Surgery

Although patients are often uncomfortable during the first few days after surgery, their pain can be controlled with medicine. Patients should feel free to discuss pain relief with the doctor or nurse. It is also common for patients to feel tired or weak for a while. The length of time it takes to recover from an operation varies for each patient.

Surgery to remove the prostate may cause permanent impotence and sometimes causes urinary incontinence. These side effects are somewhat less common than in the past. Some surgeons use new methods, especially when removing small tumors. These techniques, called nerve-sparing surgery, may prevent permanent injury to the nerves that control erection and damage to the opening of the bladder. When this surgery is fully successful, impotence and urinary incontinence are only temporary. However, men who have a prostatectomy no longer produce semen, so they have dry orgasms.

Radiation Therapy

Radiation therapy may cause patients to become very tired as treatment continues. Resting is important, but doctors usually advise patients to try to stay as active as they can. Patients may have diarrhea or frequent and uncomfortable urination. In addition, when patients receive external radiation therapy, it is common for the skin in the treated area to become red, dry, and tender. Radiation therapy can also cause hair loss in the pelvic area. The loss may be temporary or permanent, depending on the amount of radiation used.

Radiation therapy causes impotence in some men. This does not occur as often with internal radiation therapy as with external radiation therapy; internal radiation therapy is not as likely to damage the nerves that control erection.

The National Cancer Institute publication *Radiation Therapy and You* [reprinted in this volume as Chapter 66] offers helpful suggestions about coping with the side effects of this form of treatment.

Hormone Therapy

Orchiectomy, LHRH agonists, and estrogen often cause side effects such as loss of sexual desire, impotence, and hot flashes. When first taken, an LHRH agonist tends to increase tumor growth and may make the patient's symptoms worse. This temporary problem is called "tumor flare." Gradually, however, the drug causes a man's testosterone level to fall. Without testosterone, tumor growth slows down and the patient's condition improves. Prostate cancer patients who receive estrogen or an antiandrogen may have nausea, vomiting, or tenderness and swelling of the breasts. (Estrogen is used less now than in the past because it increases a man's risk of heart problems. This form of treatment is not appropriate for men who have a history of heart disease.)

Chemotherapy

The side effects of chemotherapy depend mainly on the specific drugs that are used. The National Cancer Institute publication *Chemotherapy and You* [reprinted in this volume as Chapter 63] may be helpful to patients experiencing the side effects of chemotherapy.

Biological Therapy

Biological therapy may cause flu-like symptoms such as chills, fever, muscle aches, weakness, loss of appetite, nausea, vomiting, or diarrhea. Patients may also bleed or bruise easily, and some get a rash. Some of these problems can be severe, but they go away after the treatment stops.

Nutrition for Cancer Patients

Good nutrition is important. Patients who eat well often feel better and have more energy. Eating well during cancer treatment means getting enough calories and protein to prevent weight loss, regain strength, and rebuild normal tissues.

Some patients find it hard to eat well during treatment. They may lose their appetite. In addition to loss of appetite, common side effects of treatment, such as nausea and vomiting, can make eating difficult. Foods taste different to some patients. Also, people undergoing treatment may not feel like eating when they are uncomfortable or tired.

Doctors, nurses, and dietitians can offer advice for healthy eating during cancer treatment. Patients and their families also may want to read the National Cancer Institute booklet *Eating Hints for Cancer Patients* [reprinted in this volume as Chapter 77], which has helpful information about cancer treatment and coping with side effects.

Followup Care

Regular followup exams are important for any man who has had prostate cancer. The doctor will suggest an appropriate followup schedule. The doctor will examine the patient regularly to be sure that the disease has not returned or progressed, and decide what other medical care may be needed. Followup exams may include x-rays, scans, and laboratory tests, including the PSA blood test.

Support for Cancer Patients

Living with a serious disease is not easy. People with cancer and those who care about them face many problems and challenges. Coping with these problems is often easier when people have helpful information and support services. Several useful booklets, including the National Cancer Institute booklet *Taking Time*, are available from the Cancer Information Service.

Friends and relatives can be very supportive. Also, patients may find it helpful to discuss their concerns with others who have or have had cancer. Cancer patients often get together in support groups, where they can share what they have learned about coping with cancer and the effects of treatment. It is important to keep in mind, however, that each patient is different. Treatments and ways of dealing with cancer that work for one person may not be right for another— even if they both have the same kind of cancer. It is a good idea to discuss the advice of friends and family members with the doctor.

People with cancer may worry about holding their job, caring for their family, or keeping up with daily activities. Worries about tests, treatments, hospital stays, and medical bills are common. Doctors, nurses, and other members of the health care team can answer questions about treatment, working, and other activities. Also, meeting with a social worker, counselor, or member of the clergy can be helpful to patients who want to talk about their feelings and discuss their concerns.

It is natural for a man and his partner to be concerned about the effects of prostate cancer and its treatment on their sexual relationship. They may want to talk with the doctor about possible side effects and whether these side effects are likely to be temporary or permanent. Whatever the outlook, it may be helpful for patients and their partners to talk about their concerns and to help one another find ways to be intimate during and after treatment.

Often, a social worker at the hospital or clinic can suggest local and national groups that can provide emotional support, financial aid, transportation, home care, or other services. The Cancer Information Service also has information on local resources. The American Cancer Society is one such resource. This nonprofit organization has many services for patients and their families and offers a free booklet on sexuality and cancer.

What the Future Holds

Researchers are finding better ways to treat prostate cancer, and the outlook for men with prostate cancer keeps improving. Still, it is natural for patients and their families to be concerned about what the future holds. Sometimes people use statistics to try to figure out the chances of being cured. It is important to remember, however, that statistics are averages based on large numbers of patients. They cannot be used to predict what will happen to a particular patient because no two patients are alike; treatments and responses vary greatly. The doctor who takes care of the patient is in the best position to discuss the patient's prognosis (chance of recovery or control of the disease).

When doctors talk about surviving cancer, they may use the term remission rather than cure. Even though many prostate cancer patients recover completely, doctors use this term because the disease can recur, or reappear after treatment.

Research to Understand Prostate Cancer

Prostate cancer is an important public health problem. Prostate cancer accounts for one of every three cancers among American men. Researchers are conducting studies to learn more about the causes and early detection of this common disease.

Causes and Prevention

The causes of prostate cancer are not yet understood. Researchers are looking at factors that may increase the risk of this disease.

The more they can learn about these risk factors, the better the chance of finding ways to prevent and treat prostate cancer.

Studies in the United States show that prostate cancer is found mainly in men over age 55; the average age of patients at the time of diagnosis is 72. This disease is more common in black men than in white men. In fact, black men in the United States have the highest rate of prostate cancer in the world. Doctors cannot explain why one man gets prostate cancer and another does not, but they do know that no one can "catch" prostate cancer from another person. Prostate cancer is not contagious.

Some studies have shown that a man has a higher risk for prostate cancer if his father or brother has had the disease. However, researchers are uncertain why some families have a higher incidence of prostate cancer.

Scientists are studying the effects of diet. Some evidence suggests that a diet high in fat increases the risk of prostate cancer and a diet high in fruits and vegetables decreases the risk, but these links have not been proven.

Researchers have studied whether having a vasectomy increases a man's risk for prostate cancer. Some studies suggest there may be such a link, but other studies have not supported this claim.

Other studies show that farmers and workers exposed to the metal cadmium during welding, electroplating, or making batteries may have an increased risk of getting this disease. Also, workers in the rubber industry appear to develop prostate cancer more often than members of the general public. However, more research is needed to confirm these results.

Scientists are also doing studies to determine whether BPH or a sexually transmitted virus increases the risk for prostate cancer. At this time, they do not have clear evidence of increased risk in either case.

Men over age 55 are taking part in a study of finasteride (trade name Proscar), a drug used to treat BPH. This nationwide NCI study, called the Prostate Cancer Prevention Trial, is designed to help doctors learn whether finasteride can prevent prostate cancer. The Cancer Information Service can provide information about this study.

Detection

Researchers are studying ways to screen men for prostate cancer (check for the disease in men who have no symptoms). At this time, it is not known whether screening actually saves lives. The NCI-supported

357

Prostate, Lung, Colorectal, and Ovarian Cancer Screening Trial is designed to show whether certain tests can detect these cancers early enough to reduce the number of deaths they cause. For prostate cancer, this trial is looking at the usefulness of screening with digital rectal exam and checking the PSA level in the blood in men ages 55 to 74. The results of this trial may change the way men are screened for prostate cancer. The Cancer Information Service can provide information about this trial.

Men should talk with their doctor about prostate cancer, the symptoms to watch for, and an appropriate schedule of checkups. The doctor's advice will be based on the risks and benefits of diagnosis and treatment, as well as a man's age, medical history, and other factors.

Other Federal Resources

National Institute on Aging Information Center

The National Institute on Aging, an agency of the Federal Government, is concerned with the health problems of older Americans. The Information Center can send free printed material, including fact sheets about going to the hospital and about prostate problems, sexuality, and urinary incontinence. The phone number for the Center is 1-800-222-2225.

National Kidney and Urologic Diseases Information Clearinghouse

This Clearinghouse is a service of the Federal Government's National Institute of Diabetes and Digestive and Kidney Diseases. It can supply free information about benign prostate enlargement and other noncancerous urinary tract problems. The phone number for the Clearinghouse is 301-654-4415.

For Further Information

Cancer patients, their families and friends, and others may find the following booklets useful. They are available free of charge by calling 1-800-4-CANCER or writing:

Office of Cancer Communications
National Cancer Institute
Building 31, Room 10A24
Bethesda, MD 20892

Booklets about Cancer Treatment

Radiation Therapy and You: A Guide to Self-Help During Treatment *

Chemotherapy and You: A Guide to Self-Help During Treatment *

Eating Hints: Recipes and Tips for Better Nutrition During Cancer Treatment *

Questions and Answers About Pain Control

What Are Clinical Trials All About?

Booklets about Living with Cancer

Taking Time: Support for People With Cancer and the People Who Care About Them

When Cancer Recurs: Meeting the Challenge Again *

Advanced Cancer: Living Each Day *

* Reprinted in this volume—see Table of Contents

Chapter 34

Penile Cancer

What Is Cancer of the Penis?

Cancer of the penis, a rare kind of cancer in the United States, is a disease in which cancer (malignant) cells are found on the skin and in the tissues of the penis.

Men who are not circumcised at birth may have a higher risk for getting cancer of the penis. A circumcision is an operation in which the doctor takes away part or all of the foreskin from the penis. The foreskin is the skin which covers the tip of the penis. A circumcision is done on many baby boys before they go home from the hospital.

A doctor should be seen if there are any of the following problems: growths or sores on the penis, any unusual liquid coming from the penis (abnormal discharge), or bleeding.

If there are symptoms of cancer, the doctor will examine the penis and feel for any lumps. If the penis doesn't look normal or if the doctor feels any lumps, a small sample of tissue (called a biopsy) will be cut from the penis and looked at under a microscope to see if there are any cancer cells.

The prognosis (chance of recovery) and choice of treatment depend on the stage of the cancer (whether it is just in the penis or has spread to other places), and the patient's general state of health.

PDQ Statement, National Cancer Institute (NCI), updated June 1998.

Stages of Cancer of the Penis

Once cancer of the penis is found, more tests will be done to find out if the cancer has spread from the penis to other parts of the body (staging). A doctor needs to know the stage of the disease to plan treatment. The following stages are used for cancer of the penis:

Stage I

Cancer cells are found only on the surface of the glans (the head of the penis) and on the foreskin (the loose skin that covers the head of the penis).

Stage II

Cancer cells are found in the deeper tissues of the glans and have spread to the shaft of the penis (the long, slender cylinders of tissue inside the penis that contain spongy tissue and expand to produce erections).

Stage III

Cancer cells are found in the penis and have spread to nearby lymph nodes in the groin. (Lymph nodes are small bean-shaped structures that are found throughout the body; they produce and store infection-fighting cells).

Stage IV

Cancer cells are found throughout the penis and the lymph nodes in the groin and/or have spread to other parts of the body.

Recurrent

Recurrent disease means that the cancer has come back (recurred) after it has been treated. It may come back in the same area or in another place.

How Cancer of the Penis Is Treated

There are treatments for all patients with cancer of the penis. Four kinds of treatment are used:

- surgery (taking out the cancer in an operation)

- radiation therapy (using high-dose x-rays or other high-energy rays to kill cancer cells and shrink tumors)

- chemotherapy (using drugs to kill the cancer cells)

- biological therapy (using the immune system to fight cancer)

Surgery is the most common treatment of all stages of cancer of the penis. A doctor may take out the cancer using one of the following operations:

- Wide local excision takes out only the cancer and some normal tissue on either side.

- Microsurgery is an operation that removes the cancer and as little normal tissue as possible. During this surgery, the doctor uses a microscope to look at the cancerous area to make sure all the cancer cells are removed.

- Laser surgery uses a narrow beam of light to remove cancer cells.

- Circumcision is an operation that removes the foreskin.

- Amputation of the penis is an operation that takes out the penis. It is the most common and most effective treatment of cancer of the penis. In a partial penectomy, part of the penis is taken out. In a total penectomy, the whole penis is removed. Lymph nodes in the groin may be taken out during surgery.

Radiation therapy uses x-rays or other high-energy rays to kill cancer cells and shrink tumors. Radiation may come from a machine outside the body (external radiation) or from putting materials that contain radiation through thin plastic tubes into the area where the cancer cells are (internal radiation). Radiation may be used alone or after surgery.

Chemotherapy uses drugs to kill cancer cells. Fluorouracil cream (a chemotherapy drug put on the skin of the penis) is sometimes used for very small surface cancers of the penis. Chemotherapy may also be given by pill or by a needle in a vein. When chemotherapy is given in this way, it is called a systemic treatment because the drugs enter the bloodstream, travel through the body, and can kill cancer cells outside the penis.

Biological therapy tries to get the body to fight cancer. It uses materials made by the body or made in a laboratory to boost, direct, or restore the body's natural defenses against disease. Biological treatment is sometimes called biological response modifier (BRM) therapy.

Treatment by Stage

Treatment of cancer of the penis depends on the stage of the disease, the type of disease, and the patient's age and overall condition.

Standard treatment may be considered because of its effectiveness in patients in past studies, or participation in a clinical trial may be considered. Not all patients are cured with standard therapy and some standard treatments may have more side effects than are desired. For these reasons, clinical trials are designed to find better ways to treat cancer patients and are based on the most up-to-date information. Clinical trials are ongoing on in many parts of the country for most stages of cancer of the penis. To learn more about clinical trials, call the Cancer Information Service at 1-800-4-CANCER (1-800-422-6237); TTY at 1-800-332-8615.

Stage I Penile Cancer

If the cancer is limited to the foreskin, treatment will probably be wide local excision and circumcision.

If the cancer begins in the glans and does not involve other tissues, treatment may involve:

- Fluorouracil cream

- Microsurgery

If the tumor begins in the glans and involves other tissues, treatment may involve:

- Amputation of the penis (partial penectomy). Lymph nodes in the groin may also be removed.

- External radiation therapy

- Microsurgery

Clinical trials of laser therapy for stage I penile cancer are also being conducted.

Stage II Penile Cancer

Treatment may be amputation of the penis (partial, total, or radical penectomy) or radiation therapy followed by amputation of the penis. Clinical trials of laser therapy for stage II penile cancer are also being conducted.

Stage III Penile Cancer

Treatment may be amputation of the penis, followed by removal of lymph nodes on both sides of the groin or amputation of the penis followed by radiation therapy. Clinical trials of chemotherapy and chemotherapy with radiation therapy are also being conducted.

Stage IV Penile Cancer

Treatment will be designed to reduce symptoms and may include wide local excision, microsurgery, amputation of the penis, or radiation therapy. Clinical trials of chemotherapy combined with surgery or radiation therapy are also being conducted.

Recurrent Penile Cancer

If the cancer has come back (recurred), treatment may include amputation of the penis or radiation therapy. Clinical trials of chemotherapy or biological therapy are also being conducted.

To Learn More

To learn more about cancer of the penis, call the National Cancer Institute's Cancer Information Service at 1-800-4-CANCER (1-800-422-6237); TTY at 1-800-332-8615. By dialing this toll-free number, trained information specialists can answer your questions.

Cancer patients, their families and friends, and others may find the following booklets useful. They are available free of charge by calling 1-800-4-CANCER or writing:

Office of Cancer Communications
National Cancer Institute
Building 31, Room 10A24
Bethesda, MD 20892

Booklets about Cancer Treatment

Radiation Therapy and You: A Guide to Self-Help During Treatment *

Chemotherapy and You: A Guide to Self-Help During Treatment *

Eating Hints: Recipes and Tips for Better Nutrition During Cancer Treatment *

Questions and Answers About Pain Control

What Are Clinical Trials All About?

Booklets about Living with Cancer

Taking Time: Support for People With Cancer and the People Who Care About Them

When Cancer Recurs: Meeting the Challenge Again *

Advanced Cancer: Living Each Day *

* Reprinted in this volume—see Table of Contents

Chapter 35

Adult Hodgkin's Disease

What Is Hodgkin's Disease?

Hodgkin's disease is a type of lymphoma. Lymphomas are cancers that develop in the lymph system, part of the body's immune system.

The lymph system is made up of thin tubes that branch, like blood vessels, into all parts of the body. Lymph vessels carry lymph, a colorless, watery fluid that contains white blood cells called lymphocytes. Along the network of vessels are groups of small, bean-shaped organs called lymph nodes. Clusters of lymph nodes are found in the underarm, pelvis, neck, and abdomen. The lymph nodes make and store infection-fighting cells. The spleen (an organ in the upper abdomen that makes lymphocytes and filters old blood cells from the blood), the thymus (a small organ beneath the breastbone), and the tonsils (an organ in the throat) are also part of the lymph system.

Because there is lymph tissue in many parts of the body, Hodgkin's disease can start in almost any part of the body. The cancer can spread to almost any organ or tissue in the body, including the liver, bone marrow (the spongy tissue inside the large bones of the body that makes blood cells), and spleen.

Lymphomas are divided into two general types: Hodgkin's disease and non-Hodgkin's lymphomas. The cancer cells in Hodgkin's disease look a certain way under a microscope. Non-Hodgkin's lymphomas are covered in the PDQ patient information summaries on non-Hodgkin's lymphoma (adult [see Chapter 36] or childhood).

PDQ Statement, National Cancer Institute (NCI), updated January 1999.

Adult Hodgkin's disease most commonly affects young adults and people older than 55 years of age. It may also be found in patients with acquired immunodeficiency syndrome (AIDS); these patients require special treatment. [For more information on lymphoma in patients with AIDS, see Chapter 38.] Hodgkin's disease can also occur in children and is treated differently from that in adults. (For more information on the treatment of Hodgkin's disease in children, see the PDQ patient information summary on childhood Hodgkin's disease).

A doctor should be seen if any of the following symptoms persist for longer than 2 weeks: painless swelling of the lymph nodes in the neck, underarm, or groin; fever; night sweats; tiredness; weight loss without dieting; or itchy skin.

If there are symptoms, a doctor will carefully check for swelling or lumps in the neck, underarms, and groin. If the lymph nodes don't feel normal, a doctor may need to cut out a small piece and look at it under the microscope to see if there are any cancer cells. This procedure is called a biopsy.

The chance of recovery (prognosis) and choice of treatment depend on the stage of the cancer (whether it is just in one area or has spread throughout the body), the size of the swollen areas, the results of blood tests, the type of symptoms, and the patient's age, sex, and overall condition.

Stages of Adult Hodgkin's Disease

Once Hodgkin's disease is found, more tests will be done to find out if the cancer has spread from where it started to other parts of the body. This testing is called staging. A doctor needs to know the stage of the disease to plan treatment.

A doctor may determine the stage of the disease by conducting a thorough examination which may include blood tests and different kinds of x-rays. This type of staging is called clinical staging. In some cases, the doctor may need to do an operation called a laparotomy to determine the stage of the cancer. During this operation, the doctor cuts into the abdomen and carefully looks at the organs inside to see if they contain cancer. The doctor will cut out (biopsy) small pieces of tissue during the operation and look at them under a microscope to see whether they contain cancer. This type of staging is called pathologic staging. Pathologic staging is usually done only when it is needed to help the doctor plan treatment.

Each stage for Hodgkin's disease is further divided by an "A" or "B," based on whether there are certain symptoms called B symptoms. B symptoms include the following: loss of more than 10% of weight in the previous 6 months, fever without any known cause other than Hodgkin's disease, and night sweats that leave the body soaked. For example, if a patient had stage I disease without any B symptoms, the patient would have stage IA disease; if the patient had stage I disease with B symptoms, then the patient would have stage IB disease.

The following stages are used for Hodgkin's disease.

Stage I

Cancer is found in only one lymph node area or in only one area or organ outside of the lymph nodes.

Stage II

Either of the following means the disease is stage II:

- Cancer is found in two or more lymph node areas on the same side of the diaphragm (the thin muscle under the lungs that helps us breathe).

- Cancer is found in only one area or organ outside of the lymph nodes and in the lymph nodes around it. Other lymph node areas on the same side of the diaphragm may also have cancer.

Stage III

Cancer is found in lymph node areas on both sides of the diaphragm. The cancer may also have spread to an area or organ near the lymph node areas and/or to the spleen.

Stage IV

Either of the following means the disease is stage IV:

- Cancer has spread in more than one spot to an organ or organs outside the lymph system. Cancer cells may or may not be found in the lymph nodes near these organs.

- Cancer has spread to only one organ outside the lymph system, but lymph nodes far away from that organ are involved.

Recurrent

Recurrent disease means that the cancer has come back after it has been treated. It may come back in the area where it first started or in another part of the body.

How Adult Hodgkin's Disease Is Treated

There are treatments for all patients with adult Hodgkin's disease. Two types of treatment are used:

- radiation therapy (using high-dose x-rays or other high-energy rays to kill cancer cells and shrink tumors)

- chemotherapy (using drugs to kill cancer cells and shrink tumors)

Radiation therapy is the use of high-energy x-rays to kill cancer cells and shrink tumors. Radiation for Hodgkin's disease usually comes from a machine outside the body (external-beam radiation therapy). Radiation therapy given to the neck, chest, and lymph nodes under the arms is called radiation therapy to a mantle field. Radiation therapy given to the mantle field and to the lymph nodes in the upper abdomen, the spleen, and the lymph nodes in the pelvis is called total nodal irradiation. Radiation therapy may be used alone or in addition to chemotherapy.

Chemotherapy is the use of drugs to kill cancer cells and shrink tumors. Chemotherapy may be taken by pill, or it may be put into the body by inserting a needle into a vein or muscle. Chemotherapy is called a systemic treatment because the drugs enter the bloodstream, travel through the body, and can kill cancer cells throughout the body.

Also, bone marrow transplants are being studied in clinical trials for certain patients. Bone marrow transplantation is a newer type of treatment. Sometimes Hodgkin's disease becomes resistant to treatment with radiation therapy or chemotherapy. Very high doses of chemotherapy may then be used to treat the cancer. Because the high doses of chemotherapy can destroy the bone marrow, marrow is taken from the bones before treatment. The marrow is then frozen, and the patient is given high-dose chemotherapy with or without radiation therapy to treat the cancer. The marrow is then thawed and given back to the patient through a needle in a vein to replace the marrow that was destroyed. This type of transplant is called an autologous transplant. If the marrow is taken from another person, the transplant is called an allogeneic transplant.

Another type of autologous transplant is called a peripheral blood stem cell transplant. The patient's blood is passed through a machine that removes the stem cells (immature cells from which all blood cells develop), and then returns the blood to the patient. This procedure is called leukapheresis and usually takes 3 or 4 hours to complete. The stem cells are treated with drugs to kill any cancer cells and then frozen until they are transplanted to the patient. This procedure may be done alone or with an autologous bone marrow transplant.

A greater chance for recovery occurs if a doctor chooses a hospital which does more than five bone marrow transplantations per year.

Treatment by Stage

Patients may be immunized with influenza, pneumonia, and meningitis vaccines both before and every few years after treatment in order to guard against infection.

Treatment of adult Hodgkin's disease depends on the type and stage of the disease, and the patient's age, pregnancy status, past surgery to determine the stage of the disease, symptoms, and general health.

Standard treatment may be considered based on its effectiveness in past studies, or participation in a clinical trial may be considered. Not all patients are cured with standard therapy, and some standard treatments may have more side effects than are desired. Within 5 to 15 years after treatment, some patients develop another form of cancer as a result of their treatment; you should visit your doctor regularly to be checked for this possibility. For these reasons, clinical trials are designed to find better ways to treat cancer patients and are based on the most up-to-date information. Clinical trials are ongoing in most parts of the country for most stages of adult Hodgkin's disease. To learn more about clinical trials, call the Cancer Information Service at 1-800-4-CANCER (1-800-422-6237); TTY at 1-800-332-8615.

Stage I Adult Hodgkin's Disease

Treatment depends on whether the patient has stage IA or stage IB disease and where the cancer is found.

Stage IA

If the cancer is above the diaphragm and does not involve a large part of the chest, treatment may be one of the following:

1. Combination chemotherapy and radiation therapy.

2. Radiation therapy to a mantle field and to the lymph nodes in the upper abdomen.

3. Radiation therapy to a mantle field only, after surgery to determine the stage of the tumor.

4. Clinical trials of combination chemotherapy alone.

If the cancer is above the diaphragm but involves a large part of the chest, treatment may be one of the following:

1. Radiation therapy to a mantle field plus chemotherapy.

2. Radiation therapy to a mantle field and to the lymph nodes in the upper abdomen.

If the cancer is below the diaphragm, treatment may be one of the following:

1. Radiation therapy.

2. Combination chemotherapy with radiation therapy.

3. Clinical trials of chemotherapy alone.

Stage IB

Treatment may be one of the following for patients with "B" symptoms:

1. Combination chemotherapy with radiation therapy.

2. Clinical trials of chemotherapy alone.

Stage II Adult Hodgkin's Disease

Treatment depends on whether the patient has stage IIA or stage IIB disease and where the cancer is found.

Stage IIA

If the cancer is above the diaphragm and does not involve a large part of the chest, treatment may be one of the following:

1. Combination chemotherapy and radiation therapy.

2. Radiation therapy to a mantle field and to the lymph nodes in the upper abdomen.

3. Radiation therapy to a mantle field only, after surgery to determine the stage of the tumor.

4. Clinical trials of combination chemotherapy alone.

If the cancer is above the diaphragm but involves a large part of the chest, treatment may be the following:

Radiation therapy to a mantle field plus chemotherapy.

Stage IIB

Treatment may be one of the following for patients with "B" symptoms:

1. Combination chemotherapy with or without radiation therapy.

2. Clinical trials of chemotherapy alone.

Stage III Adult Hodgkin's Disease

Treatment depends on whether the patient has stage IIIA or stage IIIB disease and where the cancer is found.

Stage IIIA

If the cancer does not involve a large part of the chest, treatment may be one of the following:

1. Combination chemotherapy alone.

2. Combination chemotherapy plus radiation therapy.

3. Total or subtotal nodal irradiation. Radiation may also be given to the liver.

4. A clinical trial of chemotherapy.

If the cancer involves a large part of the chest, treatment may be: Combination chemotherapy with radiation therapy.

Stage IIIB

Treatment may be one of the following:

1. Combination chemotherapy with radiation therapy.

2. A clinical trial of chemotherapy.

Stage IV Adult Hodgkin's Disease

Treatment may be one of the following:

1. Combination chemotherapy.

2. Combination chemotherapy and radiation therapy.

3. Clinical trials of chemotherapy with bone marrow transplantation.

Recurrent Adult Hodgkin's Disease

The treatment depends on where the disease comes back and the treatment received before. If the treatment received before was radiation therapy without chemotherapy, chemotherapy may be given. If the treatment received before was chemotherapy without radiation therapy and the cancer comes back only in the lymph nodes, radiation therapy to the lymph nodes with or without more chemotherapy may be given. If the disease comes back in more than one area, more chemotherapy may be given or a clinical trial of high doses of chemotherapy with bone marrow or peripheral stem cell transplantation may be presented as an option.

To Learn More

To learn more about adult Hodgkin's disease, call the National Cancer Institute's Cancer Information Service at 1-800-4-CANCER (1-800-422-6237); TTY at 1-800-332-8615. By dialing this toll-free number, you can speak with a trained information specialist who can answer your questions.

The Cancer Information Service also has a variety of booklets that are available to the public and can be sent on request. The following booklet about adult Hodgkin's disease may be helpful: *What You Need To Know About Hodgkin's Disease.*

Cancer patients, their families and friends, and others may find the following booklets useful. They are available free of charge by calling 1-800-4-CANCER or writing:

Office of Cancer Communications
National Cancer Institute
Building 31, Room 10A24
Bethesda, MD 20892

Booklets about Cancer Treatment

Radiation Therapy and You: A Guide to Self-Help During Treatment *

Chemotherapy and You: A Guide to Self-Help During Treatment *

Eating Hints: Recipes and Tips for Better Nutrition During Cancer Treatment *

Questions and Answers About Pain Control

What Are Clinical Trials All About?

Booklets about Living with Cancer

Taking Time: Support for People With Cancer and the People Who Care About Them

When Cancer Recurs: Meeting the Challenge Again *

Advanced Cancer: Living Each Day *

* Reprinted in this volume—see Table of Contents

Chapter 36

Non-Hodgkin's Lymphoma

Introduction

The diagnosis of cancer brings with it many questions and a need for clear, understandable answers. This chapter from the National Cancer Institute (NCI) is intended to help people with non-Hodgkin's lymphoma and their families and friends better understand this type of cancer. We hope others will read it as well to learn more about this disease.

This chapter discusses symptoms, diagnosis, and treatment. It also has information to help patients cope with non-Hodgkin's lymphoma.

Research has led to real progress against cancer—better survival and an improved quality of life. Through research, our knowledge about non-Hodgkin's lymphoma keeps increasing. For up-to-date information, call the National Cancer Institute's Cancer Information Service (CIS). The toll-free number is 1-800-4-CANCER (1-800-422-6237). The CIS provides the most current information on cancer for patients, health professionals, and the general public. Cancer information specialists can talk with callers and send information from PDQ, the NCI cancer information database, and other NCI materials about cancer. Several NCI publications are listed in the Other Booklets section. Other sources of NCI information are listed in the National Cancer Institute Information Resources section.

"What You Need To Know About Non-Hodgkin's Lymphoma," National Cancer Institute (NCI), updated April 1999.

What Is Non-Hodgkin's Lymphoma?

Non-Hodgkin's lymphoma is a type of cancer. Lymphoma is a general term for cancers that develop in the lymphatic system. Hodgkin's disease is one type of lymphoma. (It is the subject of another NCI booklet, *What You Need To Know About Hodgkin's Disease*.) All other lymphomas are grouped together and are called non-Hodgkin's lymphoma. Lymphomas account for about 5 percent of all cases of cancer in this country.

The lymphatic system is part of the body's immune system. It helps the body fight disease and infection. The lymphatic system includes a network of thin tubes that branch, like blood vessels, into tissues throughout the body. Lymphatic vessels carry lymph, a colorless, watery fluid that contains infection-fighting cells called lymphocytes. Along this network of vessels are small organs called lymph nodes. Clusters of lymph nodes are found in the underarms, groin, neck, chest, and abdomen. Other parts of the lymphatic system are the spleen, thymus, tonsils, and bone marrow. Lymphatic tissue is also found in other parts of the body, including the stomach, intestines, and skin.

To understand non-Hodgkin's lymphoma, it is helpful to know how normal cells, the body's basic unit of life, become cancerous. Cancer is a group of many different diseases that have some important things in common. They all arise in cells. Normally, cells grow and divide to produce more cells only when the body needs them. This orderly process helps keep the body healthy. Sometimes cells keep dividing when new cells are not needed, creating a mass of extra tissue. This mass is called a growth or tumor. Tumors can be either benign (not cancerous) or malignant (cancerous).

In non-Hodgkin's lymphoma, cells in the lymphatic system become abnormal. They divide and grow without any order or control, or old cells do not die as cells normally do. Because lymphatic tissue is present in many parts of the body, non-Hodgkin's lymphoma can start almost anywhere in the body. Non-Hodgkin's lymphoma may occur in a single lymph node, a group of lymph nodes, or in another organ. This type of cancer can spread to almost any part of the body, including the liver, bone marrow, and spleen.

Symptoms

The most common symptom of non-Hodgkin's lymphoma is a painless swelling of the lymph nodes in the neck, underarm, or groin.

Other symptoms may include the following:

- Unexplained fevers
- Night sweats
- Constant fatigue
- Unexplained weight loss
- Itchy skin
- Reddened patches on the skin

When symptoms like these occur, they are not sure signs of non-Hodgkin's lymphoma. They may also be caused by other, less serious conditions, such as the flu or other infections. Only a doctor can make a diagnosis. When symptoms are present, it is important to see a doctor so that any illness can be diagnosed and treated as early as possible. Do not wait to feel pain; early non-Hodgkin's lymphoma may not cause pain.

Diagnosis

If non-Hodgkin's lymphoma is suspected, the doctor asks about the person's medical history and performs a physical exam. The exam may include feeling to see if the lymph nodes in the neck, underarm, or groin are enlarged. In addition to checking general signs of health, the doctor may perform blood tests.

The doctor may also order imaging tests that produce pictures of the inside of the body. Such pictures may include:

- *X-rays:* High-energy radiation used to take pictures of areas inside the body, such as the chest, bones, liver, and spleen.

- *CT (or CAT) scan:* A series of detailed pictures of areas inside the body. The pictures are created by a computer linked to an x-ray machine.

- *MRI (magnetic resonance imaging):* Detailed pictures of areas inside the body produced with a powerful magnet linked to a computer.

- *Lymphangiogram:* Pictures of the lymphatic system taken with x-rays after a special dye is injected to outline the lymph nodes and vessels.

In most cases, a biopsy is needed to make a diagnosis. A surgeon removes a sample of tissue so that a pathologist can examine it under a microscope to check for cancer cells. A biopsy for non-Hodgkin's lymphoma is usually taken from a lymph node, but other tissues may be sampled as well. Sometimes, an operation called a laparotomy may be performed. During this operation, a surgeon cuts into the abdomen and removes samples of tissue to check under a microscope.

A patient who needs a biopsy may want to ask the doctor some of the following questions:

- How long will the biopsy take? Will it hurt?

- How soon will I know the results?

- If I do have cancer, who will talk with me about treatment? When?

Types of Non-Hodgkin's Lymphoma

Over the years, doctors have used a variety of terms to classify the many different types of non-Hodgkin's lymphoma. Most often, they are grouped by how the cancer cells look under a microscope and how quickly they are likely to grow and spread. Aggressive lymphomas, also known as intermediate and high-grade lymphomas, tend to grow and spread quickly and cause severe symptoms. Indolent lymphomas, also referred to as low-grade lymphomas, tend to grow quite slowly and cause fewer symptoms.

Staging

If non-Hodgkin's lymphoma is diagnosed, the doctor needs to learn the stage, or extent, of the disease. Staging is an attempt to determine what parts of the body the cancer has affected. Treatment decisions depend on these findings.

The doctor considers the following to determine the stage of non-Hodgkin's lymphoma:

- The number and location of affected lymph nodes.

- Whether the affected lymph nodes are above, below, or on both sides of the diaphragm (the thin muscle under the lungs and heart that separates the chest from the abdomen).

- Whether the disease has spread to the bone marrow, spleen, or to organs outside the lymphatic system such as the liver.

In staging, the doctor may use some of the same imaging tests used for diagnosis of non-Hodgkin's lymphoma. Other staging procedures may include additional biopsies of lymph nodes, the liver, bone marrow, or other tissue. A bone marrow biopsy involves removing a sample of bone marrow through a needle inserted into the hip or another large bone. A pathologist examines the sample under a microscope to check for cancer cells.

Treatment

Treatment for non-Hodgkin's lymphoma depends on the stage of the disease, the type of cells involved, whether they are indolent or aggressive, and the age and general health of the patient.

Non-Hodgkin's lymphoma is often treated by a team of specialists that includes a hematologist, medical oncologist, and/or radiation oncologist. Non-Hodgkin's lymphoma is usually treated with chemotherapy, radiation therapy, or a combination of these treatments. In some cases, bone marrow transplantation, biological therapies, or surgery may be an option. For indolent lymphomas, the doctor may decide to wait until the disease causes symptoms before starting treatment. Often, this is called "watchful waiting."

Taking part in clinical trials (research studies) to evaluate promising new ways to treat non-Hodgkin's lymphoma is an important option for many people with this disease. Such studies are designed to improve cancer treatment. For more information, see the Clinical Trials section.

Getting a Second Opinion

Before starting treatment, the patient may want a second opinion about the diagnosis and the treatment plan. Some insurance companies require a second opinion; others may cover a second opinion if the patient requests it.

There are a number of ways to find a doctor who can give a second opinion:

- The patient's doctor may be able to suggest specialists to consult.

- The Cancer Information Service, at 1-800-4-CANCER, can tell callers about cancer treatment facilities, including cancer centers and other programs supported by the National Cancer Institute.

- Patients can get the names of doctors from their local medical society, a nearby hospital, or a medical school.

- The *Official ABMS Directory of Board Certified Medical Specialists* lists doctors' names along with their specialty and their background. This resource, produced by the American Board of Medical Specialties, is available in most public libraries.

Preparing for Treatment

Many people with cancer want to learn all they can about their disease and their treatment choices so they can take an active part in decisions about their medical care. When a person is diagnosed with cancer, shock and stress are natural reactions. These feelings may make it difficult for patients to think of everything they want to ask the doctor. Often, it helps to make a list of questions. To help remember what the doctor says, patients may take notes or ask whether they may use a tape recorder. Some people also want to have a family member or friend with them when they talk to the doctor—to take part in the discussion, to take notes, or just to listen.

These are some questions a patient may want to ask the doctor before treatment begins:

- What kind of non-Hodgkin's lymphoma do I have?
- What is the stage of the disease?
- What are my treatment choices? Which do you recommend for me? Why?
- What are the risks and possible side effects of each treatment?
- What are the chances that the treatment will be successful?
- How long will treatment last?
- Will treatment affect my normal activities? If so, for how long?
- Are new treatments under study? Would a clinical trial be appropriate for me?
- What is the treatment likely to cost?

Patients do not need to ask all their questions or remember all the answers at one time. They will have other chances to ask the doctor to explain things and to get more information.

Methods of Treatment

Chemotherapy and radiation therapy are the most common treatments for non-Hodgkin's lymphoma, although bone marrow transplantation, biological therapies, or surgery are sometimes used.

Chemotherapy uses drugs to kill cancer cells. It may be given alone or with radiation therapy. Chemotherapy for non-Hodgkin's lymphoma is usually a combination of several different types of drugs.

Chemotherapy is usually given in cycles: a treatment period followed by a recovery period, then another treatment period, and so on. Most anticancer drugs are given by injection into a vein (IV); some are given by mouth. Chemotherapy is a systemic treatment because the drugs enter the bloodstream and travel throughout the body.

Usually a patient has chemotherapy as an outpatient (at the hospital, at the doctor's office, or at home). However, depending on which drugs are given and the patient's general health, a short hospital stay may be needed.

These are some questions patients may want to ask the doctor before starting chemotherapy:

- What is the goal of this treatment?

- What drugs will I be taking?

- Will the drugs cause side effects? What can I do about them?

- How long will I need to take this treatment?

- What can I do to take care of myself during treatment?

- How will we know if the drugs are working?

Radiation therapy (also called radiotherapy) uses high-energy rays to kill cancer cells. It may be given alone or with chemotherapy. Radiation therapy is local treatment; it affects cancer cells only in the treated area. Radiation therapy for non-Hodgkin's lymphoma comes from a machine that aims the rays at a specific area of the body. There is no radioactivity in the body when the treatment is over.

These are some questions a patient may want to ask the doctor before having radiation therapy:

- What is the goal of this treatment?

- How will radiation be given?

- When will the treatments begin? When will they end?

- How will I feel during therapy?

- What can I do to take care of myself during therapy?

- How will we know if the radiation therapy is working?

- How will treatment affect my normal activities?

Sometimes patients are given chemotherapy and/or radiation therapy to kill undetected cancer cells that may be present in the central nervous system (CNS). In this treatment, called central nervous system prophylaxis, the doctor injects anticancer drugs directly into the cerebrospinal fluid.

Bone marrow transplantation (BMT) may also be a treatment option, especially for patients whose non-Hodgkin's lymphoma has recurred (come back). To prepare for BMT, the body is exposed to high doses of chemotherapy and radiation in an effort to destroy all lymphoma cells. Dosages are so great that the patient's own bone marrow is destroyed and must be replaced by healthy marrow. The healthy bone marrow may come from a donor, or it may be marrow that has been removed from the patient and stored before the high-dose treatment. If the patient's own bone marrow is used, it may first be treated outside the body to remove cancerous cells. Patients who have a bone marrow transplant usually stay in the hospital for several weeks. Until the transplanted bone marrow begins to produce enough white blood cells, patients have to be carefully protected from infection.

These are some questions patients may want to ask the doctor before having a BMT:

- What are the benefits of this treatment?

- What are the risks and side effects? What can be done about them?

- How long will I be in the hospital? What care will I need after I leave the hospital?

- What changes in normal activities will be necessary?

- How will I know if the treatment is working?

Biological therapy (also called immunotherapy) is a form of treatment that uses the body's immune system, either directly or indirectly, to fight cancer or to lessen side effects that can be caused by some cancer treatments. It uses materials made by the body or made in a laboratory to boost, direct, or restore the body's natural defenses against disease. Biological therapy is sometimes also called biological response modifier therapy.

These are some questions patients may want to ask the doctor before starting biological therapy:

- What is the goal of this treatment?

- What drugs will be used?

- Will the treatment cause side effects? If so, what can I do about them?

- Will I have to be in the hospital to receive treatment?

- How long will I be on treatment?

- When will I be able to resume my normal activities?

Surgery may be performed to remove a tumor. Tissue around the tumor and nearby lymph nodes may also be removed during the operation.

These are some questions a patient may want to ask the doctor before surgery:

- What kind of operation will it be?

- How will I feel after the operation?

- If I have pain, how will you help?

- Will I need more treatment after surgery?

- When will I be able to resume my normal activities?

Clinical Trials

Many people with non-Hodgkin's lymphoma take part in clinical trials (research studies). Doctors conduct clinical trials to learn about the effectiveness and side effects of new treatments. In some cases, all patients receive the new treatment. In others, doctors compare different therapies by giving the new treatment to one group of patients and the standard therapy to another group; or they may compare one standard treatment with another. Research like this has led to significant advances in the treatment of cancer. Each achievement brings researchers closer to the eventual control of cancer.

Doctors are studying radiation therapy, new ways of giving chemotherapy, new drugs and drug combinations, biological therapies, bone marrow transplantation, peripheral blood stem cell transplantation, and new ways of combining various types of treatment. Some studies are designed to find ways to reduce the side effects of treatment and to improve the patient's quality of life.

People who take part in these studies have the first chance to benefit from treatments that have shown promise in earlier research.

They also make an important contribution to medical science. While clinical trials may pose risks for the people who take part, each study takes steps to protect patients. Patients who are interested in taking part in a clinical trial should talk with their doctor. They may want to read the National Cancer Institute booklet *Taking Part in Clinical Trials: What Cancer Patients Need To Know*, which describes how studies are carried out and explains their possible benefits and risks. NCI also has a Web site at http://cancertrials.nci.nih.gov that provides detailed information about ongoing studies for non-Hodgkin's lymphoma.

Another way to learn about clinical trials is through PDQ, a cancer information database developed by the National Cancer Institute. PDQ contains information about cancer treatment and about clinical trials in progress throughout the country. The Cancer Information Service can provide PDQ information to patients and the public. PDQ can also be accessed through other sources listed in the National Cancer Institute Information Resources section.

Side Effects of Treatment

The methods used to treat lymphomas are very powerful. It is hard to limit the effects of therapy so that only cancer cells are removed or destroyed. Because treatment also damages healthy cells and tissues, it often causes side effects.

The side effects of cancer treatment depend mainly on the type and extent of the treatment. Side effects may not be the same for everyone, and they may change from one treatment to the next. Doctors and nurses can explain the possible side effects of treatment, and they can help relieve symptoms that may occur during and after treatment.

Radiation Therapy

The side effects of radiation depend on the treatment dose and the part of the body that is treated. During radiation therapy, people are likely to become very tired, especially in the later weeks of treatment. Resting is important, but doctors usually advise patients to try to stay as active as they can.

It is common to lose hair in the treated area and for the skin to become red, dry, tender, or itchy. There may also be permanent darkening or "bronzing" of the skin in the treated area. When the chest and neck area is treated, patients may have a dry, sore throat and may have some trouble swallowing. Some patients may have tingling or numbness in their arms, legs, and lower back. Radiation therapy to the abdomen may cause nausea, vomiting, diarrhea, or urinary discomfort. Usually, the doctor can suggest certain diet changes or medicine to ease these problems.

Radiation therapy also may cause a decrease in the number of white blood cells that help protect the body against infection. Although the side effects of radiation therapy can be difficult, the doctor can usually treat or control them. The National Cancer Institute booklet *Radiation Therapy and You* [reprinted in this volume as Chapter 66] has helpful information about radiation therapy and managing its side effects. It may also help to know that, in most cases, side effects are not permanent. However, patients may want to discuss with their doctor the effect of radiation treatment on fertility (the ability to produce children) and the increased risk of second cancers after treatment is over.

Chemotherapy

The side effects of chemotherapy depend mainly on the drugs and the doses received. In addition, as with other types of treatment, side effects vary from person to person. Generally, anticancer drugs affect cells that divide rapidly. In addition to cancer cells, these include blood cells, which fight infection, help the blood to clot, or carry oxygen to all parts of the body. When blood cells are affected, people are more likely to get infections, may bruise or bleed easily, and may feel unusually weak and tired. Cells in hair roots and cells that line the digestive tract also divide rapidly. As a result, people may lose their hair and may have other side effects such as poor appetite, nausea and vomiting, or mouth and lip sores. Patients may experience dizziness and darkening of skin and fingernails. These side effects generally go away gradually during the recovery periods between treatments or after treatment is over. However, certain types of chemotherapy can increase the risk of developing a second cancer later in life.

In some men and women, chemotherapy causes a loss of fertility. Loss of fertility may be temporary or permanent depending on the drugs used and the patient's age. For men, sperm banking before treatment may be a choice. Women's menstrual periods may stop, and they may have hot flashes and vaginal dryness. Menstrual periods are more likely to return in young women. The National Cancer Institute booklet *Chemotherapy and You* [reprinted in this volume as Chapter 63] has helpful information about chemotherapy and coping with side effects.

Bone Marrow Transplantation

Patients who have a bone marrow transplant face an increased risk of infection, bleeding, and other side effects from the large doses of chemotherapy and radiation they receive. In addition, graft-versus-host disease (GVHD) may occur in patients who receive bone marrow from a donor. In GVHD, the donated marrow attacks the patient's tissues (most often the liver, the skin, and the digestive tract). GVHD can be mild or very severe. It can occur any time after the transplant (even years later). Drugs may be given to reduce the risk of GVHD and to treat the problem if it occurs. The National Cancer Institute's publication Research Report: *Bone Marrow Transplantation and Peripheral Blood Stem Cell Transplantation* [reprinted in this volume as Chapter 68] provides more information about this treatment and the possible side effects.

Biological Therapy

The side effects caused by biological therapy vary with the type of treatment. These treatments may cause flu-like symptoms such as chills, fever, muscle aches, weakness, loss of appetite, nausea, vomiting, and diarrhea. Patients also may bleed or bruise easily, get a skin rash, or have swelling. These problems can be severe, but they usually go away after treatment stops.

Surgery

The side effects of surgery depend on the location of the tumor, the type of operation, the patient's general health, and other factors. Although patients are often uncomfortable during the first few days after surgery, this pain can be controlled with medicine. People should feel free to discuss pain relief with the doctor or nurse. It is also common for patients to feel tired or weak for a while. The length of time it takes to recover from an operation varies for each patient.

Nutrition for Cancer Patients

Eating well during cancer treatment means getting enough calories and protein to help prevent weight loss and regain strength. This often helps people feel better and have more energy.

Some people with cancer find it hard to eat a balanced diet because they may lose their appetite. In addition, common side effects of treatment, such as nausea, vomiting, or mouth sores, can make eating difficult. Often, foods taste different. Also, people being treated for cancer may not feel like eating when they are uncomfortable or tired.

Doctors, nurses, and dietitians can offer advice on how to get enough calories and protein during cancer treatment. Patients and their families also may want to read the National Cancer Institute booklet *Eating Hints for Cancer Patients* [reprinted in this volume as Chapter 77], which contains many useful suggestions.

Recovery and Outlook

It is natural for anyone facing cancer to be concerned about what the future holds. Understanding the nature of cancer and what to expect can help patients and their loved ones plan treatment, anticipate lifestyle changes, and make quality of life and financial decisions.

Cancer patients frequently ask their doctors, "What is my prognosis?" Prognosis is a prediction of the future course and outcome of a disease and an indication of the likelihood of recovery. When doctors discuss a patient's prognosis, they are attempting to project what is likely to occur for that individual patient.

Sometimes patients use statistics they have heard to try to figure out their own chances of being cured. However, statistics reflect the experience of large groups of patients; they cannot be used to predict what will happen to a particular patient because no two patients are alike. The prognosis for a person with non-Hodgkin's lymphoma can be affected by many factors, particularly the stage of the cancer and the patient's age, general health, and response to treatment. The doctor who is most familiar with the patient's situation is in the best position to help interpret statistics and discuss the patient's prognosis.

When doctors talk about surviving cancer, they may use the term remission rather than cure. Although many people with non-Hodgkin's lymphoma are successfully treated, doctors use this term because cancer can return. It is important to discuss the possibility of recurrence with the doctor.

Followup Care

It is important for people who have had cancer to have regular followup examinations after their treatment is over. Regular followup care ensures that any changes in health are discussed, and any recurrent cancer can be treated as soon as possible. Generally, checkups include a careful physical exam, imaging tests, blood tests, and other laboratory tests. Patients should follow their doctor's recommendations on health care and checkups.

Support for People with Cancer

Living with a serious disease is not easy. People with cancer and those who care about them face many problems and challenges. Coping with these problems is often easier when people have helpful information and support services. Several useful National Cancer Institute booklets, including *Taking Time*, are available from the Cancer Information Service and through other sources listed in the National Cancer Institute Information Resources section.

Friends and relatives can be very supportive. It also helps many patients to discuss their concerns with others who have cancer. Cancer patients often get together in support groups, where they can share what they have learned about coping with cancer and the effects of treatment. It is important to keep in mind, however, that each person is different. Treatments and ways of dealing with cancer that work for one person may not be right for another—even if they both have the same kind of cancer. It is always a good idea to discuss the advice of friends and family members with the doctor.

Cancer patients may worry about holding their jobs, caring for their families, keeping up with daily activities, or starting new relationships. Concerns about tests, treatments, hospital stays, and medical bills are common. Doctors, nurses, social workers, and other members of the health care team can answer questions about treatment, working, or other activities. They can also discuss outlook (prognosis) and the activity level people may be able to manage. Meeting with a social worker, counselor, or member of the clergy can be helpful to people who want to talk about their feelings or discuss their concerns.

Additional information about locating support services for people with cancer and their families is available through sources described in the National Cancer Institute Information Resources section.

Risk Factors Associated with Non-Hodgkin's Lymphoma

The incidence of non-Hodgkin's lymphoma has increased dramatically over the last couple of decades. This disease has gone from being relatively rare to being the fifth most common cancer in the United States. At this time, little is known about the reasons for this increase or about exactly what causes non-Hodgkin's lymphoma.

Doctors can seldom explain why one person gets non-Hodgkin's lymphoma and another does not. It is clear, however, that lymphomas are not caused by an injury, and are not contagious; no one can "catch" non-Hodgkin's lymphoma from another person.

By studying patterns of cancer in the population, researchers have found certain risk factors that are more common in people who get non-Hodgkin's lymphoma than in those who do not get this disease. It is important to know, however, that most people with these risk factors do not get non-Hodgkin's lymphoma, and many who do get this disease have none of these risk factors.

The following are some of the factors associated with this disease:

- Sex/Age—The likelihood of getting non-Hodgkin's lymphoma increases with age and is more common in men than in women.

- Weakened Immune System—Non-Hodgkin's lymphoma is more common among people with inherited immune deficiencies, autoimmune diseases, or HIV/AIDS, and among people taking immunosuppressant drugs following organ transplants.

- Viruses—Human T-lymphotropic virus type I (HTLV-1) and Epstein-Barr virus are two infectious agents that increase the chance of getting non-Hodgkin's lymphoma.

- Environment—People who work extensively with or are otherwise exposed to some chemicals, such as pesticides, solvents, or fertilizers, have a greater chance of developing non-Hodgkin's lymphoma.

People who are concerned about non-Hodgkin's lymphoma should talk with their doctor about the disease, the symptoms to watch for, and an appropriate schedule for checkups. The doctor's advice will be based on the person's age, medical history, and other factors.

Other Booklets

Cancer patients, their families and friends, and others may find the following booklets useful. They are available free of charge by calling 1-800-4-CANCER or writing:

Office of Cancer Communications
National Cancer Institute
Building 31, Room 10A24
Bethesda, MD 20892

Booklets about Cancer Treatment

*Radiation Therapy and You: A Guide to Self-Help During Treatment ***

*Chemotherapy and You: A Guide to Self-Help During Treatment ***

*Eating Hints: Recipes and Tips for Better Nutrition During Cancer Treatment ***

Questions and Answers About Pain Control

What Are Clinical Trials All About?

Booklets about Living with Cancer

Taking Time: Support for People With Cancer and the People Who Care About Them

*When Cancer Recurs: Meeting the Challenge Again ***

*Advanced Cancer: Living Each Day ***

* Reprinted in this volume—see Table of Contents

National Cancer Institute Information Resources

You may want more information for yourself, your family, and your doctor. The following National Cancer Institute (NCI) services are available to help you.

Telephone

Cancer Information Service (CIS) Provides accurate, up-to-date information on cancer to patients and their families, health professionals, and the general public. Information specialists translate the latest scientific information into understandable language and respond in English, Spanish, or on TTY equipment.
Toll-free: 1-800-4-CANCER (1-800-422-6237)
TTY: 1-800-332-8615

Internet

http://www.nci.nih.gov—NCI's primary Web site; contains information about the Institute and its programs.

http://cancertrials.nci.nih.gov—CancerTrials; NCI's comprehensive clinical trials information center for patients, health professionals, and the public. Includes information on understanding trials, deciding whether to participate in trials, finding specific trials, plus research news and other resources.

http://cancernet.nci.nih.gov—CancerNet; contains material for health professionals, patients, and the public, including information from PDQ about cancer treatment, screening, prevention, supportive care, and clinical trials, and CANCERLIT, a bibliographic database.

E-mail

CancerMail—Includes NCI information about cancer treatment, screening, prevention, and supportive care. To obtain a contents list, send e-mail to cancermail@icicc.nci.nih.gov with the word "help" in the body of the message.

Fax

CancerFax—Includes NCI information about cancer treatment, screening, prevention, and supportive care. To obtain a contents list, dial 301-402-5874 from a fax machine hand set and follow the recorded instructions.

Chapter 37

Adult Non-Hodgkin's Lymphoma

What Is Adult Non-Hodgkin's Lymphoma?

Adult non-Hodgkin's lymphoma is a disease in which cancer (malignant) cells are found in the lymph system. The lymph system is made up of thin tubes that branch, like blood vessels, into all parts of the body. Lymph vessels carry lymph, a colorless, watery fluid that contains white blood cells called lymphocytes. Along the network of vessels are groups of small, bean-shaped organs called lymph nodes. Clusters of lymph nodes are found in the underarm, pelvis, neck, and abdomen. The lymph nodes make and store infection-fighting cells. The spleen (an organ in the upper abdomen that makes lymphocytes and filters old blood cells from the blood), the thymus (a small organ beneath the breastbone), and the tonsils (an organ in the throat) are also part of the lymph system.

Because lymph tissue is found in many parts of the body, non-Hodgkin's lymphoma can start in almost any part of the body. The cancer can spread to almost any organ or tissue in the body, including the liver, bone marrow (the spongy tissue inside the large bones of the body that makes blood cells), spleen, and nose.

Lymphomas are divided into two general types: Hodgkin's disease and non-Hodgkin's lymphomas. The cancer cells in Hodgkin's disease look a certain way under a microscope. Hodgkin's disease is discussed in the PDQ patient information summaries on Hodgkin's disease

PDQ Statement, National Cancer Institute (NCI), updated December 1999.

(adult or childhood). Non-Hodgkin's lymphoma can also occur in children and is treated differently (see the PDQ patient information summary on childhood non-Hodgkin's lymphoma for treatment of non-Hodgkin's lymphoma in children).

There are many types of non-Hodgkin's lymphomas. Some types spread more quickly than others. The type is determined by how the cancer cells look under a microscope. This determination is called the histology. The histologies for adult non-Hodgkin's lymphoma are divided into two groups: indolent lymphomas, which are slower growing and have fewer symptoms, and aggressive lymphomas, which grow more quickly.

Indolent

- follicular small cleaved cell lymphoma

- follicular mixed cell lymphoma

- follicular large cell lymphoma

- adult diffuse small cleaved cell lymphoma

- small lymphocytic (marginal zone)

Agressive

- adult diffuse mixed cell lymphoma

- adult diffuse large cell lymphoma

- adult immunoblastic large cell lymphoma

- adult lymphoblastic lymphoma

- adult small noncleaved cell lymphoma

Other types of indolent non-Hodgkin's lymphoma are lymphoplasmacytoid lymphoma, monocytoid B-cell lymphoma, mucosa-associated lymphoid tissue (MALT) lymphoma, splenic marginal zone lymphoma, hairy cell leukemia, and cutaneous T-cell lymphoma (Mycosis fungoides/ Sezary syndrome).

Other types of aggressive non-Hodgkin's lymphoma are anaplastic large-cell lymphoma, adult T-cell lymphoma/leukemia, mantle cell lymphoma, intravascular lymphomatosis, angioimmunoblastic T-cell lymphoma, angiocentric lymphoma, intestinal T-cell lymphoma, primary mediastinal B-cell lymphoma, peripheral T-cell lymphoma, lymphoblastic lymphoma, post-transplantation lymphoproliferative disorder, true histiocytic lymphoma, primary central nervous system lymphoma, and primary effusion lymphoma. Aggressive lymphomas are also seen more frequently in patients who are HIV-positive (AIDS-related lymphoma).

See specific PDQ patient information summaries for discussions of plasma cell neoplasms, hairy cell leukemia, cutaneous T-cell lymphoma, chronic lymphocytic leukemia, primary central nervous system lymphoma, and AIDS-related lymphoma, as well as childhood and adult Hodgkin's disease and acute lymphoblastic leukemia.

A doctor should be seen if any of the following symptoms persist: painless swelling in the lymph nodes in the neck, underarm, or groin; unexplained fever; drenching night sweats; tiredness; unexplained weight loss in the past 6 months; or itchy skin.

If these symptoms are present, a doctor will carefully check for swelling or lumps in the neck, underarms, and groin. If the lymph nodes don't feel normal, a doctor may need to surgically remove a small piece of tissue and look at it under a microscope to see if there are any cancer cells. This procedure is called a biopsy.

The chance of recovery (prognosis) and choice of treatment depend on the stage of the cancer (whether it is just in one area or has spread throughout the body), and the patient's age and overall condition.

Stages of Adult Non-Hodgkin's Lymphoma

Once non-Hodgkin's lymphoma is found, more tests will be done to find out if the cancer has spread from where it started to other parts of the body. This testing is called staging. A doctor needs to know the stage of the disease to plan treatment.

A doctor may determine the stage of the disease by examining the patient, doing blood and bone marrow tests, and taking x-rays called computed tomographic (CT or CAT) scans that produce an image of the inside of the body. This type of staging is called clinical staging. In some cases, the doctor may need to do a laparotomy to determine the stage of the cancer. During this operation, a doctor cuts into the abdomen and carefully looks at the organs to see if they contain cancer. A doctor will cut out (biopsy) small pieces of tissue during the operation and look at them under a microscope to see whether they contain cancer. This type of staging is called pathologic staging. Pathologic staging is usually done only when it is needed to help a doctor plan treatment.

Occasionally, specialized staging systems are used. A doctor should be aware of the system used.

A number of other factors are important in determining the staging and recovery (prognosis) of patients with non-Hodgkin's lymphoma. Some of these include the patient's age and responsiveness to treatment, tumor size, and number of places the tumor has spread outside of the lymph nodes.

The following stages are used for non-Hodgkin's lymphoma:

Stage I

Cancer is found in only one lymph node area or in only one area or organ outside the lymph nodes.

Stage II

Either of the following means that the disease is stage II:

- Cancer is found in two or more lymph node areas on the same side of the diaphragm (the thin muscle under the lungs that helps breathing).
- Cancer is found in only one area or organ outside the lymph nodes and in the lymph nodes around it. Other lymph node areas on the same side of the diaphragm may also have cancer.

In contiguous stage II cancer, the positive lymph node areas are next to one another; in non-contiguous stage II, the positive lymph nodes are not next to each other, but are still on the same side of the diaphragm.

Stage III

Cancer is found in lymph node areas on both sides of the diaphragm. The cancer may also have spread to an area or organ near the lymph node areas and/or to the spleen.

Stage IV

Either of the following means that the disease is stage IV:

- Cancer has spread to more than one organ or organs outside the lymph system. Cancer cells may or may not be found in the lymph nodes near these organs.
- Cancer has spread to only one organ outside the lymph system, but lymph nodes far away from that organ are involved.

Recurrent

Recurrent disease means that the cancer has come back after it has been treated. It may come back in the area where it first started or in another part of the body.

How Adult Non-Hodgkin's Lymphoma Is Treated

There are treatments for all patients with adult non-Hodgkin's lymphoma. Three types of treatment are used:

- radiation therapy (using high-dose x-rays or other high-energy rays to kill cancer cells and shrink tumors)

- chemotherapy (using drugs to kill cancer cells and shrink tumors)

- biological therapy (using the body's immune system to fight cancer)

Radiation therapy is the use of high-energy x-rays to kill cancer cells and shrink tumors. Radiation for non-Hodgkin's lymphoma usually comes from a machine outside the body (external-beam radiation therapy). Radiation therapy given to the neck, chest, and lymph nodes under the arms is called radiation therapy to a mantle field. Radiation therapy given to the mantle field and to the lymph nodes in the upper abdomen, the spleen, and the lymph nodes in the pelvis is called total nodal irradiation. Radiation given to the brain to keep the cancer cells from growing there is called cranial irradiation. Radiation therapy may be used alone or in addition to chemotherapy.

Chemotherapy is the use of drugs to kill cancer cells and shrink tumors. Chemotherapy may be taken by pill, or it may be put into the body by a needle in a vein or muscle. Chemotherapy is called a systemic treatment because the drugs enter the bloodstream, travel through the body, and can kill cancer cells throughout the body. To treat certain types of non-Hodgkin's lymphoma that spread to the brain, chemotherapy may be put into the fluid that surrounds the brain through a needle in the brain or back (intrathecal chemotherapy).

Biological treatment tries to help the body to fight cancer or infections. It uses materials made by the body or made in a laboratory to boost, direct, or restore the body's natural defenses against disease. Biological treatment is sometimes called biological response modifier (BRM) therapy.

Bone marrow transplantation and peripheral blood stem cell transplantation are also being tested in clinical trials for certain patients. Bone marrow transplantation is a type of treatment that uses very high doses of chemotherapy to kill resistant lymphoma cells in the body. The high doses of chemotherapy also destroy most of the bone marrow in the body. To replace the bone marrow, marrow is taken from the bones before treatment and treated with drugs or other substances to kill any cancer cells. The marrow is then frozen, and the patient is given high-dose chemotherapy with or without radiation therapy to destroy all of the remaining cancer cells. The marrow that was taken out is then thawed and given to the patient through a needle in a vein to replace the marrow that was destroyed. If the bone marrow comes from the patient, this type of transplant is called an autologous transplant. If the marrow is taken from another person, the transplant is called an allogeneic transplant. In peripheral blood stem transplantation, stem cells are removed from the patient's circulating blood before treatment and then returned after treatment. In peripheral blood stem cell transplantation, the stem cells usually come from the patient.

Other clinical trials are being conducted that are testing experimental drugs and improved therapies. Radioimmunotherapy, which is treatment with a radioactive substance that is linked to an antibody that will attach to the tumor when injected into the body, is also being performed in clinical trials.

Treatment by Stage

Treatment of adult non-Hodgkin's lymphoma depends on the stage of the disease, the histology and grade of the disease, and the patient's age and general health. Radiation therapy to the pelvis or large doses of chemotherapy may increase the risk of permanent sterility.

Standard treatment may be considered, based on its effectiveness in patients in past studies, or participation in a clinical trial. Not all patients are cured with standard therapy, and some standard treatments may have more side effects than are desired. During the 20 years after treatment, some patients develop another form of cancer, such as lung, brain, kidney, or bladder cancer; a doctor should be visited regularly to be checked for this possibility. For these reasons, clinical trials are designed to find better ways to treat cancer patients and are based on the most up-to-date information. Clinical trials are ongoing in most parts of the country for most stages of adult non-Hodgkin's lymphoma. For more information, call the Cancer Information Service at 1-800-4-CANCER (1-800-422-6237); TTY at 1-800-332-8615.

Indolent, Stage I, and Contiguous Stage II Adult NHL

Treatment options are the same whether the disease is above or below the diaphragm.

1. Radiation therapy to the area where the cancer cells are found.

2. Radiation therapy to the area where the cancer cells are found and extended to nearby lymph nodes.

3. Radiation to part or all of the lymphatic system.

4. Chemotherapy plus radiation therapy are being evaluated.

5. Chemotherapy alone or watchful waiting if radiation therapy is not possible.

Aggressive, Stage I, and Contiguous Stage II Adult NHL

If the patient had clinical staging, treatment may be one of the following:

1. Chemotherapy plus radiation therapy.

2. Chemotherapy alone.

3. Radiation therapy alone.

Indolent, Non-Contiguous Stage II/III/IV Adult NHL

Treatment may be one of the following:

1. Watchful waiting until symptoms appear.

2. Chemotherapy with a single drug.

3. Single drug chemotherapy with or without steriods.

4. Combination chemotherapy with more than one drug.

5. Chemotherapy plus radiation therapy plus bone marrow transplantation or peripheral stem cell transplantation is being tested in clinical trials.

6. A clinical trial of radioimmunotherapy with or without combination chemotherapy.

Agressive, Non-Contiguous Stage II/III/IV Adult NHL

Treatment may be one of the following:

1. Combination chemotherapy.

2. Bone marrow transplantation or peripheral stem cell transplantation is under clinical evaluation.

3. Clinical trials are evaluating new combination chemotherapies.

Adult Lymphoblastic Lymphoma

This is an aggressive form of adult non-Hodgkin's lymphoma. Treatment is usually patterned after acute lymphocytic leukemia (refer to the PDQ summary on adult acute lymphocytic leukemia for more information).
Treatment may be one of the following:

1. Combination chemotherapy including treatment of the central nervous system.

2. Combination chemotherapy plus radiation therapy.

3. Bone marrow transplantation is being evaluated in clinical trials.

Adult Diffuse Small Non-Cleaved Cell/Burkitt's Lymphoma

Treatment may be one of the following:

1. Combination chemotherapy including treatment of the central nervous system.

2. Combination chemotherapy plus bone marrow transplantation.

Indolent Recurrent Adult Non-Hodgkin's Lymphoma

Indolent lymphomas often come back (relapse) after they have been treated. Sometimes, the lymphoma will come back as a different cell type (histology), most commonly as an aggressive lymphoma. If this is the case, see the treatment section for aggressive, recurrent non-Hodgkin's lymphoma.

If the lymphoma comes back and it is still a low-grade lymphoma, treatment may be one of the following:

1. Chemotherapy with a single drug.

2. Combination chemotherapy with more than one drug.

3. Radiation therapy.

4. Radiation therapy plus chemotherapy.

5. A clinical trial of bone marrow transplantation.

6. A clinical trial of radioimmunotherapy.

Aggressive Recurrent Non-Hodgkin's Lymphoma

Treatment may be one of the following:

1. Bone marrow transplantation.

2. Bone marrow transplantation plus radiation therapy.

3. A clinical trial of chemotherapy, bone marrow transplantation or peripheral stem cell transplantation, and radiation therapy.

4. A clinical trial of radioimmunotherapy.

To Learn More

To learn more about adult non-Hodgkin's lymphoma, call the National Cancer Institute's Cancer Information Service at 1-800-4-CANCER (1-800-422-6237); TTY at 1-800-332-8615. By dialing this toll-free number, you can speak with a trained information specialist who can help answer your questions.

The Cancer Information Service also has a variety of booklets that are available on request. The following booklet about adult non-Hodgkin's lymphoma may be helpful: *What You Need To Know About non-Hodgkin's Lymphomas* *

Booklets about Cancer Treatment

Radiation Therapy and You: A Guide to Self-Help During Treatment *

Chemotherapy and You: A Guide to Self-Help During Treatment *

Eating Hints: Recipes and Tips for Better Nutrition During Cancer Treatment *

Questions and Answers About Pain Control

What Are Clinical Trials All About?

Booklets about Living with Cancer

Taking Time: Support for People With Cancer and the People Who Care About Them

When Cancer Recurs: Meeting the Challenge Again *

Advanced Cancer: Living Each Day *

* Reprinted in this volume—see Table of Contents

Chapter 38

Cutaneous T-Cell Lymphoma

What Is Cutaneous T-Cell Lymphoma?

Cutaneous T-cell lymphoma is a disease in which certain cells of the lymph system (called T-lymphocytes) become cancer (malignant) and affect the skin. Lymphocytes are infection-fighting white blood cells that are made in the bone marrow and by other organs of the lymph system. T-cells are special lymphocytes that help the body's immune system kill bacteria and other harmful things in the body.

The lymph system is part of the immune system and is made up of thin tubes that branch, like blood vessels, into all parts of the body, including the skin. Lymph vessels carry lymph, a colorless, watery fluid that contains lymphocytes. Along the network of vessels are groups of small, bean-shaped organs called lymph nodes. Clusters of lymph nodes are found in the underarm, pelvis, neck, and abdomen. The spleen (an organ in the upper abdomen that makes lymphocytes and filters old blood cells from the blood), the thymus (a small organ beneath the breastbone), and the tonsils (an organ in the throat) are also part of the lymph system.

There are several types of lymphoma. The most common types of lymphoma are called Hodgkin's disease and non-Hodgkin's lymphoma. These types of lymphoma usually start in the lymph nodes and the spleen. See the patient information summaries on adult or childhood non-Hodgkin's lymphoma or adult or childhood Hodgkin's disease for treatment of these cancers.

PDQ Statement, National Cancer Institute (NCI), updated March 1998.

Cutaneous T-cell lymphoma usually develops slowly over many years. In the early stages, the skin may itch, and dry, dark patches may develop on the skin. As the disease gets worse, tumors may form on the skin, a condition called mycosis fungoides. As more and more of the skin becomes involved, the skin may become infected. The disease can spread to lymph nodes or to other organs in the body, such as the spleen, lungs, or liver. When large numbers of the tumor cells are found in the blood, the condition is called the Sezary syndrome.

If there are symptoms of cutaneous lymphoma, a doctor may remove a growth from the skin and look at it under a microscope. This is called a biopsy.

The chance of recovery (prognosis) and choice of treatment depend on the stage of the cancer (whether it is just in the skin or has spread to other places in the body) and the patient's general state of health.

There are several other types of cancer that start in the skin. The most common are basal cell cancer and squamous cell cancer, which are covered in the PDQ patient information summary on skin cancer. Another type of skin cancer called melanoma is covered in the patient information summary on melanoma. Kaposi's sarcoma, a rare type of cancer that occurs most commonly in patients with the Acquired Immunodeficiency Syndrome (AIDS), also affects the skin. See the PDQ patient information summary on Kaposi's sarcoma for treatment of this cancer. Cancers that start in other parts of the body may also spread (metastasize) to the skin.

Stages of Cutaneous T-Cell Lymphoma

Once cutaneous T-cell lymphoma is found, more tests will be done to find out if cancer cells have spread to other parts of the body. This is called staging. A doctor needs to know the stage of the disease to plan treatment. The following stages are used for cutaneous T-cell lymphoma:

Stage I

The cancer only affects parts of the skin, which has red, dry, scaly patches, but no tumors. The lymph nodes are not larger than normal.

Stage II

Either of the following may be true:

- The skin has red, dry, scaly patches, but no tumors. Lymph nodes are larger than normal, but do not contain cancer cells.

- There are tumors on the skin. The lymph nodes are either normal or are larger than normal, but do not contain cancer cells.

Stage III

Nearly all of the skin is red, dry, and scaly. The lymph nodes are either normal or are larger than normal, but do not contain cancer cells.

Stage IV

The skin is involved, in addition to either of the following:

- Cancer cells are found in the lymph nodes.

- Cancer has spread to other organs, such as the liver or lung.

Recurrent

Recurrent disease means that the cancer has come back after it has been treated. It may come back where it started or in another part of the body.

How Cutaneous T-Cell Lymphoma Is Treated

There are treatments for all patients with cutaneous T-cell lymphoma. Three kinds of treatment are commonly used:

- radiation therapy (using high-energy rays to kill cancer cells)

- chemotherapy (using drugs to kill cancer cells)

- phototherapy (using light plus special drugs to make the cancer cells more sensitive to the light)

Biological therapy (using the body's immune system to fight cancer) is being tested in clinical trials.

Radiation therapy uses high-energy rays to kill cancer cells and shrink tumors. In cutaneous T-cell lymphoma, special rays of tiny particles called electrons are commonly used to treat all of the skin. This is called total skin electron beam radiation therapy, or TSEB radiation therapy. Electron beam radiation may also be given to smaller areas of the skin. This kind of radiation only goes into the outer layers of the skin. Another type of radiation uses x-rays to kill cancer cells. The x-rays are usually directed to only certain areas of the body, but there are studies using x-rays directed at the whole body (total body irradiation).

Chemotherapy uses drugs to kill cancer cells. Chemotherapy may be taken by pill, or it may be put into the body by a needle in a vein or muscle. Chemotherapy given in this way is called a systemic treatment because the drug enters the bloodstream, travels through the body, and can kill cancer cells throughout the body. In cutaneous T-cell lymphoma, chemotherapy drugs may be given in a cream or lotion put on the skin. This is called topical chemotherapy.

Phototherapy uses light to kill cancer cells. A drug that makes cancer cells sensitive to light is given to the patient and then a special light is used to shine on the cancer cells to kill them. In one type of phototherapy, called PUVA therapy, a patient will receive a drug called psoralen, and then ultraviolet A light will be shone on the skin. In another type of phototherapy, called extracorporeal photochemotherapy, the patient will be given drugs, and then some of the blood cells will be taken from the body, put under a special light, and put back into the body. If phototherapy is given, directions from the doctor should be followed as to the amount of sunlight the patient should receive.

Biological therapy tries to get the body to fight cancer. It uses materials made by the body or made in a laboratory to boost, direct, or restore the body's natural defenses against disease. Biological therapy is sometimes called biological response modifier (BRM) therapy or immunotherapy.

Bone marrow transplantation is used to replace the bone marrow with healthy bone marrow. First, all of the bone marrow in the body is destroyed with high doses of chemotherapy with or without radiation therapy. Healthy marrow is then taken from another person (a donor) whose tissue is the same as or almost the same as the patient's. The donor may be a twin (the best match), a brother or sister, or another person not related. The healthy marrow from the donor is given to the patient through a needle in the vein, and the marrow replaces the marrow that was destroyed. A bone marrow transplant using marrow from a relative or unrelated person is called an allogeneic bone marrow transplant.

Another type of bone marrow transplant, called autologous bone marrow transplant, is being studied in clinical trials. To do this type of transplant, bone marrow is taken from the patient and treated with drugs to kill any cancer cells. The marrow is then frozen to save it. Next, the patient is given high-dose chemotherapy with or without radiation therapy to destroy all of the remaining marrow. The frozen marrow that was saved is then thawed and given back to the patient through a needle in a vein to replace the marrow that was destroyed.

Another type of autologous transplant is called a peripheral blood stem cell transplant. The patient's blood is passed through a machine that removes the stem cells (immature cells from which all blood cells develop), then returns the blood back to the patient. This procedure is called leukapheresis and usually takes 3 or 4 hours to complete. The stem cells are treated with drugs to kill any cancer cells and then frozen until they are transplanted back to the patient. This procedure may be done alone or with an autologous bone marrow transplant.

A greater chance for recovery occurs if the doctor chooses a hospital which does more than 5 bone marrow transplantations per year.

Treatment by Stage

Treatment of cutaneous T-cell lymphoma depends on the stage of the disease, and the patient's age and overall health.

Standard treatment may be considered because of its effectiveness in patients in past studies, or participation in a clinical trial may be considered. Most patients with cutaneous T-cell lymphoma are not cured with standard therapy and some standard treatments may have more side effects than are desired. For these reasons, clinical trials are designed to find better ways to treat cancer patients and are based on the most up-to-date information. Clinical trials are ongoing in many parts of the country for most stages of cutaneous T-cell lymphoma. To learn more about clinical trials, call the Cancer Information Service at 1-800-4-CANCER (1-800-422-6237); TTY at 1-800-332-8615.

Stage I Cutaneous T-Cell Lymphoma

Treatment may be one of the following:

1. Phototherapy (PUVA therapy) with or without biological therapy.

2. Total skin electron beam radiation therapy (TSEB radiation therapy).

3. Topical chemotherapy.

4. Local electron beam or x-ray therapy to reduce the size of the tumor or to relieve symptoms.

5. Clinical trials of phototherapy.

6. Interferon alfa (biological therapy) alone or in combination with topical therapy.

Stage II Cutaneous T-Cell Lymphoma

Treatment may be one of the following:

1. Phototherapy (PUVA therapy) with or without biological therapy.

2. Total skin electron beam radiation therapy (TSEB radiation therapy).

3. Topical chemotherapy.

4. Local electron beam or x-ray therapy.

5. Interferon alfa (biological therapy) alone or in combination with topical therapy.

Stage III Cutaneous T-Cell lymphoma

Treatment may be one of the following:

1. Phototherapy (PUVA therapy) with or without biological therapy.

2. Total skin electron beam radiation therapy (TSEB radiation therapy).

3. Topical chemotherapy.

4. Local electron beam or x-ray therapy.

5. Systemic chemotherapy with or without therapy to the skin.

6. Chemotherapy for mycosis fungoides and Sezary syndrome.

7. Extracorporeal photochemotherapy.

8. Interferon alfa (biological therapy) alone or in combination with topical therapy.

9. Retinoids.

Stage IV Cutaneous T-Cell Lymphoma

Treatment may be one of the following:

1. Systemic chemotherapy.

2. Topical chemotherapy.

3. Total skin electron beam radiation therapy (TSEB radiation therapy).

4. Phototherapy (PUVA therapy) with or without biological therapy.

5. Local electron beam or x-ray therapy.

6. Chemotherapy for mycosis fungoides and Sezary syndrome.

7. Extracorporeal photochemotherapy

8. Interferon alfa (biological therapy) alone or in combination with topical therapy.

9. Monoclonal antibody therapy.

10. Retinoids.

Recurrent Cutaneous T-Cell Lymphoma

Treatment depends on many factors, including the type of treatment the patient received before. Depending on the patient's condition, treatment may be one of the following:

1. Local electron beam or x-ray therapy.

2. Total skin electron beam radiation therapy (TSEB radiation therapy).

3. Phototherapy (PUVA therapy).

4. Topical chemotherapy.

5. Systemic chemotherapy.

6. Extracorporeal photochemotherapy.

7. Clinical trials of biological therapy.

8. Clinical trials of bone marrow transplantation.

To Learn More

To learn more about cutaneous T-cell lymphoma, call the National Cancer Institute's Cancer Information Service at 1-800-4-CANCER (1-800-422-6237); TTY at 1-800-332-8615. By dialing this toll-free number, trained information specialists can answer your questions.

Cancer patients, their families and friends, and others may find the following booklets useful. They are available free of charge by calling 1-800-4-CANCER or writing:

Office of Cancer Communications
National Cancer Institute
Building 31, Room 10A24
Bethesda, MD 20892

Booklets about Cancer Treatment

Radiation Therapy and You: A Guide to Self-Help During Treatment *

Chemotherapy and You: A Guide to Self-Help During Treatment *

Eating Hints: Recipes and Tips for Better Nutrition During Cancer Treatment *

Questions and Answers About Pain Control

What Are Clinical Trials All About?

Booklets about Living with Cancer

Taking Time: Support for People With Cancer and the People Who Care About Them

When Cancer Recurs: Meeting the Challenge Again *

Advanced Cancer: Living Each Day *

* Reprinted in this volume—see Table of Contents

Chapter 39

AIDS-Related Lymphoma

What Is AIDS-Related Lymphoma?

AIDS-related lymphoma is a disease in which cancer (malignant) cells are found in the lymph system in patients who have AIDS (acquired immunodeficiency syndrome). AIDS is caused by the human immunodeficiency virus (HIV) which attacks and weakens the immune system. Infections and other diseases can then invade the body, and the immune system cannot fight against them.

The lymph system is made up of thin tubes that branch, like blood vessels, into all parts of the body. Lymph vessels carry lymph, a colorless, watery fluid that contains white blood cells called lymphocytes. Along the network of vessels are groups of small, bean-shaped organs called lymph nodes. Clusters of lymph nodes make and store infection-fighting cells. The spleen (an organ in the upper abdomen that makes lymphocytes and filters old blood cells from the blood), the thymus (a small organ beneath the breastbone), and the tonsils (an organ in the throat) are also part of the lymph system. Because there is lymph tissue in many parts of the body, the cancer can spread to almost any of the body's organs or tissues including the liver, bone marrow (the spongy tissue inside the large bones of the body that makes blood cells), spleen, or brain.

Lymphomas are divided into two general types, Hodgkin's disease and non-Hodgkin's lymphomas, which are classified by the way their cells look under a microscope. This determination is called the histology.

PDQ Statement, National Cancer Institute (NCI), updated January 1998.

Histology is also used to determine the type of non-Hodgkin's lymphoma of which there are ten. The types of non-Hodgkin's lymphomas are classified by how quickly they spread: low-grade, intermediate-grade, or high-grade. The intermediate- or high-grade lymphomas grow and spread faster than the low-grade lymphomas.

Both major types of lymphoma, Hodgkin's disease and non-Hodgkin's lymphoma, may occur in AIDS patients. Also, the intermediate- and high-grade types of non-Hodgkin's lymphoma are more commonly found in AIDS patients. Both types of lymphomas can also ocur in adults and in children (For further information about these types of lymphomas in persons who do not have AIDS, please see the PDQ patient information summaries on Hodgkin's and non-Hodgkin's lymphomas in adulthood or childhood).

A doctor should be seen if any of the following symptoms persist for longer than 2 weeks: painless swelling in the lymph nodes in the neck, underarm, or groin; fever; night sweats; tiredness; weight loss without dieting; or itchy skin.

If a patient has AIDS and symptoms of lymphoma, a doctor will carefully check for swelling or lumps in the neck, underarms, and groin. If the lymph nodes don't feel normal, the doctor may need to cut out a small piece of tissue and look at it under the microscope to see if there are any cancer cells. This procedure is called a biopsy.

In general, patients with AIDS-related lymphoma respond to treatment differently from patients with lymphoma who do not have AIDS. AIDS-related lymphoma usually grows faster and spreads outside the lymph nodes and to other parts of the body more often than lymphoma that is not related to AIDS. Because therapy can damage weak immune systems even further, patients who have AIDS-related lymphoma are generally treated with lower doses of drugs than patients who do not have AIDS.

Stages of AIDS-Related Lymphoma

Once AIDS-related lymphoma is found, more tests will be done to find out if the cancer has spread from where it started to other parts of the body. This testing is called staging. The stage of a disease, ranging from stage I to stage IV, gives an indication of how far the disease has spread. To plan treatment, a doctor needs to know the stage of the disease.

The doctor may determine the stage of the disease by conducting a thorough examination which may include blood tests and different kinds of x-rays. This testing is called clinical staging. In some cases, the doctor may need to do an operation called a laparotomy to determine the stage of the cancer. During this operation, the doctor cuts into the abdomen and carefully looks at the organs to see if they contain cancer. The doctor will cut out (biopsy) small pieces of tissue and look at them under a microscope to see whether they contain cancer. This type of staging is called pathologic staging. Pathologic staging is usually done only when it is needed to help the doctor plan treatment.

For treatment, AIDS-related lymphomas are grouped based on where they started, as follows:

Systemic/Peripheral Lymphoma

Lymphoma that has started in lymph nodes or other organs of the lymph system. The lymphoma may have spread from where it started throughout the body, including to the brain or bone marrow.

Primary Central Nervous System Lymphoma

Lymphoma that has started in the brain or spinal cord, both of which are part of the central nervous system (CNS). This type of lymphoma is called a "primary CNS lymphoma" because it starts in the CNS rather than starting somewhere else in the body and spreading to the CNS.

How AIDS-Related Lymphoma Is Treated

The treatment of AIDS-related lymphoma is difficult because of the problems caused by HIV infection, which weakens the immune system. The drug doses used are often lower than drug doses given to patients who do not have AIDS. Two types of treatment are used:

- chemotherapy (using drugs to kill cancer cells and shrink tumors)

- radiation therapy (using high-dose x-rays or other high-energy rays to kill cancer cells and shrink tumors)

Chemotherapy is the use of drugs to kill cancer cells and shrink tumors. Chemotherapy may be taken by pill, or it may be put into the body by inserting a needle into a vein or muscle. Chemotherapy is called a systemic treatment because the drugs enter the bloodstream, travel through the body, and can kill cancer cells throughout the body. Chemotherapy may be put into the fluid that surrounds the brain through a needle in the brain or back (intrathecal chemotherapy) to treat non-Hodgkin's lymphoma that has spread to the brain.

Radiation therapy is the use of high-energy x-rays to kill cancer cells and shrink tumors. Radiation for non-Hodgkin's lymphoma usually comes from a machine outside the body (external-beam radiation therapy). Radiation given to the brain is called cranial irradiation. Radiation therapy may be used alone or in addition to chemotherapy.

Additionally, clinical trials are testing the effect of giving drugs to kill the AIDS virus (antiviral therapy) in addition to treatment of lymphoma.

Treatment of AIDS-related lymphomas depends on the stage, histology, and grade of the disease, as well as the general health of the patient. A doctor must consider white blood cell count and any other diseases caused by AIDS that the patient had or currently has.

Standard treatment may be considered based on its effectiveness in past studies, or participation in a clinical trial may be considered. Not all patients are cured with standard therapy, and some standard treatments may have more side effects than are desired. For these reasons, clinical trials are designed to find better ways to treat cancer patients and are based on the most up-to-date information. To learn more about clinical trials, call the Cancer Information Service at 1-800-4-CANCER (1-800-422-6237); TTY at 1-800-332-8615 or the AIDS Clinical Trials Information Service at 1-800-342-AIDS (1-800-342-2437).

Treatment by Stage

AIDS-Related Peripheral/Systemic Lymphoma

Treatment may be one of the following:

1. Standard-dose systemic chemotherapy plus intrathecal chemotherapy.

2. Low-dose systemic chemotherapy plus intrathecal chemotherapy.

3. A clinical trial of new types of chemotherapy or new ways of giving chemotherapy.

AIDS-Related Primary CNS Lymphoma

Treatment will probably be cranial radiation therapy. A clinical trial of new types of treatment may also be an option.

To Learn More

To learn more about AIDS-related lymphoma, call the National Cancer Institute's Cancer Information Service at 1-800-4-CANCER (1-800-422-6237); TTY at 1-800-332-8615. By dialing this toll-free number, trained information specialists can help answer your questions.

Cancer patients, their families and friends, and others may find the following booklets useful. They are available free of charge by calling 1-800-4-CANCER or writing:

Office of Cancer Communications
National Cancer Institute
Building 31, Room 10A24
Bethesda, MD 20892

Booklets about Cancer Treatment

Radiation Therapy and You: A Guide to Self-Help During Treatment *

Chemotherapy and You: A Guide to Self-Help During Treatment *

Eating Hints: Recipes and Tips for Better Nutrition During Cancer Treatment *

Questions and Answers About Pain Control

What Are Clinical Trials All About?

Booklets about Living with Cancer

Taking Time: Support for People With Cancer and the People Who Care About Them

When Cancer Recurs: Meeting the Challenge Again *

Advanced Cancer: Living Each Day *

* Reprinted in this volume—see Table of Contents

Chapter 40

Leukemia

Introduction

Each year, nearly 27,000 adults and more than 2,000 children in the United States learn that they have leukemia. This chapter from the National Cancer Institute (NCI) describes the symptoms of leukemia and explains how this disease is diagnosed and treated. It also has information to help you deal with leukemia if it affects you or someone you know.

Other NCI publications are listed in the Other Booklets section. Our materials cannot answer every question you may have about leukemia. They cannot take the place of talks with doctors, nurses, and other members of the health care team. We hope our information will help with those talks.

Our knowledge about leukemia and how to treat it keeps increasing. For up-to-date information or to order this publication, call the NCI-supported Cancer Information Service (CIS) toll free at 1-800-4-CANCER (1-800-422-6237).

What Is Leukemia?

Leukemia is a type of cancer. Cancer is a group of more than 100 diseases that have two important things in common. One is that certain

"What You Need To Know About Leukemia," National Cancer Institute, updated September 1998.

cells in the body become abnormal. Another is that the body keeps producing large numbers of these abnormal cells.

Leukemia is cancer of the blood cells. To understand leukemia, it is helpful to know about normal blood cells and what happens to them when leukemia develops.

Normal Blood Cells

The blood is made up of fluid called plasma and three types of cells. Each type has special functions.

- White blood cells (also called WBCs or leukocytes) help the body fight infections and other diseases.

- Red blood cells (also called RBCs or erythrocytes) carry oxygen from the lungs to the body's tissues and take carbon dioxide from the tissues back to the lungs. The red blood cells give blood its color.

- Platelets (also called thrombocytes) help form blood clots that control bleeding.

Blood cells are formed in the bone marrow, the soft, spongy center of bones. New (immature) blood cells are called blasts. Some blasts stay in the marrow to mature. Some travel to other parts of the body to mature.

Normally, blood cells are produced in an orderly, controlled way, as the body needs them. This process helps keep us healthy.

Leukemia Cells

When leukemia develops, the body produces large numbers of abnormal blood cells. In most types of leukemia, the abnormal cells are white blood cells. The leukemia cells usually look different from normal blood cells, and they do not function properly.

Types of Leukemia

There are several types of leukemia. They are grouped in two ways. One way is by how quickly the disease develops and gets worse. The other way is by the type of blood cell that is affected.

Leukemia is either acute or chronic. In acute leukemia, the abnormal blood cells are blasts that remain very immature and cannot carry out their normal functions. The number of blasts increases rapidly, and the disease gets worse quickly. In chronic leukemia, some blast cells are present, but in general, these cells are more mature and can carry out some of their normal functions. Also, the number of blasts increases less rapidly than in acute leukemia. As a result, chronic leukemia gets worse gradually.

Leukemia can arise in either of the two main types of white blood cells—lymphoid cells or myeloid cells. When leukemia affects lymphoid cells, it is called lymphocytic leukemia. When myeloid cells are affected, the disease is called myeloid or myelogenous leukemia.

These are the most common types of leukemia:

- Acute lymphocytic leukemia (ALL) is the most common type of leukemia in young children. This disease also affects adults, especially those age 65 and older.

- Acute myeloid leukemia (AML) occurs in both adults and children. This type of leukemia is sometimes called acute non-lymphocytic leukemia (ANLL).

- Chronic lymphocytic leukemia (CLL) most often affects adults over the age of 55. It sometimes occurs in younger adults, but it almost never affects children.

- Chronic myeloid leukemia (CML) occurs mainly in adults. A very small number of children also develop this disease.

Hairy cell leukemia is an uncommon type of chronic leukemia. This and other uncommon types of leukemia are not discussed in this chapter. The Cancer Information Service can supply information about them.

Symptoms

Leukemia cells are abnormal cells that cannot do what normal blood cells do. They cannot help the body fight infections. For this reason, people with leukemia often get infections and have fevers.

Also, people with leukemia often have less than the normal amount of healthy red blood cells and platelets. As a result, there are not enough red blood cells to carry oxygen through the body. With this condition, called anemia, patients may look pale and feel weak and tired. When there are not enough platelets, patients bleed and bruise easily.

Like all blood cells, leukemia cells travel through the body. Depending on the number of abnormal cells and where these cells collect, patients with leukemia may have a number of symptoms.

In acute leukemia, symptoms appear and get worse quickly. People with this disease go to their doctor because they feel sick. In chronic leukemia, symptoms may not appear for a long time; when symptoms do appear, they generally are mild at first and get worse gradually. Doctors often find chronic leukemia during a routine checkup—before there are any symptoms.

These are some of the common symptoms of leukemia:

- Fever, chills, and other flu-like symptoms;

- Weakness and fatigue;

- Frequent infections;

- Loss of appetite and/or weight;

- Swollen or tender lymph nodes, liver, or spleen;

- Easy bleeding or bruising;

- Tiny red spots (called petechiae) under the skin;

- Swollen or bleeding gums;

- Sweating, especially at night; and/or

- Bone or joint pain.

In acute leukemia, the abnormal cells may collect in the brain or spinal cord (also called the central nervous system or CNS). The result may be headaches, vomiting, confusion, loss of muscle control, and seizures. Leukemia cells also can collect in the testicles and cause swelling. Also, some patients develop sores in the eyes or on the skin. Leukemia also can affect the digestive tract, kidneys, lungs, or other parts of the body.

In chronic leukemia, the abnormal blood cells may gradually collect in various parts of the body. Chronic leukemia may affect the skin, central nervous system, digestive tract, kidneys, and testicles.

Diagnosis

To find the cause of a person's symptoms, the doctor asks about the patient's medical history and does a physical exam. In addition to checking general signs of health, the doctor feels for swelling in the liver; the spleen; and the lymph nodes under the arms, in the groin, and in the neck.

Blood tests also help in the diagnosis. A sample of blood is examined under a microscope to see what the cells look like and to determine the number of mature cells and blasts. Although blood tests may reveal that a patient has leukemia, they may not show what type of leukemia it is.

To check further for leukemia cells or to tell what type of leukemia a patient has, a hematologist, oncologist, or pathologist examines a sample of bone marrow under a microscope. The doctor withdraws the sample by inserting a needle into a large bone (usually the hip) and removing a small amount of liquid bone marrow. This procedure is called bone marrow aspiration. A bone marrow biopsy is performed with a larger needle and removes a small piece of bone and bone marrow.

If leukemia cells are found in the bone marrow sample, the patient's doctor orders other tests to find out the extent of the disease. A spinal tap (lumbar puncture) checks for leukemia cells in the fluid that fills the spaces in and around the brain and spinal cord (cerebrospinal fluid). Chest x-rays can reveal signs of disease in the chest.

Treatment

Treatment for leukemia is complex. It varies with the type of leukemia and is not the same for all patients. The doctor plans the treatment to fit each patient's needs. The treatment depends not only on the type of leukemia, but also on certain features of the leukemia cells, the extent of the disease, and whether the leukemia has been treated before. It also depends on the patient's age, symptoms, and general health.

Whenever possible, patients should be treated at a medical center that has doctors who have experience in treating leukemia. If this is not possible, the patient's doctor should discuss the treatment plan with a specialist at such a center. Also, patients and their doctors can call the Cancer Information Service to request up-to-date treatment information from the National Cancer Institute's PDQ database.

Acute leukemia needs to be treated right away. The goal of treatment is to bring about a remission. Then, when there is no evidence of the disease, more therapy may be given to prevent a relapse. Many people with acute leukemia can be cured.

Chronic leukemia patients who do not have symptoms may not require immediate treatment. However, they should have frequent checkups so the doctor can see whether the disease is progressing. When treatment is needed, it can often control the disease and its symptoms. However, chronic leukemia can seldom be cured.

Many patients and their families want to learn all they can about leukemia and the treatment choices so they can take an active part in decisions about medical care. The doctor is the best person to answer these questions. When discussing treatment, the patient (or, in the case of a child, the patient's family) may want to talk with the doctor about research studies of new treatment methods. Such studies, called clinical trials, are designed to improve cancer treatment. More information about clinical trials is in the Clinical Trials section.

When a person is diagnosed with leukemia, shock and stress are natural reactions. These feelings may make it difficult to think of every question to ask the doctor. Also, patients may find it hard to remember everything the doctor says.

Often, it helps to make a list of questions to ask the doctor. Taking notes or, if the doctor agrees, using a tape recorder can make it easier to remember the answers. Some people find that it also helps to have a family member or friend with them—to take part in the discussion, to take notes, or just to listen. Patients do not need to ask all their questions or remember all the answers at one time. They will have other chances for the doctor to explain things that are not clear and to ask for more information.

Here are some questions patients and their families may want to ask the doctor before treatment begins:

- What type of leukemia is it?
- What are the treatment choices? Which do you recommend? Why?
- Would a clinical trial be appropriate?
- What are the expected benefits of each kind of treatment?
- What are the risks and possible side effects of each treatment?
- If I have pain, how will you help me?
- Will I have to change my normal activities?
- How long will treatment last?
- What is the treatment likely to cost? How can I find out what my insurance will cover?

Getting a Second Opinion

Sometimes it is helpful to have a second opinion about the diagnosis and treatment plan. (Many insurance companies provide coverage for a second opinion.) There are a number of ways to find a doctor who can give a second opinion:

- The patient's doctor may be able to suggest a doctor who specializes in adult or childhood leukemia. Doctors who treat adult leukemia are oncologists and hematologists. Pediatric oncologists and hematologists treat childhood leukemia.

- The Cancer Information Service, at 1-800-4-CANCER, can tell callers about cancer centers and other treatment facilities in their area, including programs that are supported by the National Cancer Institute.

- Patients can get the names of specialists from their local medical society, a nearby hospital, or a medical school.

Methods of Treatment

Most patients with leukemia are treated with chemotherapy. Some also may have radiation therapy and/or bone marrow transplantation (BMT) or biological therapy. In some cases, surgery to remove the spleen (an operation called a splenectomy) may be part of the treatment plan.

Chemotherapy is the use of drugs to kill cancer cells. Depending on the type of leukemia, patients may receive a single drug or a combination of two or more drugs.

Some anticancer drugs can be taken by mouth. Most are given by IV injection (injected into a vein). Often, patients who need to have many IV treatments receive the drugs through a catheter.

One end of this thin, flexible tube is placed in a large vein, often in the upper chest. Drugs are injected into the catheter, rather than directly into a vein, to avoid the discomfort of repeated injections and injury to the skin.

Anticancer drugs given by IV injection or taken by mouth enter the bloodstream and affect leukemia cells in most parts of the body. However, the drugs often do not reach cells in the central nervous system because they are stopped by the blood-brain barrier. This protective barrier is formed by a network of blood vessels that filter blood going to the brain and spinal cord. To reach leukemia cells in the central nervous system, doctors use intrathecal chemotherapy. In this type of treatment, anticancer drugs are injected directly into the cerebrospinal fluid.

Intrathecal chemotherapy can be given in two ways. Some patients receive the drugs by injection into the lower part of the spinal column.

Others, especially children, receive intrathecal chemotherapy through a special type of catheter called an Ommaya reservoir. This device is placed under the scalp, where it provides a pathway to the cerebrospinal fluid. Injecting anticancer drugs into the reservoir instead of into the spinal column can make intrathecal chemotherapy easier and more comfortable for the patient.

Chemotherapy is given in cycles: a treatment period followed by a recovery period, then another treatment period, and so on. In some cases, the patient has chemotherapy as an outpatient at the hospital, at the doctor's office, or at home. However, depending on which drugs are given and the patient's general health, a hospital stay may be necessary.

Here are some questions patients and their families may want to ask the doctor before starting chemotherapy:

- What drugs will be used?
- When will the treatments begin? How often will they be given? When will they end?
- Will I have to stay in the hospital?
- How will we know whether the drugs are working?
- What side effects occur during treatment? How long do the side effects last? What can be done to manage them?
- Can these drugs cause side effects later on?

Radiation therapy is used along with chemotherapy for some kinds of leukemia. Radiation therapy (also called radiotherapy) uses high-energy rays to damage cancer cells and stop them from growing. The radiation comes from a large machine.

Radiation therapy for leukemia may be given in two ways. For some patients, the doctor may direct the radiation to one specific area of the body where there is a collection of leukemia cells, such as the spleen or testicles. Other patients may receive radiation that is directed to the whole body. This type of radiation therapy, called total-body irradiation, usually is given before a bone marrow transplant.

Here are some questions patients and their families may want to ask the doctor before having radiation therapy:

- When will the treatments begin? How often are they given? When will they end?
- Can normal activities be continued?

- How will we know if the treatment is working?

- What side effects can be expected? How long will they last? What can be done about them?

- Can radiation therapy cause side effects later on?

Bone marrow transplantation also may be used for some patients. The patient's leukemia-producing bone marrow is destroyed by high doses of drugs and radiation and is then replaced by healthy bone marrow. The healthy bone marrow may come from a donor, or it may be marrow that has been removed from the patient and stored before the high-dose treatment. If the patient's own bone marrow is used, it may first be treated outside the body to remove leukemia cells. Patients who have a bone marrow transplant usually stay in the hospital for several weeks. Until the transplanted bone marrow begins to produce enough white blood cells, patients have to be carefully protected from infection. *Research Report: Bone Marrow Transplantation* provides more information about this complex treatment.

Here are some questions patients and their families may want to ask the doctor about bone marrow transplantation:

- What are the benefits of this treatment?

- What are the risks and side effects? What can be done about them?

- How long will I be in the hospital? What care will be needed after I leave the hospital?

- What changes in normal activities will be necessary?

- How will we know if the treatment is working?

Biological therapy involves treatment with substances that affect the immune system's response to cancer. Interferon is a form of biological therapy that is used against some types of leukemia.

Here are some questions patients and their families may want to ask the doctor before starting biological therapy:

- What kind of treatment will be used?

- What side effects can be expected? How long do the side effects last? What can be done to manage them?

- How will we know whether the treatment is working?

Clinical Trials

Many patients with leukemia take part in clinical trials (treatment studies). Clinical trials help doctors find out whether a new treatment is both safe and effective. They also help doctors answer questions about how the treatment works and what side effects it causes.

Patients who take part in studies may be among the first to receive treatments that have shown promise in research. In many studies, some of the patients receive the new treatment, while others receive standard treatment so that doctors can compare different treatments. Patients who take part in a trial make an important contribution to medical science. Although these patients take certain risks, they may have the first chance to benefit from improved treatment methods.

Doctors are studying new treatments for all types of leukemia. They are working on new drugs, new drug combinations, and new schedules of chemotherapy. They also are studying ways to improve bone marrow transplantation.

Many clinical trials involve various forms of biological therapy. Interleukins and colony-stimulating factors are forms of biological therapy being studied to treat leukemia. Doctors also are studying ways to use monoclonal antibodies in the treatment of leukemia. Often biological therapy is combined with chemotherapy or bone marrow transplantation.

Patients with leukemia (or their families) should talk with the doctor if they are interested in taking part in a clinical trial. They may want to read *Taking Part in Clinical Trials: What Cancer Patients Need To Know*, which explains some of the possible benefits and risks of treatment studies.

One way to learn about clinical trials is through PDQ, a computerized resource developed by the National Cancer Institute. PDQ contains information about cancer treatment and about clinical trials in progress throughout the country. The Cancer Information Service can provide PDQ information to doctors, patients, and the public.

Supportive Care

Leukemia and its treatment can cause a number of complications and side effects. Patients receive supportive care to prevent or control these problems and to improve their comfort and quality of life during treatment.

Because leukemia patients get infections very easily, they may receive antibiotics and other drugs to help protect them from infections.

They are often advised to stay out of crowds and away from people with colds and other infectious diseases. If an infection develops, it can be serious and should be treated promptly. Patients may need to stay in the hospital to treat the infection.

Anemia and bleeding are other problems that often require supportive care. Transfusions of red blood cells may be given to help reduce the shortness of breath and fatigue that anemia can cause. Platelet transfusions can help reduce the risk of serious bleeding.

Dental care also is very important. Leukemia and chemotherapy can make the mouth sensitive, easily infected, and likely to bleed. Doctors often advise patients to have a complete dental exam before treatment begins. Dentists can show patients how to keep their mouth clean and healthy during treatment.

Side Effects of Treatment

It is hard to limit the effects of therapy so that only leukemia cells are destroyed. Because treatment also damages healthy cells and tissues, it causes side effects.

The side effects of cancer treatment vary. They depend mainly on the type and extent of the treatment. Also, each person reacts differently. Side effects may even be different from one treatment to the next. Doctors try to plan the patient's therapy to keep side effects to a minimum.

Doctors and nurses can explain the side effects of treatment and can suggest medicine, diet changes, or other ways to deal with them. The National Cancer Institute booklets *Chemotherapy and You* [reprinted in this volume as Chapter 63] and *Radiation Therapy and You* [reprinted in this volume as Chapter 66] also have helpful information about cancer treatment and coping with side effects.

Chemotherapy

The side effects of chemotherapy depend mainly on the drugs the patient receives. In addition, as with other types of treatment, side effects may vary from person to person. Generally, anticancer drugs affect dividing cells. Cancer cells divide more often than healthy cells and are more likely to be affected by chemotherapy. Still, some healthy cells also may be damaged. Healthy cells that divide often, including blood cells, cells in hair roots, and cells in the digestive tract, are likely to be damaged. When chemotherapy affects healthy cells, it may lower patients' resistance to infection, and patients may have less energy and may bruise or bleed easily. They may lose their hair. The also may have nausea, vomiting, and mouth sores. Most side effects go away gradually during the recovery periods between treatments or after treatment stops.

Some anticancer drugs can affect a patient's fertility. Women's menstrual periods may become irregular or stop, and women may have symptoms of menopause, such as hot flashes and vaginal dryness. Men may stop producing sperm. Because these changes may be permanent, some men choose to have their sperm frozen and stored. Most children treated for leukemia appear to have normal fertility when they grow up. However, depending on the drugs and doses used and on the age of the patient, some boys and girls may not be able to have children when they mature.

Radiation Therapy

Patients receiving radiation therapy may become very tired. Resting is important, but doctors usually suggest that patients remain as active as they can.

When radiation is directed to the head, patients often lose their hair. Radiation can cause the scalp or the skin in the treated area to become red, dry, tender, and itchy. Patients will be shown how to keep the skin clean. They should not use any lotion or cream on the treated area without the doctor's advice. Radiation therapy also may cause nausea, vomiting, and loss of appetite. These side effects are temporary, and doctors and nurses can often suggest ways to control them until the treatment is over.

However, some side effects may be lasting. Children (especially young ones) who receive radiation to the brain may develop problems with learning and coordination. For this reason, doctors use the lowest possible doses of radiation, and they give this treatment only to children who cannot be treated successfully with chemotherapy alone.

Also, radiation to the testicles is likely to affect both fertility and hormone production. Most boys who have this form of treatment are not able to have children later on. Some may need to take hormones.

Bone Marrow Transplantation

Patients who have a bone marrow transplant face an increased risk of infection, bleeding, and other side effects of the large doses of chemotherapy and radiation they receive. In addition, graft-versus-host disease (GVHD) may occur in patients who receive bone marrow from a donor. In GVHD, the donated marrow reacts against the patient's tissues (most often the liver, the skin, and the digestive tract). GVHD can be mild or very severe. It can occur any time after the transplant (even years later). Drugs may be given to reduce the risk of GVHD and to treat the problem if it occurs.

Supportive care for bone marrow transplant patients is explained in Research Report: Bone Marrow Transplantation.

Nutrition for Cancer Patients

Some cancer patients find it hard to eat well. They may lose their appetite. In addition, the common side effects of therapy, such as nausea, vomiting, or mouth sores, can make eating difficult. For some patients, foods taste different. Also, people may not feel like eating when they are uncomfortable or tired.

Eating well means getting enough calories and protein to help prevent weight loss and regain strength. Patients who eat well during cancer treatment often feel better and have more energy. In addition, they may be better able to handle the side effects of treatment.

Doctors, nurses, and dietitians can offer advice for healthy eating during cancer treatment. Patients and their families also may want to read the National Cancer Institute booklets *Eating Hints for Cancer Patients* [reprinted in this volume as Chapter 77] and *Managing Your Child's Eating Problems During Cancer Treatment*, which contain many useful suggestions.

Followup Care

Regular followup exams are very important after treatment for leukemia. The doctor will continue to check the patient closely to be sure that the cancer has not returned. Checkups usually include exams of the blood, bone marrow, and cerebrospinal fluid. From time to time, the doctor does a complete physical exam.

Cancer treatment may cause side effects many years later. For this reason, patients should continue to have regular checkups and should also report health changes or problems to their doctor as soon as they appear.

Support for Cancer Patients

Living with a serious disease is not easy. Cancer patients and those who care about them face many problems and challenges. Coping with these problems is less difficult when people have information and support. Several useful booklets are available from the Cancer Information Service. These include *Taking Time: Support for People With Cancer and the People Who Care About Them* and *Young People With Cancer: A Handbook for Parents*. (Other booklets are listed in the Other Booklets section.)

Cancer patients may worry about holding their job, caring for their family, or keeping up with other responsibilities. Parents of children with leukemia may worry about whether their children will be able to take part in normal school or social activities, and the children themselves may be upset about not being able to join in activities with their friends. Worries about tests, treatments, hospital stays, and medical bills also are common. Doctors, nurses, and other members of the health care team can answer questions about treatment, working, or other activities. Also, meeting with a social worker, counselor, or member of the clergy can be helpful to patients who want to talk about their feelings or discuss their concerns.

Friends and relatives can be very supportive. Many patients also find it helps to discuss their concerns with others who have cancer. Cancer patients often get together in support groups, where they can share what they have learned about coping with cancer and the effects of treatment. In addition to groups for adults with cancer, special support groups for children with cancer or their parents are available in many cities. It is important to keep in mind, however, that each patient is different. Treatments and ways of dealing with cancer that work for one person may not be right for another—even if they both have the same kind of cancer. It is always a good idea to discuss the advice of friends and family members with the doctor.

Often, a social worker at the hospital or clinic can suggest groups that can help with rehabilitation, emotional support, financial aid, transportation, or home care.

What the Future Holds

Researchers are finding better ways to treat leukemia, and the chances of recovery keep improving. Still, it is natural for patients and their families to be concerned about the future.

Sometimes people use rates of survival and other statistics to try to figure out whether a patient will be cured or how long the patient will live. It is important to remember, however, that statistics are averages based on large numbers of patients. They cannot be used to predict what will happen to a certain patient because no two patients are alike; treatments and responses vary greatly. The doctor who takes care of the patient is in the best position to discuss the chance of recovery (prognosis). Patients and their families should feel free to ask the doctor about the prognosis, but they should keep in mind that not even the doctor knows exactly what will happen. Doctors often talk about surviving cancer, or they may use the term remission, rather than cure. Even though many leukemia patients are cured, doctors use these terms because the disease can recur.

Possible Causes

At this time, we do not know what causes leukemia. Researchers are trying to solve this problem. Scientists know that leukemia occurs in males more often than in females and in white people more often than in black people. However, they cannot explain why one person gets leukemia and another does not.

By studying large numbers of people all over the world, researchers have found certain risk factors that increase a person's risk of getting leukemia. For example, exposure to large amounts of high-energy radiation increases the risk of getting leukemia. Such radiation was produced by the atomic bomb explosions in Japan during World War II. In nuclear power plants, strict safety rules protect workers and the public from exposure to harmful amounts of radiation.

Some research suggests that exposure to electromagnetic fields is a possible risk factor for leukemia. (Electromagnetic fields are a type of low-energy radiation that comes from power lines and electric appliances.) However, more studies are needed to prove this link.

Certain genetic conditions can increase the risk for leukemia. One such condition is Down's syndrome; children born with this syndrome are more likely to get leukemia than other children.

Workers exposed to certain chemicals over a long period of time are at higher risk for leukemia. Benzene is one of these chemicals. Also, some of the drugs used to treat other types of cancer may increase a person's risk of getting leukemia. However, this risk is very small when compared with the benefits of chemotherapy.

Scientists have identified a virus that seems to increase the risk for one very uncommon type of leukemia. However, this virus has no known association with common forms of leukemia. Scientists throughout the world continue to study viruses and other possible risk factors for leukemia. By learning what causes this disease, researchers hope to better understand how to prevent and treat it.

Other Booklets

Cancer patients, their families and friends, and others may find the following booklets useful. They are available free of charge by calling 1-800-4-CANCER or writing:

Office of Cancer Communications
National Cancer Institute
Building 31, Room 10A24
Bethesda, MD 20892

Booklets about Cancer Treatment

Radiation Therapy and You: A Guide to Self-Help During Treatment *

Chemotherapy and You: A Guide to Self-Help During Treatment *

Eating Hints: Recipes and Tips for Better Nutrition During Cancer Treatment *

Questions and Answers About Pain Control

What Are Clinical Trials All About?

Booklets about Living with Cancer

Taking Time: Support for People With Cancer and the People Who Care About Them

When Cancer Recurs: Meeting the Challenge Again *

Advanced Cancer: Living Each Day *

* Reprinted in this volume—see Table of Contents

Chapter 41

Plasma Cell Neoplasm

What Are Plasma Cell Neoplasms?

Plasma cell neoplasms are diseases in which certain cells in the blood (called plasma cells) become cancer. Plasma cells are made by white blood cells called lymphocytes. The plasma cells make antibodies, which fight infection and other harmful things in the body. When these cells become cancer, they may make too many antibodies and a substance called M-protein is found in the blood and urine.

There are several types of plasma cell neoplasms. The most common type is called multiple myeloma. In multiple myeloma, cancerous plasma cells are found in the bone marrow. The bone marrow is the spongy tissue inside the large bones in the body. The bone marrow makes red blood cells (which carry oxygen and other materials to all tissues of the body), white blood cells (which fight infection), and platelets (which make the blood clot). The cancer cells can crowd out normal blood cells, causing anemia (too few red blood cells). The plasma cells also may cause the bone to break down. The plasma cells can collect in the bone to make small tumors called plasmacytomas.

Plasma cell neoplasms also can appear only as growths of plasma cells (plasmacytomas) in the bone and soft tissues, without cancer cells in the bone marrow or blood.

Macroglobulinemia is a type of plasma cell neoplasm in which lymphocytes that make an M-protein build up in the blood. Lymph nodes and the liver and spleen may be swollen.

PDQ Statement, National Cancer Institute (NCI), updated June 1998.

If there are symptoms, a doctor will order blood and urine tests. If the tests are not normal, the doctor may do a bone marrow biopsy. During this test, a needle is inserted into a bone and a small amount of bone marrow is taken out and looked at under the microscope. The doctor can then tell what kind of cancer the patient has and plan the best treatment. X-rays also may be done to see whether the bones are affected.

The chance of recovery (prognosis) depends on the kind of plasma cell neoplasm, and the patient's age and general health.

Stages of Plasma Cell Neoplasms

Once plasma cell neoplasm has been found, more tests will be done to see how far the cancer has spread. This is called staging. Plasma cell neoplasms are grouped together depending on the type of plasma cell cancer that is found. The following stages are used for multiple myeloma:

Multiple Myeloma

Stage I Multiple Myeloma

Relatively few cancer cells have spread throughout the body. The number of red blood cells and the amount of calcium in the blood are normal. No tumors (plasmacytomas) are found in the bone. The amount of M-protein in the blood or urine is very low. There may be no symptoms of disease.

Stage II Multiple Myeloma

A moderate number of cancer cells have spread throughout the body.

Stage III Multiple Myeloma

A relatively large number of cancer cells have spread throughout the body. There may be one or more of the following:

1. A decrease in the number of red blood cells, causing anemia.

2. The amount of calcium in the blood is very high, because the bones are being damaged.

3. More than three bone tumors (plasmacytomas) are found.

4. High levels of M-protein are found in the blood or urine.

The following groups are used to determine the treatment of plasma cell neoplasms that don't involve the bone marrow.

Isolated Plasmacytoma of Bone

Only a single plasma cell tumor is found in the bone without any other evidence of cancer. Patients may develop multiple myeloma at a later time.

Extramedullary Plasmacytoma

Plasma cell tumors are found only outside the bone and the bone marrow in the soft tissues, usually the tonsils or tissues around the nose. Patients may develop multiple myeloma at a later time.

Macroglobulinemia

Plasma cells that produce a certain type of M-protein are found in the blood. Patients usually have swollen lymph nodes and spleen or liver.

Monoclonal Gammopathy of Undetermined Significance

M-protein is found in the blood without symptoms or other signs of cancer. People with this condition may develop plasma cell neoplasms or cancer of the lymph system (lymphoma) at a later time.

Refractory Plasma Cell Neoplasms

The plasma cells do not decrease even though treatment is given.

How Plasma Cell Neoplasms Are Treated

There are treatments for all patients with plasma cell neoplasms. Three kinds of treatment are used:

- chemotherapy (using drugs to kill cancer cells)
- radiation therapy (using high-dose x-rays or other high-energy rays to kill cancer cells
- biological therapy (using the body's immune system to fight cancer)

Surgery may be used in certain cases.

Chemotherapy uses drugs to kill cancer cells. Chemotherapy may be taken by pill, or it may be put into the body by a needle in the vein or muscle. Chemotherapy is called a systemic treatment because the drug enters the bloodstream, travels through the body, and can kill cancer cells throughout the body.

Radiation therapy uses x-rays or other high-energy rays to kill cancer cells and shrink tumors. Radiation for plasma cell neoplasms usually comes from a machine outside the body (external radiation therapy).

Biological therapy tries to get the body to fight cancer. It uses materials made by the body or made in a laboratory to boost, direct, or restore the body's natural defenses against disease. Biological therapy is sometimes called biological response modifier (BRM) therapy or immunotherapy.

Bone marrow transplantation is used to replace the bone marrow with healthy bone marrow. First, all of the bone marrow in the body is destroyed with high doses of chemotherapy with or without radiation therapy. Healthy marrow is then taken from another person (a donor) whose tissue is the same as or almost the same as the patient's. The donor may be a twin (the best match), a brother or sister, or an unrelated person. The healthy marrow from the donor is given to the patient through a needle in the vein to replace the marrow that was destroyed. A bone marrow transplant using marrow from a relative or unrelated person is called an allogeneic bone marrow transplant.

Another type of bone marrow transplant, called autologous bone marrow transplant, is being studied in clinical trials. To do this type of transplant, bone marrow is taken from the patient and treated with drugs to kill any cancer cells. The marrow is then frozen to save it. Next, the patient is given high-dose chemotherapy with or without radiation therapy to destroy all of the remaining marrow. The frozen marrow that was saved is then thawed and given back to the patient through a needle in a vein to replace the marrow that was destroyed.

Another type of autologous transplant is called a peripheral blood stem cell transplant. The patient's blood is passed through a machine that removes the stem cells (immature cells from which all blood cells develop). The machine then returns the blood back to the patient. This procedure is called leukapheresis and usually takes 3 or 4 hours to complete. The stem cells are treated with drugs to kill any cancer cells and then frozen until they are transplanted back to the patient. This procedure may be done alone or with an autologous bone marrow transplant.

A greater chance for recovery occurs if a doctor chooses a hospital which does more than five bone marrow transplantations per year.

If the spleen is swollen, the doctor may take out the spleen in an operation called a splenectomy.

If too many M-proteins build up in the blood, the patient's blood may need to be filtered through a special machine. This is called plasmapheresis.

Treatment by Stage

Treatment of plasma cell neoplasms depends on the type and stage of the disease, and the patient's age and overall health.

Standard treatment may be considered because of its effectiveness in patients in past studies, or participation in a clinical trial may be considered. Not all patients are cured with standard therapy and some standard treatments may have more side effects than are desired. For these reasons, clinical trials are designed to find better ways to treat cancer patients and are based on the most up-to-date information. Clinical trials are ongoing in most parts of the country for most stages of plasma cell neoplasms. To learn more about clinical trials, call the Cancer Information Service at 1-800-4-CANCER (1-800-422-6237); TTY at 1-800-332-8615.

Multiple Myeloma

If there are no symptoms, treatment may not be needed. A doctor will follow the patient closely so treatment can be started if symptoms develop. If there are symptoms, treatment will probably be chemotherapy. Clinical trials are testing new chemotherapy drugs and dose regimens.

Isolated Plasmacytoma of Bone

Treatment will probably be external radiation therapy to the tumor. If other symptoms appear, patients may receive chemotherapy.

Extramedullary Plasmacytoma

Treatment may be one of the following:

1. External radiation therapy to the tumor.

2. Surgery to remove the tumor, usually followed by external radiation therapy. If other symptoms appear, patients may receive chemotherapy.

Macroglobulinemia

If there are no symptoms, treatment may not be needed. A doctor will follow the patient closely so treatment can be started if symptoms develop. If there are symptoms, treatment will probably be chemotherapy. Clinical trials are testing new chemotherapy drugs and combinations of drugs. If the blood becomes too thick, patients may have plasmapheresis to filter cells from the blood.

Monoclonal Gammopathy of Undetermined Significance

A doctor will follow the patient closely to see if symptoms of plasma cell neoplasm or lymphoma develop.

Refractory Plasma Cell Neoplasm

Treatment will probably be chemotherapy. Clinical trials are testing new drugs and combinations of drugs.

To Learn More

To learn more about plasma cell neoplasms, call the National Cancer Institute's Cancer Information Service at 1-800-4-CANCER (1-800-422-6237); TTY at 1-800-332-8615. By dialing this toll-free number, trained information specialists can answer your questions.

Cancer patients, their families and friends, and others may find the following booklets useful. They are available free of charge by calling 1-800-4-CANCER or writing:

Office of Cancer Communications
National Cancer Institute
Building 31, Room 10A24
Bethesda, MD 20892

Booklets about Cancer Treatment

Radiation Therapy and You: A Guide to Self-Help During Treatment *

Chemotherapy and You: A Guide to Self-Help During Treatment *

Eating Hints: Recipes and Tips for Better Nutrition During Cancer Treatment *

Questions and Answers About Pain Control

What Are Clinical Trials All About?

Booklets about Living with Cancer

Taking Time: Support for People With Cancer and the People Who Care About Them

When Cancer Recurs: Meeting the Challenge Again *

Advanced Cancer: Living Each Day *

* Reprinted in this volume—see Table of Contents

Chapter 42

Myelodysplastic Syndrome

What Are Myelodysplastic Syndromes?

Myelodysplastic syndromes, also called pre-leukemia or "smoldering" leukemia, are diseases in which the bone marrow does not function normally and not enough normal blood cells are made. The bone marrow is the spongy tissue inside the large bones in the body. The bone marrow makes red blood cells (which carry oxygen and other materials to all tissues of the body), white blood cells (which fight infection), and platelets (which make the blood clot). Normally, bone marrow cells called blasts develop (mature) into several different types of blood cells that have specific jobs in the body.

Myelodysplastic syndromes occur most often in older people, but they can occur in younger people. The most common sign is anemia, which means there are too few mature red blood cells to carry oxygen. There may also be too few white blood cells in the blood to fight infections. If the number of platelets in the blood is lower than normal, this may cause people to bleed or bruise more easily. A doctor should be seen if a person bleeds without any reason, bruises more easily than normal, has an infection that won't go away, or feels tired all the time.

If there are symptoms, a doctor may order blood tests to count the number of each kind of blood cell. If the results of the blood test are not normal, the doctor may do a bone marrow biopsy. During this test, a needle is inserted into a bone and a small amount of bone marrow

PDQ Statement, National Cancer Institute (NCI), updated March 1998.

is taken out and looked at under the microscope. The doctor can then determine the kind of disease and plan the best treatment.

A myelodysplastic syndrome may develop following treatment with drugs or radiation therapy for other diseases, or it may develop without any known cause. The myelodysplastic syndromes may change into acute myeloid leukemia, a form of cancer in which too many white blood cells are made.

Myelodysplastic syndromes are grouped together based on how the bone marrow cells and blood cells look under a microscope. There are five types of myelodysplastic syndromes: refractory anemia, refractory anemia with ringed sideroblasts, refractory anemia with excess blasts, refractory anemia with excess blasts in transformation, and chronic myelomonocytic leukemia.

Stages of Myelodysplastic Syndromes

There is no staging for the myelodysplastic syndromes. Treatment depends on whether or not the disease developed following other treatments, or whether the patient has been treated for the myelodysplastic syndrome. Myelodysplastic syndromes are grouped as follows:

De Novo Myelodysplastic Syndromes

De novo myelodysplastic syndromes develop without any known cause. The patient has not received radiation therapy or chemotherapy for other diseases.

Secondary Myelodysplastic Syndromes

Secondary myelodysplastic syndromes develop following treatment with radiation therapy or chemotherapy for other diseases.

Previously Treated Myelodysplastic Syndromes

Previously treated myelodysplastic syndrome means the disease has been treated but has gotten worse.

How Myelodysplastic Syndromes Are Treated

There are treatments for all patients with myelodysplastic syndromes. Often the main treatment is giving red blood cells or platelets by a needle in a vein (transfusion) to control anemia or bleeding. Vitamins or other drugs may also be given to treat anemia.

Chemotherapy and biological therapy are being tested in clinical trials. Chemotherapy uses drugs to treat disease. Chemotherapy may be taken by pill, or it may be put into the body by a needle in the vein or muscle. Chemotherapy is called a systemic treatment because the drug enters the bloodstream, travels through the body, and affects cells throughout the body. Biological therapy tries to get the body to fight disease. It uses materials made by the body or made in a laboratory to boost, direct, or restore the body's natural defenses against disease. Biological therapy is sometimes called biological response modifier (BRM) therapy or immunotherapy.

Bone marrow transplantation is a newer type of treatment that uses high doses of chemotherapy and/or radiation therapy (high doses of x-rays or other high-energy rays) to destroy all of the bone marrow in the body, then transplants healthy bone marrow back into the body. Healthy marrow is then taken from another person (a donor) whose tissue is the same or almost the same as the patient's. The donor may be a twin (the best match), a brother, sister, or other relative, or another person not related. The healthy marrow is given to the patient through a needle in the vein, and the marrow replaces the marrow that was destroyed. A bone marrow transplant using marrow from a relative or person not related to the patient is called an allogeneic bone marrow transplant.

Treatment by Stage

The choice of treatment depends on the type of myelodysplastic syndrome, and the patient's age and general health.

Standard treatment may be considered because of its effectiveness in patients in past studies, or participation in a clinical trial may be considered. Most patients with myelodysplastic syndromes are not cured with standard therapy and some standard treatments may have more side effects than are desired. For these reasons, clinical trials are designed to find better ways to treat cancer patients and are based on the most up-to-date information. Clinical trials are ongoing in most parts of the country for patients with myelodysplastic syndromes. To learn more about clinical trials, call the Cancer Information Service at 1-800-4-CANCER (1-800-422-6237); TTY at 1-800-332-8615.

De Novo Myelodysplastic Syndrome

Treatment may be one of the following:

1. Treatment to relieve symptoms of the disease, such as anemia or bleeding.

2. Allogeneic bone marrow transplantation.

3. Clinical trials of chemotherapy or biological therapy.

Secondary Myelodysplastic Syndrome

Patients will probably receive treatment to relieve symptoms of the disease, such as anemia or bleeding. They may also choose to take part in a clinical trial of chemotherapy or biological therapy.

Previously Treated Myelodysplastic Syndrome

Patients will probably receive treatment to relieve symptoms of the disease, such as anemia or bleeding. They may also choose to take part in a clinical trial of chemotherapy or biological therapy.

To Learn More

To learn more about myelodysplastic syndromes, call the National Cancer Institute's Cancer Information Service at 1-800-4-CANCER (1-800-422-6237); TTY at 1-800-332-8615. By dialing this toll-free number, trained information specialists can answer your questions.

Cancer patients, their families and friends, and others may find the following booklets useful. They are available free of charge by calling 1-800-4-CANCER or writing:

Office of Cancer Communications
National Cancer Institute
Building 31, Room 10A24
Bethesda, MD 20892

Booklets about Cancer Treatment

Radiation Therapy and You: A Guide to Self-Help During Treatment *

Chemotherapy and You: A Guide to Self-Help During Treatment *

Eating Hints: Recipes and Tips for Better Nutrition During Cancer Treatment *

Questions and Answers About Pain Control

What Are Clinical Trials All About?

Booklets about Living with Cancer

Taking Time: Support for People With Cancer and the People Who Care About Them

When Cancer Recurs: Meeting the Challenge Again *

Advanced Cancer: Living Each Day *

* Reprinted in this volume—see Table of Contents

Chapter 43

Adrenocortical Carcinoma

What Is Cancer of the Adrenal Cortex?

Cancer of the adrenal cortex, a rare cancer, is a disease in which cancer (malignant) cells are found in the adrenal cortex, which is the outside layer of the adrenal gland. Cancer of the adrenal cortex is also called adrenocortical carcinoma. There are two adrenal glands, one above each kidney in the back of the upper abdomen. The adrenal glands are also called the suprarenal glands. The inside layer of the adrenal gland is called the adrenal medulla. Cancer that starts in the adrenal medulla is called pheochromocytoma and is discussed in a separate PDQ patient information statement.

The cells in the adrenal cortex make important hormones that help the body work properly. When cells in the adrenal cortex become cancerous, they may make too much of one or more hormones, which can cause symptoms such as high blood pressure, weakening of the bones, or diabetes. If male or female hormones are affected, the body may go through changes such as a deepening of the voice, growing hair on the face, swelling of the sex organs, or swelling of the breasts. Cancers that make hormones are called functioning tumors. Many cancers of the adrenal cortex do not make extra hormones and are called nonfunctioning tumors.

PDQ Statement, National Cancer Institute (NCI), updated October 1997.

A doctor should be seen if the following symptoms appear and won't go away: pain in the abdomen, loss of weight without dieting, and weakness. If there is a functioning tumor, there may be symptoms or signs caused by too many hormones.

If there are symptoms, a doctor will order blood and urine tests to see whether the amounts of hormones in the body are normal. A doctor may also order a computed tomography scan of your abdomen, a special x-ray that uses a computer to make a picture of the inside of the abdomen. Other special x-rays may also be done to tell what kind of tumor is present.

The chance of recovery (prognosis) depends on how far the cancer has spread (stage) and on whether a doctor was able to surgically remove all of the cancer.

Stages of Cancer of the Adrenal Cortex

Once cancer of the adrenal cortex has been found, more tests will be done to see how far the cancer has spread. This is called staging. A doctor needs to know the stage of of the cancer to plan treatment. The following stages are used for cancer of the adrenal cortex:

Stage I

The cancer is less than 5 centimeters (less than 2 inches) and has not spread into tissues around the adrenal gland.

Stage II

The cancer is more than 5 centimeters (less than 2 inches) and has not spread into tissues around the adrenal gland.

Stage III

The cancer has spread into tissues around the adrenal gland or has spread to the lymph nodes around the adrenal gland. Lymph nodes are part of the lymph system and are small, bean shaped organs that make and store infection-fighting cells.

Stage IV

The cancer has spread to tissues or organs in the area and to lymph nodes around the adrenal cortex, or the cancer has spread to other parts of the body.

Recurrent

The cancer has come back (recurred) after it has been treated. It may come back in the adrenal cortex or in another part of the body.

How Cancer of the Adrenal Cortex Is Treated

There are treatments for all patients with cancer of the adrenal cortex. Three kinds of treatment are used:

- surgery (taking out the cancer)

- chemotherapy (using drugs to kill cancer cells)

- radiation therapy (using high-dose x-rays or other high-energy rays to kill cancer cells).

A doctor may take out the adrenal gland in an operation called an adrenalectomy. Tissues around the adrenal glands that contain cancer may be removed. Lymph nodes in the area may also be removed (lymph node dissection).

Chemotherapy uses drugs to kill cancer cells. Chemotherapy may be taken by pill, or it may be put into the body by a needle in a vein or muscle. Chemotherapy is called a systemic treatment because the drug enters the bloodstream, travels through the body, and kills cancer cells throughout the body.

Radiation therapy uses high-energy x-rays to kill cancer cells and shrink tumors. Radiation for cancer of the adrenal cortex usually comes from a machine outside the body (external radiation therapy).

Besides treatment for cancer (chemotherapy, radiation therapy, and/or surgery), a patient may also receive therapy to prevent or treat symptoms caused by the extra hormones that are made by the cancer.

Treatment by Stage

Treatment depends on how far the cancer has spread, and a patient's age and overall health.

Standard treatment may be considered because of its effectiveness in past studies, or participation in a clinical trial may be considered. Not all patients are cured with standard therapy, and some standard treatments may have more side effects than are desired. For these reasons, clinical trials are designed to find better ways to treat cancer patients and are based on the most up-to-date information. Clinical trials are ongoing in some parts of the country for patients with cancer of the adrenal cortex. For more information, call the Cancer Information Service at 1-800-4-CANCER (1-800-422-6237); TTY at 1-800-332-8615.

Stage I Adrenocortical Carcinoma

Treatment will probably be surgery to remove the cancer.

Stage II Adrenocortical Carcinoma

Treatment will probably be surgery to remove the cancer. Clinical trials are testing new treatments.

Stage III Adrenocortical Carcinoma

Treatment may be one of the following:

1. Surgery to remove the cancer. Lymph nodes in the area may also be removed (lymph node dissection).

2. A clinical trial of radiation therapy.

3. A clinical trial of chemotherapy if the size of the tumor can be measured with x-rays and/or if the tumor is making hormones.

Stage IV Adrenocortical Carcinoma

Treatment may be one of the following:

1. Chemotherapy. Clinical trials are testing new drugs.

2. Radiation therapy to bones where the cancer has spread.

3. Surgery to remove the cancer in places where it has spread.

Recurrent Adrenocortical Carcinoma

Treatment depends on many factors, including where the cancer came back and what treatment has already been received. In some cases, surgery can be effective in decreasing the symptoms of the disease by removing some of the tumor. Clinical trials are testing new treatments.

To Learn More

To learn more about cancer of the adrenal cortex, call the National Cancer Institute's Cancer Information Service at 1-800-4-CANCER

(1-800-422-6237); TTY at 1-800-332-8615. By dialing this toll-free number, trained information specialists can help answer your questions.

Cancer patients, their families and friends, and others may find the following booklets useful. They are available free of charge by calling 1-800-4-CANCER or writing:

Office of Cancer Communications
National Cancer Institute
Building 31, Room 10A24
Bethesda, MD 20892

Booklets about Cancer Treatment

Radiation Therapy and You: A Guide to Self-Help During Treatment *

Chemotherapy and You: A Guide to Self-Help During Treatment *

Eating Hints: Recipes and Tips for Better Nutrition During Cancer Treatment *

Questions and Answers About Pain Control

What Are Clinical Trials All About?

Booklets about Living with Cancer

Taking Time: Support for People With Cancer and the People Who Care About Them

When Cancer Recurs: Meeting the Challenge Again *

Advanced Cancer: Living Each Day *

* Reprinted in this volume—see Table of Contents

Chapter 44

Pituitary Tumor

What Are Pituitary Tumors?

Pituitary tumors are tumors found in the pituitary gland, a small organ about the size of a pea in the center of the brain just above the back of the nose. The pituitary gland makes hormones that affect the growth and the functions of other glands in the body.

Most pituitary tumors are benign. This means that they grow very slowly and do not spread to other parts of the body. This patient information summary covers several types of pituitary tumors. Another type of pituitary tumor, called craniopharyngioma, is covered in the patient information summaries on adult or childhood brain tumors.

If a pituitary tumor is found, the pituitary gland may be making too many hormones. This can cause other problems in the body. Tumors that make hormones are called functioning tumors, while those that do not make hormones are called nonfunctioning tumors.

Certain pituitary tumors can cause a disease called Cushing's disease, in which too many hormones called glucocorticoids are released into the bloodstream. This causes fat to build up in the face, back, and chest, and the arms and legs to become very thin. Other symptoms include too much sugar in the blood, weak muscles and bones, a flushed face, and high blood pressure. Other pituitary tumors can cause a condition called acromegaly. Acromegaly means that the hands, feet, and face are larger than normal; in very young people,

PDQ Statement, National Cancer Institute (NCI), updated June 1998.

the whole body may grow much larger than normal. Another type of pituitary tumor can cause the breasts to make milk, even though a woman may not be pregnant; periods may stop as well.

A doctor should be seen if there are symptoms such as headaches, trouble seeing, nausea or vomiting, or any of the symptoms caused by too many hormones.

If there are symptoms, a doctor may order laboratory tests to see what the hormone levels are in the blood. The doctor may also order an MRI (magnetic resonance imaging) scan, which uses magnetic waves to make a picture of the inside of the brain. Other special x-rays may also be done.

The prognosis (chance of recovery) and choice of treatment depend on the type of tumor, and the patient's age and general state of health.

Types of Pituitary Tumors

Once a pituitary tumor is found, more tests will be done to find out how far the tumor has spread and whether or not it makes hormones. A doctor needs to know the type of tumor to plan treatment. The following types of pituitary tumors are found:

ACTH-Producing Tumors

These tumors make a hormone called adrenocorticotropic hormone (ACTH), which stimulates the adrenal glands to make glucocorticoids. When the body makes too much ACTH, it causes Cushing's disease.

Prolactin-Producing Tumors

These tumors make prolactin, a hormone that stimulates a woman's breasts to make milk during and after pregnancy. Prolactin-secreting tumors can cause the breasts to make milk and menstrual periods to stop when a woman is not pregnant. In men, prolactin-producing tumors can cause impotence.

Growth Hormone-Producing Tumors

These tumors make growth hormone, which can cause acromegaly or gigantism when too much is made.

Nonfunctioning Pituitary Tumors

Nonfunctioning tumors do not produce hormones.

Recurrent Pituitary Tumors

Recurrent disease means that the tumor has come back (recurred) after it has been treated. It may come back in the pituitary gland or in another part of the body.

How Pituitary Tumors Are Treated

There are treatments for all patients with pituitary tumors. Three kinds of treatment are used:

- surgery (taking out the tumor in an operation)
- radiation therapy (using high-dose x-rays to kill tumor cells)
- drug therapy

Surgery is a common treatment of pituitary tumors. A doctor may remove the tumor using one of the following operations:

- A transphenoidal hypophysectomy removes the tumor through a cut in the nasal passage.
- A craniotomy removes the tumor through a cut in the front of the skull.

Radiation therapy uses high-energy x-rays to kill cancer cells and shrink tumors. Radiation for pituitary tumors usually comes from a machine outside the body (external radiation therapy). Radiation therapy may be used alone or in addition to surgery or drug therapy.

Certain drugs can also block the pituitary gland from making too many hormones.

Treatment by Type

Treatments for pituitary tumors depend on the type of tumor, how far the tumor has spread into the brain, and the patient's age and overall health.

Standard treatment may be considered because of its effectiveness in patients in past studies, or participation in a clinical trial may be considered. Not all patients are cured with standard therapy and some standard treatments may have more side effects than are desired. For these reasons, clinical trials are designed to find better ways to treat cancer patients and are based on the most up-to-date information. Clinical trials are ongoing in some parts of the country for patients with pituitary tumors. To learn more about clinical trials, call the Cancer Information Service at 1-800-4-CANCER (1-800-422-6237); TTY at 1-800-332-8615.

ACTH-Producing Pituitary Tumors

Treatment may be one of the following:

1. Surgery to remove the tumor (transphenoidal hypophysectomy or craniotomy

2. Radiation therapy. Clinical trials may be testing new types of radiation therapy.

3. Surgery plus radiation therapy.

4. Radiation therapy plus drug therapy to stop the tumor from making ACTH.

Prolactin-Producing Pituitary Tumors

Treatment may be one of the following:

1. Surgery to remove the tumor (transphenoidal hypophysectomy or craniotomy).

2. Radiation therapy.

3. Surgery, radiation therapy, and drug therapy.

4. Drug therapy to stop the tumor from making prolactin. Clinical trials are testing new drugs for this purpose.

Growth Hormone-Producing Pituitary Tumors

Treatment may be one of the following:

1. Surgery to remove the tumor (transphenoidal hypophysectomy or craniotomy).

2. Radiation therapy.

3. Drug therapy to stop the tumor from making growth hormone.

Nonfunctioning Pituitary Tumors

Treatment may be one of the following:

1. Surgery to remove the tumor (transphenoidal hypophysectomy or craniotomy).

2. Radiation therapy alone or in addition to surgery.

Recurrent Pituitary Tumor

Treatment of recurrent pituitary tumor depends on the type of
tumor, the type of treatment the patient has already had, and other
factors such as the patient's general condition. Patients may want to
take part in a clinical trial of new treatments.

To Learn More

To learn more about pituitary tumor, call the National Cancer
Institute's Cancer Information Service at 1-800-4-CANCER (1-800-
422-6237); TTY at 1-800-332-8615. By dialing this toll-free number,
trained information specialists can answer your questions.

Cancer patients, their families and friends, and others may find
the following booklets useful. They are available free of charge by
calling 1-800-4-CANCER or writing:

Office of Cancer Communications
National Cancer Institute
Building 31, Room 10A24
Bethesda, MD 20892

Booklets about Cancer Treatment

Radiation Therapy and You: A Guide to Self-Help During Treatment *

Chemotherapy and You: A Guide to Self-Help During Treatment *

*Eating Hints: Recipes and Tips for Better Nutrition During Cancer
Treatment* *

Questions and Answers About Pain Control

What Are Clinical Trials All About?

Booklets about Living with Cancer

*Taking Time: Support for People With Cancer and the People Who Care
About Them*

When Cancer Recurs: Meeting the Challenge Again *

Advanced Cancer: Living Each Day *

* Reprinted in this volume—see Table of Contents

Chapter 45

Thyroid Cancer

What Is Cancer of the Thyroid?

Cancer of the thyroid is a disease in which cancer (malignant) cells are found in the tissues of the thyroid gland. The thyroid gland is at the base of the throat. It has two lobes, one on the right side and one on the left. The thyroid gland makes important hormones that help the body function normally.

Cancer of the thyroid is more common in women than in men. Most patients are between 25 and 65 years old. People who have been exposed to large amounts of radiation, or who have had radiation treatment for medical problems in the head and neck have a higher chance of getting thyroid cancer. The cancer may not occur until 20 years or longer after radiation treatment.

A doctor should be seen if there is a lump or swelling in the front of the neck or in other parts of the neck.

If there are symptoms, a doctor will feel the patient's thyroid and check for lumps in the neck. The doctor may order blood tests and special scans to see whether a lump in the thyroid is making too many hormones. The doctor may want to take a small amount of tissue from the thyroid. This is called a biopsy. To do this, a small needle is inserted into the thyroid at the base of the throat and some tissue is drawn out. The tissue is then looked at under a microscope to see whether it contains cancer.

PDQ Statement, National Cancer Institute (NCI), updated July 1998.

461

There are four main types of cancer of the thyroid (based on how the cancer cells look under a microscope): papillary, follicular, medullary, and anaplastic. The chance of recovery (prognosis) depends on the type of thyroid cancer, whether it is just in the thyroid or has spread to other parts of the body (stage), and the patient's age and overall health. Some types of thyroid cancer grow much faster than others.

The genes in our cells carry the hereditary information from our parents. An abnormal gene has been found in patients with some forms of thyroid cancer. If medullary thyroid cancer is found, the patient may have been born with a certain abnormal gene which may have led to the cancer. Family members may have also inherited this abnormal gene. Tests have been developed to determine who has the genetic defect long before any cancer appears. It is important that the patient and his or her family members (children, grandchildren, parents, brothers, sisters, nieces and nephews) see a doctor about tests that will show if the abnormal gene is present. These tests are confidential and can help the doctor help patients. Family members, including young children, who don't have cancer, but do have this abnormal gene, may reduce the chance of developing medullary thyroid cancer by having surgery to safely remove the thyroid gland (thyroidectomy).

Stages of Cancer of the Thyroid

Once cancer of the thyroid is found (diagnosed), more tests will be done to find out if cancer cells have spread to other parts of the body. This is called staging. A doctor needs to know the stage of the disease to plan treatment.

The following stages are used for papillary cancers of the thyroid:

Stage I Papillary

Cancer is only in the thyroid and may be found in one or both lobes.

Stage II Papillary

In patients younger than 45 years of age:

- Cancer has spread beyond the thyroid.

In patients older than 45 years of age:

- Cancer is only in the thyroid and larger than 1 centimeter (about 1/2 inch).

Stage III Papillary

Cancer is found in patients older than 45 years of age and has spread outside the thyroid (but not outside of the neck) or has spread to the lymph nodes.

Stage IV Papillary

Cancer is found in patients older than 45 years of age and has spread to other parts of the body, such as the lungs and bones.

The following stages are used for follicular cancers of the thyroid:

Stage I Follicular

Cancer is only in the thyroid and may be found in one or both lobes.

Stage II Follicular

In patients younger than 45 years of age:

* Cancer has spread beyond the thyroid.

In patients older than 45 years of age:

* Cancer is only in the thyroid and larger than 1 centimeter (about 1/2 inch).

Stage III Follicular

Cancer is found in patients older than 45 years of age and has spread outside the thyroid (but not outside of the neck) or to the lymph nodes.

Stage IV Follicular

Cancer is found in patients older than 45 years of age and has spread to other parts of the body, such as the lungs and bones.

Other types or stages of thyroid cancer include the following:

Stage I Medullary

Cancer is less than 1 centimeter (about 1/2 inch) in size.

Stage II Medullary

Cancer is between 1 and 4 centimeters (about 1/2" to 1 1/2") in size.

Stage III Medullary

Cancer has spread to the lymph nodes.

Stage IV Medullary

Cancer has spread to other parts of the body.

Anaplastic

There is no staging system for anaplastic cancer of the thyroid. This type of cancer of the thyroid grows faster than the other types.

Recurrent

Recurrent disease means that the cancer has come back (recurred) after it has been treated. It may come back in the thyroid or in another part of the body.

How Cancer of the Thyroid Is Treated

There are treatments for all patients with cancer of the thyroid. Four types of treatment are used:

- surgery (taking out the cancer)
- radiation therapy (using high-dose x-rays or other high-energy rays to kill cancer cells)
- hormone therapy (using hormones to stop cancer cells from growing)
- chemotherapy (using drugs to kill cancer cells)

Surgery is the most common treatment of cancer of the thyroid. A doctor may remove the cancer using one of the following operations:

- Lobectomy removes only the side of the thyroid where the cancer is found. Lymph nodes in the area may be taken out (biopsied) to see if they contain cancer.
- Near-total thyroidectomy removes all of the thyroid except for a small part.

- Total thyroidectomy removes the entire thyroid.

- Lymph node dissection removes lymph nodes in the neck that contain cancer.

Radiation therapy uses high-energy x-rays to kill cancer cells and shrink tumors. Radiation for cancer of the thyroid may come from a machine outside the body (external radiation therapy) or from drinking a liquid that contains radioactive iodine. Because the thyroid takes up iodine, the radioactive iodine collects in any thyroid tissue remaining in the body and kills the cancer cells.

Hormone therapy uses hormones to stop cancer cells from growing. In treating cancer of the thyroid, hormones can be used to stop the body from making other hormones that might make cancer cells grow. Hormones are usually given as pills.

Chemotherapy uses drugs to kill cancer cells. Chemotherapy may be taken by pill, or it may be put into the body by a needle in the vein or muscle. Chemotherapy is called a systemic treatment because the drug enters the bloodstream, travels through the body, and can kill cancer cells outside the thyroid.

Treatment by Stage

Treatment of cancer of the thyroid depends on the type and stage of the disease, and the patient's age and overall health.

Standard treatment may be considered because of its effectiveness in patients in past studies, or participation in a clinical trial may be considered. Not all patients are cured with standard therapy and some standard treatments may have more side effects than are desired. For these reasons, clinical trials are designed to find better ways to treat cancer patients and are based on the most up-to-date information. Clinical trials are ongoing in many parts of the country for some patients with cancer of the thyroid. To learn more about clinical trials, call the Cancer Information Service at 1-800-4-CANCER (1-800-422-6237); TTY at 1-800-332-8615.

Stage I Papillary Thyroid Cancer

Treatment may be one of the following:

1. Surgery to remove one lobe of the thyroid (lobectomy), followed by hormone therapy. Radioactive iodine also may be given following surgery.

2. Surgery to remove the thyroid (total thyroidectomy).

Stage I Follicular Thyroid Cancer

Treatment may be one of the following:

1. Surgery to remove the thyroid (total thyroidectomy).

2. Surgery to remove one lobe of the thyroid (lobectomy), followed by hormone therapy. Radioactive iodine also may be given following surgery.

Stage II Papillary Thyroid Cancer

Treatment may be one of the following:

1. Surgery to remove one lobe of the thyroid (lobectomy) and lymph nodes that contain cancer, followed by hormone therapy. Radioactive iodine also may be given following surgery.

2. Surgery to remove the thyroid (total thyroidectomy).

Stage II Follicular Thyroid Cancer

Treatment may be one of the following:

1. Surgery to remove the thyroid (total thyroidectomy).

2. Surgery to remove one lobe of the thyroid (lobectomy) and lymph nodes that contain cancer, followed by hormone therapy. Radioactive iodine also may be given following surgery.

Stage III Papillary Thyroid Cancer

Treatment may be one of the following:

1. Surgery to remove the entire thyroid (total thyroidectomy) and lymph nodes where cancer has spread.

2. Total thyroidectomy followed by radiation therapy with radioactive iodine or external beam radiation therapy.

Stage III Follicular Thyroid Cancer

Treatment may be one of the following:

1. Surgery to remove the entire thyroid (total thyroidectomy) and lymph nodes or other tissues around the thyroid where the cancer has spread.

2. Total thyroidectomy followed by radioactive iodine or external beam radiation therapy.

Stage IV Papillary Thyroid Cancer

Treatment may be one of the following:

1. Radioactive iodine.

2. External beam radiation therapy.

3. Hormone therapy.

4. A clinical trial of chemotherapy.

Stage IV Follicular Thyroid Cancer

Treatment may be one of the following:

1. Radioactive iodine.

2. External beam radiation therapy.

3. Hormone therapy.

4. A clinical trial of chemotherapy.

Medullary Thyroid Cancer

Treatment will probably be surgery to remove the entire thyroid (total thyroidectomy) unless the cancer has spread to other parts of the body. If lymph nodes in the neck contain cancer, the lymph nodes in the neck will be removed (lymph node dissection). If the cancer has spread to other parts of the body, chemotherapy may be given.

Anaplastic Thyroid Cancer

Treatment may be one of the following:

1. Surgery to remove the thyroid and the tissues around it. Because this cancer often spreads very quickly to other tissues, a doctor may have to take out part of the tube through which a person breathes. The doctor will then make an airway in the

throat so the patient can breathe. This is called a tracheo-stomy.

2. Total thyroidectomy to reduce symptoms if the disease remains in the area of the thyroid.

3. External beam radiation therapy.

4. Chemotherapy.

5. Clinical trials studying new methods of treatment of thyroid cancer.

Recurrent Thyroid Cancer

The choice of treatment depends on the type of thyroid cancer the patient has, the kind of treatment the patient had before, and where the cancer comes back. Treatment may be one of the following:

1. Surgery with or without radioactive iodine.

2. External beam radiation therapy to relieve symptoms caused by the cancer.

3. Chemotherapy.

4. Radioactive iodine.

5. Radiation therapy given during surgery.

6. Clinical trials.

To Learn More

To learn more about cancer of the thyroid, call the National Cancer Institute's Cancer Information Service at 1-800-4-CANCER (1-800-422-6237); TTY at 1-800-332-8615. By dialing this toll-free number, you can speak with a trained information specialist who can answer your questions.

The Cancer Information Service also has booklets about cancer that are available to the public and can be sent on request. The following booklet about thyroid cancer may be helpful: *In Answer to Your Questions About Thyroid Cancer.*

Cancer patients, their families and friends, and others may find the following booklets useful. They are available free of charge by calling 1-800-4-CANCER or writing:

Office of Cancer Communications
National Cancer Institute
Building 31, Room 10A24
Bethesda, MD 20892

Booklets about Cancer Treatment

Radiation Therapy and You: A Guide to Self-Help During Treatment *

Chemotherapy and You: A Guide to Self-Help During Treatment *

Eating Hints: Recipes and Tips for Better Nutrition During Cancer Treatment *

Questions and Answers About Pain Control

What Are Clinical Trials All About?

Booklets about Living with Cancer

Taking Time: Support for People With Cancer and the People Who Care About Them

When Cancer Recurs: Meeting the Challenge Again *

Advanced Cancer: Living Each Day *

* Reprinted in this volume—see Table of Contents

Chapter 46

Parathyroid Cancer

What Is Parathyroid Cancer?

Parathyroid cancer, a very rare cancer, is a disease in which cancer (malignant) cells are found in the tissues of the parathyroid gland. The parathyroid gland is at the base of the neck, near the thyroid gland. The parathyroid gland makes a hormone called parathyroid hormone (PTH), or parathormone, which helps the body store and use calcium.

Problems with the parathyroid gland are common and are usually not caused by cancer. If parathyroid cancer is found, the parathyroid gland may be making too much PTH. This causes too much calcium to be found in the blood. The extra PTH also takes calcium from the bones, which causes pain in the bones, kidney problems, and other types of problems. There are other conditions that can cause the parathyroid gland to make too much PTH. It is important for a doctor to determine what is causing the extra PTH. Hyperparathyroidism is a condition which can cause the body to make extra PTH. If hyperparathyroidism runs in the family, there is a greater chance of getting this type of cancer.

A doctor should be seen if there are the following symptoms: bone pain, a lump in the neck, pain in the upper part of the back, weak muscles, difficulty speaking, or vomiting.

If there are symptoms, the doctor will conduct a physical examination and feel for lumps in the throat. The doctor may also order blood tests and other tests to check for cancer or other types of tumors that may not be cancer (benign tumors).

PDQ Statement, National Cancer Institute (NCI), updated June 1998.

The chance of recovery (prognosis) depends on whether the cancer is just in the parathyroid gland or has spread to other parts of the body (stage) and the patient's general health.

Stages of Parathyroid Cancer

Once parathyroid cancer is found, more tests will be done to find out if cancer cells have spread to other parts of the body. This is called staging. A doctor needs to know the stage of the disease to plan treatment. The following stages are used for parathyroid cancer.

Localized

The cancer is only on the parathyroid gland and has not spread to tissues next to the parathyroid.

Metastatic

The cancer has spread to lymph nodes in the area or to other parts of the body, such as the lungs (lymph nodes are small bean-shaped structures that are found throughout the body; they produce and store infection-fighting cells).

Recurrent

Recurrent disease means that the cancer has come back (recurred) after it has been treated. It may come back in the original place or in another part of the body.

How Parathyroid Cancer Is Treated

There are treatments for all patients with parathyroid cancer. Two kinds of treatment are used:

- surgery (taking out the cancer)
- radiation therapy (using high-dose x-rays or other high-energy rays to kill cancer cells)

Surgery is the most common treatment of parathyroid cancer. A doctor may remove the parathyroid gland (parathyroidectomy) and the half of the thyroid on the same side as the cancer (ipsilateral thyroidectomy).

Radiation therapy uses high-energy x-rays to kill cancer cells and shrink tumors. Radiation may come from a machine outside the body (external radiation therapy) or from putting materials that produce radiation (radioisotopes) through thin plastic tubes in the area where the cancer cells are found (internal radiation therapy).

Chemotherapy (using drugs to kill cancer cells) is being studied in clinical trials. Chemotherapy uses drugs to kill cancer cells. Chemotherapy may be taken by pill, or it may be put into the body by a needle in the vein or muscle. Chemotherapy is called a systemic treatment because the drug enters the bloodstream, travels through the body, and can kill cancer cells outside the parathyroid gland.

Treatment by Stage

Treatment for parathyroid cancer depends on the type and stage of the disease and the patient's age and overall health.

Standard treatment may be considered because of its effectiveness in patients in past studies, or participation in a clinical trial may be considered. Not all patients are cured with standard therapy and some standard treatments may have more side effects than are desired. For these reasons, clinical trials are designed to find better ways to treat cancer patients and are based on the most up-to-date information. Clinical trials are ongoing in some parts of the country for patients with parathyroid cancer. To learn more about clinical trials, call the Cancer Information Service at 1-800-4-CANCER (1-800-422-6237); TTY at 1-800-332-8615.

Localized Parathyroid Cancer

Treatment may be one of the following:

1. Surgery to remove the parathyroid gland (parathyroidectomy) and the half of the thyroid on the same side as the cancer (ipsilateral thyroidectomy).

2. A clinical trial of surgery followed by radiation therapy.

3. A clinical trial of radiation therapy.

Metastatic Parathyroid Cancer

Treatment may be one of the following:

1. Surgery to remove the parathyroid gland (parathyroidectomy) and other tissues around the thyroid if they contain cancer.

2. Surgery to remove as much of the parathyroid gland as possible in order to reduce production of PTH.

3. Medical treatment to reduce the amount of calcium in the blood.

4. A clinical trial of surgery followed by radiation therapy.

5. A clinical trial of radiation therapy.

6. A clinical trial of chemotherapy.

Recurrent Parathyroid Cancer

Recurrent disease can occur as late as 34 years after the first tumor. Treatment may be one of the following:

1. Surgery to remove the parathyroid gland (parathyroidectomy) and other tissues around the thyroid if they contain cancer.

2. Surgery to remove as much of the parathyroid gland as possible in order to reduce production of PTH.

3. Medical treatment to reduce the amount of calcium in the blood.

4. A clinical trial of surgery followed by radiation therapy.

5. A clinical trial of radiation therapy.

6. A clinical trial of chemotherapy.

To Learn More

To learn more about parathyroid cancer, call the National Cancer Institute's Cancer Information Service at 1-800-4-CANCER (1-800-422-6237); TTY at 1-800- 332-8615. By dialing this toll-free number, trained information specialists can answer your questions.

Cancer patients, their families and friends, and others may find the following booklets useful. They are available free of charge by calling 1-800-4-CANCER or writing:

Office of Cancer Communications
National Cancer Institute
Building 31, Room 10A24
Bethesda, MD 20892

Booklets about Cancer Treatment

Radiation Therapy and You: A Guide to Self-Help During Treatment *

Chemotherapy and You: A Guide to Self-Help During Treatment *

Eating Hints: Recipes and Tips for Better Nutrition During Cancer Treatment *

Questions and Answers About Pain Control

What Are Clinical Trials All About?

Booklets about Living with Cancer

Taking Time: Support for People With Cancer and the People Who Care About Them

When Cancer Recurs: Meeting the Challenge Again *

Advanced Cancer: Living Each Day *

* Reprinted in this volume—see Table of Contents

Chapter 47

Pheochromocytoma

What Is Pheochromocytoma?

Pheochromocytoma, a rare cancer, is a disease in which cancer (malignant) cells are found in special cells in the body called chromaffin cells. Most pheochromocytomas start inside the adrenal gland (the adrenal medulla) where most chromaffin cells are located. There are two adrenal glands, one above each kidney in the back of the upper abdomen. Cells in the adrenal glands make important hormones that help the body work properly. Usually pheochromocytoma affects only one adrenal gland. Pheochromocytoma may also start in other parts of the body, such as the area around the heart or bladder.

Most tumors that start in the chromaffin cells do not spread to other parts of the body and are not cancer. These are called benign tumors. If a tumor is found, the doctor will need to determine whether it is cancer or benign.

Pheochromocytomas often cause the adrenal glands to make too many hormones called catecholamines. The extra catecholamines cause high blood pressure (hypertension), which can cause headaches, sweating, pounding of the heart, pain in the chest, and a feeling of anxiety. High blood pressure that goes on for a long time without treatment can lead to heart disease, stroke, and other major health problems.

If there are symptoms, a doctor may order blood and urine tests to see if there are extra hormones in the body. A patient may also have

PDQ Statement, National Cancer Institute (NCI), updated June 1998.

a special nuclear medicine scan. A CT scan, an x-ray that uses a computer to make a picture of the inside of a part of the body or an MRI scan, which uses magnetic waves to make a picture of the abdomen, may also be done.

Pheochromocytoma is sometimes part of a condition called multiple endocrine neoplasia syndrome (MEN). People with MEN often have other cancers (such as thyroid cancer) and other hormonal problems.

The chance of recovery (prognosis) depends on how far the cancer has spread, and the patient's age and general health.

Stages of Pheochromocytoma

Once pheochromocytoma is found, more tests will be done to see how far the cancer has spread. This is called staging. A doctor needs to know the stage of the disease to plan treatment. The following stages are used for pheochromocytoma:

Localized Benign Pheochromocytoma

Tumor is found in only one area and has not spread to other tissues. Most pheochromocytomas do not spread to other parts of the body and are not cancer.

Regional Pheochromocytoma

Cancer has spread to lymph nodes in the area or to other tissues around the original cancer. (Lymph nodes are small bean-shaped structures that are found throughout the body. They produce and store infection-fighting cells.)

Metastatic Pheochromocytoma

The cancer has spread to other parts of the body.

Recurrent Pheochromocytoma

Recurrent disease means that the cancer has come back (recurred) after it has been treated. It may come back in the area where it started or in another part of the body.

How Pheochromocytoma Is Treated

There are treatments for all patients with pheochromocytoma. Three kinds of treatment are used:

- surgery (taking out the cancer)

- radiation therapy (using high-dose x-rays or other high-energy rays to kill cancer cells)

- chemotherapy (using drugs to kill cancer cells)

Surgery is the most common treatment of pheochromocytoma. A doctor may remove one or both adrenal glands in an operation called adrenalectomy. The doctor will look inside the abdomen to make sure all the cancer is removed. If the cancer has spread, lymph nodes or other tissues may also be taken out.

Chemotherapy uses drugs to kill cancer cells. Chemotherapy may be taken by pill, or it may be put into the body by a needle in the vein or muscle. Chemotherapy is called a systemic treatment because the drug enters the bloodstream, travels through the body, and can kill cancer cells throughout the body.

Radiation therapy uses high-energy x-rays to kill cancer cells and shrink tumors. Radiation comes from a machine outside the body (external radiation therapy).

Treatment by Stage

Treatments for pheochromocytoma depend on the stage of the disease, and the patient's age and overall health. For more information, call the Cancer Information Service at 1-800-4-CANCER (1-800-422-6237); TTY at 1-800-332-8615.

Localized Benign Pheochromocytoma

Treatment will probably be surgery to remove one or both adrenal glands (adrenalectomy). After surgery the doctor will order blood and urine tests to make sure hormone levels return to normal.

Regional Pheochromocytoma

Treatment may be one of the following:

1. Surgery to remove one or both adrenal glands (adrenalectomy) and as much of the cancer as possible. If cancer remains after surgery, drugs will be given to control high blood pressure.

2. External radiation therapy to relieve symptoms (in rare cases).

3. Chemotherapy.

Metastatic Pheochromocytoma

Treatment may be one of the following:

1. Surgery to remove as much of the cancer as possible. If cancer remains after surgery, drugs will be given to control high blood pressure.

2. External radiation therapy to relieve symptoms.

3. Chemotherapy

Recurrent Pheochromocytoma

Treatment may be one of the following:

1. Surgery to remove as much of the cancer as possible. If cancer remains after surgery, drugs will be given to control high blood pressure.

2. External radiation therapy to relieve symptoms.

3. Chemotherapy.

To Learn More

To learn more about pheochromocytoma, call the National Cancer Institute's Cancer Information Service at 1-800-4-CANCER (1-800-422-6237); TTY at 1-800-332-8615. By dialing this toll-free number, trained information specialists can answer your questions.

Cancer patients, their families and friends, and others may find the following booklets useful. They are available free of charge by calling 1-800-4-CANCER or writing:

Office of Cancer Communications
National Cancer Institute
Building 31, Room 10A24
Bethesda, MD 20892

Booklets about Cancer Treatment

Radiation Therapy and You: A Guide to Self-Help During Treatment *

Chemotherapy and You: A Guide to Self-Help During Treatment *

Eating Hints: Recipes and Tips for Better Nutrition During Cancer Treatment *

Questions and Answers About Pain Control

What Are Clinical Trials All About?

Booklets about Living with Cancer

Taking Time: Support for People With Cancer and the People Who Care About Them

When Cancer Recurs: Meeting the Challenge Again *

Advanced Cancer: Living Each Day *

* Reprinted in this volume—see Table of Contents

Chapter 48

Malignant Thymoma

What Is Malignant Thymoma?

Malignant thymoma is a disease in which cancer (malignant) cells are found in the tissues of the thymus. The thymus is a small organ that lies under the breastbone. It makes white blood cells called lymphocytes, which travel through the body and fight infection. People with malignant thymoma often have other diseases of their immune system. The most common disease in people with thymoma is one in which the muscles are weak, called myasthenia gravis.

A doctor should be seen if a person has a cough that won't go away, weakness in the muscles, or pain in the chest.

If there are symptoms, the doctor may take an x-ray of the chest. The doctor may also do a CT scan, a special x-ray that uses a computer to make a picture of part of the body.

The chance of recovery (prognosis) and choice of treatment depend on the stage of the cancer (whether it is just in the thymus or has spread to other places), the types of cells found in the cancer, and the patient's general state of health.

Stages of Malignant Thymoma

Once malignant thymoma is found, more tests will be done to find out if cancer cells have spread to other parts of the body. This is called

PDQ Statement, National Cancer Institute (NCI), updated February 1999.

staging. A doctor needs to know the stage of the disease to plan treatment. The following staging system may be used for malignant thymoma:

- Stage I—cancer found only within the thymus gland and its sac
- Stage II—cancer invasion into surrounding fat or lining of lung cavity
- Stage III—cancer invasion into organs near the thymus
- Stage IVa—greater spread of cancer into sac around heart or lungs
- Stage IVb—greater spread of cancer through vessels carrying blood or lymph

Stage I malignant thymoma may be referred to as noninvasive malignant thymoma. Stages II through IVb malignant thymoma may be referred to as invasive malignant thymoma.

- Recurrent—Recurrent disease means that the cancer has come back (recurred) after it has been treated. It may come back in the thymus or in another part of the body.

How Malignant Thymoma Is Treated

There are treatments for all patients with malignant thymoma. Three kinds of treatment are used:

- surgery (taking out the cancer in an operation)
- radiation therapy (using high-dose x-rays or other high-energy rays to kill cancer cells)
- hormone therapy (using hormones to stop cancer cells from growing)

Chemotherapy (using drugs to kill cancer cells) is being studied in clinical trials.

Surgery to remove the tumor is the most common treatment of malignant thymoma. A doctor also may take out lymph nodes or tissue around the cancer.

Radiation therapy uses x-rays or other high-energy rays to kill cancer cells and shrink tumors. Radiation for thymoma usually comes from a machine outside the body (external beam radiation therapy). Radiation therapy can be used alone or in addition to surgery.

If the doctor removes all the cancer that can be seen at the time of the operation, the patient may be given radiation therapy after surgery to kill any cancer cells that are left. Radiation therapy given after an operation when no cancer cells can be seen is called adjuvant radiation therapy.

Hormone therapy uses hormones to stop cancer cells from growing. Hormones called steroids may be given to stop the tumor from growing.

Chemotherapy uses drugs to kill cancer cells. Chemotherapy may be taken by pill, or it may be put into the body by a needle in the vein or muscle. Chemotherapy is called a systemic treatment because the drug enters the bloodstream, travels through the body, and can kill cancer cells outside the thymus.

Treatment by Stage

Treatment of malignant thymoma depends on the stage of the disease, and the patient's age and overall condition.

Standard treatment may be considered because of its effectiveness in patients in past studies, or participation in a clinical trial may be considered. Not all patients are cured with standard therapy and some standard treatments may have more side effects than are desired. For these reasons, clinical trials are designed to find better ways to treat cancer patients and are based on the most up-to-date information. Clinical trials are ongoing in many parts of the country for patients with malignant thymoma. To learn more about clinical trials, call the Cancer Information Service at 1-800-4-CANCER (1-800-422-6237); TTY at 1-800-332-8615.

Noninvasive Malignant Thymoma

Treatment may be one of the following:

1.   Surgery to remove the cancer.

2.   Radiation therapy in rare cases.

Invasive Malignant Thymoma

Treatment may be one of the following:

1.   Surgery to remove the cancer followed by adjuvant radiation therapy.

2. Radiation therapy alone, if the cancer cannot be removed by surgery.

3. A clinical trial of chemotherapy.

4. A clinical trial of chemotherapy followed by surgery.

5. A clinical trial of both chemotherapy and radiation therapy if the cancer cannot be removed by surgery.

Recurrent Malignant Thymoma

Treatment may be one of the following:

1. Surgery to remove the cancer with or without radiation therapy.

2. Radiation therapy.

3. Hormone therapy with steroids.

4. A clinical trial of chemotherapy.

To Learn More

To learn more about malignant thymoma, call the National Cancer Institute's Cancer Information Service at 1-800-4-CANCER (1-800-422-6237); TTY at 1-800-332-8615. By dialing this toll-free number, trained information specialists can answer your questions.

Cancer patients, their families and friends, and others may find the following booklets useful. They are available free of charge by calling 1-800-4-CANCER or writing:

Office of Cancer Communications
National Cancer Institute
Building 31, Room 10A24
Bethesda, MD 20892

Booklets about Cancer Treatment

Radiation Therapy and You: A Guide to Self-Help During Treatment *

Chemotherapy and You: A Guide to Self-Help During Treatment *

Eating Hints: Recipes and Tips for Better Nutrition During Cancer Treatment *

Questions and Answers About Pain Control

What Are Clinical Trials All About?

Booklets about Living with Cancer

Taking Time: Support for People With Cancer and the People Who Care About Them

*When Cancer Recurs: Meeting the Challenge Again ***

*Advanced Cancer: Living Each Day ***

* Reprinted in this volume—see Table of Contents

Chapter 49

Skin Cancer

Each year, more than 600,000 people in the United States learn that they have skin cancer. This chapter will give you some important information about this disease. It explains how skin cancer is diagnosed and treated and has information about preventing this disease.

Other National Cancer Institute (NCI) publications are listed below, in the section entitled "For Further Information." NCI materials cannot answer every question you may have about skin cancer. They cannot take the place of talks with doctors, nurses, and other members of the health care team. We hope our information will help with those talks.

Research has led to better methods of diagnosing and treating this disease. It is encouraging to know that skin cancer is now almost 100 percent curable if found early and treated promptly.

Our knowledge about skin cancer and other types of cancer is increasing rapidly. For up-to-date information, call the NCI-supported Cancer Information Service (CIS) toll free at 1-800-4-CANCER (1-800-422-6237). The CIS is described in the "Resources" section.

The Skin

The skin is the body's outer covering. It protects us against heat and light, injury, and infection. It regulates body temperature and

"What You Need To Know About Skin Cancer," National Cancer Institute. National Institutes of Health Publication 94-1563, April 1993. Updated 28 September 1998.

stores water, fat, and vitamin D. Weighing about 6 pounds, the skin is the body's largest organ. It is made up of two main layers: the outer epidermis and the inner dermis.

The epidermis (outer layer of the skin) is mostly made up of flat, scale-like cells called squamous cells. Under the squamous cells are round cells called basal cells. The deepest part of the epidermis also contains melanocytes. These cells produce melanin, which gives the skin its color.

The dermis (inner layer of skin) contains blood and lymph vessels, hair follicles, and glands. These glands produce sweat, which helps regulate body temperature, and sebum, an oily substance that helps keep the skin from drying out. Sweat and sebum reach the skin's surface through tiny openings called pores.

What Is Cancer?

Cancer is a group of more than 100 diseases. Although each type of cancer differs from the others in many ways, every cancer is a disease of some of the body's cells.

Healthy cells that make up the body's tissues grow, divide, and replace themselves in an orderly way. This process keeps the body in good repair. Sometimes, however, normal cells lose their ability to limit and direct their growth. They divide too rapidly and grow without any order. Too much tissue is produced, and tumors begin to form. Tumors can be benign or malignant.

- Benign tumors are not cancer. They do not spread to other parts of the body and are seldom a threat to life. Often, benign tumors can be removed by surgery, and they are not likely to return.

- Malignant tumors are cancer. They can invade and destroy nearby healthy tissues and organs. Cancer cells also can spread, or metastasize, to other parts of the body and form new tumors.

Skin Cancer

The two most common kinds of skin cancer are basal cell carcinoma and squamous cell carcinoma. (Carcinoma is cancer that begins in the cells that cover or line an organ.) Basal cell carcinoma accounts for more than 90 percent of all skin cancers in the United States. It is a slow-growing cancer that seldom spreads to other parts of the body. Squamous cell carcinoma also rarely spreads, but it does so more often than basal cell carcinoma. However, it is important that skin cancers are found and treated early because they can invade and destroy nearby tissue.

Basal cell carcinoma and squamous cell carcinoma are sometimes called non-melanoma skin cancer. Another type of cancer that occurs in the skin is melanoma, which begins in the melanocytes. More information about this disease can be found in the booklet *What You Need To Know About Melanoma* [reprinted in this volume as Chapter 50].

Cause and Prevention

Skin cancer is the most common type of cancer in the United States. According to current estimates, 40 to 50 percent of Americans who live to age 65 will have skin cancer at least once.

Several risk factors increase the chance of getting skin cancer. Ultraviolet (UV) radiation from the sun is the main cause of skin cancer. Artificial sources of UV radiation, such as sunlamps and tanning booths, can also cause skin cancer. Although anyone can get skin cancer, the risk is greatest for people who have fair skin that freckles easily—often those with red or blond hair and blue or light-colored eyes.

The risk of developing skin cancer is also affected by where a person lives. People who live in areas that get high levels of UV radiation from the sun are more likely to get skin cancer. In the United States, for example, skin cancer is more common in Texas than it is in Minnesota, where the sun is not as strong. Worldwide, the highest rates of skin cancer are found in South Africa and Australia, areas that receive high amounts of UV radiation.

In addition, skin cancer is related to lifetime exposure to UV radiation. Most skin cancers appear after age 50, but the sun's damaging effects begin at an early age. Therefore, protection should start in childhood to prevent skin cancer later in life.

Whenever possible, people should avoid exposure to the midday sun (from 10 a.m. to 2 p.m. standard time, or from 11 a.m. to 3 p.m. daylight saving time). Keep in mind that protective clothing, such as sun hats and long sleeves, can block out the sun's harmful rays. Also, lotions that contain sunscreens can protect the skin. Sunscreens are rated in strength according to a sun protection factor (SPF), which ranges from 2 to 30 or higher. Those rated 15 to 30 block most of the sun's harmful rays.

The NCI is supporting research to try to find new ways to prevent skin cancer. This research involves people who have a high risk of developing skin cancer—those who have already had the disease and those who have certain other rare skin diseases that increase their risk of skin cancer.

Symptoms

The most common warning sign of skin cancer is a change on the skin, especially a new growth or a sore that doesn't heal. Skin cancers don't all look the same. For example, the cancer may start as a small, smooth, shiny, pale, or waxy lump. Or it can appear as a firm red lump. Sometimes, the lump bleeds or develops a crust. Skin cancer can also start as a flat, red spot that is rough, dry, or scaly.

Both basal and squamous cell cancers are found mainly on areas of the skin that are exposed to the sun—the head, face, neck, hands, and arms. However, skin cancer can occur anywhere.

Actinic keratosis, which appears as rough, red or brown, scaly patches on the skin, is known as a precancerous condition because it sometimes develops into squamous cell cancer. Like skin cancer, it usually appears on sun exposed areas but can be found elsewhere.

Changes in the skin are not sure signs of cancer; however, it is important to see a doctor if any symptom lasts longer than 2 weeks. Don't wait for the area to hurt—skin cancers seldom cause pain.

Detection

The cure rate for skin cancer could be 100 percent if all skin cancers were brought to a doctor's attention before they had a chance to spread. Therefore, people should check themselves regularly for new growths or other changes in the skin. Any new, colored growths or any changes in growths that are already present should be reported to the doctor without delay. (See the end of this chapter for a simple guide on how to do a skin self-exam.)

Doctors should also look at the skin during routine physical exams. People who have already had skin cancer should be sure to have regular exams so that the doctor can check the skin—both the treated areas and other places where cancer may develop.

Diagnosis

Basal cell carcinoma and squamous cell carcinoma are generally diagnosed and treated in the same way. When an area of skin does not look normal, the doctor may remove all or part of the growth. This is called a biopsy. To check for cancer cells, the tissue is examined under a microscope by a pathologist or a dermatologist. A biopsy is the only sure way to tell if the problem is cancer.

Doctors generally divide skin cancer into two stages: local (affecting only the skin) or metastatic (spreading beyond the skin). Because skin cancer rarely spreads, a biopsy often is the only test needed to determine the stage. In cases where the growth is very large or has been present for a long time, the doctor will carefully check the lymph nodes in the area. In addition, the patient may need to have additional tests, such as special x-rays, to find out whether the cancer has spread to other parts of the body. Knowing the stage of a skin cancer helps the doctor plan the best treatment.

Treatment Planning

In treating skin cancer, the doctor's main goal is to remove or destroy the cancer completely with as small a scar as possible. To plan the best treatment for each patient, the doctor considers the location and size of the cancer, the risk of scarring, and the person's age, general health, and medical history.

It is sometimes helpful to have the advice of more than one doctor before starting treatment. It may take a week or two to arrange for a second opinion, but this short delay will not reduce the chance that treatment will be successful. There are a number of ways to find a doctor for a second opinion:

- The patient's doctor may be able to suggest a doctor, such as a dermatologist or a plastic surgeon, who has a special interest in skin cancer.

- The American Academy of Dermatology and the American Society of Plastic and Reconstructive Surgeons can provide the names of specialists in local areas. These organizations are listed in the "Resources" section below.

- The Cancer Information Service, at 1-800-4-CANCER, can tell callers about treatment facilities, including cancer centers and other programs that are supported by the National Cancer Institute.

- Patients can get the names of doctors from their local medical society, a nearby hospital, or a medical school.

- The *Directory of Medical Specialists* lists doctors' names and gives their background. It is in most public libraries.

Treating Skin Cancer

Treatment for skin cancer usually involves some type of surgery. In some cases, doctors suggest radiation therapy or chemotherapy. Sometimes a combination of these methods is used.

Surgery. Many skin cancers can be cut from the skin quickly and easily. In fact, the cancer is sometimes completely removed at the time of the biopsy, and no further treatment is needed.

Curettage and Electrodesiccation. Doctors commonly use a type of surgery called curettage. After a local anesthetic numbs the area, the cancer is scooped out with a curette, an instrument with a sharp, spoon shaped end. The area is also treated by electrodesiccation. An electric current from a special machine is used to control bleeding and kill any cancer cells remaining around the edge of the wound. Most patients develop a flat, white scar.

Mohs' Surgery. Mohs' technique is a special type of surgery used for skin cancer. Its purpose is to remove all of the cancerous tissue and as little of the healthy tissue as possible. It is especially helpful when the doctor is not sure of the shape and depth of the tumor. In addition, this method is used to remove large tumors, those in hard-to-treat places, and cancers that have recurred. The patient is given a local anesthetic, and the cancer is shaved off one thin layer at a time. Each layer is checked under a microscope until the entire tumor is removed. The degree of scarring depends on the location and size of the treated area. This method should be used only by doctors who are specially trained in this type of surgery.

Cryosurgery. Extreme cold may be used to treat precancerous skin conditions, such as actinic keratosis, as well as certain small skin cancers. In cryosurgery, liquid nitrogen is applied to the growth to freeze and kill the abnormal cells. After the area thaws, the dead tissue falls off. More than one freezing may be needed to remove the growth completely. Cryosurgery usually does not hurt, but patients may have pain and swelling after the area thaws. A white scar may form in the treated area.

Laser Therapy. Laser therapy uses a narrow beam of light to remove or destroy cancer cells. This approach is sometimes used for cancers that involve only the outer layer of skin.

Grafting. Sometimes, especially when a large cancer is removed, a skin graft is needed to close the wound and reduce the amount of scarring. For this procedure, the doctor takes a piece of healthy skin from another part of the body to replace the skin that was removed.

Radiation. Skin cancer responds well to radiation therapy (also called radiotherapy), which uses high-energy rays to damage cancer cells and stop them from growing. Doctors often use this treatment for cancers that occur in areas that are hard to treat with surgery. For example, radiation therapy might be used for cancers of the eyelid, the tip of the nose, or the ear. Several treatments may be needed to destroy all of the cancer cells. Radiation therapy may cause a rash or make the skin in the area dry or red. Changes in skin color and/or texture may develop after the treatment is over and may become more noticeable many years later.

Topical Chemotherapy. Topical chemotherapy is the use of anticancer drugs in a cream or lotion applied to the skin. Actinic keratosis can be treated effectively with the anticancer drug fluorouracil (also called 5-FU). This treatment is also useful for cancers limited to the top layer of skin. The 5-FU is applied daily for several weeks. Intense inflammation is common during treatment, but scars usually do not occur.

Clinical Trials

In clinical trials (research studies with patients), doctors are studying new treatments for skin cancer. For example, they are exploring the value of injecting interferon directly into the tumor. They are also testing photodynamic therapy, the use of laser light and drugs that make the cancer cells sensitive to light so the laser can destroy them.

Followup Care

Even though most skin cancers are cured, people who have been treated for skin cancer have a higher-than-average risk of developing a new cancer of the skin. That's why it's so important for them to continue to examine themselves regularly, to visit their doctor for regular checkups, and to follow their doctor's instructions on how to reduce their risk of developing skin cancer again.

Questions to Ask the Doctor

Skin cancer has a better prognosis, or outcome, than most other types of cancer; it is curable in over 95 percent of cases. But any diagnosis of cancer can be frightening, and it's natural to have concerns about medical tests, treatments, and doctors' bills.

Patients have many important questions to ask about cancer, and their doctor is the best person to provide answers. Most people want to know exactly what kind of cancer they have, how it can be treated, and how successful the treatment is likely to be. The following are some other questions that patients might want to ask their doctor:

- What types of treatment are available?

- Are there any risks or side effects of treatment?

- Will there be a scar?

- Will I have to change my normal activities?

- How can I protect myself from getting skin cancer again?

- How often are checkups needed?

Some patients become concerned that treatment may change their appearance, especially if the skin cancer is on their face. Patients should discuss this important concern with their doctor. And they may want to have a second opinion before treatment. (See "Treatment Planning" above.)

Skin Cancer Research

Scientists at hospitals and research centers are studying the causes of skin cancer and looking for new ways to prevent the disease. They are also exploring ways to improve treatment.

When laboratory research shows that a new prevention or treatment method has promise, doctors use it with people in clinical trials. These trials are designed to answer scientific questions and to find out whether the new approach is both safe and effective. People who take part in clinical trials make an important contribution to medical science and may have the first chance to benefit from improved methods.

People interested in taking part in a trial should discuss this option with their doctor. *What Are Clinical Trials All About?* is an NCI booklet that explains some of the possible benefits and risks of such studies.

One way to learn about clinical trials is through PDQ, a computerized resource developed by NCI. PDQ contains information about cancer treatment and an uptodate list of trials all over the country.

The Cancer Information Service can provide PDQ information to doctors, patients, and the public.

Resources

Information about skin cancer is available from the sources listed below. You may wish to check for additional information at your local library or bookstore and from support groups in your community.

Cancer Information Service (CIS)

The Cancer Information Service, a program of the National Cancer Institute, is a nationwide telephone service for cancer patients and their families and friends, the public, and health care professionals. The staff can answer questions (in English or Spanish) and can send free National Cancer Institute booklets about cancer. They also know about local resources and services. One toll-free number, 1-800-4-CANCER (1-800-422-6237), connects callers all over the country with the office that serves their area.

American Cancer Society (ACS)

The American Cancer Society is a voluntary organization with a national office and local units all over the country. It supports research, conducts educational programs, and offers many services to patients and their families. To obtain information about services and activities in local areas, call the Society's toll-free number, 1-800-ACS-2345 (1-800-227-2345), or the number listed under "American Cancer Society" in the white pages of the telephone book.

Skin Cancer Foundation
Suite 2402
245 Fifth Avenue
New York, NY 10016
212-725-5176

This nonprofit organization provides publications and audiovisual materials on the prevention, early detection, and treatment of skin cancer. The Foundation also publishes *Sun and Skin News* and *The Skin Cancer Foundation Journal*, which have nontechnical articles on skin cancer. Send a stamped, self-addressed envelope to receive free printed information.

American Academy of Dermatology
Post Office Box 4014
Schaumburg, IL 60168-4014
708-330-0230

The American Academy of Dermatology is an organization of doctors who specialize in diagnosing and treating skin problems. It provides free booklets on skin cancer and can refer people to dermatologists in their local area.

American Society of Plastic and Reconstructive Surgeons
444 East Algonquin Road
Arlington Heights, IL 60005
1-800-635-0635

This Society sends free information about various surgical procedures. It can also provide the names of board-certified plastic surgeons in a patient's area.

For Further Information

The National Cancer Institute booklets listed below are available free of charge by calling 1-800-4-CANCER.

- *Facing Forward: A Guide For Cancer Survivors* *

- *Radiation Therapy and You: A Guide to Self-Help During Treatment* *

- *Taking Time: Support for People With Cancer and the People Who Care About Them*

- *What Are Clinical Trials All About?*

- *What You Need To Know About Melanoma* *

- *What You Need To Know About Moles and Dysplastic Nevi* *

- *When Cancer Recurs: Meeting the Challenge Again* *

* Reprinted in this volume—see Table of Contents.

How to Do a Skin Self-Exam

You can improve your chances of finding skin cancer promptly by performing a simple skin self-exam regularly.

The best time to do this self-exam is after a shower or bath. You should check your skin in a well-lighted room using a full-length mirror and a hand-held mirror. It's best to begin by learning where your birthmarks, moles, and blemishes are and what they usually look like. Check for anything new—a change in the size, texture, or color of a mole, or a sore that does not heal.

Check all areas, including the back, the scalp, between the buttocks, and the genital area.

- Look at the front and back of your body in the mirror, then raise your arms and look at the left and right sides.

- Bend your elbows and look carefully at the palms, the forearms, including the undersides, and the upper arms.

- Examine the back and front of the legs. Also look between the buttocks and around the genital area.

- Sit and closely examine the feet, including the soles and the spaces between the toes.

- Look at your face, neck, and scalp. You may want to use a comb or a blow dryer to move hair so that you can see better.

By checking your skin regularly, you will become familiar with what is normal. If you find anything unusual, see your doctor right away. Remember, the earlier skin cancer is found, the better the chance for cure.

Chapter 50

Melanoma

Melanoma is the most serious cancer of the skin. In some parts of the world, especially among Western countries, the number of people who develop melanoma is increasing faster than any other cancer. In the United States, for example, the incidence rate of melanoma has more than doubled in the past 20 years. The National Cancer Institute (NCI) has written this chapter to help people with melanoma and their families and friends better understand this disease. We hope others will read it as well to learn more about melanoma.

This chapter discusses prevention strategies, detection, symptoms, diagnosis, treatment, and followup care. It also has information about resources and sources of support to help patients cope with melanoma.

Two more common and less serious types of skin cancer, squamous cell and basal cell cancer, are discussed in another NCI booklet, *What You Need To Know About Skin Cancer*. This and other NCI booklets are listed in the Other Booklets section.

Cancer research has led to real progress against cancer—better survival and an improved quality of life. Through research, our knowledge about melanoma and other cancers keeps increasing. We are finding new ways to detect and treat melanoma. The Cancer Information Service (CIS) and other NCI resources listed under the National Cancer Institute Information Resources section can provide the latest, most accurate information on melanoma. To order this publication,

"What You Need To Know About Melanoma," National Cancer Institute publication, updated: 10/21/98.

501

call the Cancer Information Service toll free at 1-800-4-CANCER (1-800-422-6237).

What Is Melanoma?

Melanoma is a type of skin cancer. It begins in certain cells in the skin called melanocytes. To understand melanoma, it is helpful to know about the skin and about melanocytes—what they do, how they grow, and what happens when they become cancerous.

The Skin

The skin is the body's largest organ. It protects us against heat, sunlight, injury, and infection. It helps regulate body temperature, stores water and fat, and produces vitamin D. The skin has two main layers: the outer epidermis and the inner dermis.

The epidermis is mostly made up of flat, scalelike cells called squamous cells. Round cells called basal cells lie under the squamous cells in the epidermis. The lower part of the epidermis also contains melanocytes.

The dermis contains blood vessels, lymphatic vessels, hair follicles, and glands. Some of these glands produce sweat, which helps regulate body temperature, and some produce sebum, an oily substance that helps keep the skin from drying out. Sweat and sebum reach the skin's surface through tiny openings called pores.

Melanocytes and Moles

Melanocytes are spread throughout the lower part of the epidermis. They produce melanin, the pigment that gives our skin its natural color. When skin is exposed to the sun, melanocytes produce more pigment, causing the skin to tan, or darken.

Sometimes, clusters of melanocytes and surrounding tissue form benign (noncancerous) growths called moles. (Doctors also call a mole a nevus; the plural is nevi.) Moles are very common. Most people have between 10 and 40 of these flesh-colored, pink, tan, or brown areas on the skin. Moles can be flat or raised. They are usually round or oval and smaller than a pencil eraser. They may be present at birth or may appear later on—usually before age 40. Moles generally grow or change only slightly over a long period of time. They tend to fade away in older people. When moles are surgically removed, they normally do not return.

Cancer

Cancer is actually a group of many different diseases. What all cancers have in common is that each type develops from our normal cells, the body's basic unit of life. To understand cancer it is helpful to know how cancer cells are different from normal cells.

The body is made up of many types of cells. Normally cells grow, divide, and produce more cells to keep the body healthy and functioning properly. Sometimes, however, the process goes astray—cells keep dividing when new cells are not needed. The mass of extra cells forms a growth or tumor. Tumors can be benign or malignant.

- Benign tumors are not cancer. They often can be removed and, in most cases, they do not come back. Cells in benign tumors do not spread to other parts of the body. Most importantly, benign tumors are rarely a threat to life.

- Malignant tumors are cancer. Cells in malignant tumors are abnormal and divide without control or order. These cancer cells can invade and destroy the tissue around them. Cancer cells can also break away from a malignant tumor and enter the bloodstream or lymphatic system (the tissues and organs that produce and store cells that fight infection and disease). This process, called metastasis, is how cancer spreads from the original tumor to form new tumors in other parts of the body. When cancer spreads (metastasizes) to another part of the body, the new tumor has the same kind of abnormal cells and the same name as the original tumor.

Melanoma

Melanoma occurs when melanocytes (pigment cells) become malignant. Most pigment cells are in the skin; when melanoma starts in the skin, the disease is called cutaneous melanoma. Melanoma may also occur in the eye and is called ocular melanoma or intraocular melanoma. Rarely, melanoma may arise in the meninges, the digestive tract, lymph nodes, or other areas where melanocytes are found. Melanomas arising in areas other than the skin are not discussed in this chapter. (This chapter focuses on melanoma that begins in the skin. The Cancer Information Service can provide more specific information about intraocular melanoma and its treatment.)

Melanoma can occur on any skin surface. In men, it is often found on the trunk (the area from the shoulders to the hips) or the head and neck. In women, melanoma often develops on the lower legs. Melanoma is rare in black people and others with dark skin. When it does develop in dark-skinned people, it tends to occur under the fingernails or toenails or on the palms or soles. The chance of developing melanoma increases with age, but this disease affects people of all age groups. Melanoma is one of the most common cancers in young adults.

When melanoma spreads, cancer cells are also found in the lymph nodes (sometimes called lymph glands). If the cancer has reached the lymph nodes, it may mean that cancer cells have spread to other parts of the body such as the liver, lungs, or brain. In such cases, the cancer cells in the new tumor are still melanoma cells, and the disease is called metastatic melanoma rather than liver, lung, or brain cancer.

Signs and Symptoms of Melanoma

Often, the first sign of melanoma is a change in the size, shape, color, or feel of an existing mole. Most melanomas have a black or blue-black area. Melanoma also may appear as a new, black, abnormal, or "ugly-looking" mole.

If you have a question or concern about something on your skin, do not use pictures to try to diagnose it yourself. Pictures are useful examples, but they cannot take the place of a doctor's examination.

Thinking of "ABCD" can help you remember what to watch for:

- Asymmetry—The shape of one half does not match the other.

- Border—The edges are often ragged, notched, blurred, or irregular in outline; the pigment may spread into the surrounding skin.

- Color—The color is uneven. Shades of black, brown, and tan may be present. Areas of white, grey, red, pink, or blue also may be seen.

- Diameter—There is a change in size, usually an increase. Melanomas are usually larger than the eraser of a pencil (5 mm or 1/4 inch).

Melanomas can vary greatly in the ways they look. Many show all of the ABCD features. However, some may show changes or abnormalities in only one or two of the ABCD features.

Early melanomas may be found when a pre-existing mole changes slightly—such as forming a new black area. Other frequent findings are newly formed fine scales or itching in a mole. In more advanced melanoma, the texture of the mole may change. For example, it may become hard or lumpy. Although melanomas may feel different and more advanced tumors may itch, ooze, or bleed, melanomas usually do not cause pain.

Melanoma can be cured if it is diagnosed and treated when the tumor is thin and has not deeply invaded the skin. However, if a melanoma is not removed at its early stages, cancer cells may grow downward from the skin surface, invading healthy tissue. When a melanoma becomes thick and deep, the disease often spreads to other parts of the body and is difficult to control.

A skin examination is often part of a routine checkup by a doctor, nurse specialist, or nurse practitioner. People also can check their own skin for new growths or other changes. (The How To Do a Skin Self-Exam section, below, has a simple guide on how to do a skin self-exam.) Changes in the skin or a mole should be reported to the doctor or nurse without delay. The person may be referred to a dermatologist, a doctor who specializes in diseases of the skin.

People who have had melanoma have a high risk of developing a new melanoma. Also, those with relatives who have had this disease have an increased risk. Doctors may advise people at risk to check their skin regularly and to have regular skin exams by a doctor or nurse specialist.

Some people have certain abnormal-looking moles, called dysplastic nevi or atypical moles, that may be more likely than normal moles to develop into melanoma. Most people with dysplastic nevi have just a few of these abnormal moles; others have many. They and their doctor should examine these moles regularly to watch for changes. Additional information about moles and dysplastic nevi and melanoma risk is available in the NCI booklet *What You Need To Know About Moles and Dysplastic Nevi* [reprinted in this volume—see Chapter 52].

Dysplastic nevi often look very much like melanoma. Doctors with special training in skin diseases are in the best position to decide whether an abnormal-looking mole should be closely watched or should be removed and checked for cancer.

In some families, many members have a large number of dysplastic nevi, and some have had melanoma. Members of these families have a very high risk for melanoma. Doctors often recommend that they have frequent checkups (every 3 to 6 months) so that any problems can be detected early. The doctor may take pictures of a person's skin to help in detecting any changes that occur.

Diagnosis and Staging

If the doctor suspects that a spot on the skin is melanoma, the patient will need to have a biopsy. A biopsy is the only way to make a definite diagnosis. In this procedure, the doctor tries to remove all of the suspicious-looking growth. If the growth is too large to be removed entirely, the doctor removes a sample of the tissue. A biopsy can usually be done in the doctor's office using a local anesthetic. A pathologist then examines the tissue under a microscope to check for cancer cells. Sometimes it is helpful for more than one pathologist to look at the tissue to determine whether melanoma is present.

A person who needs a biopsy may want to ask the doctor some of the following questions:

- Why do I need to have a biopsy?

- How long will it take? Will it hurt?

- Will the entire tumor be removed?

- What side effects can I expect?

- How soon will I know the results?

- If I do have cancer, who will talk with me about treatment? When?

If melanoma is found, the doctor needs to learn the extent, or stage, of the disease before planning treatment. The treatment plan takes into account the location and thickness of the tumor, how deeply the melanoma has invaded the skin, and whether melanoma cells have spread to nearby lymph nodes or other parts of the body. Removal of nearby lymph nodes for examination under a microscope is sometimes necessary. (Such surgery may be considered part of the treatment because removing cancerous lymph nodes may help control the disease.) The doctor also does a careful physical exam and, depending on the thickness of the tumor, may order chest x-rays; blood tests; and scans of the liver, bones, and brain.

Treatment

After diagnosis and staging, the doctor develops a treatment plan to fit each patient's needs. Treatment for melanoma depends on the extent of the disease, the patient's age and general health, as well as other factors.

People with melanoma are often treated by a team of specialists, which may include a dermatologist, surgeon, medical oncologist, and plastic surgeon. The standard treatment for melanoma is surgery; in some cases, doctors may also use chemotherapy, biological therapy, or radiation therapy. The doctors may decide to use one treatment method or a combination of methods.

Some patients take part in a clinical trial, which is a research study using new treatment methods. Such trials are designed to improve cancer treatment. (The Clinical Trials section has more information about clinical trials.)

Getting a Second Opinion

Before starting treatment, the patient may want a second specialist to review the diagnosis and treatment plan. It may take a week or two to arrange for a second opinion. A short delay will not reduce the chance that treatment will be successful. Some insurance companies require a second opinion; many others will cover a second opinion if the patient requests it.

There are a number of ways to find a doctor who can give a second opinion:

- One doctor may refer the patient to another who has special interest and training in treating melanoma.

- The Cancer Information Service, at 1-800-4-CANCER, can tell callers about treatment facilities, including cancer centers and other programs supported by the National Cancer Institute.

- Patients can get the names of doctors from their local medical society, a nearby hospital, or a medical school.

- The *Official ABMS Directory of Board Certified Medical Specialists* lists doctors' names along with their specialty and their background. This resource is in most public libraries.

Preparing for Treatment

Many people with cancer want to learn all they can about their disease and their treatment choices so they can take an active part in decisions about their medical care. When a person is diagnosed with cancer, shock and stress are natural reactions. These feelings may make it difficult for patients to think of everything they want to ask the doctor. Often, it helps to make a list of questions. To help remember

507

what the doctor says, patients may take notes or ask whether they may use a tape recorder. Some people also want to have a family member or friend with them when they talk to the doctor—to take part in the discussion, to take notes, or just to listen.

These are some questions a patient may want to ask the doctor before treatment begins:

- What is my diagnosis?
- What is the stage of the disease?
- What are the treatment choices? Which do you recommend? Why?
- What are the chances that the treatment will be successful?
- What new treatments are being studied? Would a treatment study be appropriate for me?
- What are the risks and possible side effects of each treatment?
- How will I feel after the operation?
- If I have pain, how can it be controlled?
- Will I need more treatment after surgery?
- Will I need a skin graft or plastic surgery? Will there be a scar?
- Will treatment affect my normal activities? If so, for how long?
- How often will I need checkups?
- What is the treatment likely to cost?

Patients do not need to ask all their questions or remember all the answers at one time. They will have other chances to ask the doctor to explain things and to get more information.

Methods of Treatment

Surgery to remove (excise) a melanoma is the standard treatment for this disease. It is necessary to remove not only the tumor but also some normal tissue around it in order to minimize the chance that any cancer will be left in the area.

The width and depth of surrounding skin that needs to be removed depends on the thickness of the melanoma and how deeply it has invaded the skin. In cases in which the melanoma is very thin, enough tissue is often removed during the biopsy, and no further surgery is necessary. If the melanoma was not completely removed during the biopsy, the doctor also takes out the remaining tumor. In most cases, additional surgery is performed to remove normal-looking tissue around the tumor to make sure all melanoma cells are removed. This is necessary, even for thin melanomas, to provide adequate surgical margins around the removed tumors. For thick melanomas, it may be necessary to do a wider excision to take out a larger margin of tissue.

If a large area of tissue is removed, a skin graft may be done at the same time. For this procedure, the doctor uses skin from another part of the body to replace the skin that was removed.

Lymph nodes near the tumor may be removed during surgery because cancer can spread through the lymphatic system. If the pathologist finds cancer cells in the lymph nodes, it may mean that the disease has spread to other parts of the body.

Surgery is generally not effective in controlling melanoma that is known to have spread to other parts of the body. In such cases, doctors may use other methods of treatment, such as chemotherapy, biological therapy, radiation therapy, or a combination of these methods. When therapy is given after surgery (primary therapy), the treatment is called adjuvant therapy. The goal of adjuvant therapy is to kill any undetected cancer cells that may remain in the body.

Chemotherapy is the use of anticancer drugs to kill cancer cells. It is generally a systemic treatment, meaning that it can affect cancer cells throughout the body. In chemotherapy, one or more anticancer drugs are given by mouth or by injection into a vein (intravenous). Either way, the drugs enter the bloodstream and travel through the body.

Chemotherapy is usually given in cycles: a treatment period followed by a recovery period, then another treatment period, and so on. Usually a patient has chemotherapy as an outpatient (at the hospital, at the doctor's office, or at home). Depending on which drugs are given, however, and the patient's general health, a short hospital stay may be needed.

One method of giving chemotherapy drugs currently under investigation is called limb perfusion. It is being tested for use when melanoma occurs only on an arm or leg. In limb perfusion the flow of blood to and from the limb is stopped for a while with a tourniquet. Anticancer drugs are then put into the blood of the limb. The patient receives high doses of drugs directly into the area where the melanoma occurred. Since most of the anticancer drugs remain in one limb, limb perfusion is not truly systemic therapy.

Biological therapy (also called biotherapy or immunotherapy) helps the body's immune system fight disease more effectively. Biological therapy is also a systemic therapy and involves the use of substances called biological response modifiers (BRMs). The body normally produces these substances in small amounts in response to infection and disease. Using modern laboratory techniques, scientists can produce BRMs in large amounts for use in cancer treatment. In some cases, biological therapy given after surgery can help prevent melanoma from recurring. For patients with a high risk of recurrence, interferon-alfa is sometimes recommended after surgery to decrease this risk. Interleukin-2 and tumor vaccines are other BRMs under study.

In some cases, radiation therapy (also called radiotherapy) is used to relieve some of the symptoms caused by melanoma. Radiation therapy is the use of high-energy rays to damage cancer cells and stop them from growing. Like surgery, radiation therapy is a local therapy; it affects only the cells in the treated area. Radiation therapy is most commonly used to help control melanoma that has spread to the brain, bones, and other parts of the body.

Clinical Trials

Many people with melanoma take part in clinical trials (treatment studies). Doctors conduct clinical trials to learn about the effectiveness and side effects of new treatments. In some trials, all patients receive the new treatment. In others, doctors compare different therapies by giving the new treatment to one group of patients and the standard therapy to another group; or they may compare one standard treatment with another.

Research has led to significant advances in the treatment of melanoma. Through research, doctors learn new ways to treat melanoma that may be more effective than standard therapies. People who take part in these trials have the first chance to benefit from treatments that have shown promise in earlier research. They also make an important contribution to medical science.

Doctors are studying new ways of treating melanoma. Clinical trials involve chemotherapy, biological therapies, and radiation therapy; new drugs and drug combinations; and new ways of combining various types of treatment. Some trials are designed to explore ways to reduce the side effects of treatment and to improve the quality of life.

Patients who are interested in taking part in a clinical trial should talk with their doctor. They may want to read the National Cancer Institute booklet *Taking Part in Clinical Trials: What Cancer Patients Need To Know* [reprinted in this volume as Chapter 72], which explains the possible benefits and risks of clinical trials.

One way to learn about clinical trials is through PDQ, a cancer information database developed by the National Cancer Institute. PDQ contains information about cancer treatment and about clinical trials in progress throughout the country. The Cancer Information Service can provide PDQ information to patients and the public. Online sources of NCI information, including PDQ, are listed under the National Cancer Institute Information Resources section.

Side Effects of Treatment

Doctors plan treatment to keep side effects to a minimum. For example, to avoid causing large scars, they remove as little tissue as they can without increasing the chance of recurrence. In general, the scar from surgery to remove an early stage melanoma is a small line (often 1 to 2 inches long), and it fades with time. How noticeable the scar is depends on where the melanoma was located, how well the person heals, and whether the person develops raised scars called keloids. When a tumor is large and thick, more surrounding skin and tissue (including muscle) are removed. Although skin grafts reduce scarring from the removal of large growths, these scars will still be quite noticeable.

Surgery to remove the lymph nodes from the underarm or groin may damage the lymphatic system and slow the flow of lymph in the arm or leg. Lymph may build up in a limb and cause swelling (lymphedema). The doctor or nurse can suggest exercises or other ways to reduce swelling if it becomes a problem. Also, it is harder for the body to fight infection in a limb after nearby lymph nodes have been removed, so the patient will need to protect the arm or leg from cuts, scratches, bruises, or burns that may lead to infection. If an infection does develop, the patient should see the doctor right away.

Although doctors plan chemotherapy, biological therapy, and radiation therapy very carefully, it is hard to limit the effects of these treatments so that only cancer cells are destroyed. Because healthy cells also may be damaged, cancer treatment often causes unwanted side effects.

The side effects of cancer treatment depend mainly on the type and extent of the treatment. Also, they may not be the same for each person, and they may even change from one treatment to the next. Doctors and nurses can explain the possible side effects of treatment, and they can help relieve symptoms that may occur during and after treatment.

The side effects of chemotherapy depend mainly on the drugs and the doses received. In addition, as with other types of treatment, side effects vary from person to person. Generally, anticancer drugs affect cells that divide rapidly. These include blood cells, which fight infection, help the blood to clot, or carry oxygen to all parts of the body. When blood cells are affected, people are more likely to get infections, may bruise or bleed easily, and may have shortness of breath and less energy. Cells in hair roots and cells that line the digestive tract also divide rapidly. As a result, people may lose their hair and may have other side effects, such as poor appetite, nausea and vomiting, or mouth sores.

Usually, these side effects go away gradually during the recovery periods between treatments or after treatment is over. However, some side effects may continue even after chemotherapy is over. The National Cancer Institute booklet *Chemotherapy and You* [reprinted in this volume as Chapter 63] has helpful information about chemotherapy and coping with side effects.

The side effects caused by biological therapy vary with the type of treatment. These treatments may cause flu-like symptoms, such as chills, fever, muscle aches, weakness, loss of appetite, nausea, vomiting, and diarrhea. Patients may also have bruising, skin rashes, swelling, or shortness of breath. These problems can be severe, but they go away after the treatment stops.

The side effects of radiation therapy depend on the amount of radiation given and the area being treated. Side effects that may occur during treatment include fatigue and hair loss in the treated area. Although the side effects of radiation therapy can be unpleasant, the doctor can usually treat or control them. It also helps to know that, in most cases, side effects are not permanent. The National Cancer Institute booklet *Radiation Therapy and You* [reprinted in this volume as Chapter 66] has helpful information about radiation therapy and managing its side effects.

Nutrition for Cancer Patients

Eating well during cancer treatment means getting enough calories and protein to help prevent weight loss and regain strength. Eating well often helps people feel better and have more energy.

Some people with cancer find it hard to eat well. They may lose their appetite. In addition, common side effects of treatment, such as nausea, vomiting, or mouth sores, can make eating difficult. Foods may taste different. Also, people being treated for cancer may not feel like eating when they are uncomfortable or tired.

Doctors, nurses, and dietitians can offer advice on how to eat well during cancer treatment. Patients and their families also may want to read the National Cancer Institute booklet *Eating Hints for Cancer Patients* [reprinted in this volume as Chapter 77], which contains many useful suggestions.

Followup Care

Melanoma patients have a high risk of developing separate new melanomas. Some also are at risk for a recurrence of the original melanoma in nearby skin or in other parts of the body.

To increase the chance that a new melanoma will be detected as early as possible, patients should follow their doctor's schedule for regular checkups. It is especially important for patients who have dysplastic nevi and a family history of melanoma to have frequent checkups. Patients also should examine their skin monthly (keeping in mind the "ABCD" guidelines in the Signs and Symptoms of Melanoma section and the skin self-exam guide described in How To Do a Skin Self-Exam) and follow their doctor's advice about how to reduce their chance of developing another melanoma. General information about preventing melanoma is described in the Causes, Risk Factors, and Prevention section.

The chance of recurrence is greater for patients whose melanoma was thick or had spread to nearby tissue than for patients with very thin melanomas. Followup care for those who have a high risk of recurrence may include x-rays; blood tests; and scans of the chest, liver, bones, and brain.

Recovery and Outlook

People with melanoma and their families are naturally concerned about their recovery from cancer and their outlook for the future. Sometimes people use statistics to try to figure out their chances of being cured. However, statistics reflect the experience of large groups of patients, not individuals. Statistics cannot be used to predict what will happen to a particular patient because no two patients are alike, and treatments and responses vary greatly. The doctor who takes care of the patient and knows his or her medical history is in the best position to talk about the chance of recovery (prognosis). People should feel free to ask the doctor about their prognosis, while keeping in mind that not even the doctor knows exactly what will happen.

When doctors discuss a patient's prognosis, they may talk about surviving cancer rather than a cure. Although many patients with melanoma are actually cured, the disease can return. It is important to discuss the possibility of recurrence with the doctor.

Support for People with Cancer

Living with a serious disease is not easy. People with cancer and those who care about them face many problems and challenges. Coping with these problems is often easier when people have helpful information and support services. Several useful booklets, including *Taking Time*, are available from the Cancer Information Service.

Friends and relatives can be very supportive. Also, it helps many patients to discuss their concerns with others who have cancer. Cancer patients often get together in support groups, where they can share what they have learned about coping with cancer and the effects of treatment. It is important to keep in mind, however, that each person is different. Treatments and ways of dealing with cancer that work for one person may not be right for another—even if they both have the same kind of cancer. It is always a good idea to discuss the advice of friends and family members with the doctor.

People living with cancer may worry about what the future holds. They may worry about caring for their family, holding their job, or keeping up with daily activities. Concerns about tests, treatments, hospital stays, and medical bills are also common. Doctors, nurses, and other members of the health care team can answer questions about treatment, working, or other activities. Meeting with a social worker, counselor, or member of the clergy can be helpful to people who want to talk about their feelings or discuss their concerns.

Often, a social worker can suggest groups that can help with rehabilitation, emotional support, financial aid, transportation, or home care. The Cancer Information Service can supply information about melanoma and about programs and services for patients and their families.

Causes, Risk Factors, and Prevention

Researchers at hospitals and medical centers all across the country are studying melanoma. They are trying to learn what causes the disease and how to prevent it.

At this time, the causes of melanoma are not fully understood. It is clear, however, that this disease is not contagious; no one can "catch" cancer from another person.

Researchers study patterns of cancer in the population to look for factors that are more common in people who develop melanoma than in people who don't develop this disease. It is important to know that most people with these risk factors do not get cancer, and people who do develop melanoma may have none of these factors.

Risk Factors for Melanoma

- Family history of melanoma
- Dysplastic nevi
- Previous melanoma
- Immunosuppressive therapy
- Many ordinary moles (more than 50)
- Severe, blistering sunburns
- Many freckles
- Fair skin, light eyes

Scientists have observed that certain factors increase a person's chance of developing melanoma. For example, having two or more close relatives who have had this disease is a risk factor because melanoma sometimes runs in families. In fact, about 10 percent of all patients with melanoma have family members who also have had this disease. When melanoma runs in a family, the family members should be checked regularly by a doctor.

Certain types of mole patterns are associated with an increased risk of developing melanoma, such as having dysplastic nevi (atypical moles). As described in the Signs and Symptoms of Melanoma section, dysplastic nevi are more likely than ordinary moles to become cancerous. Many people have only a few of these abnormal moles; the risk of melanoma is greater for people with a large number of dysplastic nevi. The risk is especially high for people who have a family history of both dysplastic nevi and melanoma. Having an unusually high number of moles (more than 50) is another risk factor for melanoma. Also, people whose immune system is weakened by certain cancers, by drugs given following organ transplants, or by AIDS are at increased risk of developing melanoma.

The number of people who develop melanoma is increasing. Researchers believe that the number of melanomas may be increasing because people are spending more time in the sun. They know that ultraviolet (UV) radiation from the sun causes premature aging of the skin and skin damage that can lead to melanoma. (Two types of ultraviolet radiation—UVA and UVB—are explained in the Glossary section.) Artificial sources of UV radiation, such as sunlamps and tanning booths, also can cause skin damage and probably an increased risk of melanoma.

People who have had one or more severe, blistering sunburns as a child or teenager are at increased risk for melanoma. Because of this, doctors advise protecting children's skin from the sun, which they hope will help prevent, or at least reduce the risk of melanoma later in life. Sunburns in adulthood are also a risk factor for melanoma.

Melanoma occurs more frequently in people who have fair skin that burns or freckles easily (these people also usually have red or blond hair and blue eyes) than in people with dark skin. White people get melanoma far more often than do black people, probably because light skin is more easily damaged by the sun. In addition, this disease is more common in people who live in areas that get large amounts of UV radiation from the sun. In the United States, for example, melanoma is more common in Texas than it is in Minnesota, where the sun is not as strong.

To help prevent and reduce the risk of melanoma, people should avoid exposure to the midday sun (from 10 a.m. to 2 p.m. standard time, or from 11 a.m. to 3 p.m. daylight saving time) whenever possible. Another simple rule is to protect yourself from the sun when your shadow is shorter than you are. Wearing a hat and long sleeves offers protection. Also, lotions or creams that contain sunscreens help prevent sunburn. Many doctors believe sunscreens may help prevent melanoma, especially those that block or absorb both types of ultraviolet radiation. Sunscreens are rated in strength according to a sun protection factor (SPF). Those rated 15 or higher give the best protection. Sunglasses that have UV-absorbing lenses should also be worn. The label should specify that the lenses block at least 99 percent of UVA and UVB radiation.

People who think they may be at risk for developing melanoma should discuss this concern with their doctor. The doctor may suggest ways to reduce the risk and can plan an appropriate schedule for checkups.

How to Do a Skin Self-Exam

Your doctor or nurse may recommend that you do a regular skin self-exam. If your doctor has taken photos of your skin, you can use these pictures when looking for changes.

The best time to do a skin self-exam is after a shower or bath. You should check your skin in a well-lighted room using a full-length mirror and a hand-held mirror. It's best to begin by learning where your birthmarks, moles, and blemishes are and what they usually look and feel like. Check for anything new, especially a change in the size, shape, texture, or color of a mole or a sore that does not heal.

Check yourself from head to toe. Don't forget to check all areas of the skin, including the back, the scalp, between the buttocks, and the genital area.

1. Look at the front and back of your body in the mirror, then raise your arms and look at your left and right sides.

2. Bend your elbows and look carefully at your fingernails, palms, forearms (including the undersides), and upper arms.

3. Examine the back, front, and sides of your legs. Also look between the buttocks and around the genital area.

4. Sit and closely examine your feet, including the toenails, the soles, and the spaces between the toes.

5. Look at your face, neck, ears, and scalp. You may want to use a comb or a blow dryer to move hair so that you can see better. You also may want to have a relative or friend check through your hair because this is difficult to do yourself.

By checking your skin regularly, you will become familiar with what is normal for you. It may be helpful to record the dates of your skin exams and to write notes about the way your skin looks. If you find anything unusual, see your doctor right away.

National Cancer Institute Information Resources

You may want more information for yourself, your family, and your doctor. The following National Cancer Institute (NCI) services are available to help you.

Telephone

Cancer Information Service (CIS) Provides accurate, up-to-date information on cancer to patients and their families, health professionals, and the general public. Information specialists translate the latest scientific information into understandable language and respond in English, Spanish, or on TTY equipment.

Toll-free: 1-800-4-CANCER (1-800-422-6237)
TTY: 1-800-332-8615

Internet

These Web sites may be useful:

http://www.nci.nih.gov NCI's primary Web site; contains information about the Institute and its programs.

http://cancertrials.nci.nih.gov CancerTrials; NCI's comprehensive clinical trials information center for patients, health professionals, and the public. Includes information on understanding trials, deciding whether to participate in trials, finding specific trials, plus research news and other resources.

http://cancernet.nci.nih.gov CancerNet; contains material for health professionals, patients, and the public, including information from PDQ about cancer treatment, screening, prevention, supportive care, and clinical trials, and CANCERLIT, a bibliographic database.

E-mail

CancerMail— Includes NCI information about cancer treatment, screening, prevention, and supportive care. To obtain a contents list, send e-mail to cancermail@icicc.nci.nih.gov with the word "help" in the body of the message.

Fax

CancerFax—Includes NCI information about cancer treatment, screening, prevention, and supportive care. To obtain a contents list, dial 301-402-5874 from a fax machine hand set and follow the recorded instructions.

Other Booklets

The National Cancer Institute booklets listed below and others are available from the Cancer Information Service by calling 1-800-4-CANCER.

Booklets about Skin Conditions

What You Need To Know About Moles and Dysplastic Nevi *

What You Need To Know About Skin Cancer *

Booklets about Cancer Treatments

Helping Yourself During Chemotherapy: 4 Steps for Patients

Chemotherapy and You: A Guide to Self-Help During Treatment *

Radiation Therapy and You: A Guide to Self-Help During Treatment *

Eating Hints for Cancer Patients *

Get Relief From Cancer Pain

Questions and Answers About Pain Control

Taking Part in Clinical Trials: What Cancer Patients Need To Know *

Booklets about Living with Cancer

Taking Time: Support for People With Cancer and the People Who Care About Them

Facing Forward: A Guide for Cancer Survivors *

Young People With Cancer: A Handbook For Parents

When Someone in Your Family Has Cancer

When Cancer Recurs: Meeting the Challenge Again *

Advanced Cancer: Living Each Day *

* Reprinted in this volume—see Table of Contents

Chapter 51

Nonmelanoma

What Is Nonmelanoma?

Nonmelanoma (skin cancer) is a disease in which cancer (malignant) cells are found in the outer layers of the skin. The skin protects the body against heat, light, infection, and injury. It also stores water, fat, and vitamin D.

The skin has two main layers and several kinds of cells. The top layer of skin is called the epidermis. It contains three kinds of cells: flat, scaly cells on the surface called squamous cells; round cells called basal cells; and cells called melanocytes, which give the skin its color.

The inner layer of skin is called the dermis. This layer is thicker, and contains blood vessels, nerves, and sweat glands. The hair on the skin also grows from tiny pockets in the dermis, called follicles. The dermis makes sweat, which helps to cool the body, and oils that keep the skin from drying out.

There are several types of cancer that start in the skin. The most common are basal cell cancer and squamous cell cancer, which are covered in this chapter. These types of skin cancer are called nonmelanoma skin cancer. Melanoma is a type of skin cancer that starts in the melanocytes. It is not as common as basal cell or squamous cell skin cancer, but it is much more serious.

Nonmelanoma skin cancer is more common in people with light colored skin who have spent a lot of time in the sunlight. Skin cancer can occur anywhere on the body, but it is most common in places that

PDQ statement, National Cancer Institute, revised July 1999

have been exposed to more sunlight, such as the face, neck, hands, and arms.

Nonmelanoma skin cancer can look many different ways. The most common sign of skin cancer is a change on the skin, such as a growth or a sore that won't heal. Sometimes there may be a small lump. This lump can be smooth, shiny and waxy looking, or it can be red or reddish brown. Skin cancer may also appear as a flat red spot that is rough or scaly. Not all changes in the skin are cancer, but a doctor should be seen if changes in the skin are noticed.

If there is a spot or lump on the skin, a doctor may remove the growth and look at the tissue under a microscope. This is called a biopsy. A biopsy can usually be done in a doctor's office. Before the biopsy, the patient will be given a local anesthetic to numb the area for a short period of time.

Most nonmelanoma skin cancers can be cured. The chance of recovery (prognosis) and choice of treatment depend on the type of skin cancer and how far it has spread.

Other kinds of cancer that may affect the skin include cutaneous T-cell lymphoma, a cancer of the lymph system, and Kaposi's sarcoma. Cancers that start in other parts of the body may also spread (metastasize) to the skin.

Stage Explanation: Types of Melanoma Skin Cancer

Once skin cancer is found, more tests may be done to see if the cancer has spread. This is called staging. A doctor needs to know the stage and type of skin cancer to plan treatment. The following types are used to plan treatment:

Basal cell cancer. Basal cell cancer is the most common type of nonmelanoma skin cancer. It usually occurs on areas of the skin that have been in the sun. Often this cancer appears as a small raised bump that has a smooth, pearly appearance. Another type looks like a scar, and it is firm to the touch. Basal cell cancers may spread to tissues around the cancer, but it usually does not spread to other parts of the body.

Squamous cell carcinoma. Squamous cell tumors also occur on areas of the skin that have been in the sun, often on the top of the nose, forehead, lower lip, and hands. They may also appear on areas of the skin that have been burned, exposed to chemicals, or had x-ray therapy. Often this cancer appears as a firm red bump. Sometimes the tumor may feel scaly or bleed or develop a crust. Squamous cell tumors may spread to the lymph nodes in the area (lymph nodes are small bean-shaped structures that are found throughout the body; they produce and store infection-fighting cells).

Actinic keratosis. Actinic keratosis is a skin condition that is not cancer, but can change into basal cell or squamous cell skin cancer in some people. It appears as rough, red or brown, scaly patches on the skin, usually in areas that have been exposed to the sun.

Recurrent. Recurrent disease means that the cancer has come back (recurred) after it has been treated.

Treatment

There are treatments for all patients with nonmelanoma skin cancer. Three kinds of treatments are used:

- surgery (taking out the cancer)

- chemotherapy (using drugs to kill cancer cells)

- radiation therapy (using x-rays to kill cancer cells)

Many skin cancers are treated by doctors who treat skin diseases (dermatologists). Often, the cancer can be treated in a doctor's office.

Surgery is the most common treatment of skin cancer. A doctor may remove the cancer using one of the following:

- Electrodesiccation and curettage burns the lesion and removes it with a sharp instrument.

- Cryosurgery freezes the tumor and kills it.

- Simple excision cuts the cancer from the skin along with some of the healthy tissue around it.

- Micrographic surgery removes the cancer and as little normal tissue as possible. During this surgery, the doctor removes the cancer and then uses a microscope to look at the cancerous area to make sure no cancer cells remain.

- Laser therapy uses a narrow beam of light to remove cancer cells.

Surgery may leave a scar on the skin. Depending on the size of the cancer, skin may be taken from another part of the body and put on the area where the cancer was removed. This is called a skin graft. New ways of doing surgery and grafting may reduce scarring.

Radiation therapy uses x-rays to kill cancer cells and shrink tumors. Radiation therapy for skin cancer comes from a machine outside the body (external radiation therapy).

Chemotherapy uses drugs to kill cancer cells. In treating skin cancer, chemotherapy is often given as a cream or lotion placed on the skin to kill cancer cells (topical chemotherapy). Chemotherapy may also be taken by pill, or it may be put into the body by a needle in a vein or muscle. Chemotherapy given in this way is called a systemic treatment because the drug enters the bloodstream, travels through the body, and can kill cancer cells outside the skin. Systemic chemotherapy is being tested in clinical trials.

Biological therapy (using the body's immune system to fight cancer) is being tested in clinical trials. Biological therapy tries to get the body to fight cancer. It uses materials made by the body or made in a laboratory to boost, direct, or restore the body's natural defenses against disease. Biological therapy is sometimes called biological response modifier (BRM) therapy or immunotherapy.

Photodynamic therapy uses a certain type of light and a special chemical to kill cancer cells.

Treatment by Type

Treatment of skin cancer depends on the type and stage of the disease, and the patient's age and overall health.

Standard treatment may be considered because of its effectiveness in patients in past studies, or participation in a clinical trial may be considered. Not all patients are cured with standard therapy and some standard treatments may have more side effects than are desired. For these reasons, clinical trials are designed to find better ways to treat cancer patients and are based on the most up-to-date information. Clinical trials are ongoing in some parts of the country for patients with skin cancer. To learn more about clinical trials, call the Cancer Information Service at 1-800-4-CANCER (1-800-422-6237); TTY at 1-800-332-8615.

Basal Cell Carcinoma of the Skin

Treatment may be one of the following:

1. Micrographic surgery.
2. Simple excision.

3. Electrodesiccation and curettage.
4. Cryosurgery.
5. Radiation therapy.
6. Laser therapy.
7. Topical chemotherapy.
8. Clinical trials of chemoprevention.
9. Clinical trials of biological therapy.
10. Photodynamic therapy.

It is important to have the skin examined regularly so the cancer can be treated if it comes back (recurs).

Squamous Cell Carcinoma of the Skin

Treatment may be one of the following:

1. Micrographic surgery.
2. Simple excision.
3. Electrodesiccation and curettage.
4. Cryosurgery.
5. Radiation therapy.
6. Topical chemotherapy.
7. Laser therapy.
8. Clinical trials of biological therapy with or without chemoprevention.

It is important to have the skin examined regularly so the cancer can be treated if it comes back (recurs).

Actinic Keratosis

Treatment may be one of the following:

1. Topical chemotherapy.
2. Cryosurgery.
3. Electrodesiccation and curettage.
4. Removing the top layer of skin with a special machine (dermabrasion).
5. Shaving the very top layer of skin (shave excision).

6.   Laser therapy.

To Learn More

To learn more about skin cancer, call the National Cancer Institute's Cancer Information Service at 1-800-4-CANCER (1-800-422-6237); TTY at 1-800-332-8615. By dialing this toll-free number, you can speak with a trained information specialist who can answer your questions.

The Cancer Information Service also has booklets about cancer that are available to the public and can be sent on request. The following booklet about skin cancer may be helpful: *What You Need To Know About Skin Cancer* *

The following general booklets on questions related to cancer may also be helpful:

Taking Time: Support for People with Cancer and the People Who Care About Them

What Are Clinical Trials All About?

Chemotherapy and You: A Guide to Self-Help During Treatment *

Radiation Therapy and You: A Guide to Self-Help During Treatment *

Eating Hints for Cancer Patient *

What You Need To Know About Cancer *

Reprinted in this volume—see Table of Contents

There are many other places where people can get material and information about cancer treatment and services. The social service office at a hospital can be checked for local and national agencies that can help with getting information about finances, getting to and from treatment, getting care at home, and dealing with problems.

For more information from the National Cancer Institute, please write to this address:

National Cancer Institute
Office of Cancer Communications
31 Center Drive, MSC 2580
Bethesda, MD 20892-2580

Chapter 52

Moles and Dysplastic Nevi

Moles

Moles are growths on the skin. Doctors call moles nevi (one mole is a nevus). These growths, which are usually pink, tan, brown, or flesh-colored, occur when cells in the skin called melanocytes grow in a cluster with tissue around them. Melanocytes are also spread evenly throughout the skin and make the pigment that gives skin its natural color. When skin is exposed to the sun, melanocytes produce more pigment, causing the skin to darken, or tan.

Most people have between 10 and 40 moles. A person may develop new moles from time to time, usually until about age 40. Many moles begin as a small, flat spot and slowly become larger in diameter and raised. Over many years, they may flatten again, become flesh-colored, and go away.

Dysplastic Nevi

About one out of every ten people has at least one unusual (or atypical) mole that looks different from an ordinary mole. The medical term for these unusual moles is dysplastic nevi. Table 52.1 describes the differences between ordinary moles and dysplastic nevi.

Doctors believe that dysplastic nevi are more likely than ordinary moles to develop into a type of skin cancer called melanoma. Because

"What You Need To Know About Moles and Dysplastic Nevi," National Cancer Institute publication, updated October 21, 1998.

of this, moles should be checked regularly by a doctor or nurse specialist, especially if they look unusual; grow larger; or change in color, outline, or in any other way.

Melanoma

Melanoma is a type of skin cancer—one of the most serious types because advanced melanomas have the ability to spread to other parts of the body. (Melanoma can also develop in the eye, called intraocular melanoma, or rarely in other parts of the body where pigment cells are found. The CIS can provide information about the diagnosis and treatment of intraocular melanoma.) Melanoma begins when melanocytes (pigment cells) gradually become more abnormal and keep dividing without control, moving into nearby normal tissue. The abnormal cells form a growth of malignant tissue (a cancerous tumor) on the surface of the skin. Melanoma can begin either in an existing mole or as a new growth on the skin. Table 52.2 describes melanoma. A doctor or nurse specialist can tell whether an abnormal-looking mole should be closely watched or should be removed and checked for melanoma cells. The purpose of routine skin exams is to identify and follow such moles.

The removal of a mole to look for cancer cells is called a biopsy. If possible, it is best to remove moles by an excisional biopsy, rather than a shave biopsy.

If the biopsy results in a diagnosis of melanoma, the patient and the doctor should work together to make treatment decisions. In many cases, melanoma can be cured by minimal surgery if the tumor is discovered when it is thin (before it has grown downward from the skin surface) and before the cancer cells have begun to spread to other places in the body. However, if melanoma is not found early, the cancer cells can spread through the bloodstream and lymphatic system to form tumors in other parts of the body. Melanoma is much harder to control when it has spread. The spread of cancer is called metastasis.

Doctors and scientists believe that it is possible to prevent many melanomas and to detect most others early, when the disease is more likely to be cured with minimal surgery. In the past several decades, an increasing percentage of melanomas have been diagnosed at very early stages when they are quite thin. Learning about prevention and early detection, while important for everyone, is especially important for people who have an increased risk for melanoma. Some of those at an increased risk are people who have dysplastic nevi or a very large number of ordinary moles.

Table 52.1. Descriptions of Ordinary Moles and Dysplastic Nevi

	Ordinary Moles	**Dysplastic Nevi**
Color	Evenly tan or brown; all typical moles on one person tend to look similar	Mixture of tan, brown, and red/pink. A person's moles often look quite different from one another.
Shape	Round or oval, with a distinct edge that separates the mole from the rest of the skin.	Have irregular, sometimes notched edges. May fade into the skin around it. The flat portion of the mole may be level with the skin.
Surface	Begin as flat, smooth spots on skin; may become raised and form a smooth bump.	May have a smooth, slightly scaly, or rough, irregular, "pebbly" appearance.
Size	Usually less than 5 millimeters (about 1/4 inch) across (size of a pencil eraser).	Often larger than 5 millimeters (about 1/4 inch) across and sometimes larger than 10 millimeters (about ½ inch).
Number	Between 10 and 40 typical moles may be present on an adult's body.	May be present in large numbers (more than 100 on same person). However, some people have only a few dysplastic nevi.
Location	Usually found above the waist on sun-exposed surfaces of the body. Scalp, breasts, and buttocks rarely have normal moles.	May occur anywhere on the body but most frequently on the back and areas exposed to the sun. May also appear below the waist and on the scalp, breasts, and buttocks.

Risk Factors for Melanoma

- Family history of melanoma
- Dysplastic nevi
- Previous melanoma
- Immunosuppressive therapy
- Many ordinary moles (more than 50)
- Severe blistering sunburns
- Freckles (many)
- Fair skin, light eyes

Chapter 50 on Melanoma has more information about risk factors for this disease.

It is important to remember that not everyone who has dysplastic nevi or other risk factors for melanoma gets the disease. In fact, most do not. Also, about half the people who develop melanoma do not have dysplastic nevi, and they may not have any other known risk factor for the disease. At this time, no one can explain why one person gets melanoma while another does not, but sun exposure, especially bad, blistering sunburns, is an important, avoidable risk factor. Scientists are continuing their studies of risk factors for this disease.

Prevention of Melanoma

The number of people in the world who develop melanoma is increasing each year. In the United States, the number has more than doubled in the past 20 years.

Ultraviolet (UV) radiation from the sun and from sunlamps and tanning booths damages the skin and can lead to melanoma and other types of skin cancer. Experts believe that much of the worldwide increase in melanoma is related to an increase in the amount of time people spend in the sun. Everyone, especially those who have dysplastic nevi or other risk factors, should try to reduce the risk of developing melanoma by protecting the skin from UV radiation. The intensity of UV radiation from the sun is greatest in the summer, particularly during midday hours (between 10 a.m. and 2 p.m. standard time, or 11 a.m. and 3 p.m. daylight saving time). A simple rule is to avoid the sun or protect your skin whenever your shadow is shorter than you are.

People who work or play in the sun should wear protective clothing, such as a hat and long sleeves. Also, a lotion that contains a sunscreen can help protect the skin. Some lotions protect the skin against both UVA and UVB radiation.

Sunscreens are rated in strength according to an SPF (sun protection factor). Sunscreens with an SPF of 15 or higher provide the best protection by blocking out most of the sun's harmful rays. It is important to use a sunscreen that blocks both UVA and UVB rays.

Sunglasses that have UV-absorbing lenses should also be worn. The label should specify that the lenses block at least 99 percent of UVA and UVB radiation.

Early Detection of Melanoma

Because melanoma usually begins on the surface of the skin, it often can be detected at an early stage with a total skin examination by a trained health care worker. Checking the skin regularly for any signs of the disease increases the chance of finding melanoma early. A monthly skin self-exam is very important for people who have any of the known risk factors, but doing skin self-exams routinely is a good idea for everyone.

How to Do a Skin Self-Exam

1. After a shower or bath, stand in front of a full-length mirror in a well-lighted room. Use a hand-held mirror to look at hard-to-see areas.

2. Begin with the face and scalp and go downward, checking the head, neck, shoulders, back, chest, and so on. Be sure to check the front, back, and sides of the arms and legs. Also, check the groin, the palms, the fingernails, the soles of the feet, the toenails, and the area between the toes.

3. Be sure to check the hard-to-see areas of the body, such as the scalp and neck. A friend or relative may be able to help inspect these areas. A comb or a blow dryer can help move hair so you can see better.

4. Be aware of where your moles are and how they look. By checking your skin regularly, you will become familiar with what your moles look like. Look for any signs of change in a mole, particularly a new black area or a change in outline, shape, size, color, or feel of a mole. Also, note any new, unusual, or "ugly-looking" moles. If your doctor has taken photos

of your skin, you can compare these pictures with the way your skin looks on self-examination.

5.   Check moles carefully during times of hormone changes, such as adolescence, pregnancy, and menopause. As hormone levels vary, moles may change.

6.   It may be helpful to record the dates of your skin exams and to write notes about the way your skin looks. If you find anything unusual, see your doctor right away. Remember, the earlier a melanoma is found, the better the chance for a cure.

In addition to doing routine skin self-exams, people should have their skin checked regularly by a doctor or nurse specialist. The family doctor can do a skin exam during visits for regular checkups. People who think they have dysplastic nevi should point them out to the doctor. It is also important to tell the doctor about any new, changing, or "ugly-looking" moles.

Sometimes it is necessary to see a specialist. A dermatologist (skin doctor) is likely to have the most training in diseases of the skin. Some plastic surgeons, general surgeons, oncologists, internists, and family doctors also have a special interest and training in moles and melanoma.

Doctors have found that melanoma runs in some families and that some members of these families are at high risk for the disease. In some of these families, certain members also have a large number of dysplastic nevi, often more than 100. These people have an especially high risk of developing melanoma. When two or more family members develop melanoma, it is important for all of the patients' close relatives (parents, brothers, sisters, and children above the age of 10) to see a doctor and be examined carefully for dysplastic nevi or any signs of melanoma. The doctor will then decide how often each person needs to be seen. (Doctors often recommend that these family members have checkups every 6 months.) Anyone who has a large number of dysplastic nevi also should be examined regularly.

A doctor may want to watch a slightly abnormal mole closely to see whether it changes over time. Pictures taken at one visit may be compared with the appearance of the mole at the next visit. Sometimes a doctor decides that a mole should be removed so that the tissue can be examined under a microscope. This surgery, called a biopsy, is usually done in the doctor's office using local anesthesia. It generally takes only a few minutes. The patient may require stitches, and a small scar will remain after healing. A pathologist examines the tissue under a microscope to see whether the melanocytes are normal, dysplastic, or cancerous.

Because most moles, including most dysplastic nevi, do not develop into melanoma, removing all of them is not necessary. A doctor can recommend when and when not to remove moles. Usually, only moles that look like melanoma, those that change, or those that are both new and look abnormal need to be removed.

Other Booklets

The National Cancer Institute booklets listed below and others are available from the Cancer Information Service by calling 1-800-4-CANCER.

What You Need To Know About Cancer

What You Need To Know About Melanoma *

What You Need To Know About Skin Cancer *

* Reprinted in this volume—see Table of Contents

Table 52.2. Descriptions of Melanoma

Large size	Most melanomas are at least 5 millimeters (about 1/4 inch) across when they are found; many are much larger. An unusually large mole may be melanoma.
Many colors	A mixture of tan, brown, white, pink, red, gray, blue, and especially black in a mole suggests melanoma.
Irregular border	If a mole has an edge that is irregular or notched, it may be melanoma.
Abnormal surface	If a mole is scaly, flaky, oozing, or bleeding, has an open sore that does not heal, or has a hard lump in it, it may be melanoma.
Unusual sensation	If a mole itches or is painful or tender, melanoma may be present.
Abnormal skin around mole	If color from the mole spreads into the skin around it or if this skin becomes red or loses its color (becomes white or gray), melanoma may be present.

Chapter 53

Kaposi's Sarcoma

What Is Kaposi's Sarcoma?

Kaposi's sarcoma (KS) is a disease in which cancer (malignant) cells are found in the tissues under the skin or mucous membranes that line the mouth, nose, and anus. KS causes red or purple patches (lesions) on the skin and/or mucous membranes and spreads to other organs in the body, such as the lungs, liver, or intestinal tract.

Until the early 1980's, Kaposi's sarcoma was a very rare disease that was found mainly in older men, patients who had organ transplants, or African men. With the Acquired Immunodeficiency Syndrome (AIDS) epidemic in the early 1980's, doctors began to notice more cases of Kaposi's sarcoma in Africa and in gay men with AIDS. Kaposi's sarcoma usually spreads more quickly in these patients.

If there are signs of KS, a doctor will examine the skin and lymph nodes carefully (lymph nodes are small bean-shaped structures that are found throughout the body; they produce and store infection-fighting cells). The doctor also may order other tests to see if the patient has other diseases.

The chance of recovery (prognosis) depends on what type of Kaposi's sarcoma the patient has, the patient's age and general health, and whether or not the patient has AIDS.

PDQ Statement, National Cancer Institute (NCI), updated April 1999.

Stages of Kaposi's Sarcoma

There is no accepted staging system for Kaposi's sarcoma. Patients are grouped depending on which type of Kaposi's sarcoma they have. There are three types of Kaposi's sarcoma:

Classic

Classic Kaposi's sarcoma usually occurs in older men of Jewish, Italian, or Mediterranean heritage. This type of Kaposi's sarcoma progresses slowly, sometimes over 10 to 15 years. As the disease gets worse, the lower legs may swell and the blood may not be able to flow properly. After some time, the disease may spread to other organs. Many patients with classic Kaposi's sarcoma may develop another type of cancer later on in their lives.

Immunosuppressive Treatment-Related

Kaposi's sarcoma may occur in people who are taking drugs to make their immune systems weaker (immunosuppressants). The immune system helps the body fight off infection. People who have had an organ transplant (such as a liver or kidney transplant) have to take drugs to prevent their immune system from attacking the new organ.

Epidemic

Kaposi's sarcoma in patients who have Acquired Immunodeficiency Syndrome (AIDS) is called epidemic Kaposi's sarcoma. AIDS is caused by a virus called the Human Immunodeficiency Virus (HIV), which attacks and weakens the immune system. Infections and other diseases can then invade the body, and the immune system cannot fight against them. Kaposi's sarcoma in people with AIDS usually spreads more quickly than other kinds of Kaposi's sarcoma and often is found in many parts of the body.

Recurrent

Recurrent disease means that the KS has come back (recurred) after it has been treated. It may come back in the area where it first started or in another part of the body.

How Kaposi's Sarcoma Is Treated

There are treatments for all patients with Kaposi's sarcoma. Four kinds of treatment are used:

- surgery (taking out the cancer)

- chemotherapy (using drugs to kill cancer cells)

- radiation therapy (using high-dose x-rays to kill cancer cells)

- biological therapy (using the body's immune system to fight cancer)

Radiation therapy is a common treatment of Kaposi's sarcoma. Radiation therapy uses high-dose x-rays or other high-energy rays to kill cancer cells and shrink tumors. Radiation for Kaposi's sarcoma comes from a machine outside the body (external beam radiation therapy).

Surgery means taking out the cancer. A doctor may remove the cancer using one of the following:

- Local excision cuts out the lesion and some of the tissue around it.

- Electrodesiccation and curettage burns the lesion and removes it with a sharp instrument.

- Cryotherapy freezes the tumor and kills it.

Chemotherapy uses drugs to kill cancer cells. Chemotherapy may be taken by pill, or it may be put into the body by a needle in a vein or muscle. Chemotherapy is called a systemic treatment because the drug enters the bloodstream, travels through the body, and can kill cancer cells outside the original site. Chemotherapy for Kaposi's sarcoma also may be injected into the lesion (intralesional chemotherapy).

Biological therapy tries to get the body to fight the cancer. It uses materials made by the body or made in a laboratory to boost, direct, or restore the body's natural defenses against disease. Biological therapy is sometimes called biological response modifier (BRM) therapy or immunotherapy.

Treatment by Stage

Treatment of Kaposi's sarcoma depends on the type of Kaposi's sarcoma the patient has, and the patient's age and general health.

Standard treatment may be considered because of its effectiveness in patients in past studies, or participation in a clinical trial may be considered. Not all patients are cured with standard therapy and some standard treatments may have more side effects than are desired. For these reasons, clinical trials are designed to find better ways to treat cancer patients and are based on the most up-to-date information. Clinical trials are ongoing in most parts of the country for most stages of Kaposi's sarcoma. To learn more about clinical trials, call the Cancer Information Service at 1-800-4-CANCER (1-800-422-6237); TTY at 1-800-332-8615.

Classic Kaposi's Sarcoma

Treatment may be one of the following:

1. Radiation therapy.

2. Local excision.

3. Systemic or intralesional chemotherapy.

4. Chemotherapy plus radiation therapy.

Immunosuppressive Treatment-Related Kaposi's Sarcoma

Depending on the patient's condition, the cancer may be controlled if immunosuppressive drugs are stopped. If the patient cannot stop taking these drugs or if this does not work, treatment may be one of the following:

1. Radiation therapy.

2. A clinical trial of chemotherapy.

Epidemic Kaposi's Sarcoma

Treatment may be one of the following:

1. Surgery (local excision, electrodesiccation and curettage, or cryotherapy) with or without radiation therapy.

2. Systemic chemotherapy. Clinical trials are testing new drugs and drug combinations.

3. Biological therapy.

4. A clinical trial evaluating new treatments.

Recurrent Kaposi's Sarcoma

Treatment of recurrent Kaposi's sarcoma depends on the type of Kaposi's sarcoma, and the patient's general health and response to earlier treatments. The patient may want to take part in a clinical trial.

To Learn More

To learn more about Kaposi's sarcoma, call the National Cancer Institute's Cancer Information Service at 1-800-4-CANCER (1-800-422-6237); TTY at 1-800-332-8615. By dialing this toll-free number, trained information specialists can answer your questions.

Cancer patients, their families and friends, and others may find the following booklets useful. They are available free of charge by calling 1-800-4-CANCER or writing:

Office of Cancer Communications
National Cancer Institute
Building 31, Room 10A24
Bethesda, MD 20892

Booklets about Cancer Treatment

Radiation Therapy and You: A Guide to Self-Help During Treatment *

Chemotherapy and You: A Guide to Self-Help During Treatment *

Eating Hints: Recipes and Tips for Better Nutrition During Cancer Treatment *

Questions and Answers About Pain Control

What Are Clinical Trials All About?

Booklets about Living with Cancer

Taking Time: Support for People With Cancer and the People Who Care About Them

When Cancer Recurs: Meeting the Challenge Again *

Advanced Cancer: Living Each Day *

* Reprinted in this volume—see Table of Contents

Chapter 54

Adult Soft Tissue Sarcoma

What Is Adult Soft Tissue Sarcoma?

Adult soft tissue sarcoma is a disease in which cancer (malignant) cells are found in the soft tissue of part of the body. The soft tissues of the body include the muscles, connective tissues (tendons), vessels that carry blood or lymph, joints, and fat.

A lump or swelling in part of the body may appear if a person has a soft tissue sarcoma. The lump may not be painful. If there are symptoms, a doctor may cut out a piece of tissue from the swollen area. This is called a biopsy. The tissue will be looked at under a microscope to see if there are any cancer cells. A patient may need to go to the hospital for this test.

The chance of recovery (prognosis) and choice of treatment depend on the size and stage of the cancer (how far the cancer has spread), and the patient's age and general health.

Stages of Adult Soft Tissue Sarcoma

Once adult soft tissue sarcoma is found, more tests will be done to find out if cancer cells have spread to other parts of the body. This testing is called staging. A doctor needs to know the stage of the disease to plan treatment. Unlike most other cancers, the size of a soft tissue sarcoma is not as important as how the cancer cells look under a microscope. The more different the cancer cells look from normal

PDQ Statement, National Cancer Institute (NCI), updated September 1999.

cells, the higher the stage. The following stages are used for adult soft tissue sarcoma:

Stage IA

The cancer cells look either very much like or somewhat different from normal cells (well-differentiated or moderately well-differentiated). The cancer is either near the surface or deep and is less than 5 centimeters in size (about 2 inches), but it has not spread to lymph nodes or other parts of the body (lymph nodes are small bean-shaped structures that are found throughout the body; they produce and store infection-fighting cells).

Stage IB

The cancer cells look either very much like or somewhat different from normal cells (well-differentiated or moderately well-differentiated). The cancer is near the surface and more than 5 centimeters in size, but it has not spread to lymph nodes or other parts of the body.

Stage IIA

The cancer cells look either very much like or somewhat different from normal cells (well-differentiated or moderately well-differentiated). The cancer is deep and more than 5 centimeters in size, but it has not spread to lymph nodes or other parts of the body.

Stage IIB

The cancer cells look very different from normal cells (poorly differentiated or undifferentiated). The cancer is either near the surface or deep and is less than 5 centimeters in size, but it has not spread to lymph nodes or other parts of the body.

Stage IIC

The cancer cells look very different from normal cells (poorly differentiated or undifferentiated). The cancer is near the surface and is more than 5 centimeters in size, but it has not spread to lymph nodes or other parts of the body.

Stage III

The cancer cells look very different from normal cells (poorly differentiated or undifferentiated). The cancer is deep and is more than

5 centimeters in size, but it has not spread to lymph nodes or other parts of the body.

Stage IV

The cancer may have spread to lymph nodes in the area or may have spread to other parts of the body, such as the lungs, head, or neck.

Recurrent

Recurrent disease means that the cancer has come back (recurred) after it has been treated. It may come back in the tissues where it first started, or it may come back in another part of the body.

How Adult Soft Tissue Sarcoma Is Treated

There are treatments for all patients with adult soft tissue sarcoma. Three kinds of treatment are used:

- surgery (taking out the cancer in an operation)
- radiation therapy (using high-dose x-rays to kill cancer cells)
- chemotherapy (using drugs to kill cancer cells)

Surgery is the most common treatment of adult soft tissue sarcoma. A doctor may remove the cancer and some of the healthy tissue around the cancer. Sometimes all or part of an arm or leg may have to be removed (amputated) to make sure that all of the cancer is taken out. If cancer has spread to lymph nodes, the lymph nodes will be removed (lymph node dissection).

Radiation therapy uses x-rays or other high-energy rays to kill cancer cells and shrink tumors. Radiation may come from a machine outside the body (external-beam radiation therapy) or from putting materials that produce radiation (radioisotopes) through thin plastic tubes in the area where the cancer cells are found (internal radiation therapy).

Chemotherapy uses drugs to kill cancer cells. Chemotherapy may be taken by pill, or it may be put into the body by a needle in a vein or muscle. Chemotherapy is called a systemic treatment because the drug enters the blood stream, travels through the body, and kills cancer cells throughout the body. Chemotherapy that is given after surgery when no cancer cells can be seen is called adjuvant chemotherapy.

In soft tissue sarcoma, chemotherapy is sometimes injected directly into the blood vessels in the area where the cancer is found. This treatment is called regional chemotherapy.

Chemotherapy and/or radiation therapy may be used to shrink the cancer so it can be removed without taking off an entire arm or leg.

Treatment by Stage

Treatments for adult soft tissue sarcoma depend on the stage of the disease, and the patient's age and general health.

Patients may consider standard therapy, because of its effectiveness in past studies, or participation in a clinical trial. Not all patients are cured with standard therapy, and some standard treatments may have more side effects than are desired. For these reasons, clinical trials are designed to find better ways to treat cancer patients and are based on the most up-to-date information. For more information about clinical trials, call the Cancer Information Service at 1-800-4-CANCER (1-800-422-6237); TTY at 1-800-332-8615.

Stage IA, IB, and IIA Adult Soft Tissue Sarcoma

Treatment may be one of the following:

1. Surgery to remove the cancer.

2. Surgery with radiation therapy, before or after the surgery.

3. High-dose radiation therapy followed by surgery and radiation therapy.

If cancer is found in the head or neck or in the abdomen or chest, treatment may be one of the following:

1. Surgery to remove the cancer possibly followed by radiation therapy.

2. Radiation therapy followed by surgery.

Stage IIB, IIC, and III Adult Soft Tissue Sarcoma

Treatment may be one of the following:

1. Surgery to remove the cancer.

2. Surgery to remove the cancer followed by radiation therapy.

3. Radiation therapy alone.

4. Radiation therapy and/or chemotherapy before surgery, possibly followed by radiation therapy.

Stage IV adult Soft Tissue Sarcoma

If the cancer has spread to the lymph nodes, treatment may be one of the following:

1. Surgery to remove the cancer and removal of the lymph nodes where the cancer has spread (lymph node dissection), possibly followed by radiation therapy.

2. Radiation therapy before and after surgery to remove the cancer and lymph node dissection.

3. A clinical trial of surgery and/or radiation therapy followed by chemotherapy

If the cancer has spread to the lungs, treatment may be one of the following:

1. Surgery to remove the primary cancer followed by radiation therapy followed by surgery to remove the cancer from the lungs.

2. Surgery to remove the primary cancer.

3. Surgery to remove the primary cancer followed by radiation therapy.

4. Radiation therapy, possibly followed by chemotherapy.

If the cancer has spread to other parts of the body, treatment may be one of the following:

1. Surgery to remove the cancer with radiation therapy before or after the surgery, possibly followed by chemotherapy

2. Chemotherapy to reduce the pain and discomfort caused by the cancer.

Recurrent Adult Soft Tissue Sarcoma

Treatment depends on the kind of treatment the patient had before. Treatment may be one of the following:

1. Surgery to remove the cancer.

2. Surgery to remove the cancer followed by radiation therapy.

3. Chemotherapy alone.

To Learn More

To learn more about adult soft tissue sarcoma, call the National Cancer Institute's Cancer Information Service at 1-800-4-CANCER (1-800-422-6237); TTY at 1-800-332-8615. By dialing this toll-free number, trained information specialists can help answer your questions.

Cancer patients, their families and friends, and others may find the following booklets useful. They are available free of charge by calling 1-800-4-CANCER or writing:

Office of Cancer Communications
National Cancer Institute
Building 31, Room 10A24
Bethesda, MD 20892

Booklets about Cancer Treatment

Radiation Therapy and You: A Guide to Self-Help During Treatment *

Chemotherapy and You: A Guide to Self-Help During Treatment *

Eating Hints: Recipes and Tips for Better Nutrition During Cancer Treatment *

Questions and Answers About Pain Control

What Are Clinical Trials All About?

Booklets about Living with Cancer

Taking Time: Support for People With Cancer and the People Who Care About Them

When Cancer Recurs: Meeting the Challenge Again *

Advanced Cancer: Living Each Day *

* Reprinted in this volume—see Table of Contents

Chapter 55

Synovial Sarcoma

Synovial Sarcoma

Synovial sarcoma, also called synovioma, is a rare cancer that begins in synovial tissue. Synovial tissue can be found in tendons (tissues that connect muscle to bone), bursae (fluid-filled, cushioning sacs found in spaces between tendons, ligaments, and bones), and the cavity (hollow enclosed area) that separates the bones of a freely movable joint, such as the knee or elbow.

Synovial sarcomas occur mainly in the arms and legs, where they tend to arise in the area of large joints, especially the knee region. Less frequently, the disease develops in the head and neck and in the trunk. This cancer occurs mostly in adolescents and young adults, and it affects more males than females.

The most common symptom of synovial sarcoma is a deep-seated swelling or a mass that may be accompanied by pain or tenderness. In a few cases, pain or tenderness is present for several years even though a mass cannot be felt. These cases can be easily mistaken for arthritis, bursitis, or synovitis. Sometimes synovial sarcoma causes other symptoms related to the location of the tumor. The diagnosis of synovial sarcoma is made by biopsy (removal of tissue for examination under a microscope).

The type of treatment selected depends on the extent (stage) of the disease and the location of the sarcoma. The most common treatment for this type of cancer is surgery to remove the entire tumor, nearby

PDQ Statement, National Cancer Institute (NCI), updated August 1998.

muscle, and lymph nodes. Some patients have radiation, chemotherapy, or a combination of treatment methods. Biological therapy (treatment to stimulate or restore the ability of the immune system to fight the disease) and new types of chemotherapy are currently being studied in clinical trials.

Synovial sarcoma tends to recur locally and to involve regional lymph nodes. Distant metastasis (spreading to other areas of the body) occurs in about one-half of the cases, sometimes many years after the initial diagnosis.

Information about ongoing clinical trials is available from the Cancer Information Service (see below), or from the National Cancer Institute's clinical trials website at http://cancertrials.nci.nih.gov via the Internet. At this website, trials for patients with synovial sarcoma are included with "sarcoma, soft tissue, adult" and "sarcoma, soft tissue, childhood."

National Cancer Institute Information Resources

You may want more information for yourself, your family, and your doctor. The following National Cancer Institute (NCI) services are available to help you.

Telephone

Cancer Information Service (CIS) Provides accurate, up-to-date information on cancer to patients and their families, health professionals, and the general public. Information specialists translate the latest scientific information into understandable language and respond in English, Spanish, or on TTY equipment.

Toll-free: 1-800-4-CANCER (1-800-422-6237)
TTY: 1-800-332-8615

Internet

These Web sites may be useful:

http://www.nci.nih.gov—NCI's primary Web site; contains information about the Institute and its programs.

http://cancertrials.nci.nih.gov—CancerTrials; NCI's comprehensive clinical trials information center for patients, health professionals, and the public. Includes information on understanding trials, deciding whether to participate in trials, finding specific trials, plus research news and other resources.

http://cancernet.nci.nih.gov—CancerNet; contains material for health professionals, patients, and the public, including information from PDQ about cancer treatment, screening, prevention, supportive care, and clinical trials, and CANCERLIT, a bibliographic database.

E-mail

CancerMail—Includes NCI information about cancer treatment, screening, prevention, and supportive care. To obtain a contents list, send e-mail to cancermail@icicc.nci.nih.gov with the word "help" in the body of the message.

Fax

CancerFax—Includes NCI information about cancer treatment, screening, prevention, and supportive care. To obtain a contents list, dial 301-402-5874 from a fax machine hand set and follow the recorded instructions.

Chapter 56

Osteosarcoma

What Is Osteosarcoma?

Osteosarcoma is a disease in which cancer (malignant) cells are found in the bone. It is the most common type of bone cancer. In children, it occurs most commonly in the bones around the knee. Osteosarcoma most often occurs in adolescents and young adults.

Ewing's sarcoma is another kind of bone cancer, but the cancer cells look different under a microscope than osteosarcoma cancer cells. If you want information on Ewing's sarcoma, see the PDQ patient information summary on Ewing's sarcoma.

If a patient has symptoms (such as pain and swelling of a bone or a bone region), a doctor may order x-rays and blood tests. If it is suspected that the problem is osteosarcoma, your doctor may recommend seeing a specialist called an orthopedic oncologist. The orthopedic oncologist may cut out a piece of tissue from the affected area. This is called a biopsy. The tissue will be looked at under a microscope to see if there are any cancer cells. This test may be done in the hospital.

The chance of recovery (prognosis) and choice of treatment depend on the size, location, type, and stage of the cancer (how far the cancer has spread), how long the patient had symptoms, how much of the cancer is taken out by surgery and/or killed by chemotherapy, and the patient's age, blood and other test results, and general health.

PDQ Statement, National Cancer Institute (NCI), updated December 1999.

Stages of Osteosarcoma

Once osteosarcoma has been found, more tests may be done to find out if cancer cells have spread to other parts of the body. This is called staging. At present, there is no staging system for osteosarcoma. Instead, most patients are grouped depending on whether cancer is found in only one part of the body (localized disease) or whether the cancer has spread from one part of the body to another (metastatic disease). Your doctor needs to know where the cancer is located and how far the disease has spread to plan treatment. The following groups are used for osteosarcoma:

Localized

The cancer cells have not spread beyond the bone or nearby tissue in which the cancer began. In young patients most tumors occur around the knee.

Metastatic

The cancer cells have spread from the bone in which the cancer began to other parts of the body. The cancer most often spreads to the lungs. It may also spread to other bones.

Recurrent

Recurrent disease means that the cancer has come back (recurred) after it has been treated. It may come back in the tissues where it first started or it may come back in another part of the body.

How Osteosarcoma Is Treated

If it is suspected that the problem is osteosarcoma, before the first biopsy, your doctor may recommend a specialist called an orthopedic oncologist.

There are treatments for all patients with osteosarcoma. Three kinds of treatment are used:

- surgery (taking out the cancer in an operation)
- chemotherapy (using drugs to kill cancer cells)
- radiation therapy (using high-dose x-rays to kill cancer cells)

Surgery is a common treatment for osteosarcoma. The doctor may remove the cancer and some of the healthy tissue around the cancer.

Sometimes all or part of an arm or leg may have to be removed (amputated) to make sure that all of the cancer is taken out. If cancer has spread to lymph nodes, the lymph nodes will be removed (lymph node dissection).

In patients with osteosarcoma that has not spread beyond the bone, researchers are studying whether surgery without amputation of the arm or leg (limb-sparing procedures) can be done without the cancer coming back. Sometimes the cancer can be taken out without amputation, and artificial devices or bones from other places in the body can be used to replace the bone that was removed.

Chemotherapy uses drugs to kill cancer cells. Chemotherapy may be taken by pill or put into the body by a needle in a vein or muscle. Chemotherapy is called systemic treatment because the drug enters the blood stream, travels through the body, and can kill cancer cells throughout the body. Chemotherapy with more than one drug is called combination chemotherapy.

Sometimes chemotherapy is injected directly into the area where the cancer is found (regional chemotherapy). In osteosarcoma, surgery is often used to remove the local tumor and chemotherapy is then given to kill any cancer cells that remain in the body. Chemotherapy given after surgery has removed the cancer is called adjuvant chemotherapy. Chemotherapy can also be given before surgery to shrink the cancer so that it can be removed during surgery; this is called neoadjuvant chemotherapy.

Radiation therapy uses x-rays or other high-energy rays to kill cancer cells and shrink tumors. Radiation for osteosarcoma usually comes from a machine outside the body (external radiation therapy).

Treatment by Stage

Treatment for osteosarcoma depends on the stage of the disease, where the cancer is found, and the patient's age and general health.

A patient may receive treatment that is considered standard based on its effectiveness in a number of patients in past studies, or may choose to go into a clinical trial. Not all patients are cured with standard therapy, and some standard treatments may have more side effects than are desired. For these reasons, clinical trials are designed to find better ways to treat cancer patients and are based on the most up-to-date information. Clinical trials for osteosarcoma are ongoing in many parts of the country. If you want more information, call the Cancer Information Service at 1-800-4-CANCER (1-800-422-6237); TTY at 1-800-332-8615.

Localized Osteosarcoma

Treatment may be the following:

- Chemotherapy followed by surgery followed by adjuvant chemotherapy.

Clinical trials are evaluating new methods of giving chemotherapy and new schedules of treatment. The use of radiation therapy is also under study.

Metastatic Osteosarcoma

Treatment may be one of the following:

1. Chemotherapy followed by surgery to remove the cancer followed by adjuvant chemotherapy.

2. Surgery to remove the cancer followed by adjuvant chemotherapy. Surgery often includes removal of cancer that has spread to the lungs.

Recurrent Osteosarcoma

Treatment depends on where the cancer recurred, what kind of treatment was given before, as well as other factors. A clinical trial may be a reasonable treatment option.

If the cancer has come back only in the lungs, treatment may be surgery to remove the cancer in the lungs with or without chemotherapy. If the cancer has come back in other places besides the lungs, treatment may be combination chemotherapy. Clinical trials are evaluating new chemotherapy drugs.

To Learn More

To learn more about osteosarcoma, call the National Cancer Institute's Cancer Information Service at 1-800-4-CANCER (1-800-422-6237); TTY at 1-800-332-8615. The call is toll-free and a trained information specialist can answer your questions.

Cancer patients, their families and friends, and others may find the following booklets useful. They are available free of charge by calling 1-800-4-CANCER or writing:

Office of Cancer Communications
National Cancer Institute
Building 31, Room 10A24
Bethesda, MD 20892

Booklets about Cancer Treatment

Radiation Therapy and You: A Guide to Self-Help During Treatment *

Chemotherapy and You: A Guide to Self-Help During Treatment *

Eating Hints: Recipes and Tips for Better Nutrition During Cancer Treatment *

Questions and Answers About Pain Control

What Are Clinical Trials All About?

Booklets about Living with Cancer

Taking Time: Support for People With Cancer and the People Who Care About Them

When Cancer Recurs: Meeting the Challenge Again *

Advanced Cancer: Living Each Day *

* Reprinted in this volume—see Table of Contents

Chapter 57

Multiple Myeloma

Introduction

Each year, nearly 13,000 people in the United States learn that they have multiple myeloma. This chapter describes symptoms, diagnosis, and treatment of this type of cancer. It also has information to help you deal with this disease if it affects you or someone you know.

Other NCI publications are listed in the Other Booklets section. Our materials cannot answer every question you may have about multiple myeloma and its treatment. They cannot take the place of talks with doctors, nurses, and other members of the health care team. We hope our information will help with those talks.

Researchers continue to look for better ways to diagnose and treat multiple myeloma, and our knowledge is growing. For up-to-date information or to order this publication, call the NCI-supported Cancer Information Service (CIS) toll free at 1-800-4-CANCER (1-800-422-6237).

What Is Multiple Myeloma?

Multiple myeloma is a type of cancer. It affects certain white blood cells called plasma cells. To understand multiple myeloma, it is helpful to know about normal cells, especially plasma cells, and what happens when they become cancerous.

"What You Need To Know About Multiple Myeloma," National Cancer Institute (NCI), updated September 1998.

Normal Cells

The body is made up of many kinds of cells. Each type of cell has special functions. Normal cells are produced in an orderly, controlled way as the body needs them. This process keeps us healthy.

Plasma cells and other white blood cells are part of the immune system, which helps protect the body from infection and disease. All white blood cells begin their development in the bone marrow, the soft, spongy tissue that fills the center of most bones. Certain white blood cells leave the bone marrow and mature in other parts of the body. Some of these develop into plasma cells when the immune system needs them to fight substances that cause infection and disease.

Plasma cells produce antibodies, proteins that move through the bloodstream to help the body get rid of harmful substances. Each type of plasma cell responds to only one specific substance by making a large amount of one kind of antibody. These antibodies find and act against that one substance. Because the body has many types of plasma cells, it can respond to many substances.

Cancer Cells

Cancer is a group of diseases with one thing in common: Cells become abnormal and are produced in large amounts. Cancerous cells interfere with the growth and functions of normal cells. In addition, they can spread from one part of the body to another.

Myeloma Cells

When cancer involves plasma cells, the body keeps producing more and more of these cells. The unneeded plasma cells—all abnormal and all exactly alike—are called myeloma cells.

Myeloma cells tend to collect in the bone marrow and in the hard, outer part of bones. Sometimes they collect in only one bone and form a single mass, or tumor, called a plasmacytoma. In most cases, however, the myeloma cells collect in many bones, often forming many tumors and causing other problems. When this happens, the disease is called multiple myeloma. This chapter deals mainly with multiple myeloma. (It is important to keep in mind that cancer is classified by the type of cell or the part of the body in which the disease begins. Although plasmacytoma and multiple myeloma affect the bones, they begin in cells of the immune system. These cancers are different from bone cancer, which actually begins in cells that form the hard, outer part of the bone. This fact is important because the diagnosis and treatment of plasmacytoma and multiple myeloma are different from the diagnosis and treatment of bone cancer.)

Because people with multiple myeloma have an abnormally large number of identical plasma cells, they also have too much of one type of antibody. These myeloma cells and antibodies can cause a number of serious medical problems:

- As myeloma cells increase in number, they damage and weaken bones, causing pain and sometimes fractures. Bone pain can make it difficult for patients to move.

- When bones are damaged, calcium is released into the blood. This may lead to hypercalcemia—too much calcium in the blood. Hypercalcemia can cause loss of appetite, nausea, thirst, fatigue, muscle weakness, restlessness, and confusion.

- Myeloma cells prevent the bone marrow from forming normal plasma cells and other white blood cells that are important to the immune system. Patients may not be able to fight infection and disease.

- The cancer cells also may prevent the growth of new red blood cells, causing anemia. Patients with anemia may feel unusually tired or weak.

- Multiple myeloma patients may have serious problems with their kidneys. Excess antibody proteins and calcium can prevent the kidneys from filtering and cleaning the blood properly.

Symptoms

Symptoms of multiple myeloma depend on how advanced the disease is. In the earliest stage of the disease, there may be no symptoms. When symptoms do occur, patients commonly have bone pain, often in the back or ribs. Patients also may have broken bones, weakness, fatigue, weight loss, or repeated infections. When the disease is advanced, symptoms may include nausea, vomiting, constipation, problems with urination, and weakness or numbness in the legs. These are not sure signs of multiple myeloma; they can be symptoms of other types of medical problems. A person should see a doctor if these symptoms occur. Only a doctor can determine what is causing a patient's symptoms.

Diagnosis

Multiple myeloma may be found as part of a routine physical exam before patients have symptoms of the disease. When patients do have symptoms, the doctor asks about their personal and family medical history and does a complete physical exam. In addition to checking general signs of health, the doctor may order a number of tests to determine the cause of the symptoms. If a patient has bone pain, x-rays can show whether any bones are damaged or broken. Samples of the patient's blood and urine are checked to see whether they contain high levels of antibody proteins called M proteins. The doctor also may do a bone marrow aspiration and/or a bone marrow biopsy to check for myeloma cells. In an aspiration, the doctor inserts a needle into the hip bone or breast bone to withdraw a sample of fluid and cells from the bone marrow. To do a biopsy, the doctor uses a larger needle to remove a sample of solid tissue from the marrow. A pathologist examines the samples under a microscope to see whether myeloma cells are present.

To plan a patient's treatment, the doctor needs to know the stage, or extent, of the disease. Staging is a careful attempt to find out what parts of the body are affected by the cancer. Treatment decisions depend on these findings. Results of the patient's exam, blood tests, and bone marrow tests can help doctors determine the stage of the disease. In addition, staging usually involves a series of x-rays to determine the number and size of tumors in the bones. In some cases, a patient will have MRI if closeup views of the bones are needed.

Treatment

Treatment depends on the extent of the cancer and the patient's symptoms. The doctor also considers the person's age and general health. The doctor may want to discuss the patient's case with other doctors who treat multiple myeloma. Also, the patient may want to talk with the doctor about taking part in a research study of new treatment methods. Such studies, called clinical trials, are designed to improve the treatment of this type of cancer. These studies are discussed in the Treatment Studies section.

Many patients want to learn all they can about their disease and their treatment choices so they can take an active part in decisions about their medical care. Patients have many important questions about their health, and the doctor is the best person to answer them. Most people want to know the extent of their cancer, how it can be treated, how effective the treatment is likely to be, and how much it is expected to cost. These are some questions patients may want to ask the doctor:

- What are my treatment choices?

- Would a clinical trial be appropriate for me?

- What are the expected benefits of treatment?

- What are the risks and possible side effects of treatment?

- If I have pain, how will you help me?

- Will I need to change my normal activities?

- How often will I need to have checkups?

Many people find it helpful to make a list of their questions before they see the doctor. Taking notes can make it easier to remember what the doctor says. Some patients also find that it helps to have a family member or friend with them when they see the doctor—to take part in the discussion or just to listen.

There is a lot to learn about cancer and its treatment. Patients do not need to ask all their questions or remember all the answers at one time. They will have other chances to ask the doctor to explain things and to get more information.

Before Treatment

Treatment decisions for multiple myeloma are complex. Before starting treatment, the patient might want a second doctor to review the diagnosis and treatment plan. A short delay usually does not reduce the chance that treatment will be effective. There are a number of ways to find a doctor for a second opinion:

- The patient's doctor may be able to suggest a doctor who treats multiple myeloma. Doctors who specialize in treating this disease include oncologists, hematologists, and radiation oncologists.

- The Cancer Information Service, at 1-800-4-CANCER, can tell callers about treatment facilities, including cancer centers and other NCI-supported programs in their area.

- Patients can get the names of doctors from their local medical society, a nearby hospital, or a medical school.

Treatment Methods

Plasmacytoma and multiple myeloma are very hard to cure. Although patients who have a plasmacytoma may be free of symptoms for a long time after treatment, many eventually develop multiple myeloma. For those who have multiple myeloma, treatment can improve the quality of a patient's life by controlling the symptoms and complications of the disease.

People who have multiple myeloma but do not have symptoms of the disease usually do not receive treatment. For these patients, the risks and side effects of treatment are likely to outweigh the possible benefits. However, these patients are watched closely, and they begin treatment when symptoms appear. Patients who need treatment for multiple myeloma usually receive chemotherapy and sometimes radiation therapy.

Chemotherapy is the use of drugs to treat cancer. It is the main treatment for multiple myeloma. Doctors may prescribe two or more drugs that work together to kill myeloma cells. Many of these drugs are taken by mouth; others are injected into a blood vessel. Either way, the drugs travel through the bloodstream, reaching myeloma cells all over the body. For this reason, chemotherapy is called systemic therapy.

Anticancer drugs often are given in cycles—a treatment period followed by a rest period, then another treatment and rest period, and so on. Most patients take their chemotherapy at home, as outpatients at the hospital, or at the doctor's office. However, depending on their health and the drugs being given, patients may need to stay in the hospital during treatment.

Radiation therapy (also called radiotherapy) uses high-energy rays to damage cancer cells and stop them from growing. In this form of treatment, a large machine aims the rays at a tumor and the area close to it. Treatment with radiation is local therapy; it affects only the cells in the treated area.

Radiation therapy is the main treatment for people who have a single plasmacytoma. They usually receive radiation therapy every weekday for 4 to 5 weeks in the outpatient department of a hospital or clinic.

People who have multiple myeloma sometimes receive radiation therapy in addition to chemotherapy. The purpose of the radiation therapy is to help control the growth of tumors in the bones and relieve the pain that these tumors cause. Treatment usually lasts for 1 to 2 weeks.

Treatment Studies

Because multiple myeloma is so hard to control, many researchers are looking for more effective treatments. They also are looking for treatments that have fewer side effects and for better ways to care for patients who have complications caused by this disease. When laboratory research shows that a new method has promise, doctors use it to treat cancer patients in clinical trials. These trials are designed to find out whether the new approach is both safe and effective and to answer scientific questions. Patients who take part in clinical trials may have the first chance to benefit from improved treatment methods, and they make an important contribution to medical science.

Many clinical trials of new treatments for multiple myeloma are under way. In some studies, doctors are testing new drugs and new drug combinations. In others, they are using chemotherapy along with biological therapy, treatment with substances that boost the immune system's response to cancer.

Researchers also are testing new approaches to cancer treatment that allow the use of very high doses of anticancer drugs, sometimes along with radiation. Doctors believe that higher doses of anticancer drugs and radiation might be more effective than the usual doses in destroying myeloma cells. However, higher doses also cause greater damage to healthy bone marrow. New approaches to treatment may help the healthy marrow recover or may allow doctors to replace marrow that is destroyed. These approaches (bone marrow transplantation, peripheral stem cell support, and treatment with colony-stimulating factors) are described in the Glossary.

Patients interested in taking part in a clinical trial should discuss this option with their doctor. *Taking Part in Clinical Trials: What Cancer Patients Need To Know* is a National Cancer Institute booklet that explains some of the risks and possible benefits of treatment studies.

One way to learn about clinical trials is through PDQ, a computerized resource developed by the National Cancer Institute. This resource contains information about cancer treatment and about clinical trials in progress all over the country. The Cancer Information Service can provide PDQ information to patients and the public.

Side Effects of Treatment

The methods used to treat multiple myeloma are very powerful. Treatment can help patients feel better by relieving symptoms such as bone pain. However, it is hard to limit the effects of therapy so that only cancer cells are destroyed. Because healthy cells also may be damaged, treatment can cause unpleasant side effects.

The side effects that patients have during cancer treatment vary for each person. They may even be different from one treatment to the next. Doctors try to plan treatment to keep side effects to a minimum. They also monitor patients very carefully so they can help with any problems that occur.

The side effects of chemotherapy depend on the drugs that are given. In general, anticancer drugs affect rapidly growing cells, such as blood cells that fight infection, cells that line the digestive tract, and cells in hair follicles. As a result, patients may have lower resistance to infection, loss of appetite, nausea, vomiting, or mouth sores. Patients also may have less energy and may lose their hair. One drug used to treat multiple myeloma, called prednisone, may cause swelling of the face and feet, burning indigestion, mood swings, restlessness, and acne. The side effects of chemotherapy usually go away over time after treatment stops.

During radiation therapy, the patient may be more tired than usual. Resting is important, but doctors usually advise patients to stay as active as they can. Also, the skin in the treated area may become red or dry. The skin should be exposed to the air but protected from the sun, and patients should avoid wearing clothes that rub the treated area. They should not use any lotion or cream on the skin without the doctor's advice. Patients may have other side effects, depending upon the areas treated. For example, radiation to the lower back may cause nausea, vomiting, or diarrhea because the lower digestive tract is exposed to radiation. The doctor often can prescribe medicine or suggest changes in diet to ease these problems. Side effects usually disappear gradually after radiation therapy is over.

Loss of appetite can be a problem for patients with multiple myeloma. People may not feel hungry when they are uncomfortable or tired. Some of the common side effects of cancer treatment, such as nausea and vomiting, can also make it hard to eat. Yet patients who eat well often feel better and have more energy, so good nutrition is important. Eating well means getting enough calories and protein to prevent weight loss, regain strength, and rebuild normal tissues. Many patients find that having several small meals and snacks during the day works better than having three regular meals.

Doctors, nurses, and dietitians can explain the side effects of cancer treatment and can suggest ways to deal with them. In addition, the National Cancer Institute publications *Chemotherapy and You* [reprinted in this volume as Chapter 63], *Radiation Therapy and You* [Chapter 66], and *Eating Hints for Cancer Patients*[Chapter 77] contain helpful information about cancer treatment and coping with side effects.

Supportive Care

The complications of multiple myeloma can affect many parts of the body. Chemotherapy and radiation therapy often can help control complications such as pain, bone damage, and kidney problems. However, from time to time, most patients need additional treatment to manage these and other problems caused by the disease. This type of treatment, called supportive care, is given to improve patients' comfort and quality of life.

Patients with multiple myeloma frequently have pain caused by bone damage or by tumors pressing on nerves. Doctors often suggest that patients take pain medicine and/or wear a back or neck brace to help relieve their pain. Some patients find that techniques such as relaxation and imagery can reduce their pain. These and other methods of relieving pain are discussed in the booklet *Questions and Answers About Pain Control*.

Preventing or treating bone fractures is another important part of supportive care. Because exercise can reduce the loss of calcium from the bones, doctors and nurses encourage patients to be active, if possible. They may suggest appropriate forms of exercise. If a patient has a fracture or a breakdown of certain bones, especially those in the spine, a surgeon may need to operate to remove as much of the cancer as possible and to strengthen the bone.

Patients who have hypercalcemia may be given medicine to reduce the level of calcium in the blood. They also are encouraged to drink large amounts of fluids every day; some may need intravenous (IV) fluids. Getting plenty of fluids helps the kidneys get rid of excess calcium in the blood. It also helps prevent problems that occur when calcium collects in the kidneys.

If the kidneys aren't working well, dialysis or plasmapheresis may be necessary. In dialysis, the patient's blood passes through a machine that removes wastes, and the blood is then returned to the patient. Plasmapheresis is used to remove excess antibodies produced by the myeloma cells. This process thins the blood, making it easier for the kidneys and the heart to function.

Multiple myeloma weakens the immune system. Patients must be very careful to protect themselves from infection. It is important that they stay out of crowds and away from people with colds or other infectious diseases. Any sign of infection (fever, sore throat, cough) should be reported to the doctor right away. Patients who develop infections are treated with antibiotics or other drugs.

Patients who have anemia may have transfusions of red blood cells. Transfusions can help reduce the shortness of breath and fatigue that can be caused by anemia.

Followup Care

Regular followup is very important for anyone who has multiple myeloma. Checkups generally include a physical exam, x-rays, and blood and urine tests. Regular followup exams help doctors detect and treat problems promptly if they should arise. It is also important for the patient to tell the doctor about any new symptoms or problems that develop between checkups.

Living with Cancer

The diagnosis of multiple myeloma can change the lives of patients and the people who care about them. These changes can be hard to handle. It is common for patients and their families and friends to have many different and sometimes confusing emotions.

At times, patients and their loved ones may feel frightened, angry, or depressed. These are normal reactions when people face a serious health problem. Most people handle their problems better if they can share their thoughts and feelings with those close to them. Sharing can help everyone feel more at ease and can open the way for people to show one another their concern and offer their support.

Worries about tests, treatments, hospital stays, and medical bills are common. Doctors, nurses, social workers, and other members of the health care team may help calm fears and ease confusion. They also can provide information and suggest resources.

Patients and their families are naturally concerned about what the future holds. Sometimes people use statistics to try to figure out whether a cure is possible or how long the patient will live. It is important to remember, however, that statistics are averages based on large numbers of patients. They can't be used to predict what will happen to a certain patient because no two cancer patients are alike. The doctor who takes care of the patient and knows his or her history is in the best position to discuss the person's outlook (prognosis).

People should feel free to ask the doctor about their prognosis, but not even the doctor knows for sure what will happen. Doctors may talk about the chances of remission. They also may talk about managing or controlling multiple myeloma rather than curing it, even when patients respond well to treatment. They use these terms because the disease may get worse at a later time.

Services for Cancer Patients

Living with a serious disease isn't easy. Cancer patients and those who care about them face many problems and challenges. Finding the strength to cope with these difficulties is easier when people have helpful information and support services.

The doctor can explain the disease and give advice about treatment, working, or other activities. Patients also may want to discuss concerns about the future, family relationships, and finances. It may help to talk with a nurse, social worker, counselor, or member of the clergy.

Friends and relatives can be very supportive. Also, it helps many patients to meet and talk with others who are facing problems like theirs. Cancer patients often get together in support groups, where they can share what they have learned about cancer, its treatment, and coping with the disease. It's important to keep in mind, however, that each patient is different. Treatments and ways of dealing with cancer that work for one person may not be right for another—even if they both have the same kind of cancer. It is always a good idea to discuss the advice of friends and family members with the doctor.

Often, a social worker at the hospital or clinic can suggest local and national groups that help with rehabilitation, emotional support, financial aid, transportation, or home care. Cancer patients and their families also can find helpful suggestions in the National Cancer Institute booklet *Taking Time*.

Possible Causes

Scientists at hospitals, medical schools, and research laboratories across the country are studying multiple myeloma. At this time, we do not know what causes this disease or how to prevent it. However, we do know that no one can "catch" multiple myeloma from another person; cancer is not contagious.

Although scientists cannot explain why one person gets multiple myeloma and another doesn't, we do know that most multiple myeloma patients are between 50 and 70 years old. This disease affects blacks more often than whites and men more often than women.

Some research suggests that certain risk factors increase a person's chance of getting multiple myeloma. For example, a person's family background appears to affect the risk of developing multiple myeloma; children and brothers and sisters of patients who have this disease have a slightly increased risk. Farmers and petroleum workers exposed to certain chemicals also seem to have a higher-than-average chance of getting multiple myeloma. In addition, people exposed to large amounts of radiation (such as survivors of the atomic bomb explosions in Japan) have an increased risk for this disease. Scientists have some concern that smaller amounts of radiation (such as those radiologists and workers in nuclear plants are exposed to) also may increase the risk. At this time, however, scientists do not have clear evidence that large numbers of medical x-rays increase the risk for multiple myeloma. In fact, most people receive a fairly small number of x-rays, and scientists believe that the benefits of medical x-rays far outweigh the possible risk for multiple myeloma.

In most cases, people who develop multiple myeloma have no clear risk factors. The disease may be the result of several factors (known and/or unknown) acting together.

Other Booklets

Cancer patients, their families and friends, and others may find the following booklets useful. They are available free of charge by calling 1-800-4-CANCER or writing:

Office of Cancer Communications
National Cancer Institute
Building 31, Room 10A24
Bethesda, MD 20892

Booklets about Cancer Treatment

Radiation Therapy and You: A Guide to Self-Help During Treatment *

Chemotherapy and You: A Guide to Self-Help During Treatment *

Eating Hints: Recipes and Tips for Better Nutrition During Cancer Treatment *

Questions and Answers About Pain Control

What Are Clinical Trials All About?

Booklets about Living with Cancer

Taking Time: Support for People With Cancer and the People Who Care About Them

When Cancer Recurs: Meeting the Challenge Again *

Advanced Cancer: Living Each Day *

* Reprinted in this volume—see Table of Contents

National Cancer Institute Information Resources

You may want more information for yourself, your family, and your doctor. The following National Cancer Institute (NCI) services are available to help you.

Telephone

Cancer Information Service (CIS) Provides accurate, up-to-date information on cancer to patients and their families, health professionals, and the general public. Information specialists translate the latest scientific information into understandable language and respond in English, Spanish, or on TTY equipment.

Toll-free: 1-800-4-CANCER (1-800-422-6237)
TTY: 1-800-332-8615

Internet

http://www.nci.nih.gov—NCI's primary Web site; contains information about the Institute and its programs.

http://cancertrials.nci.nih.gov—CancerTrials; NCI's comprehensive clinical trials information center for patients, health professionals, and the public. Includes information on understanding trials, deciding whether to participate in trials, finding specific trials, plus research news and other resources.

http://cancernet.nci.nih.gov—CancerNet; contains material for health professionals, patients, and the public, including information from PDQ about cancer treatment, screening, prevention, supportive care, and clinical trials, and CANCERLIT, a bibliographic database.

E-mail

CancerMail—Includes NCI information about cancer treatment, screening, prevention, and supportive care. To obtain a contents list, send e-mail to cancermail@icicc.nci.nih.gov with the word "help" in the body of the message.

Fax

CancerFax—Includes NCI information about cancer treatment, screening, prevention, and supportive care. To obtain a contents list, dial 301-402-5874 from a fax machine hand set and follow the recorded instructions.

Chapter 58

Myeloproliferative Disorders

What Are Myeloproliferative Disorders?

Myeloproliferative disorders are diseases in which too many of certain types of blood cells are made in the bone marrow. The bone marrow is the spongy tissue inside the large bones in the body. The bone marrow makes red blood cells (which carry oxygen to all the tissues in the body), white blood cells (which fight infection), and platelets (which make the blood clot).

There are four types of myeloproliferative disorders: chronic myelogenous leukemia, polycythemia vera, agnogenic myeloid metaplasia, and essential thrombocythemia. Chronic myelogenous leukemia affects the cells that are developing into white blood cells, called granulocytes. See the PDQ patient information summary on chronic myelogenous leukemia for treatment of that disease.

Polycythemia vera means too many red blood cells are made in the bone marrow and build up in the blood. The spleen (the organ in the upper abdomen that filters the blood to remove old cells) may swell because the extra blood cells collect there. Also, a person may have itching all over the body.

Agnogenic myeloid metaplasia means red blood cells and certain white blood cells called granulocytes do not mature properly. The red blood cells look like teardrops instead of discs. The spleen may swell and there may be too few mature red blood cells to carry oxygen, causing anemia.

PDQ Statement, National Cancer Institute (NCI), updated January 1999.

Essential thrombocythemia means the number of platelets in the blood is much higher than normal without any known cause, but other cells in the blood are normal. The extra platelets make it hard for the blood to flow normally.

If there are symptoms, a doctor will order blood tests to count the numbers of each of the different cells in the blood. If the results of the tests are not normal, more blood tests may be done. The doctor may also do a bone marrow biopsy. During this test, a needle is inserted into a bone to take out some of the marrow. The marrow is then looked at under a microscope. The doctor can then tell what kind of disease the patient has and plan the best treatment.

The chance of recovery (prognosis) depends on the type of myeloproliferative disorder, and the patient's age and general health. The diseases usually vary from person to person, often progressing slowly and requiring little treatment. In some people, the disease may turn into an acute leukemia, in which too many white blood cells are made.

Stages of Myeloproliferative Disorders

There is no staging for these diseases. Treatment depends on the type of myeloproliferative disorder the patient has.

How Myeloproliferative Disorders Are Treated

There are treatments for all patients with myeloproliferative disorders. Usually the diseases cannot be cured, but the symptoms can be controlled and the number of blood cells can be reduced with treatment. Sometimes there are few symptoms and no treatment is needed.

Chemotherapy uses drugs to kill extra blood cells in the body. Chemotherapy may be taken by pill, or it may be put into the body by a needle in the vein or muscle. Chemotherapy is called a systemic treatment because the drug enters the bloodstream, travels through the body, and can kill cells throughout the body.

Phlebotomy is taking blood from the body by a needle in a vein. This treatment is used in polycythemia vera to lower the amount of blood in the body.

Sometimes a special machine is used to filter platelets from the blood. This is called plateletpheresis.

Radiation therapy can be used to relieve symptoms. Radiation therapy uses high-energy x-rays to kill cells. Radiation therapy for the myeloproliferative disorders is usually given from a machine outside the body (external beam radiation therapy). A radioactive drug called P32 can also be given by a needle in a vein to lower the number of red blood cells made by the bone marrow.

Hormones can also be used in certain instances to treat side effects of the disease. In patients with agnogenic myeloid metaplasia, hormones called glucocorticoids may be given to help the red blood cells live longer. Hormones called androgens are also sometimes used in this disease to make the bone marrow produce more blood cells.

Surgery to remove the spleen (splenectomy) may be done if the spleen is swollen.

Biological therapy is being tested for the treatment of myeloproliferative disorders. Biological therapy tries to get the body to fight disease. It uses materials made by the body or made in a laboratory to boost, direct, or restore the body's natural defenses against disease. Biological therapy is sometimes called biological response modifier (BRM) therapy or immunotherapy.

Treatment by Type

Treatment for myeloproliferative disorders depends on the type of myeloproliferative disorder, whether the patient has symptoms or not, and the patient's age and overall health.

Standard treatment may be considered because of its effectiveness in patients in past studies, or participation in a clinical trial may be considered. Most patients with myeloproliferative disorders are not cured with standard therapy and some standard treatments may have more side effects than are desired. For these reasons, clinical trials are designed to find better ways to treat cancer patients and are based on the most up-to-date information. Clinical trials are ongoing in most parts of the country for the myeloproliferative disorders. To learn more about clinical trials, call the Cancer Information Service at 1-800-4-CANCER (1-800-422-6237); TTY at 1-800-332-8615.

Polycythemia Vera

Treatment may be one or more of the following:

1. Phlebotomy from time to time to lower the amount of blood in the body.

2. Chemotherapy or P32 radiation therapy to lower the number of red blood cells.

3. Biological therapy.

Agnogenic Myeloid Metaplasia

Treatment may be one or more of the following:

1. If there are no symptoms, treatment may not be needed. The doctor will follow the patient closely so treatment can be started if symptoms develop.

2. External radiation therapy to the spleen.

3. Chemotherapy to reduce swelling of the spleen.

4. Hormone therapy to increase the number of red blood cells.

5. Surgery to remove the spleen (splenectomy).

6. A clinical trial of biological therapy.

Essential Thrombocythemia

Treatment may be one or more of the following:

1. Chemotherapy to lower the number of platelets in the blood.

2. Plateletpheresis to remove extra platelets from the blood.

3. A clinical trial of biological therapy.

To Learn More

To learn more about myeloproliferative disorders, call the National Cancer Institute's Cancer Information Service at 1-800-4-CANCER (1-800-422-6237); TTY at 1-800-332-8615. By dialing this toll-free number, trained information specialists can answer your questions.

Cancer patients, their families and friends, and others may find the following booklets useful. They are available free of charge by calling 1-800-4-CANCER or writing:

Office of Cancer Communications
National Cancer Institute
Building 31, Room 10A24
Bethesda, MD 20892

Booklets about Cancer Treatment

Radiation Therapy and You: A Guide to Self-Help During Treatment *

Chemotherapy and You: A Guide to Self-Help During Treatment *

Eating Hints: Recipes and Tips for Better Nutrition During Cancer Treatment *

Questions and Answers About Pain Control

What Are Clinical Trials All About?

Booklets about Living with Cancer

Taking Time: Support for People With Cancer and the People Who Care About Them

When Cancer Recurs: Meeting the Challenge Again *

Advanced Cancer: Living Each Day *

* Reprinted in this volume—see Table of Contents

Chapter 59

Carcinoma of Unknown Primary

What Is Carcinoma of Unknown Primary?

Carcinoma of unknown primary (CUP) is a disease in which cancer (malignant) cells are found somewhere in the body, but the place where they first started growing (the origin or primary site) cannot be found. This occurs in about 2 to 4 percent of cancer patients.

Actually, CUP can be described as a group of different types of cancer all of which have become known by the place or places in the body where the cancer has spread (metastasized) from another part of the body. Because all of these diseases are not alike, chance of recovery (prognosis) and choice of treatment may be different for each patient.

If CUP is suspected, a doctor will order several tests, one of which may be a biopsy. This means a small piece of tissue is cut from the tumor and looked at under a microscope. The doctor may also do a complete history and physical examination, and order chest x-rays along with blood, urine, and stool tests. A cancer can be called CUP when the doctor cannot tell from the test results where the cancer began.

The pattern of how CUP has spread may also give the doctor information to help determine where it started. For example, lung metastases are more common when cancer begins above the diaphragm (the thin muscle under the lungs that helps the breathing process). Most large studies have shown that CUP often starts in the lungs or pancreas. Less often, it may start in the colon, rectum, breast, or prostate.

PDQ statement, National Cancer Institute, revised February 1999.

577

An important part of trying to find out where the cancer started is to see how the cancer cells look under a microscope (histology). Other special tests may also be done that help the doctor find out where the cancer started and choose the best type of treatment.

Stages of Carcinoma of Unknown Primary

When cancer is diagnosed, more tests are usually done to find out if cancer cells have spread to other parts of the body. This is called staging. But, when CUP is diagnosed, the number and type of tests done may be different for each patient. The treatment options in this summary are based on whether the cancer has just been found (newly diagnosed) or the cancer has come back after it has been treated (recurrent).

The treatment options are also based on where the cancer is found or what it looks like. A doctor may find that the cancer fits into one of the following groups:

- Cancer in the cervical lymph nodes: cancer in the small, bean-shaped organs that make and store infection-fighting cells (lymph nodes) in the neck area

- Poorly differentiated carcinomas: the cancer cells look very different from normal cells

- Metastatic melanoma to a single nodal site: cancer of the cells that color the skin (melanocytes) that has spread to lymph nodes in only one part of the body

- Isolated axillary metastasis: cancer that has spread only to lymph nodes in the area of the armpits

- Inguinal node metastasis: cancer that has spread to lymph nodes in the groin area

- Multiple involvement: cancer that has spread to several different areas of the body

How Carcinoma of Unknown Primary Is Treated

Many different treatments are used either alone or in combination to treat CUP. Some of the treatments that are used are:

- surgery (taking out the cancer in an operation)

- radiation therapy (using high-dose x-rays to kill cancer cells)

- chemotherapy (using drugs to kill cancer cells)
- hormone therapy (using hormones to stop the cancer cells from growing)

Surgery is a common treatment for CUP. A doctor may remove the cancer and some of the healthy tissue around it. Different operations are used depending on where the cancer is found. If the cancer has spread to lymph nodes, the lymph nodes may be removed (lymph node dissection). If the nodes involved are in the groin, this operation is called a superficial groin dissection. If the cancer has spread to lymph nodes and also to some surrounding areas, the doctor may have to remove a larger portion of tissue around the nodes. When muscles, nerves, and other tissue in the neck are removed, this is called a radical neck dissection.

Radiation therapy uses x-rays or other high-energy rays to kill cancer cells and shrink tumors. Radiation may be used alone or before or after surgery.

Chemotherapy uses drugs to kill cancer cells. Chemotherapy may be taken by mouth or it may be put into the body by a needle in a vein or muscle. Chemotherapy is called a systemic treatment because the drugs enter the bloodstream, travel through the body, and can kill cancer cells throughout the body. Chemotherapy may be used alone or after surgery. Therapy given after an operation when there are no cancer cells that can be seen is called adjuvant therapy.

Hormone therapy is used to stop the hormones in the body that help cancer cells grow. This may be done by using drugs that change the way hormones work or by surgery that takes out organs that make hormones, such as the testicles (orchiectomy).

Treatment by Stage

Treatment of CUP depends on where the doctor thinks the cancer started, what the cancer cells look like under a microscope, and other factors. Surgery and tests may be done to find where the cancer started.

Standard treatment may be considered because of its effectiveness in patients in past studies, or participation in a clinical trial may be considered. Not all patients are cured with standard therapy and some standard treatments may have more side effects than are desired. For these reasons, clinical trials are designed to find better ways to treat cancer patients and are based on the most up-to-date information. Clinical trials are ongoing in most parts of the country for CUP. To learn more about clinical trials, call the Cancer Information Service at 1-800-4-CANCER (1-800-422-6237); TTY at 1-800-332-8615.

Newly Diagnosed Carcinoma of Unknown Primary

If the cancer is in the neck area (cervical lymph nodes), treatment may be one of the following:

1. Surgery to remove the tonsils (tonsillectomy).

2. Radiation therapy.

3. Radiation therapy followed by surgery.

4. Neck surgery (radical neck dissection).

5. Neck surgery followed by radiation therapy.

More information is available in the PDQ patient information summary for metastatic squamous neck cancer with occult primary.

If the cancer is a poorly differentiated carcinoma (the cancer cells look very different than normal cells), the treatment will probably be chemotherapy. Surgery or radiation therapy has also been used for patients with neuroendocrine (nervous system and hormonal system) cancer.

If the cancer is peritoneal adenocarcinomatosis (the tumor is in the lining inside the abdomen), the treatment will probably be chemotherapy.

If the cancer is an isolated axillary nodal metastasis, it is likely that the cancer started in the lung or breast. If female, a mammogram (an x-ray picture of the breast) will be used to check for breast cancer. After tests to check for lung and breast cancer, the treatment may be one of the following:

1. Surgery to remove the lymph nodes with or without surgery to remove the breast (mastectomy) or radiation therapy to the breast.

2. Treatment as described above plus chemotherapy that is used for breast cancer.

If the cancer is in the inguinal nodes, the treatment may be one of the following:

1. Surgery to remove the cancer.

2. Groin surgery (superficial groin dissection).

3. Surgery to remove some of the tumor (biopsy) with or without radiation therapy, surgery to remove the lymph nodes, or chemotherapy.

If the cancer is melanoma that has spread to a single nodal site, the treatment will probably be surgery to remove the lymph nodes.

If there is cancer in several different areas of the body and the doctor thinks that the origin of the cancer is one for which there is standard systemic therapy, then that therapy should be given. The following are examples:

1. Hormone therapy for prostate cancer.

2. Chemotherapy or hormone therapy for breast cancer.

3. Chemotherapy for ovarian cancer.

If the source of the cancer cannot be found, then the best treatment may not be known. Patients may want to consider taking part in a clinical trial.

Recurrent Carcinoma of Unknown Primary

Treatment of recurrent CUP depends on the type of cancer, what treatment was received before, the part of the body where the cancer has come back, and other factors. A patient may want to consider taking part in a clinical trial.

To Learn More

To learn more about carcinoma of unknown primary, call the National Cancer Institute's Cancer Information Service at 1-800-4-CAN-CER (1-800-422-6237); TTY at 1-800-332-8615. By dialing this toll-free number, trained information specialists can answer your questions.

The Cancer Information Service also has booklets about cancer that are available to the public and can be sent on request. The following general booklets on questions related to cancer may be helpful:

What You Need To Know About Cancer

Taking Time: Support for People with Cancer and the People Who Care About Them

What Are Clinical Trials All About?

Chemotherapy and You: A Guide to Self-Help During Treatment *

Radiation Therapy and You: A Guide to Self-Help During Treatment *

Eating Hints for Cancer Patients *

Advanced Cancer: Living Each Day *

When Cancer Recurs: Meeting the Challenge Again *

* Reprinted in this volume—see Table of Contents

There are many other places where people can get material and information about cancer treatment and services. The social service office at a hospital can be checked for local and national agencies that help with getting information about finances, getting to and from treatment, getting care at home, and dealing with problems.

For more information from the National Cancer Institute, please write to this address:

National Cancer Institute
Office of Cancer Communications
31 Center Drive, MSC 2580
Bethesda, MD 20892-2580

Chapter 60

Malignant Mesothelioma

What Is Malignant Mesothelioma?

Malignant mesothelioma, a rare form of cancer, is a disease in which cancer (malignant) cells are found in the sac lining the chest (the pleura) or abdomen (the peritoneum). Most people with malignant mesothelioma have worked on jobs where they breathed asbestos.

A doctor should be seen if a person has shortness of breath, pain in the chest, or pain or swelling in the abdomen. If there are symptoms, the doctor may order an x-ray of the chest or abdomen.

The doctor may look inside the chest cavity with a special instrument called a thoracoscope. A cut will be made through the chest wall and the thoracoscope will be put into the chest between two ribs. This test, called thoracoscopy, is usually done in the hospital. Before the test, the patient will be given a local anesthetic (a drug that causes a loss of feeling for a short period of time). Some pressure may be felt, but usually there is no pain.

The doctor may also look inside the abdomen (peritoneoscopy) with a special tool called a peritoneoscope. The peritoneoscope is put into an opening made in the abdomen. This test is also usually done in the hospital. Before the test is done, a local anesthetic will be given.

If tissue that is not normal is found, the doctor will need to cut out a small piece and have it looked at under a microscope to see if there

PDQ statement, National Cancer Institute, revised March 1998.

are any cancer cells. This is called a biopsy. Biopsies are usually done during the thoracoscopy or peritoneoscopy.

The chance of recovery (prognosis) depends on the size of the cancer, where the cancer is, how far the cancer has spread, how the cancer cells look under the microscope, how the cancer responds to treatment, and the patient's age.

Stages of Malignant Mesothelioma

Once malignant mesothelioma is found, more tests will be done to find out if cancer cells have spread to other parts of the body. This is called staging. A doctor needs to know the stage of the cancer to plan treatment. The following stages are used for malignant mesothelioma.

Localized Malignant Mesothelioma

Stage I: The cancer is found in the lining of the chest cavity near the lung and heart or in the diaphragm or the lung.

Advanced Malignant Mesothelioma

Stage II: The cancer has spread beyond the lining of the chest to lymph nodes in the chest.

Stage III: Cancer has spread into the chest wall, center of the chest, heart, through the diaphragm, or abdominal lining, and in some cases into nearby lymph nodes.

Stage IV: Cancer has spread to distant organs or tissues.

Recurrent Malignant Mesothelioma

Recurrent disease means that the cancer has come back (recurred) after it has been treated. It may come back in the lining of the chest or abdomen or in another part of the body.

How Malignant Mesothelioma Is Treated

There are treatments for all patients with malignant mesothelioma. Three kinds of treatment are used:

- surgery (taking out the cancer)

- radiation therapy (using high-dose x-rays or other high-energy rays to kill cancer cells)

- chemotherapy (using drugs to fight the cancer)

Surgery is a common treatment of malignant mesothelioma. The doctor may remove part of the lining of the chest or abdomen and some of the tissue around it. Depending on how far the cancer has spread, a lung also may be removed in an operation called a pneumonectomy. Sometimes part of the diaphragm, the muscle below the lungs that helps with breathing, is also removed.

Radiation therapy uses high-energy x-rays to kill cancer cells and shrink tumors. Radiation may come from a machine outside the body (external radiation therapy) or from putting materials that produce radiation (radioisotopes) through thin plastic tubes in the area where the cancer cells are found (internal radiation therapy).

If fluid has collected in the chest or abdomen, the doctor may drain the fluid out of the body by putting a needle into the chest or abdomen and using gentle suction to remove the fluid. If fluid is removed from the chest, this is called thoracentesis. If fluid is removed from the abdomen, this is called paracentesis. The doctor may also put drugs through a tube into the chest to prevent more fluid from accumulating.

Chemotherapy uses drugs to kill cancer cells. Chemotherapy may be taken by pill, or it may be put into the body by a needle in the vein or muscle. Chemotherapy is called a systemic treatment because the drug enters the bloodstream, travels through the body, and can kill cancer cells throughout the body. In mesothelioma, chemotherapy may be put directly into the chest (intrapleural chemotherapy).

Intraoperative photodynamic therapy is a new type of treatment that uses special drugs and light to kill cancer cells during surgery. A drug that makes cancer cells more sensitive to light is injected into a vein several days before surgery. During surgery to remove as much of the cancer as possible, a special light is used to shine on the pleura. This treatment is being studied for early stages of mesothelioma in the chest.

Treatment by Stage

Treatment depends on where the cancer is, how far it has spread, and the patient's age and general health.

Standard treatment may be considered because of its effectiveness in patients in past studies, or participation in a clinical trial may be considered. Not all patients are cured with standard therapy and some standard treatments may have more side effects than are desired. For these reasons, clinical trials are designed to find better ways to treat cancer patients and are based on the most up-to-date information. Clinical trials are ongoing in many parts of the country for many patients with malignant mesothelioma. To learn more about clinical trials, call the Cancer Information Service at 1-800-4-CANCER (1-800-422-6237); TTY at 1-800-332-8615.

Localized Malignant Mesothelioma (Stage I)

If the cancer is only in one place in the chest or abdomen, treatment will probably be surgery to remove part of the pleura and some of the tissue around it.

If the cancer is found in a larger part of the pleura, treatment may be one of the following:

1. Surgery to remove the pleura and the tissue near it to relieve symptoms, with or without radiation therapy after surgery.

2. Surgery to remove sections of the pleura, the lung, part of the diaphragm, and part of the lining around the heart.

3. External beam radiation therapy to relieve symptoms.

4. A clinical trial of surgery followed by chemotherapy given inside the chest.

5. A clinical trial of surgery, radiation therapy, and/or chemotherapy.

Advanced Malignant Mesothelioma (Stages II, III, and IV)

Treatment may be one of the following:

1. Draining of fluid in the chest or abdomen (thoracentesis or paracentesis) to reduce discomfort. Drugs also may be put into the chest or abdomen to prevent further collection of fluid.

2. Surgery to relieve symptoms.

3. Radiation therapy to relieve symptoms.

4. Chemotherapy.

5. A clinical trial of surgery, radiation therapy, and chemotherapy.

6. Chemotherapy given in the chest or abdomen.

Recurrent Malignant Mesothelioma

Treatment depends on many factors, including where the cancer came back and what treatment the patient received before. Clinical trials are testing new treatments.

To Learn More

To learn more about malignant mesothelioma, call the National Cancer Institute's Cancer Information Service at 1-800-4-CANCER (1-800-422-6237); TTY at 1-800-332-8615. By dialing this toll-free number, trained information specialists can answer your questions.

The Cancer Information Service also has booklets about cancer that are available to the public and can be sent on request. The following general booklets on questions related to cancer may be helpful:

What You Need To Know About Cancer

Taking Time: Support for People with Cancer and the People Who Care About Them

What Are Clinical Trials All About?

Chemotherapy and You: A Guide to Self-Help During Treatment *

Radiation Therapy and You: A Guide to Self-Help During Treatment *

Eating Hints for Cancer Patients *

Advanced Cancer: Living Each Day *

When Cancer Recurs: Meeting the Challenge Again *

* Reprinted in this volume—see Table of Contents

There are many other places where people can get material and information about cancer treatment and services. The social service office at a hospital can be checked for local and national agencies that help with getting information about finances, getting to and from treatment, getting care at home, and dealing with problems.

For more information from the National Cancer Institute, please write to this address:

National Cancer Institute
Office of Cancer Communications
31 Center Drive, MSC 2580
Bethesda, MD 20892-2580

Chapter 61

Neuroblastoma

Neuroblastoma

Neuroblastoma is a solid cancerous tumor that begins in nerve tissue in the neck, chest, abdomen, or pelvis but usually originates in the abdomen in the tissues of the adrenal gland. By the time it is diagnosed, the cancer usually has spread (metastasized), most commonly to the lymph nodes, liver, lungs, bones, and bone marrow. Neuroblastoma is predominantly a tumor of early childhood; two thirds of children with neuroblastoma are diagnosed when they are younger than 5 years of age. It is often present at birth but usually is not detected until later; in rare cases, neuroblastoma can be detected before birth by fetal ultrasound.

The most common symptoms of neuroblastoma are the result of pressure by the tumor or bone pain from cancer that has spread to the bone. Protruding eyes and dark circles around the eyes are common and are caused by cancer that has spread to the area behind the eye. Neuroblastomas may compress the spinal cord, causing paralysis. Fever, anemia, and high blood pressure are found occasionally. Rarely, children may have severe watery diarrhea, uncoordinated or jerky muscle movements, or uncontrollable eye movement.

If your child has symptoms that may be caused by neuroblastoma, his or her doctor will conduct a careful examination and order laboratory tests and special x-rays. A computed tomographic (CT) scan, a diagnostic test that uses computers and x-rays to create pictures of

PDQ Statement, National Cancer Institute, revised February 1999.

the body, may be performed. A magnetic resonance imaging (MRI) scan, a diagnostic test similar to a CT scan but which uses magnetic waves instead of x-rays, may also be performed.

Often, removal of tissue from the tumor and/or bone marrow is required to determine whether neuroblastoma exists. A small sample of the tissue may be surgically removed and examined under a microscope. This is called a biopsy. Sometimes a biopsy is done by making a small hole and using a needle to extract a sample of the tissue.

Your child's chance of recovery (prognosis) and choice of treatment depend on the stage of your child's cancer (how far your child's cancer has spread), your child's age at diagnosis, the location of the tumor, and evaluation of the tumor cells under a microscope.

Stage Explanation

Once neuroblastoma is found, more tests will be done to find out if the cancer has spread from where it started to surrounding tissues or other parts of the body. This is called staging. Your child's doctor needs to know the stage of the disease to plan treatment. Although there are several staging systems currently available for neuroblastoma, for the purposes of treatment the disease is categorized as follows:

Localized Resectable

The cancer is confined to the site of origin, there is no evidence of spread, and the cancer can be surgically removed.

Localized Unresectable

The cancer is confined to the site of origin but the cancer cannot be completely removed surgically.

Regional

The cancer has extended beyond the site of origin to regional lymph nodes and/or surrounding organs or tissues, but has not spread to distant parts of the body.

Disseminated

The cancer has spread from the site of origin to distant lymph nodes, bone, liver, skin, bone marrow, and/or other organs (except as defined for stage IVS).

Stage IVS

Stage IVS neuroblastoma is also called "special" neuroblastoma because it is treated differently. The cancer is localized, with dissemination (spread) limited to liver, skin, and/or, to a very limited extent, bone marrow.

Recurrent

Recurrent neuroblastoma means that the cancer has come back (recurred) or continued to spread (progressed) after it has been treated. It may come back in the original site or in another part of the body.

Treatment Option Overview

There are treatments for all children with neuroblastoma. Treatment options are related to age at diagnosis, tumor location, stage of disease, regional lymph node involvement, and tumor biology. Four types of treatment are used:

- surgery (removing the tumor in an operation).

- radiation therapy (using high-dose x-rays or other high-energy rays to kill cancer cells and shrink tumors).

- chemotherapy (using drugs to kill cancer cells and shrink tumors).

- bone marrow transplantation (replacing the patient's bone marrow with healthy bone marrow).

More than one method of treatment may be used, depending on the needs of the patient. Surgery is used when possible to remove as much of the cancer as possible. If the cancer cannot be removed, surgery may be limited to a biopsy of the cancer.

Radiation therapy uses high-energy rays (radiation) to damage or kill cancer cells and shrink tumors. Radiation usually comes from a machine outside the body (external beam radiation therapy).

Chemotherapy is the use of drugs to kill cancer cells and shrink tumors. Chemotherapy drugs may be taken by mouth or injected into a vein (intravenous) or a muscle. Chemotherapy is called a systemic treatment because the drug enters the bloodstream, travels through the body, and can kill cancer cells throughout the body. Chemotherapy may be given after the tumor has been surgically removed to kill any remaining cancer cells; this is called adjuvant chemotherapy. Chemotherapy can also be given before surgery to shrink the cancer so that it can be removed during surgery; this is called neoadjuvant chemotherapy.

Bone marrow transplantation is a procedure in which healthy bone marrow is given to replace bone marrow destroyed by treatment with high doses of anticancer drugs or radiation. Transplantation may be autologous (the patient's own marrow saved earlier and possibly treated with drugs to kill any cancer cells), allogeneic (marrow from a healthy "matched" donor, usually a brother or sister), or syngeneic (marrow from an identical twin).

Treatment by Stage

For the purposes of treatment presented here, neuroblastoma is categorized as localized resected, localized unresected, regional, disseminated, and special.

Your child may receive treatment that is considered standard based on its effectiveness in a number of people in past studies, or you may choose to enter your child in a clinical trial. Not all patients are cured with standard therapy and some standard treatments may have more side effects than are desired. For these reasons, clinical trials are designed to test new treatments and to find better ways to treat people with cancer. Clinical trials are ongoing in most parts of the country for most stages of neuroblastoma. If you want more information, call the Cancer Information Service at 1-800-4-CANCER (1-800-422-6237); TTY at 1-800-332-8615.

Localized Resectable Neuroblastoma

Your child's treatment may be one of the following:

1. Surgery to remove the cancer.

2. Surgery plus adjuvant chemotherapy.

3. Surgery plus radiation therapy.

Localized Unresectable Neuroblastoma

Initial treatment generally consists of surgical removal of as much of the cancer as possible followed by chemotherapy. A second surgery may be performed to remove any cancer that remains, and radiation therapy may then be given.

Regional Neuroblastoma

Treatment depends on your child's age.

If your child is younger than 1 year of age, treatment may include the following:

1. Surgery to remove the cancer.
2. Chemotherapy.

If your child is older than 1 year of age, treatment may be one of the following:

1. Surgery to remove the cancer.
2. Surgery followed by chemotherapy.
3. Chemotherapy with or without radiation therapy to reduce the tumor, followed by surgery.
4. Multi-drug chemotherapy.
5. Radiation therapy.
6. A clinical trial of new methods of treatment. Listings of current clinical trials are available on PDQ or by calling the National Cancer Institute's Cancer Information Service at 1-800-4-CANCER.

Disseminated Neuroblastoma

Your child's treatment may be one of the following:

1. Multi-drug chemotherapy with or without surgery and/or radiation therapy.
2. A clinical trial of new methods of treatment. Listings of current clinical trials are available on PDQ or by calling the National Cancer Institute's Cancer Information Service at 1-800-4-CANCER.

Stage IVS Neuroblastoma

Children with this special type of neuroblastoma may not require therapy. You may want to have your child take part in a clinical trial of new methods of treatment. Listings of current clinical trials are available on PDQ or by calling the National Cancer Institute's Cancer Information Service at 1-800-4-CANCER.

Recurrent Neuroblastoma

The selection of treatment of recurrent or progressive neuroblastoma depends on the location and extent of the recurrence or progression and on the previous therapy as well as individual patient considerations.

A clinical trial may be appropriate. Listings of current clinical trials are available on PDQ or by calling the National Cancer Institute's Cancer Information Service at 1-800-4-CANCER.

To Learn More

To learn more about neuroblastoma, call the National Cancer Institute's Cancer Information Service at 1-800-4-CANCER (1-800-422-6237); TTY at 1-800-332-8615. The call is toll-free and a trained information specialist can answer your questions.

The Cancer Information Service can also send you booklets. The following booklets on childhood cancer may be helpful to you:

Young People with Cancer: A Handbook for Parents

Talking with Your Child About Cancer

Managing Your Child's Eating Problems During Cancer Treatment

When Someone in Your Family Has Cancer

The following general booklets on topics related to cancer may also be helpful:

Taking Time: Support for People with Cancer and the People Who Care About Them

What Are Clinical Trials All About?

Chemotherapy and You: A Guide to Self-Help During Treatment *

Radiation Therapy and You: A Guide to Self-Help During Treatment *

What You Need To Know About Cancer *

* Reprinted in this volume—see Table of Contents

There are many other places where material about cancer treatment and information about services are available. Check the hospital social service office for local and national agencies that help with finances, getting to and from treatment, care at home, and dealing with other problems. Write to the National Cancer Institute at this address:

National Cancer Institute
Office of Cancer Communications
31 Center Drive, MSC 2580
Bethesda, MD 20892-2580

Part Three

Treatments and Therapies

Chapter 62

Your Health Care Team: Your Doctor Is Only the Beginning

Coping with cancer is not an easy thing. The physical effects of illness and treatment can be quite severe, and the emotional and psychological impact of having cancer can be equally challenging. However, the good news is that there are many different kinds of help available to you through the different members of your health care team.

Below is a description of the health care professionals who are usually accessible to someone who has cancer. Each of these people can play a vital role in helping you obtain the best treatment possible and maintain the highest quality of life throughout your diagnosis and treatment.

First Things First: Your Own Role

It may seem obvious, but it is very important to remember that you are the most important person on your health care team. As with any type of health care you receive, you are a consumer of services, and you should not be afraid to ask questions about what you are getting and who is providing it.

You might consider these tips:

- When you are going to meet with someone (a doctor, nurse, or specialist), bring someone else with you. It helps to have another person hear what is said and think of questions to ask.

"Your Health Care Team: Your Doctor Is Only the Beginning," National Cancer Institute (NCI), February 1998.

- Write out your questions beforehand to make sure you don't forget to discuss any.

- Write down the answers you get, and make sure you understand what you are hearing.

- Don't be afraid to ask your questions or ask where you can find more information about what you are discussing. Being well-informed is your most important task on the health care team.

Social Workers: Lots of Help from One Place

Social workers are professionally trained in counseling and practical assistance. They provide the broadest range of help to people with cancer, and are a good place to start if you have recently been diagnosed with cancer and aren't sure what to do next. Oncology social workers specialize in cancer; most hospitals that treat cancer patients have certified oncology social workers on staff. Clinical or psychiatric social workers have an advanced degree or Ph.D. in social work and are trained to provide family therapy, marital counseling, or counseling focused on coping with chronic illness. A hospital social worker can also refer you to a clinical social worker in private practice in the community.

The hospital social worker can also provide counseling, find a support group for you, locate services in your community that can help you with home care or transportation, and guide you through the process of applying to the government for Social Service Disability or other forms of assistance. They can also help you understand your diagnosis and talk to you about treatment, side effects, and what to expect. If you need help finding a social worker in your area, start at your local hospital.

Psychiatrists: If You Need Medication or Feel Depressed

A psychiatrist is a medical doctor who specializes in providing psychotherapy, or general psychological help. A psychiatrist specializes in helping people who are depressed, anxious, or otherwise unable to cope psychologically. Because they are medical doctors, psychiatrists can also prescribe medication, such as anti-depressants or medication to help you sleep. To find a psychiatrist, you can ask your doctor for a referral, ask if your hospital has a psychiatric department, call your Health Maintenance Organization (HMO) or other managed care plan, or ask a social worker to help.

Psychologists: Providing Therapy and Counseling

A psychologist is also someone who can assist you if you are feeling depressed, anxious, or sad. While not medical doctors, psychologists have obtained a doctoral degree in psychology and counseling; many specialize in marital counseling or chronic illness. Some cancer centers have psychologists on staff but if you are looking for one, ask your doctor, your HMO, your hospital, or a social worker for a referral.

Nurses: A Very Important Role in Care

Nurses are an extremely important part of your health care team. Nurses have a wide range of skills, and are usually in charge of actually implementing the plan of care your doctor has set up for you. They are trained to administer medication and monitor side effects, and all major medical centers have nurses who specialize in cancer. Whether you are staying in the hospital for care or receive it on an outpatient basis (which means you go home after each treatment), you will benefit from seeking assistance, asking questions, or getting tips and advice from your nurse or nurse-practitioner. Nurses are often aware of support services in your community and can usually provide you with educational materials and pamphlets.

You may also arrange or request a registered nurse to visit you at home if needed. If the visit is approved by your doctor, it will usually be covered by insurance. Another option is to hire a private duty nurse who doesn't work for your hospital or health care service. This can be expensive and often is not covered by insurance, but can ease the burden of care on your family or loved ones.

Home Health Aides: Care at Home

Another form of home care is from a home health aide. Home health aides assist people who are ill and need help moving around, bathing, cooking, or doing household chores. Some state Medicaid programs will pay for home health aide care, provided they are supervised by a nurse. However, private insurance or managed care plans rarely pay for a home health aide unless there is also a need for skilled nursing care. To find home health aide care, ask your physician, nurse, or social worker, and remember to ask if the charges vary based on income. Also, the National Association of Home Care (202-547-7424) publishes a free booklet, *How to Select a Home Care Agency*. The telephone yellow pages are another source, but be sure to check credentials, find out whether the agency is bonded, and ask for references.

Rehabilitation Specialists: Help for Recovery

Rehabilitation services help people recover from physical changes caused by cancer or cancer treatment. It includes the services of physical therapists, occupational therapists, counselors, speech therapists, and other professionals who help you physically recover from cancer. For example, physical therapy can help you rebuild the muscles in your arm and shoulder if you have had chest surgery.

Most physicians will refer you to rehabilitation services if you need them; be sure to ask if you think you might want them. Also, check to see if these types of services are covered under your insurance plan (some may be, others may not). Additionally, some cancer or social service organizations may provide you with free rehabilitation services if you are not insured for them.

Dietary or Nutritional Services

Cancer and cancer treatment can cause people to lose weight. For this reason, dietary or nutrition counseling or services are commonly prescribed for people with cancer. A dietitian can suggest ways to get enough calories, vitamins, and protein to help you feel better and control your weight, and can give you tips about increasing your appetite if you experience nausea, heartburn, or fatigue from your illness or treatment.

Most hospitals have registered dietitians on staff, and you can ask your doctor about meeting with them. If you are trying to locate a dietitian in your community, be sure to ask about experience and training. Remember to check if the services of a dietitian are covered under your insurance; if not, ask your doctor, nurse, or social worker about community-based programs that offer free services.

Clergy: Spiritual Support Is Important

Prayer and spiritual counseling can be very important in coping with a serious illness such as cancer. Many people find it useful to get help from clergy or other spiritual leaders, and there is no question that a strong sense of spirituality can help people face difficult challenges with courage and a sense of hope. Some studies show that people with cancer have less anxiety and depression, even pain, when they feel spiritually connected. Even if your beliefs are challenged by your illness, don't be afraid to reach out to others for help. It is important to remember that you are not alone at this time.

Hospice Care: Help with Terminal Illness

Hospice care focuses on the special needs of people who have terminal cancer. Sometimes called palliative care, this type of care centers around providing comfort, controlling physical symptoms like pain, and giving emotional or spiritual support. Hospice care is usually provided at home, although there are hospice centers that operate much like hospitals and provide full-time care. Your doctor or social worker can refer you for hospice care.

Home hospice care is usually coordinated through a nurse, who then sends a home health aide, social worker, occupational therapist, clergy, or the type of specialist that is appropriate for the needs of the hospice patient. Hospice care is not for everyone. It is important to discuss this option carefully and get guidance from your doctor, nurse, or social worker.

Putting the Team Together: Find Help and Hope

A diagnosis of cancer may be the most difficult challenge you or your loved ones will ever face. That is why it is important to find help and try to maintain your sense of hope no matter what your situation. Your team of health care professionals is knowledgeable about the many different aspects of cancer: medical, physical, emotional, social, and spiritual. They are available to you as much or as little as you need, but it is difficult for them to know if you need help unless you ask for it. Don't be afraid, embarrassed, or hesitant to ask questions; voice your opinion, and seek the care you feel you need and deserve.

This chapter was adapted with permission from Cancer Care, Inc., a nonprofit social service agency whose mission is to help people with cancer and their families. Cancer Care's toll-free telephone number is 1-800-813-HOPE. The National Cancer Institute and Cancer Care, Inc. are in partnership to increase awareness of the psychosocial issues faced by cancer patients and to provide resources to cancer patients and their families. Cancer Information from the Office of Cancer Communications National Cancer Institute news releases are available via the Internet through the World Wide Web (http://rex.nci.nih.gov). Click on Mass Media.

Resources

Cancer Information Service: The Cancer Information Service (CIS), a national information and education network, is a free public service of the NCI, the Nation's primary agency for cancer research. The CIS meets the information needs of patients, the public, and health professionals. Specially trained staff provide the latest scientific information in understandable language. CIS staff answer questions in English and Spanish and distribute NCI materials.

Toll-free phone number: 1-800-4-CANCER (1-800-422-6237)
TTY: 1-800-332-8615 CancerFax-R

CancerFax-R: For NCI information by fax, dial (301) 402-5874 from the telephone on a fax machine and listen to recorded instructions.

Internet: For NCI information by computer:

CancerMail (via E-mail) To obtain a contents list, send E-mail to cancernet@icicc.nci.nih.gov with the word "help" in the body of the message.

CancerNet-R CancerNet is also accessible via the Internet through the World Wide Web (http://cancernet.nci.nih.gov).

Chapter 63

Chemotherapy and You:
A Guide to Self-Help during
Treatment

Introduction

This chapter will help you, your family, and your friends understand chemotherapy, the use of drugs to treat cancer. It will answer many
of the questions you may have about this method of cancer treatment.
It also will show you how you can help yourself during chemotherapy.

Taking care of yourself during chemotherapy is important for several reasons. For one thing, it can lessen some of the physical side
effects you may have from your treatment. As you will see, some
simple tips can make a big difference in how you feel. But the benefits of self-help aren't just physical; they're psychological, too. Knowing some ways to take care of yourself can give your emotions a boost
at a time when you may be feeling that much of what's happening to
you is out of your control. This feeling can be easier to deal with when
you discover how you can contribute to your own well-being, in partnership with your doctors and nurses.

Chemotherapy and You will help you become an informed partner
in your care. Remember, though, it is only a guide. Self-help is never
a substitute for professional medical care. Be sure to ask your doctor
and nurse any questions you may have about chemotherapy, and tell
them about any side effects you may have.

You will find several helpful sections at the end of this chapter. The
section on "Paying for Chemotherapy" gives you information about

"Chemotherapy and You: A Guide to Self-Help During Treatment," National Cancer Institute (NCI), NIH publication 94-856, February 1994.

603

insurance and other payment methods. The section called "Resources" tells you how to get more information about Cancer and how to find many services available to cancer patients and their families.

Understanding Chemotherapy

What Is Chemotherapy?

Chemotherapy is the use of drugs to treat cancer. The drugs often are called anticancer drugs.

How Does Chemotherapy Work?

Normal cells grow and die in a controlled way. But cancer occurs when cells become abnormal and keep dividing and forming more cells without control or order. Anticancer drugs destroy cancer cells by stopping them from growing or multiplying at one or more points in their life cycle. Because some drugs work better together than alone, chemotherapy often may consist of more than one drug. This is called combination chemotherapy.

In addition to chemotherapy other methods sometimes are used to treat cancer. For example, your doctor may recommend that you have surgery to remove a tumor or to relieve certain symptoms that may be caused by your cancer. You also may receive radiation therapy to treat your cancer or its symptoms. Sometimes, as described below, your doctor may suggest a combination of chemotherapy, surgery, and/or radiation therapy.

Other types of drugs may be used to treat your cancer. These may include certain drugs that can block the effect of hormones. Doctors also may use biological therapy to boost the body's natural defenses against cancer.

Depending on the type of cancer and its stage of development, chemotherapy can be used:

- To cure cancer.

- To keep the cancer from spreading.

- To slow the cancer's growth.

- To kill cancer cells that may have spread to other parts of the body from the original tumor.

- To relieve symptoms that may be caused by the cancer.

Chemotherapy also can help people live more comfortably; this is known as palliative care.

Will Chemotherapy Be My Only Treatment for Cancer?

Sometimes chemotherapy is the only therapy a patient receives. More often, however, chemotherapy is used in addition to surgery and/ or radiation therapy; when it is used for this purpose it is called adjuvant therapy. There are several reasons why chemotherapy may be given in addition to other treatment methods. For instance, chemotherapy may be used to shrink a tumor before surgery or radiation therapy. It also may be used after surgery and/or radiation therapy to help destroy any cancer cells that may remain.

Which Drugs Will I Get?

Your doctor decides which drug or drugs will work best for you. The decision depends on what kind of cancer you have, where it is, the extent of its growth, how it is affecting your normal body functions, and your general health.

Your doctor also may suggest that you join a clinical trial for chemotherapy, or you may want to bring up this option with your doctor. Clinical trials are carefully designed research studies that test promising new cancer treatments. Patients who take part in research may be the first to benefit from improved treatment methods. These patients also can make an important contribution to medical care because the results of the studies may help many people. Patients participate in clinical trials only if they choose to and are free to withdraw at any time.

To learn more about clinical trials, call the National Cancer Institute's Cancer Information Service and ask for the booklet *What Are Clinical Trials All About?* You also may want to ask about the videotape "Patient to Patient: Cancer Clinical Trials and You." This videotape can put to rest fears you may have about taking part in clinical trials. The Cancer Information Service can be reached by dialing 1-800-4-CANCER (1-800-422-6237).

Where Will I Get Chemotherapy?

You may get your chemotherapy at home, in your doctor's office, in a clinic, in your hospital's outpatient department, or in a hospital. The choice of where you get chemotherapy depends on which drug or drugs you are getting, your hospital's policies, and your doctor's preferences.

When you first start chemotherapy, you may need to stay at the hospital for a short time so that your doctor can watch the medicine's effects closely and make any adjustments that are needed.

How Often Will I Get Chemotherapy, and How Long Will I Get It?

How often and for how long you get chemotherapy depends on the kind of cancer you have, the goals of the treatment, the drugs that are used, and how your body responds to them. You may get chemotherapy every day, every week, or every month. Chemotherapy is often given in on-and-off cycles that include rest periods so that your body has a chance to build healthy new cells and regain its strength. Your doctor should be able to estimate how long you will be getting chemotherapy.

Whatever schedule your doctor prescribes, it is very important to stay with it. Otherwise, the anticancer drugs might not have their desired effect. If you miss a treatment session or skip a dose of medication, contact your doctor for instructions about what to do.

Sometimes, your doctor may delay a treatment based on the results of certain blood tests. Your doctor will let you know what to do during this time and when it's okay to start your treatment sessions again.

Depending on the type of cancer you have and the drug or drugs you are getting, your chemotherapy may be given in one or more of the following ways:

- Into a vein (intravenously, or IV). You will get the drug through a thin needle inserted into a vein, usually on your hand or lower arm. Another way to get IV chemotherapy is by means of a catheter, a thin tube that is placed into a large vein in your body and remains there as long as it is needed. This type of catheter is known as a central venous catheter. Sometimes, a central venous catheter is attached to a port, a small plastic or metal container placed surgically under the skin.

- By mouth (orally, or PO) in pill, capsule, or liquid form. You will swallow the drug, just as you do many other medications.

- Into a muscle (intramuscularly, or IM), under the skin (subcutaneously, or SQ or SC), or directly into a cancerous area in the skin (intralesionally, or IL). You will get an injection with a needle.

- Topically. The medication will be applied onto the skin.

Chemotherapy also may be delivered to specific areas of the body using a catheter (or a catheter plus a port). Catheters may be placed directly into the spinal fluid, abdominal cavity, bladder, or liver. Your doctor or nurse may use specific terms when talking about certain types of catheters. For example, an intrathecal (IT) catheter is used to deliver drugs into the spinal fluid. Intracavitary (IC) catheters can be placed in the abdomen, pelvis, or chest.

Two kinds of pumps—external and internal—may be used to control the rate of delivery of chemotherapy. External pumps remain outside of the body. Some are portable and allow a person to move around while the pump is in use. Other external pumps are not portable and may restrict activity. Internal pumps are placed surgically inside the body, usually right under the skin. They contain a small reservoir (storage area) that delivers the drugs into the catheter. Internal pumps allow people to go about most of their daily activities.

Does Chemotherapy Hurt?

Getting chemotherapy by mouth on the skin, or by injection generally feels the same as taking other medications by these methods. Having an IV started usually feels like having blood drawn for a blood test. Some people feel a coolness or other unusual sensation in the area of the injection when the IV is started. Report these feelings to your doctor or nurse. Be sure that you also report any pain, burning, or discomfort that occurs during or after an IV treatment.

Many people have little or no trouble having the IV needle in their hand or lower arm. However, if a person has a hard time for any reason, or if it becomes difficult to insert the needle into a vein for each treatment, it may be possible to use a central venous catheter or port. This avoids repeated insertion of the needle into the vein.

Central venous catheters and ports cause no pain or discomfort if they are properly placed and cared for, although a person usually is aware that they are there. It is important to report any pain or discomfort with a catheter or port to your doctor or nurse.

Can I Take Other Medicines while I Am Getting Chemotherapy?

Some medicines may interact with the effects of your chemotherapy. That is why you should take a list of all your medications to your doctor before you start chemotherapy. Your list should include the name of each drug, how often you take it, the reason you take it, and the dosage. Remember to include over-the-counter drugs such as laxatives, cold pills, pain relievers, and vitamins. Your doctor will tell you if you should stop taking any of these medications before you start chemotherapy. After your treatments begin, be sure to check with your doctor before taking any new medicines or stopping the ones you already are taking.

Most people are able to continue working while they are being treated with anticancer drugs. It may be possible to schedule your treatments late in the day or right before the weekend, so they interfere with work as little as possible.

If your chemotherapy makes you very tired, you might want to think about adjusting your work schedule for a while. Speak with your employer about your needs and wishes at this time. You may be able to agree on a part-time schedule, or perhaps you can do some of your work at home.

Will I Be Able to Work During Chemotherapy?

Under Federal and state laws, some employers may be required to allow you to work a flexible schedule to meet your treatment needs. To find out about your on-the-job protections, check with your local American Cancer Society, a social worker, or your congressional or state representative. The National Cancer Institute's publication *Facing Forward: A Guide for Cancer Survivors* also has information on work-related concerns.

How Will I Know If My Chemotherapy Is Working?

Your doctor and nurse will use several methods to measure how well your treatments are working. You will have frequent physical exams, blood tests, scans, and x-rays. Don't hesitate to ask the doctor about the test results and what they show about your progress.

While tests and exams can tell a lot about how chemotherapy is working, side effects tell very little. (Side effects—such as nausea or hair loss—occur because chemotherapy harms some normal cells as well as cancer cells.) Sometimes people think that if they don't have side effects, the drugs aren't working, or that, if they do have side effects, the drugs are working well. But side effects vary so much from person to person, and from drug to drug, that having them or not having them usually isn't a sign of whether the treatment is effective.

If you do have side effects, there is a lot you can do to help relieve them. The next section of this booklet describes some of the most common side effects of chemotherapy and gives you some hints for coping with them.

Coping with Side Effects

If you have questions about side effects, you are not alone. Before chemotherapy starts, most people are concerned about whether they will have side effects and, if so, what they will be like. Once treatments begin, people who have side effects want to know the best ways to cope with them. This section will answer some of your questions.

If you are reading this section before you start chemotherapy you may feel overwhelmed by the wide range of side effects it describes. But remember: Every person doesn't get every side effect, and some people get few, if any. In addition, the severity of side effects varies greatly from person to person. Whether you have a particular side effect, and how severe it will be, depends on the kind of chemotherapy you get and how your body reacts. Be sure to talk to your doctor and nurse about which side effects are most likely to occur with your chemotherapy, how long they might last, how serious they might be, and when you should seek medical attention for them.

What Causes Side Effects?

Because cancer cells grow and divide rapidly, anticancer drugs are made to kill fast-growing cells. But certain normal, healthy cells also multiply quickly, and chemotherapy can affect these cells, too. When it does, side effects may result. The fast-growing, normal cells most likely to be affected are blood cells forming in the bone marrow and cells in the digestive tract, reproductive system, and hair follicles. Anticancer drugs also can damage cells of the heart, kidney, bladder, lungs, and nervous system. The most common side effects of chemotherapy include nausea and vomiting, hair loss, and fatigue.

Other common side effects include an increased chance of bleeding, getting an infection or developing anemia. These side effects result from changes in blood cells during chemotherapy.

How Long Do Side Effects Last?

Most normal cells recover quickly when chemotherapy is over, so most side effects gradually disappear after treatment ends, and the healthy cells have a chance to grow normally. The time it takes to get over some side effects and regain energy varies from person to person. How soon you will feel better depends on many factors, including your overall health and the kinds of drugs you have been taking.

While many side effects go away fairly rapidly, certain ones may take months or years to disappear completely. Sometimes the side effects can last a lifetime as when chemotherapy causes permanent damage to the heart lungs kidneys or reproductive organs. And certain types of chemotherapy occasionally may cause delayed effects, such as a second cancer, that show up many years later.

It is important to remember that many people have no long-term problems due to chemotherapy. It also is reassuring to know that doctors are making great progress in preventing some of chemotherapy's more serious side effects. For instance, they are using many new drugs and techniques that increase chemotherapy's powerful effects on cancer cells while decreasing its harmful effects on the body's healthy cells.

The side effects of chemotherapy can be unpleasant but they must be measured against the treatment's ability to destroy cancer. People getting chemotherapy sometimes become discouraged about the length of time their treatment is taking or the side effects they are having. If that happens to you talk to your doctor. It may be that your medication or the treatment schedule can be changed. Or your doctor may be able to suggest ways to reduce side effects or make them easier to tolerate. Remember though, your doctor will not ask you to continue treatments unless the expected benefits outweigh any problems you might have.

On the pages that follow, you will find suggestions for dealing with some of the more common side effects of chemotherapy.

Nausea and Vomiting

Chemotherapy can cause nausea and vomiting by affecting the stomach, the area of the brain that controls vomiting, or both. This reaction to chemotherapy varies from person to person and from drug to drug. For example, some people never vomit or feel nauseous. Others feel mildly nauseated most of the time, while some become severely nauseated for a limited time during or after a treatment. Their symptoms may start soon after a treatment or hours later. They may feel sick for just a few hours or for about a day. Be sure to tell your doctor or nurse if you are very nauseated and/or have vomited for more than a day or if your nausea is so bad that you cannot even keep liquids down.

610

Nausea and vomiting almost always can be controlled or at least lessened. If you experience this side effect, your doctor can choose from a range of drugs known as antiemetics which help curb nausea and vomiting. Different drugs work for different people, and it may be necessary to use more than one drug to get relief. Don't give up. Continue to work with your doctor and nurse to find the drug or drugs that work best for you.

You can also try the following ideas:

- Avoid big meals so your stomach won't feel too full. Eat small meals throughout the day, instead of one, two, or three large meals.

- Drink liquids at least an hour before mealtime, instead of with your meals.

- Eat and drink slowly.

- Stay away from sweet, fried, or fatty foods.

- Eat foods cold or at room temperature so you won't be bothered by strong smells.

- Chew your food well for easier digestion.

- If nausea is a problem in the morning, try eating dry foods like cereal, toast, or crackers before getting up. (Don't try this if you have mouth or throat sores or if you are troubled by a lack of saliva.)

- Drink cool, clear, unsweetened fruit juices, such as apple or grape juice, or light-colored sodas, such as ginger ale, that have lost their fizz.

- Suck on ice cubes, mints, or tart candies. (Don't use tart candies if you have mouth or throat sores.)

- Try to avoid odors that bother you, such as cooking smells, smoke, or perfume.

- Prepare and freeze meals in advance for days when you don't feel like cooking.

- Rest in a chair after eating, but don't lie flat for at least 2 hours after you've finished your meal.

- Wear loose-fitting clothes.

- Breathe deeply and slowly when you feel nauseated.

611

- Distract yourself by chatting with friends or family members, listening to music, or watching a movie or TV show.

- Use relaxation techniques.

- Avoid eating for at least a few hours before treatment if nausea usually occurs during chemotherapy.

Hair Loss

Hair loss (alopecia) is a common side effect of chemotherapy, but it doesn't always happen. Your doctor can tell you whether hair loss is likely to occur with the drug or drugs you are taking. When hair loss does occur, the hair may become thinner or may fall out entirely. The hair usually grows back after the treatments are over. Some people even start to get their hair back while they are still having treatments. In some cases, hair may grow back in a different color or texture.

Hair loss can occur on all parts of the body, not just the head. Facial hair, arm and leg hair, underarm hair, and pubic hair all may be affected.

Hair loss usually doesn't happen right away; more often, it begins after a few treatments. At that point, hair may fall out gradually or in clumps. Any hair that is still growing may become dull and dry.

To care for your scalp and hair during chemotherapy:

- Use mild shampoos.

- Use soft hair brushes.

- Use low heat when drying your hair.

- Don't use brush rollers to set your hair.

- Don't dye your hair or get a permanent.

- Have your hair cut short. A shorter style will make your hair look thicker and fuller. It also will make hair loss easier to manage if it occurs.

- Use a sunscreen, sunblock, hat, or scarf to protect your scalp from the sun if you lose a lot of the hair on your head.

Some people who lose all or most of their hair choose to wear turbans, scarves, caps, wigs, or hairpieces. Others leave their head uncovered. Still others switch back and forth, depending on whether they are in public or at home with friends and family members. There are no "right" or "wrong" choices; do whatever feels comfortable for you.

Here are some tips if you choose to cover your head:

- Get your wig or hairpiece before you lose a lot of hair. That way, you can match your natural color and current hair style if you wish. You may be able to buy a wig or hairpiece at a specialty shop just for cancer patients. Someone even may come to your home to help you. You also can buy a wig or hairpiece through a catalog or by phone. Call the American Cancer Society for more information.

- Consider borrowing a wig or hairpiece, rather than buying one. Check with the local chapter of the American Cancer Society or with the social work department at your hospital.

Remember that a hairpiece needed because of cancer treatment is a tax-deductible expense and may be at least partially covered by your health insurance. Be sure to check your policy.

Losing hair from your head, face, or body can be hard to accept. It's common—and perfectly all right—to feel angry or depressed about this loss. Talking about your feelings can help.

Fatigue/Anemia

Chemotherapy can reduce the bone marrow's ability to make red blood cells, which carry oxygen to all parts of your body. When there are too few red blood cells, body tissues don't get enough oxygen to do their work. This condition is called anemia.

Anemia can make you feel very weak and tired. Other symptoms of anemia include dizziness, chills. or shortness of breath. Be sure to report any of these symptoms to your doctor.

Your doctor will check your blood cell count often during your treatment. If your red count falls too low, you may need a blood transfusion to increase the number of red blood cells in your body.

Here are some things you can do to help yourself feel better if you develop anemia:

- Get plenty of rest. Sleep more at night and take naps during the day if you can.

- Limit your activities: Do only the things that are most important to you.

- Don't be afraid to get help when you need it. Ask family and friends to pitch in with things like child care, shopping, housework, or driving.

- Eat a well balanced diet.

- When sitting or lying down, get up slowly. This will help prevent dizziness.

Chemotherapy can make you more likely to get infections. This happens because most anticancer drugs affect the bone marrow and decrease its ability to produce white blood cells, the cells that fight many types of infections. An infection can begin in almost any part of your body, including your mouth, skin, lungs, urinary tract, rectum, and reproductive tract.

Your doctor will check your blood cell count often while you are getting chemotherapy. Your doctor also may add colony stimulating factors to your treatment to keep your blood count from getting too far below normal. In spite of these extra steps, however, your white blood cell count still may drop. If this happens, your doctor may postpone your next treatment or give you a lower dose of drugs for a while.

When your white count is lower than normal, it is very important to try to prevent infections by taking the following steps:

- Wash your hands often during the day. Be sure to wash them extra well before you eat and before and after you use the bathroom.

- Clean your rectal area gently but thoroughly after each bowel movement. Ask your doctor or nurse for advice if the area becomes irritated or if you have hemorrhoids. Also, check with your doctor before using enemas or suppositories.

- Stay away from people who have diseases you can catch, such as a cold, the flu, measles, or chickenpox. Also try to avoid crowds.

- Stay away from children who recently have received immunizations, such as vaccines for polio, measles, mumps and rubella (German measles).

- Don't cut or tear the cuticles of your nails.

- Be careful not to cut or nick yourself when using scissors, needles, or knives.

- Use an electric shaver instead of a razor to prevent breaks or cuts in your skin.

- Use a soft toothbrush that won't hurt your gums.

- Don't squeeze or scratch pimples.

- Take a warm (not hot) bath, shower, or sponge bath every day. Pat your skin dry using a light touch. Don't rub.

- Use lotion or oil to soften and heal your skin if it becomes dry and cracked.

- Clean cuts and scrapes right away with warm water, soap, and an antiseptic.

- Wear protective gloves when gardening or cleaning up after animals and others, especially small children.

- Do not get any immunization shots without checking first with your doctor to see if it's all right.

Most infections come from the bacteria normally found on the skin and in the intestines and genital tract. In some cases, the cause of an infection may not be known. When your white blood cell count is low, your body may not be able to fight off infections. So, even if you take extra care, you still may get an infection.

Be alert to the signs that you might have an infection and check your body regularly for its signs, paying special attention to your eyes, nose, mouth, and genital and rectal areas. The symptoms of infection include:

- Fever over 100 degrees F.

- Chills.

- Sweating.

- Loose bowels. (This also can be a side effect of chemotherapy.)

- A burning feeling when you urinate.

- A severe cough or sore throat.

- Unusual vaginal discharge or itching.

- Redness, swelling, or tenderness, especially around a wound, sore, pimple, or intravenous catheter site.

Report any signs of infection to your doctor right away. This is especially important when your white blood cell count is low. If you have a fever, don't use aspirin, acetaminophen, or any other medicine to bring your temperature down without first checking with your doctor.

Blood Clotting Problems

Anticancer drugs can affect the bone marrow's ability to make platelets, the blood cells that help stop bleeding by making your blood clot. If your blood does not have enough platelets, you may bleed or bruise more easily than usual, even from a minor injury.

Be sure to let your doctor know if you have unexpected bruising, small red spots under the skin, reddish or pinkish urine, or black or bloody bowel movements. Also report any bleeding from your gums or nose. Your doctor will check your platelet count often while you are having chemotherapy. If your platelet count falls too low, the doctor may give you a transfusion to build up the count. Here are some ways to avoid problems if your platelet count is low:

- Don't take any medicine without first checking with your doctor or nurse. This includes aspirin or aspirin-free pain relievers, including acetaminophen, and ibuprofen, and any other medicines you can buy without a prescription. These drugs may affect platelet function.

- Don't drink any alcoholic beverages unless your doctor says it's all right.

- Use a very soft toothbrush to clean your teeth.

- Clean your nose by blowing gently into a soft tissue.

- Take care not to cut or nick yourself when using scissors, needles, knives, or tools.

- Be careful not to burn yourself when ironing or cooking. Use a padded glove when you reach into the oven.

- Avoid contact sports and other activities that might result in injury.

Mouth, Gum, and Throat Problems

Good oral care is important during cancer treatment. Anticancer drugs can cause sores in the mouth and throat. They also can make these tissues dry and irritated or cause them to bleed. In addition to being painful, mouth sores can become infected by the many germs that live in the mouth. Because infections can be hard to fight during chemotherapy and can lead to serious problems, it's important to take every possible step to prevent them.

Here are some suggestions for keeping your mouth, gums, and throat healthy:

- If possible, see your dentist before you start chemotherapy to have your teeth cleaned and to take care of any problems such as cavities, abscesses, gum disease, or poorly fitting dentures. Ask your dentist to show you the best ways to brush and floss your teeth during chemotherapy. Chemotherapy can make you more likely to get cavities, so your dentist may suggest using a fluoride rinse or gel each day to help prevent decay.

- Brush your teeth and gums after every meal. Use a soft toothbrush and a gentle touch; brushing too hard can damage soft mouth tissues. Ask your doctor, nurse, or dentist to suggest a special type of toothbrush and/or toothpaste if your gums are very sensitive.

- Rinse your toothbrush well after each use and store it in a dry place.

- Avoid commercial mouthwashes that contain a large amount of salt or alcohol. Ask your doctor or nurse about a mild mouthwash that you might use.

If you develop sores in your mouth, be sure to contact your doctor or nurse because you may need medical treatment for the sores. If the sores are painful or keep you from eating, you also can try these ideas:

- Ask your doctor if there is anything you can apply directly to the sores. You also may ask your doctor to prescribe a medicine you can use to ease the pain.

- Eat foods cold or at room temperature. Hot and warm foods can irritate a tender mouth and throat.

- Choose soft, soothing foods, such as ice cream, milkshakes, baby food, soft fruits (bananas and applesauce), mashed potatoes, cooked cereals, soft-boiled or scrambled eggs, cottage cheese, macaroni and cheese, custards, puddings, and gelatin.

- You also can puree cooked foods in the blender to make them smoother and easier to eat.

- Avoid irritating, acidic foods, such as tomatoes, citrus fruit, and fruit juice (orange, grapefruit, and lemon); spicy or salty foods; and rough, coarse, or dry foods such as raw vegetables, granola, and toast.

If mouth dryness bothers you or makes it hard for you to eat, try these tips:

- Ask your doctor if you should use an artificial saliva product to moisten your mouth.

- Drink plenty of liquids.

- Suck on ice chips, popsicles, or sugarless hard candy. You can also chew sugarless gum.

- Moisten dry foods with butter, margarine, gravy, sauces, or broth.

- Dunk crisp, dry foods in mild liquids.

- Eat soft and pureed foods like those listed above.

- Use lip balm if your lips become dry.

Diarrhea

When chemotherapy affects the cells lining the intestine, the result can be diarrhea (loose stools). If you have diarrhea that continues for more than 24 hours, or if you have pain and cramping along with the diarrhea, call your doctor. In severe cases, the doctor may prescribe an antidiarrheal medicine. However, you should not take any over-the-counter antidiarrheal medicines without asking your doctor first.

You also can try these ideas to help control diarrhea:

- Eat smaller amounts of food, but eat more often.

- Avoid high-fiber foods, which can lead to diarrhea and cramping. High-fiber foods include whole grain breads and cereals, raw vegetables, beans, nuts, seeds, popcorn, and fresh and dried fruit. Eat low fiber foods instead. Low-fiber foods include white bread, white rice or noodles creamed cereals, ripe bananas, canned or cooked fruit without skins, cottage cheese, yogurt, eggs, mashed or baked potatoes without the skin, pureed vegetables, chicken or turkey without the skin, and fish.

- Avoid coffee, tea, alcohol, and sweets. Stay away from fried, greasy, or highly spiced foods, too. They are irritating and can cause diarrhea and cramping.

- Avoid milk and milk products if they make your diarrhea worse.

- Unless your doctor has told you otherwise, eat more potassium-rich foods because diarrhea can cause you to lose this important mineral. Bananas, oranges, potatoes, and peach and apricot nectars are good sources of potassium.

- Drink plenty of fluids to replace those you have lost through diarrhea. Mild, clear liquids, such as apple juice, water, weak tea, clear broth, or ginger ale, are best. Drink them slowly and make sure they are at room temperature. Let carbonated drinks lose their fizz before you drink them.

If your diarrhea is severe, it is important to let your doctor know. Ask your doctor if you should try a clear liquid diet to give your bowels time to rest. As you feel better, you gradually can add the low-fiber foods listed above. A clear liquid diet doesn't provide all the nutrients you need, so don't follow one for more than 3 to 5 days.

If your diarrhea is very severe, you may need to get intravenous fluids to replace the water and nutrients you have lost.

Constipation

Some people who get chemotherapy become constipated because of the drugs they are taking. Others may become constipated because they are less active or less nourished than usual. Tell your doctor if you have not had a bowel movement for more than a day or two. You may need to take a laxative or stool softener or use an enema, but don't use these remedies unless you have checked with your doctor, especially if your white blood cell count is low. You also can try these ideas to deal with constipation:

- Drink plenty of fluids to help loosen the bowels. Warm and hot fluids work especially well.

- Eat a lot of high-fiber foods. High-fiber foods include bran, whole-wheat breads and cereals, raw or cooked vegetables, fresh and dried fruit, nuts, and popcorn.

- Get some exercise. Simply getting out for a walk can help, as can a more structured exercise program. Be sure to check with your doctor before becoming more active.

Nerve and Muscle Effects

Your nervous system affects just about all your body's organs and tissues. So it's not surprising that when chemotherapy affects the cells of the nervous system—as the drugs sometimes do—a wide range of

side effects can result. For example, certain drugs can cause peripheral neuropathy, a condition that may make you feel a tingling, burning, weakness, or numbness in the hands and/or feet. Other nerve
related symptoms include loss of balance, clumsiness, difficulty picking up objects and buttoning clothing, walking problems, jaw pain,
hearing loss, stomach pain, and constipation. In addition to affecting
the nerves, certain anticancer drugs also can affect the muscles and
make them weak, tired, or sore.

In some cases, nerve and muscle effects—though annoying—may
not be serious. In other cases, nerve and muscle symptoms may indicate serious problems that need medical attention. Be sure to report
any suspected nerve or muscle symptoms to your doctor.

Caution and common sense can help you deal with nerve and
muscle problems. For example, if your fingers become numb, be very
careful when grasping objects that are sharp, hot, or otherwise dangerous. If your sense of balance or muscle strength is affected, avoid
falls by moving carefully, using handrails when going up or down
stairs and using bathmats in the bathtub or shower. Do not wear slippery shoes.

Effects on Skin and Nails

You may have minor skin problems while you are having chemotherapy. Possible side effects include redness, itching, peeling, dryness, and acne. Your nails may become darkened, brittle, or cracked.
They also may develop vertical lines or bands.

You will be able to take care of most of these problems yourself. If
you develop acne, try to keep your face clean and dry and use over-
the-counter medicated creams or soaps. For itching, apply cornstarch
as you would a dusting powder. To help avoid dryness, take quick
showers or sponge baths rather than long, hot baths. Apply cream and
lotion while your skin is still moist and avoid perfume, cologne, or
aftershave lotion that contains alcohol. You can strengthen your nails
with the remedies sold for this purpose, but be alert to signs of a wors-
ening problem because these products can be irritating to some people.
Protect your nails by wearing gloves when washing dishes, gardening, or performing other work around the house. Get further advice
from your doctor if these skin and nail problems don't respond to your
efforts. Be sure to let your doctor know if you have redness, pain, or
changes around the cuticles.

Certain anticancer drugs, when given intravenously, may produce
a fairly dramatic darkening of the skin all along the vein. Some people

use makeup to cover the area, but this can become difficult and time-consuming if several veins are affected, which sometimes happens. The darkened areas usually will fade on their own a few months after treatment ends.

Exposure to the sun may increase the effects some anticancer drugs have on your skin. Check with your doctor or nurse about using a sunscreen lotion with a skin protection factor of 15 to protect against the sun's effects. They may even suggest that you avoid being in direct sunlight or that you use a product, such as zinc oxide, that blocks the sun's rays completely. Long-sleeve cotton shirts, hats, and pants also will block the sun.

Some people who have had radiation therapy develop "radiation recall" during their chemotherapy. During or shortly after certain anticancer drugs are given, the skin over the area that was treated with radiation turns red, a shade anywhere from light to very bright, and may itch or burn. This reaction may last hours or even days. You can soothe the itching and burning by putting a cool, wet compress over the affected area. Radiation recall reactions should be reported to your doctor or nurse.

Most skin problems are not serious, but a few demand immediate attention. For example, certain drugs given intravenously can cause serious and permanent tissue damage if they leak out of the vein. Tell your doctor or nurse right away if you feel any burning or pain when you are getting IV drugs.

These symptoms don't always mean there's a problem, but they always must be checked out at once.

You should also let your doctor or nurse know right away if you develop sudden or severe itching, if your skin breaks out in a rash or hives, or if you have wheezing or any other trouble breathing. These symptoms may mean you are having an allergic reaction that may need to be treated at once.

Kidney and Bladder Effects

Some anticancer drugs can irritate the bladder or cause temporary or permanent damage to the kidneys. Be sure to ask your doctor if your anticancer drugs are among the ones that have this effect, and notify the doctor if you have any symptoms that might indicate a problem. Signs to watch for include:

- Pain or burning when you urinate.
- Frequent urination.

- A feeling that you must urinate right away ("urgency").
- Reddish or bloody urine.
- Fever.
- Chills.

In general, it's a good idea to drink plenty of fluids to ensure good urine flow and help prevent problems; this is especially important if your drugs are among those that affect the kidney and bladder. Water, juice, coffee, tea, soup, soft drinks, broth, ice cream, soup, popsicles, and gelatin are all considered fluids. Your doctor will let you know if you must increase your fluid intake.

You also should be aware that some anticancer drugs cause the urine to change color (orange, red, or yellow) or to take on a strong or medicine-like odor. For a short time, the color and odor of semen may be affected as well. Check with your doctor to see if the drugs you are taking have this effect.

Flu-Like Syndrome

Some people report feeling as though they have the flu a few hours to a few days after chemotherapy. Flu-like symptoms—muscle aches, headache, tiredness, nausea, slight fever, chills, and poor appetite—may last from 1 to 3 days. These symptoms also can be caused by an infection or by the cancer itself, so it's important to check with your doctor if you have flu-like symptoms.

Fluid Retention

Your body may retain fluid when you are having chemotherapy. This may be due to hormonal changes from your therapy, to the effect of the drugs themselves, or to your cancer. Check with your doctor or nurse if you notice swelling or puffiness in your face, hands, feet, or abdomen. You may need to avoid table salt and foods with a high sodium content. If the problem is severe, your doctor may prescribe diuretics, medicine to help your body get rid of excess fluids. However, don't take any over-the-counter diuretics without asking your doctor first.

Sexual Effects: Physical and Psychological

Chemotherapy may—but does not always—affect sexual organs and functioning in both men and women. The side effects that might occur depend on the drugs used and the person's age and general health.

Men

Chemotherapy drugs may lower the number of sperm cells, reduce their ability to move, or cause other abnormalities. These changes can result in infertility, which may be temporary or permanent. Infertility affects a man's ability to father a child but does not affect his ability to have sexual intercourse.

Because permanent sterility may occur, it's important to discuss this issue with your doctor before you begin chemotherapy. If you wish, you might consider sperm banking, a procedure that freezes sperm for future use.

Men undergoing chemotherapy should use an effective means of birth control with their partners during treatment because of the harmful effects of the drugs on chromosomes. Ask your doctor when you can stop using birth control for this purpose.

Women

Anticancer drugs can damage the ovaries and reduce the amount of hormones they produce. As a result, some women find that their menstrual periods become irregular or stop completely while they are having chemotherapy.

The hormonal effects of chemotherapy also may cause menopause-like symptoms such as hot flashes and itching, burning, or dryness of vaginal tissues. These tissue changes can make intercourse uncomfortable, but the symptoms often can be relieved by using a water-based vaginal lubricant. The tissue changes also can make a woman more likely to get vaginal infections. To help prevent infection, avoid oil-based lubricants such as petroleum jelly, wear cotton underwear and pantyhose with a ventilated cotton lining, and don't wear tight slacks or shorts. Your doctor also may prescribe a vaginal cream or suppository to reduce the chances of infection. If infection does occur, it should be treated right away.

Damage to the ovaries may result in infertility, the inability to become pregnant. In some cases, the infertility is a temporary condition; in other cases, it may be permanent. Whether infertility occurs, and how long it lasts, depends on many factors, including the type of drug, the dosage given, and the woman's age.

Although pregnancy may be possible during chemotherapy, it still is not advisable because some anticancer drugs may cause birth defects.

Doctors advise women of childbearing age—from the teens through the end of menopause—to use birth control throughout their treatment.

If a woman is pregnant when her cancer is discovered, it may be possible to delay chemotherapy until after the baby is born. For a woman who needs treatment sooner, the doctor may suggest starting chemotherapy after the 12th week of pregnancy when the fetus is beyond the stage of greatest risk. In some cases, termination of the pregnancy may be considered.

Sexuality

Sexual feelings and attitudes vary among people during chemotherapy. Some people find that they feel closer than ever to their partners and have an increased desire for sexual activity. Others experience little or no change in their sexual desire and energy level. Still others find that their sexual interest declines because of the physical and emotional stresses of having cancer and getting chemotherapy. These stresses may include worries about changes in appearance; anxiety about health family or finances; or side effects including fatigue and hormonal changes.

A partner's concerns or fears also can affect the sexual relationship. Some may worry that physical intimacy will harm the person who has cancer; others may fear that they might catch the cancer or be affected by the drugs. Many of these issues can be cleared up by talking about misunderstandings. Both you and your partner should feel free to discuss sexual concerns with your doctor, nurse, or other counselor who can give you the information and the reassurance you need.

You and your partner also should try to share your feelings with one another. If it's difficult for you to talk to each other about sex, or cancer, or both, you may want to speak to a counselor who can help you communicate more openly. People who can help include psychiatrists, psychologists, social workers, marriage counselors, sex therapists, and members of the clergy.

If you were comfortable with and enjoyed sexual relations before starting therapy, chances are you will still find pleasure in physical intimacy during your treatment. You may discover, however, that intimacy takes on a new meaning and character. Hugging, touching, holding, and cuddling may become more important, while sexual intercourse may become less important. Remember that what was true before you started chemotherapy remains true now: There is no one 'right way' to express your sexuality. It's up to you and your partner to determine together what is pleasurable and satisfying to you both.

The American Cancer Society has two free booklets on sexuality that may be helpful, one for women and one for men. Contact your local unit or the national office for copies.

Eating Well during Chemotherapy

It is very important to eat as well as you can while you are undergoing treatment. People who eat well can cope with side effects better and are able to fight infection more easily. In addition, their bodies can rebuild healthy tissues faster.

Eating well during chemotherapy means choosing a balanced diet that contains all the nutrients the body needs. A good way to do this is to eat foods from each of the following food groups: fruits and vegetables; poultry, fish, and meat; cereals and breads; and dairy products. Eating well also means having a diet high enough in calories to keep your weight up and, most important, high enough in protein to build and repair skin, hair, muscles, and organs.

You also may need to drink extra amounts of fluid to protect your bladder and kidneys during your treatment.

What If I Don't Feel Like Eating?

Even when you know it's important to eat well, there may be days when you feel you just can't. This may happen because side effects such as nausea or mouth and throat problems make it difficult or painful to eat. You also can lose your appetite if you feel depressed or tired. If this is the case, be sure to read the sections in this booklet on your particular discomforts. They will give you tips that can make it easier for you to eat.

When a poor appetite is the problem, try these hints:

- Eat small meals or snacks whenever you want. You don't have to eat three regular meals each day.

- When possible, take a walk before meals; this may make you feel hungrier.

- Try changing your mealtime routine. For example, eat by candlelight or in a different location.

- Eat with friends or family members. When eating alone, listen to the radio or watch TV.

If you live alone, you might want to arrange for "Meals on Wheels" or a similar program to bring food to you. Ask your doctor, nurse, local American Cancer Society office, or the Cancer Information Service about these programs, which are provided in many communities.

The National Cancer Institute's booklet *Eating Hints* [reprinted in this volume as Chapter 77] provides more tips about how to make eating easier and more enjoyable. It also gives many ideas about how to eat well and increase your protein and calorie intake during cancer treatment. For a free copy of *Eating Hints*, call the Cancer Information Service at 1-800-4-CANCER.

Can I Drink Alcoholic Beverages?

Small amounts of alcohol can help you relax and increase your appetite. On the other hand, alcohol may interact with some drugs to reduce their effectiveness or worsen their side effects. For this reason, some people must drink less alcohol or avoid alcohol completely during chemotherapy. Be sure to ask your doctor if it's okay for you to drink beer, wine, or other alcoholic beverages.

Should I Take Vitamin or Mineral Supplements?

There is no single answer to this question, but one thing is clear: No diet or nutritional plan can "cure" cancer, and taking vitamin and mineral supplements should never be considered a substitute for medical care. You should not take any supplements without your doctor's knowledge and consent.

Talking With Your Doctor and Nurse

Some people with cancer want to know every detail about their condition and their treatment. Others prefer only general information. The choice of how much information to seek is yours, but there are questions that every person getting chemotherapy should ask. These include:

- Why do I need chemotherapy?
- What are the benefits of chemotherapy?
- What are the risks of chemotherapy?
- What drug or drugs will I be taking?
- How will the drugs be given?
- Where will I get my treatments?

- How long will my treatment last?
- What are the possible side effects?
- Are there any side effects that I should report right away?
- Are there any other possible treatment methods for my type of cancer?

This list is just a start. You always should feel free to ask your doctor, nurse, and pharmacist as many questions as you want. If you don't understand their answers, keep asking until you do. Remember, when it comes to cancer and cancer treatment there is no such thing as a "stupid" question. To make sure you get all the answers you want, you may find it helpful to draw up a list of questions before your appointment. Some people even keep a "running list" and jot down each new question as it occurs to them.

To help remember your doctor's answers, you may want to take notes during your appointment. Don't feel shy about asking your doctor to slow down when you need more time to write. You might also ask if you can use a tape recorder during your visit. That way, you can review your conversation later as many times as you wish. Some doctors like this idea and others don't, so be sure to check before you try it. Another way to help you remember is to bring a friend or family member to sit with you while you talk to your doctor. This person can help you understand what your doctor says during your visit and help refresh your memory afterward.

Chemotherapy and Your Emotions

Chemotherapy can bring major changes to a person's life. It can affect overall health, threaten a sense of well-being, disrupt day-to-day schedules, and put a strain on personal relationships. No wonder then, that many people feel fearful, anxious, angry, or depressed at some point during their chemotherapy.

These emotions are perfectly normal and understandable, but they also can be disturbing. Fortunately, there are ways to cope with these emotional "side effects," just as there are ways to cope with the physical side effects of chemotherapy.

How Can I Get the Support I Need?

There are many sources of support you can draw on. Here are some of the most important:

Doctors and Nurses

If you have questions or worries about your cancer treatment, talk with members of your health care team.

Counseling Professionals

There are many kinds of counselors who can help you express, understand, and cope with the emotions cancer treatment can cause. Depending on your preferences and needs, you might want to talk with a psychiatrist, psychologist, social worker, sex therapist, or member of the clergy.

Friends and Family Members

Talking with friends or family members can help you feel a lot better. Often, they can comfort and reassure you in ways that no one else can. You may find, though, that you'll need to help them help you. At a time when you might expect that others will rush to your aid, you may have to make the first move.

Many people do not understand cancer, and they may withdraw from you because they're afraid of your illness. Others may worry that they will upset you by saying "the wrong thing."

You can help relieve these fears by being open in talking with others about your illness, your treatment, your needs, and your feelings. By talking openly, you can correct mistaken ideas about cancer. You can also let people know that there's no single "right" thing to say, so long as their caring comes through loud and clear. Once people know they can talk with you honestly, they may be more willing and able to open up and lend their support.

The National Cancer Institute's booklet *Taking Time* offers useful advice to help cancer patients and their families and friends communicate with one another.

Support Groups

Support groups are made up of people who are going through the same kinds of experiences as you. Many people with cancer find they can share thoughts and feelings with group members that they don't feel comfortable sharing with anyone else. Support groups also can serve as an important source of practical information about living with cancer.

Support can also be found in one-to-one programs that put you in touch with another person very similar to you in terms of age, sex, type of cancer, and so forth. In some programs, this person comes to visit you. In others, a "hotline" puts you in touch with someone you can talk with on the telephone.

Sources for information about support programs include your hospital's social work department, the local office of your American Cancer Society, and the National Cancer Institute's Cancer Information Service.

How Can I Make My Daily Life Easier?

Here are some tips to help yourself while you are getting chemotherapy:

- Try to keep your treatment goals in mind. This will help you keep a positive attitude on days when the going gets rough.

- Remember that eating well is very important. Your body needs food to rebuild tissues and regain strength.

- Learn as much as you want to know about your disease and its treatment. This can lessen your fear of the unknown and increase your feeling of control.

- Keep a journal or diary while you're in treatment. A record of your activities and thoughts can help you understand the feelings you have as you go through treatment and highlight questions you need to ask your doctor or nurse. You also can use your journal to record the steps you take to cope with side effects and how well those steps work. That way, you'll know which methods worked best for you in case you have the same side effects again.

- Set realistic goals and don't be too hard on yourself. You may not have as much energy as usual, so try to get as much rest as you can, let the "small stuff" slide, and only do the things that are most important to you.

- Try new hobbies and learn new skills. Exercise if you can. Using your body cam make you feel better about yourself, help you get rid of tension or anger, and build your appetite. Ask your doctor or nurse about a safe and practical exercise program.

How Can I Relieve Stress?

You can use a number of methods to cope with the stresses of cancer and its treatment. The techniques described here can help you

629

relax. Try some of these methods to find the one (or ones) that work best for you. You may want to check with your doctor before using these techniques, especially if you have lung problems.

Muscle Tension and Release

Lie down in a quiet room. Take a slow, deep breath. As you breathe in, tense a particular muscle or group of muscles. For example you can squeeze your eyes shut, frown, clench your teeth, make a fist, or stiffen your arms or legs. Hold your breath and keep your muscles tense for a second or two. Then breathe out, release the tension, and let your body relax completely. Repeat the process with another muscle or muscle group.

You also can try a variation of this method, called "progressive relaxation." Start with the toes of one foot and, working upward, progressively tense and relax all the muscles of one leg. Next, do the same with the other leg. Then tense and relax the rest of the muscle groups in your body, including those in your scalp. Remember to hold your breath while tensing your muscles and to breathe out when releasing the tension.

Rhythmic Breathing

Get into a comfortable position and relax all your muscles. If you keep your eyes open, focus on a distant object. If you close your eyes, imagine a peaceful scene or simply clear your mind and focus on your breathing.

Breathe in and out slowly and comfortably through your nose. If you like, you can keep the rhythm steady by saying to yourself, "In, one two; Out, one two." Feel yourself relax and go limp each time you breathe out.

You can do this technique for just a few seconds or for up to 10 minutes. End your rhythmic breathing by counting slowly and silently to three.

Biofeedback

With training in biofeedback, you can control body functions such as heart rate, blood pressure, and muscle tension. A machine will sense when your body shows signs of tension and will let you know in some way such as making a sound or flashing a light. The machine will also give you feedback when you relax your body. Eventually, you will be able to control your relaxation responses without having to depend on feedback from the machine. Your doctor or nurse can refer you to someone trained in teaching biofeedback.

Imagery

Imagery is a way of daydreaming that uses all your senses. It usually is done with your eyes closed. To begin, breathe slowly and feel yourself relax. Imagine a ball of healing energy—perhaps a white light—forming somewhere in your body. When you can "see" the ball of energy, imagine that as you breathe in you can blow the ball to any part of the body where you feel pain, tension, or discomfort such as nausea. When you breathe out, picture the air moving the ball away from your body, taking with it any painful or uncomfortable feelings. (Be sure to breathe naturally; don't blow.) Continue to picture the ball moving toward you and away from you each time you breathe in and out. You may see the ball getting bigger and bigger as it takes away more and more tension and discomfort.

To end the imagery, count slowly to three, breathe in deeply, open your eyes, and say to yourself, "I feel alert and relaxed."

If you choose to use imagery as a relaxation technique, please be sure to read the caution in the following section.

Visualization

Visualization is a method that is similar to imagery. With visualization, you create an inner picture that represents your fight against cancer. Some people getting chemotherapy use images of rockets blasting away their cancer cells or of knights in armor battling their cancer cells. Others create an image of their white blood cells or their drugs attacking the cancer cells.

Visualization and imagery may help relieve stress and increase your sense of self-control. But it is very important to remember that they cannot take the place of the medical care your doctor prescribes to treat your cancer.

Hypnosis

Hypnosis puts you in a trance-like state that can help reduce discomfort and anxiety. You can be hypnotized by a qualified person, or you can learn how to hypnotize yourself. If you are interested in learning more, ask your doctor or nurse to refer you to someone trained in the technique.

Distraction

You use distraction any time an activity takes your mind off your worries or discomforts. Try watching TV, listening to the radio, reading, going to the movies, or working with your hands by doing needlework or puzzles, building models, or painting. You may be surprised how comfortably the time passes.

Paying for Chemotherapy

The cost of chemotherapy varies with the kinds and dose of drugs used, how long and how often they are given, and whether you get them at home, in a clinic or offices or in the hospital. Most health insurance policies (including Medicare Part B, which helps pay for doctors bills and many other medical services) cover at least part of the cost of many kinds of chemotherapy.

Sometimes, however, an insurer may not pay for the use of certain drugs for certain kinds of cancers—at least not at first. If your insurer denies payment for your treatment, don't give up. Most people do get payment eventually.

Teamwork with your doctor and the office staff is important. Be sure to let them know if you have been denied payment. They can consult with your insurer and help answer any questions your insurer may have. They also can consult with the company that makes the drug or drugs you are taking. Often, these companies can provide information or other services that will help you get payment.

In some states, Medicaid (which makes health care services available for people with financial need) may help pay for certain treatments. Contact the office that handles social services in your city or county to find out whether you are eligible for Medicaid and whether your chemotherapy is a covered expense.

If you need help paying for treatments, contact your hospital's social service office, the Cancer Information Service, or the local office of the American Cancer Society. They may be able to direct you to other sources of help. Another possibility is the Leukemia Society of America; to find a chapter near you, check the white pages of your local telephone book.

Resources

Information about cancer is available from many sources, including the ones listed below. You may want to check for additional information at your local library or bookstore and from support groups in your community.

Cancer Information Service 1-800-4-CANCER

The Cancer Information Service, a program of the National Cancer Institute, is a nationwide telephone service for cancer patients and their families and friends, the public, and health care professionals. The staff can answer questions in English or Spanish and can send free National Cancer Institute booklets about cancer. They also know about local resources and services. One toll-free number, 1-800-4-CANCER (1-800-422-6237), connects callers with the office that serves their area.

PDQ

People who have cancer, those who care about them, and doctors need up-to-date and accurate information about cancer treatment. To meet these needs, PDQ was developed by NCI. PDQ contains an up-to-date list of clinical trials all over the country. The Cancer Information Service, at 1-800-4-CANCER, can provide PDQ information to doctors, patients, and the public.

American Cancer Society

1599 Clifton Road, N.E.
Atlanta, GA 30329
1-800-ACS-2345

The American Cancer Society is a voluntary organization with a national office (at the above address) and local units all over the country. To obtain further information about services and activities in local areas, call the Society's toll-free number, 1-800-ACS-2345 (1-800-227-2345), or the number listed under American Cancer Society in the white pages of the telephone book.

Other Booklets

National Cancer Institute printed materials, including the booklets listed below, are available from the Cancer Information Service free of charge by calling 1-800-4-CANCER.

Advanced Cancer: Living Each Day *

Eating Hints: Tips for Better Nutrition During Cancer Treatment *

Facing Forward: A Guide for Cancer Survivors *

Questions and Answers About Pain Control

Radiation Therapy and You: A Guide to Self-Help During Treatment *

Taking Time: Support for People With Cancer and the People Who Care About Them

What are Clinical Trials All About?

What You Need To Know About Cancer. A series of booklets about different types of cancer.

When Cancer Recurs: Meeting the Challenge Again *

* Reprinted in this volume—see Table of Contents

A Final Word

The National Cancer Institute hopes *Chemotherapy and You* helps you and your family, whether you are waiting to begin chemotherapy or already have begun your treatment. Discuss the information in this booklet with your doctor and nurse, and take good care of yourself during your chemotherapy. By working together, you, your family, and your health care providers will make the strongest possible team in your fight against cancer.

Acknowledgments: The National Cancer Institute is grateful to the numerous health professionals and patients who contributed to the development and review of this publication.

Chapter 64

Chemotherapy Drug Approvals

This alphabetic list of drugs contains the medications that have been approved by the Food and Drug Administration (FDA) from June 1996 through December 1999 for use as cancer therapies or for side effects of cancer treatment.

Actiq (fentanyl citrate), flavored sugar lozenge on a stick, by Anesta Corporation received approval on November 4, 1998, for management of chronic pain in cancer patients that are experiencing breakthrough pain on their regular narcotic (opioid) therapy.

Anzemet (dolasetron mesylate Tablet) sponsored by Hoechst Marion Roussel, Inc., received approval on September 11, 1997, for the prevention of chemotherapy-induced nausea and vomiting, and prevention of postoperative nausea and vomiting.

Aredia (pamidronate disodium) for Injection, sponsored by Ciba Geigy Corporation Pharmaceuticals Division, received an additional indication on July 16, 1996, for the treatment of osteolytic bone metastases of breast cancer. Aredia was previously indicated for hypercalcemia associated with malignancy, osteolytic bone lesions of multiple myeloma, and Paget's disease of bone.

Aromasin (exemestane) Tablets, from Pharmacia & Upjohn Company, received approval on October 21, 1999, for the treatment of advance

"Drug Approvals for Cancer Indications," Food and Drug Administration (FDA), December 1999.

breast cancer in postmenopausal women whose disease has progressed following tamoxifen therapy.

Blenoxane (bleomycin sulfate), from Bristol-Myers Squibb, received approval on February 20, 1996, as a sclerosing agent for the treatment of malignant pleural effusion and prevention of recurrent pleural effusions.

Busulfex (busulfan), by Orphan Medical Inc received approval on February 4, 1999, for use in combination with cyclophosphamide as a conditioning regiment prior to allogeneic hematopoietic progenitor cell transplantation for chronic myelogenous leukemia.

Camptosar (irinotecan hydrochlorise) by Pharmacia & Upjohn received additional approval on October 22, 1998, for the treatment of patients with metastatic carcinoma of the colon or rectum whose disease has recurred or progressed following 5-FU-based therapy.

Camptosar (irinotecan HCL) sponsored by Pharmacia and Upjohn, received accelerated approval on June 14, 1996, for treatment of metastatic carcinoma of the colon or rectum which has progressed or recurred after treatment with 5-fluorouracil (5FU).

Ceprate SC Stem Cell Concentration System, from CellPro Incorporated received additional approval for processing peripheral blood progenitor cells to obtain a CD34 positive cell enriched population which is intended for hematopoietic support after myeloablative chemotherapy in patients with CD34 negative tumors.

Daunorubicin HCL (daunorubicin hydrochloride) by Bedford Laboratories, Div. Ben Venue Laboratories, Inc., received approval on January 30, 1998, to provide a new 5 mg/mL, 4 mL ready-to-use solution which can be immediately used in an IV infusion without the possibility of reconstitution error. Daunorubicin HCL's indication is for use in combination with other approved anticancer drugs for remission induction in acute nonlymphocytic leukemia (myelogenous, monocytic, erythroid) of adults and for remission induction in acute lymphocytic leukemia of children and adults.

DaunoXome (daunorubicin citrate liposome) from NeXstar, received approval on April 8, 1996, for the first line cytotoxic treatment of advanced HIV-associated Kaposi's sarcoma.

DepoCyt (cytarabine liposomal injection, 10 mg/mL), by DepoTech Corporation, received accelerated approval on April 1, 1999, for the intrathecal treatment of lymphomatous meningitis. This indication is based on demonstration of increased complete response rate compared to unencapsulated cytarabine. There are no controlled trials that demonstrate a clinical benefit resulting from this treatment, such as improvement in disease-related symptoms, or increased time to disease progression, or increased survival. (Labeling)

Dostinex (cabergoline) Tablets, sponsored by Pharmacia & Upjohn Company, received approval on December 23, 1996, for the treatment of hyperprolactinemic disorders, either idiopathic (i.e. of unknown cause) or due to pituitary adenomas.

Doxil (doxorubicin HCL liposome injection), from Alza Corporation, received accelerated approval on June 28, 1999, for a supplemental indication for the treatment of metastatic carcinoma of the ovary in patients with disease that is refractory to both paclitaxel- and platinum-based chemotherapy regimens. Refractory disease is defined as disease that has progressed while on treatment, or within 6 months of completing treatment.(Labeling)

Doxil (doxorubicin HCL liposome injection), from Sequus received approval on December 29, 1998, for the treatment of metastatic carcinoma of the ovary in patients with disease that is refractory to both paclitaxel and platinum based chemotherapy regimens.

Duraclon (clonidine hydrochloride) for Injection, sponsored by Fujisawa USA Incorporated, was approved on October 2, 1996, for continuous epidural administration (a type of injection) as additional therapy with intraspinal opiates (pain medication injected into the spinal column) for the treatment of severe pain in cancer patients that is not adequately relieved by opioid pain relievers alone.

Ellence (epirubicin hydrochloride), from Pharmacia & Upjohn received approval on September 15, 1999, for use as a component of adjuvant therapy in patients with evidence of axillary node tumor involvement following resection of primary breast cancer.

Elliotts B Solution (calcium chloride, dextrose, magnesium sulfate, potassium chloride, sodium bicarbonate, sodium chloride, sodium phosphate, dibasic) for Injection, sponsored by Orphan Medical Incorporated, was approved on September 27, 1996, for use in mixing methotrexate sodium and/or cytarabine for intrathecal administration (a type of injection) to prevent or treat meningeal leukemia or lymphocytic lymphoma.

Ethyol (amifostine) for Injection, by US Bioscience, received additional approval on June 24, 1999, to reduce the incidence of moderate to severe xerostomia in patients undergoing post-operative radiation treatment for head and neck cancer, where the radiation port includes a substantial portion of the parotid glands. Ethyol is also marketed by Alza Pharmaceuticals. (Labeling)

Ethyol (amifostine), from Alza, received approval on March 15, 1996, for chemoprotectant/ cisplatin non-small cell lung cancer (NSCLC).

Etopophos (etoposide phosphate) from Bristol-Myers Squibb, received approval on May 17, 1996, for the management of small cell lung cancer, firstline and refractory testicular tumors, in combination with other approved chemotherapeutic agents.

Fareston (toremifene citrate) Tablets, sponsored by Orion Corporation, received approval on May 29, 1997, for the treatment of metastatic breast cancer in postmenopausal women with estrogen receptor positive or receptor unknown tumors.

Femara (letrozole) Tablets, sponsored by Novartis Pharmaceuticals Corporation, received approval on July 25, 1997, for the treatment of advanced breast cancer in postmenopausal women.

Gemzar (gemcitabine HCL) for injection by Eli Lilly & Co. received additional approval on August 26, 1998, for use in combination with cisplatin for the first-line treatment of patients with inoperable, locally advanced (Stage IIIA or IIIB) or metastatic (Stage IV) non-small cell lung cancer.

Gemzar (gemcitabine HCL), from Lilly, received approval on May 16, 1996, for first line treatment for locally advanced (nonresectable stage II or III) or metastatic (stage IV) pancreatic cancer; second-line treatment for pancreatic cancer previously treated with 5-fluorouracil.

Gliadel (carmustine wafer) for Implantation, sponsored by Guilford Pharmaceuticals Incorporated, was approved on September 23, 1996, for use in addition to surgery to prolong survival in patients with recurrent glioblastoma multiforme who qualify for surgery.

Herceptin (trastuzumab) intravenous injection by Genentech, Inc., received approval on September 25, 1998, for use alone for certain patients who have tried chemotherapy with little success or as a first-line treatment for metastatic disease when used in combination with paclitaxel (trade name Taxol)(additional information)

Hycamtin (topotecan hydrochloride) for injection, by SmithKline Beecham Pharmaceuticals received additional approval on November 30, 1998, for the use of Hycamtin in the treatment of small cell lung cancer sensitive disease after failure of first-line chemotherapy. In clinical studies submitted to support approval, sensitive disease was defined as disease responding to chemotherapy but subsequently progressing at least 60 days (in the phase 3 study) or at least 90 days (in the phase 2 studies) after chemotherapy. (Labeling)

Hycamtin (topotecan HCL), from SmithKline Beecham, received approval on May 28, 1996, for the treatment of metastatic ovarian cancer after failure of first line chemotherapy.

Intron A (interferon alfa-2a) sponsored by Schering Corp., received approval on November 6, 1997, for use in conjunction with chemotherapy in patients with follicular lymphoma.

Kytril (granisetron), from SmithKline Beecham, received additional approval on June 27, 1999, for the prevention of nausea and vomiting associated with radiation, including total body irradiation (TBI) and fractionated abdominal radiation.

Levulan Kerastick (aminolevulinic acid HCL) for Topical Solution, 20%, received approval on December 3, 1999, to be used in conjunction with photodyamic therapy for treatment of actinic keratoses (AKs) (pre-cancerous skin lesiions) of the face or scalp. This is the first combined drug and device treatment designed for targeted treatment that can be limited just to the lesion site(s). Aminolevulinic acid HCL is marketed by DUSA Pharmaceuticals, Inc. of Valhalla, NY and will be marketed under the trade number Levulan Kerastick for Topical solution, 20%. It is to be marketed in combination with the light source BLU-U Blue Light Photodynamic Therapy Illuminator. (Approval Letter, Labeling)

Lupron Depot (leuprolide acetate) for Injection, sponsored by TAP Holdings Incorporated, received an additional indication on May 30, 1997, to help relieve the symptoms associated with advanced prostate cancer. Lupron was previously indicated for management of endometriosis, preoperative hematologic improvement of anemia caused by uterine leiomyomata, palliative treatment of advanced prostate cancer and central precocious puberty.

Neupogen (filgrastim) by Amgen, Inc. received additional approval on April 2, 1998, for use in patients with acute myeloid leukemia.

Neumega (oprelvekin) sponsored by Genetics Institute, Inc., received approval on November 25, 1997, for the prevention of severe thrombocytopenia and the reduction of the need for platelet transfusion following myelosuppressive chemotherapy in patients with nonmyeloid malignancies who are at high risk of severe thrombocytopenia.

Nilandron (nilutamide) Tablets, sponsored by GH Besselaar Associates Incorporated, was approved on September 19, 1996, for use in combination with surgical castration for the treatment of stage D2 metastatic prostate cancer.

Nolvadex (tamoxifen citrate) by Zeneca Pharmaceuticals received additional approval on October 29, 1998, to reduce the incidence of breast cancer in women at high risk for breast cancer.

Novantrone (mitoxantrone hydrochloride) for Injection, sponsored by Immunex Corporation, received an additional indication on November 13, 1996, for use in combination with corticosteroids as initial chemotherapy for the treatment of patients with pain related to advanced hormone refractory prostate cancer. Novantrone was previously indicated for use in combination with other approved drugs in the initial therapy of acute nonlymphocytic leukemia (ANLL) in adults. This category includes myelogenous, promyelocytic, monocytic, and erythroid acute leukemias.

Ontak (denileukin diftitox), marketed by Ligand Pharmaceuticals and manufactured by Seragen, Inc., received accelerated approval (based on tumor reduction) on February 5, 1999, for the treatment of persistent or recurrent cutaneous t-cell lymphoma, (CTCL), a rare slow-growing form of non-Hodgkin's lymphoma, whose malignant cells express the CD25 component of the IL-2 receptor.

Photofrin (porfimer sodium), by QLT Phototherapeutics, Inc., received additional approval on December 22, 1998, for use in photodynamic therapy (PDT) for reduction of obstruction and palliation of symptoms in patients with completely or partially obstructing endobroncial nonsmall cell lung cancer (NSCLC).

Proleukin (aldesleukin) sponsored by Chiron Corporation received an additional indication on January 9, 1998, for treatment of adults with metastatic melanoma and updated response data for metastatic renal cell carcinoma patients, as well as revised package insert information.

Photofrin (porfimer sodium) sponsored by QLT Phototherapeutics, Inc., received an additional indication on January 9, 1998, for treatment in photodynamic therapy for treatment of microinvasive endobronchial nonsmall cell lung cancer in patients for whom surgery and radiotherapy are not indicated.

Quadramet (samarium sm 153 edtmp) for Injection, sponsored by Cytogen Corporation, received approval on March 28, 1997, for the relief of pain in patients with confirmed osteoblastic metastatic bone lesions that enhance on radionuclide bone scan.

Rituxan (rituximab) sponsored by Genentech, Inc., received approval on November 26, 1997, for the treatment of patients with relapsed or refractory low-grade or follicular, B-cell non-Hodgkin's lymphoma.

Sandostatin LAR® Depot (octreotide acetate for injectable suspension), by Novartis Pharmaceuticals, was approved on November 25, 1998, for the reduction of growth hormone and IGF-1 in acromegaly, the suppression of severe diarrhea and flushing associated with malignant carcinoid syndrome and for the treatment of the profuse watery diarrhea associated with VIPoma (vasoactive intestinal peptide tumor). (Labeling)

Taxol (paclitaxel) injection, from Bristol-Myers Squibb, received additional approval on October 25, 1999, for adjuvant treatment of node-positive breast cancer administered sequentially to standard doxorubicin-containing combination chemotherapy. In the clinical trial, there was an overall favorable effect on disease-free and overall survival in the total population of patients with receptor-positive and receptor-negative tumors, but the benefit has been specifically demonstrated by available data (median follow up 30 months) only in the patients with estrogen and progesterone receptor negative tumors.

Taxol (paclitaxel) injection by Bristol-Myers Squibb Pharmaceutical Research Institute received additional approval on June 30, 1998, for use in combination with cisplatin, for the first-line treatment of non-small cell lung cancer in patients who are not candidates for potentially curative surgery and/or radiation therapy.

Taxol (paclitaxel) injection by Bristol-Myers Squibb Pharmaceutical Research Institute received additional approval on April 9, 1998, for first-line therapy for the treatment of advanced carcinoma of the ovary in combination with cisplatin.

Taxol (paclitaxel) for Injection, sponsored by Bristol Myers Squibb Co. Pharmaceutical Research Institute, received an additional indication on August 4, 1997, for the second line treatment of AIDS-related Kaposi's sarcoma. Taxol was previously indicated, after failure of first-line or subsequent chemotherapy for the treatment of metastatic carcinoma of the ovary, and for treatment of breast cancer after failure of combination chemotherapy for metastatic disease or relapse within 6 months of adjuvant chemotherapy.

Taxotere (docetaxel) injection concentrate (20 mg and 80 mg) by Rhone-Poulenc Rorer received additional approval on June 22, 1998, for the treatment of patients with locally advanced or metastatic breast cancer after failure of prior chemotherapy.

Taxotere (docetaxel) from Rhone-Poulenc Rorer, received approval on May 14, 1996, for the treatment of locally advanced or metastatic breast cancer which has progressed during anthracycline-based treatment or relapsed during anthracycline-based adjuvant therapy.

Temodar (temozolomide), from Schering-Plough Corporation received accelerated approval on August 11, 1999, for the treatment of adult patients with refractory anaplastic astrocytoma, (i.e. patients at first relapse who have experienced disease progression on a drug regimen containing a nitgrosourea and procarbazine).

Urowave Microwave Thermotherapy System by Dornier Medical Systems, Inc., received approval on May 29, 1998, as a non-surgical treatment alternative to transurethral resection of the prostate (TURP). To treat symptomatic benign prostatic hyperplasia (BPH) in men withprostatic lengths between 30 mm and 55 mm.

UVADEX (methoxsalen sterile solution, 20 mcg/mL), by Therakos, Inc. received approval on February 25, 1999, for the use of UVADEX with the UVAR Photopheresis System in the palliative treatment of the skin manifestations of cutaneous T-cell lymphoma (CTCL) that is unresponsive to other forms of treatment.(Labeling)

Valstar (valrubicin) Sterile Solution for Intravesical Instillation, 5 mL, Single-Use Vials (40 mg/mL) by Anthra Pharmaceuticals received approval on September 25, 1998, for intravesical therapy of BCG-refractory carcinoma in situ (CIS) of the urinary bladder in patients for whom immediate cystectomy would be associated with unacceptable morbidity or mortality.

Xeloda (capecitabine) tablets by Hoffman-La Roche received accelerated approval on April 30, 1998, for treatment of patients with metastatic breast cancer resistant to both paclitaxel and an anthracycline containing chemotherapy regimen or resistant to paclitaxel and for whom further anthracycline therapy may be contraindicated, e.g., patients who have received cumulative doses of 400 mg/m2 of doxorubicin or doxorubicin equivalents.

Zofran (ondansetron), from Glaxo Wellcome received additional approval on August 27, 1999, for the prevention of nausea and vomiting associated with highly emetogenic cancer chemotherapy, including cisplatin.

Zofran ODT (odansetron) orally disintegrating tablets, by Glaxo Wellcome, Inc., received additional approval on January 27, 1999, for prevention of chemotherapy and radiation-induced nausea and vomiting, and prevention of postoperative nausea and vomiting (new dosage form).

Zofran (ondanstron hydrochloride) sponsored by Glaxo Wellcome Inc., received approval on October 31, 1997, for intramuscular administration as an alternative to intravenous administration in the prevention of postoperative nausea and vomiting (new route of administration.)

Zofran (ondansetron hydrochloride) Oral Solution, sponsored by Glaxo Wellcome Incorporated, received approval on January 24, 1997, for the prevention of chemotherapy, radiotherapy, and postoperative induced nausea and vomiting. Zofran was previously available in oral tablet and injectable formulations.

Zoladex, (goserelin acetate implant) by Zeneca Pharmaceuticals received additional approval on July 27, 1998, for use of 3.6 mg and 10.8 mg depots in combination with flutamide for the management of locally confined Stage T2b-T4 (Stage B2-C) carcinoma of the prostate. [New dosage and Administration]

Zoladex (goserelin acetate implant) by Zeneca Pharmaceuticals, Inc., received additional approval on April 9, 1998, for palliative treatment of advanced carcinoma of the prostate. [New Route of Administration]

Zyloprim (allopurinol sodium) from Glaxo Wellcome, received approval on May 17, 1996, for the management of patients with leukemia, lymphoma, and solid tumor malignancies who are receiving cancer therapy which causes elevation of uric acid levels and who cannot tolerate oral therapy.

Prepared by: Cancer Liaison Program Office of Special Health Issues, Office of International and Constituents Relations. Last revised December 9, 1999. E-mail: oshi@oc.fda.gov

Chapter 65

List of Chemotherapy Drugs

Older Drugs

Adriamycin (Doxorubicin)

Adriamycin, an active medicine against many cancers, is one of the older chemotherapy drugs, having been in use for decades. Adriamycin is a clear, orange-red colored powder or liquid, which is administered intravenously only. It is most commonly used in treatment of the following cancers:

- Breast Stomach Lymphomas
- Multiple myeloma
- Sarcomas
- Bone tumors

The type and extent of a cancer will determine the method and schedule of administration of this drug. This decision is made by the medical oncologist. Adriamycin may be administered as a continuous intravenous infusion over a span of four to five days, or given on a scheduled basis, i.e., once a week or once every three to four weeks, etc.

Side Effects

The degree and severity of the side effects depend on the amount and schedule of the administration of Adriamycin. It is imperative that

---

Reprinted with permission from Tirgan Oncology Associates, M. Hossein Tirgan, MD, http://www.tirgan.com/chemolst.htm, November 1998.

patients relay any side effects or problems to their medical oncologist. Some of the significant side effects are:

- Soreness of the mouth, difficulty swallowing
- Diarrhea
- Low white blood counts
- Low platelet count
- Anemia
- Heart problems
- Damage to the veins (it can cause redness and irritation at the site of injection, despite proper injection)
- Severe damage to the tissues if it leaks from the injection site (extravasation)
- Red urine, which is due to excretion of the medicine by the kidneys

Alkeran (Melphalan)

Alkeran is one of the older chemotherapy drugs. It has been in use for many years. Alkeran is administered orally in pill form. The most common conditions for which this drug is administered are:

- Multiple Myeloma
- Breast cancer
- Ovarian cancer
- Bone marrow transplantation

The type and extent of a cancer will determine the method and schedule of administration of this drug. This decision is made by the medical oncologist. Alkeran is normally prescribed once a day for up to two to three weeks at a time.

Side Effects

The degree and severity of the side effects depend on the amount and schedule of the administration of Alkeran. It is imperative that patients relay any side effects or problems to their medical oncologist. Some of the most common adverse effects are as follows:

- Low white blood counts
- Low platelet count
- Anemia
- Diarrhea
- Loss of appetite

Ara-C (Cytarabine)

Ara-C is one of the older chemotherapy drugs which has been around and in use for many years. Ara-C is a clear, colorless liquid given by intravenous route. It is most commonly used in treatment of the following cancers:

- Acute Myeloid Leukemia and Chronic Myeloid Leukemia
- Acute Lymphoid Leukemia
- Lymphomas

The type and extent of a cancer will determine the method and schedule of administration of this drug. This decision is made by the medical oncologist. Ara-C is normally given on a daily basis for five to seven days. It can also be given inside the spinal fluid in patients with Leukemias or Lymphomas.

Side Effects

The degree and severity of the side effects depend on the amount and schedule of the administration of Ara-C. It is imperative that patients relay any side effects or problems to their medical oncologist. Following are some of the most common and important ill effects:

- Low white blood counts
- Low platelet count
- Anemia
- Hair loss
- Soreness of the mouth, difficulty swallowing
- Diarrhea
- Damage to the brain when used in very high doses, causing an imbalance and inability to perform highly coordinated movements, poor handwriting, etc.

BiCNU (Carmustine)

BiCNU is one of the older chemotherapy drugs which has been around and in use for many years. BiCNU is a white powder, desolved in an alcohol based, colorless solution, and is given by intravenous route only. It has to be mixed in a high volume of solution, otherwise can cause pain in the arm, if it is given in an arm vein, and also damage to the veins. It is most commonly used in treatment of the following cancers:

- Brain
- Multiple Myeloma
- Melanoma
- Lymphomas
- Bone Marrow Transplantation

647

The type and extent of a cancer will determine the method and schedule of administration of this drug. This decision is made by the medical oncologist. BiCNU is normally given once, every 6-8 weeks.

Side Effects

The degree and severity of the side effects depend on the amount and schedule of the administration of BiCNU. It is imperative that patients relay any side effects or problems to their medical oncologist. Following are some of the most common and important ill effects:

- Low white blood counts
- Low platelet count
- Anemia
- Hair Loss
- Soreness of the mouth, difficulty swallowing
- Diarrhea
- Kidney and Lung damage when used in very high doses

Busulfan (Myleran)

Busulfan is one of the older chemotherapy drugs which has been around and in use for many years. Busulfan is a pill which is taken orally. It is most commonly used in the following situations:

- Chronic Myeloid Leukemia • Bone Marrow Transplantation

The type and extent of a cancer will determine the method and schedule of administration of this drug. This decision is made by the medical oncologist. Busulfan is normally prescribed on a daily basis for a long period of time—until a remission is achieved. In a bone marrow transplant setting, it is given orally for a few days in very high doses.

Side Effects

The degree and severity of the side effects depend on the amount and schedule of the administration of Busulfan. It is imperative that patients relay any side effects or problems to their medical oncologist. Following are some of the most common and significant ill effects:

- Low white blood counts
- Low platelet count
- Anemia

- Hair Loss
- Soreness of the mouth, difficulty swallowing
- Diarrhea
- Lung damage is a serious side effect of this medicine. It may manifest itself by shortness of breath or cough after lengthy or high dose treatments with Busulfan.

CCNU *(Lomustine)*

CCNU is one of the older chemotherapy drugs which has been around and in use for many years. CCNU is a capsule taken orally. It is most commonly used in treatment of the following cancers:

- Lung
- Multiple Myeloma
- Brain tumors

The type and extent of a cancer will determine the method and schedule of administration of this drug. This decision is made by the medical oncologist. CCNU is normally administered once every six to eight weeks.

Side Effects

The degree and severity of the side effects depend on the amount and schedule of the administration of CCNU. It is imperative that patients relay any side effects or problems to their medical oncologist. Following are some of the most common and significant ill effects:

- Low white blood counts
- Low platelet count
- Anemia
- Hair Loss
- Lung damage
- Diarrhea

Cisplatinum *(Platinol)*

Cisplatinum is one of the older chemotherapy drugs which has been around and in use for decades. It is an active medicine against many cancers. Cisplatinum is a white powder which, when prepared for use, becomes a clear, colorless liquid. It is given by intravenous route only. It is most commonly used in treatment of the following cancers:

- Ovarian
- Endometrial
- Head and Neck
- Lung
- Testis
- Breast
- Stomach
- Lymphomas
- Leukemias

The type and extent of a cancer will determine the method and schedule of administration of this drug. This decision is made by the medical oncologist. Cisplatinum is given by intravenous infusion, over one to five days, every three to four weeks.

Side Effects

The degree and severity of the side effects depend on the amount and schedule of the administration of Cisplatinum. It is imperative that patients relay any side effects or problems to their medical oncologist. Following are some of the most common and significant ill effects:

- Kidney damage
- Diarrhea
- Low Platelet count
- Anemia
- Hair Loss
- Nausea and vomiting
- Damage to ears and hearing problems

In order to prevent damage to kidneys and hearing, patients receive plenty of fluids prior to the administration of Cisplatinum. A new drug called, Amifostine (Ethyol) seems to be able to counteract the side effects and protect the kidneys against the ill effects of Cisplatinum. Anti-nausea medications are also used beforehand.

Cytoxan (Cyclophosphamide)

Cytoxan is one of the older chemotherapy drugs which has been available for use for decades. Cytoxan comes in pill form, as well as a white powder, which, when made ready for use, is a clear color liquid. It is given by intravenous route. It is most commonly used in treatment of the following cancers:

- Breast
- Lymphomas
- Leukemias
- Multiple myeloma
- Ovarian
- Lung
- Bladder
- Soft tissue sarcomas
- Bone

The type and extent of a cancer will determine the method and schedule of administration of this drug. This decision is made by the medical oncologist. Cytoxan may be given as intravenous infusion or orally.

Side Effects

The degree and severity of the side effects depend on the amount and schedule of the administration of Cytoxan. It is imperative that patients relay any side effects or problems to their medical oncologist. Following are some of the most common and significant ill effects:

- Soreness of the mouth, difficulty swallowing
- Diarrhea
- Low white blood counts
- Anemia
- Low platelet count
- Hair Loss
- Irritation and bleeding of bladder

Daunorubicin

Daunorubicin is one of the older chemotherapy drugs which has been in use for many years. Daunorubicin, when prepared for use, becomes a clear, red liquid, and is given by intravenous route only. It is most commonly used in treatment of the following cancers:

- Acute Myeloid Leukemia
- Acute Lymphocytic Leukemia

The type and extent of a cancer will determine the method and schedule of administration of this drug. This decision is made by the medical oncologist. Daunorubicin is normally administered daily for three consecutive days.

Side Effects

The degree and severity of the side effects depend on the amount and schedule of the administration of Daunorubicin. It is imperative that patients relay any side effects or problems to their medical oncologist. Following are some of the most common and significant ill effects:

- Low white blood counts
- Low platelet count
- Anemia
- Hair Loss
- Soreness of the mouth, difficulty swallowing

- Diarrhea
- Heart damage
- Skin rash
- Red urine, which is due to excretion of the medicine by the kidneys into the urine.

DTIC (Dacarbazine)

DTIC is one of the older chemotherapy drugs which has been around and in use for many years. DTIC is a white powder and when prepared for use, it becomes a clear and colorless liquid and is given by intravenous route only. It is most commonly used in treatment of the following cancers:

- Melanoma
- Soft tissue sarcoma
- Hodgkin's Disease
- Neuroblastoma

The type and extent of a cancer will determine the method and schedule of administration of this drug. This decision is made by the medical oncologist. DTIC is normally given daily for 5-10 days.

Side Effects

The degree and severity of the side effects depend on the amount and schedule of the administration of DTIC. It is imperative that patients relay any side effects or problems to their medical oncologist. Following are some of the most common and important ill effects:

- Low white blood counts
- Low platelet count
- Anemia
- Hair Loss
- Soreness of the mouth, difficulty swallowing
- Diarrhea
- Transient Liver Damage

5 Fluorouracil (5-FU)

5-FU is one of the oldest chemotherapy drugs, and has been around and in use for decades. It is an active medicine against many cancers. 5-FU is a clear and colorless liquid, and is given by intravenous route. It is also available in a creme form for treatment of skin cancer. It is most commonly used in treatment of the following cancers:

- Colon
- Breast
- Stomach
- Pancreas

The type and extent of a cancer will determine the method and schedule of administration of this drug. This decision is made by the medical oncologist. 5-FU may be given as a continuous intravenous infusion, over 4-5 days, or given on a scheduled basis, (e.g., once a week, or once every 3-4 weeks, etc.)

Side Effects

5-FU is normally administered by intravenous route. The life span of 5-FU in blood and body tissues is very short and limited to minutes. 5-FU binds to an enzyme inside of the cancer cells called *Thymidilate Synthetase* and thereby exerts its anti-cancer effect on the cells. Leucovorin enhances the binding of 5-FU to this enzyme and as a result prolongs the life span of 5-FU within the cancer cells, resulting in a greater anti-cancer effect. The degree and severity of the side effects depend on the amount and schedule of the administration of 5-FU. It is imperative that patients relay any side effects or problems to their medical oncologist. Following are some of the most common and important ill effects:

- Soreness of the mouth, difficulty swallowing
- Diarrhea
- Stomach pain
- Low white blood counts
- Low platelet counts
- Anemia
- Sensitive skin (to sun exposure)
- Excessive tear formation from the eyes

Hydroxyurea (Hydrea)

Hydrea is one of the older chemotherapy drugs which has been around and in use for many years. Hydrea is a capsule and is given orally. It is most commonly used in treatment of the following cancers:

- Chronic Myelocytic Leukemia
- Polycythemia
- Increased platelets
- Head and neck cancer
- Sickle cell disease

The type and extent of a cancer will determine the method and schedule of administration of this drug. This decision is made by the medical oncologist. Hydrea is normally given orally, daily for many days, until a response is achieved.

Side Effects

The degree and severity of the side effects depend on the amount and schedule of the administration of Hydrea. It is imperative that patients relay any side effects or problems to their medical oncologist. Following are some of the most common and important ill effects:

- Low white blood counts
- Low platelet count
- Anemia
- Hair loss (after prolonged use)

ldarubicin (Idamycin)

Idarubicin is one of the older chemotherapy drugs which has been around and in use for decades. It is an active medicine against certain cancers. Idarubicin is given by intravenous route only, being most commonly used in treatment of the following cancers:

- Acute Myeloid Leukemia
- Chronic Myeloid Leukemia
- Acute Lymphoid Leukemia

The type and extent of a cancer will determine the method and schedule of administration of this drug. This decision is made by the medical oncologist. Idarubicin may be given as a continuous intravenous infusion over four to five days, or given on a scheduled basis, (i.e., once a week, or once every three to four weeks, etc.)

Side Effects

The degree and severity of the side effects depend on the amount and schedule of the administration of ldarubicin. It is imperative that patients relay any side effects or problems to their medical oncologist. Following are some of the most common and important ill effects:

- Low white blood counts
- Low platelet counts
- Anemia

- Hair loss
- Soreness of the mouth; difficulty swallowing
- Diarrhea

Ifosfamide

Ifosfamide is one of the newer chemotherapy drugs which has been around and in use for many years. Ifosfamide is a white powder which, when prepared for use becomes a clear, colorless liquid. It is given by intravenous route only and is most commonly used in treatment of the following cancers:

- Lung
- Testis
- Lymphomas
- Bone
- Soft tissue sarcomas

The type and extent of a cancer will determine the method and schedule of administration of this drug. This decision is made by the medical oncologist. Ifosfamide is normally given over three to four days, every three to four weeks.

Side Effects

The degree and severity of the side effects depend on the amount and schedule of the administration of Ifosfamide. It is imperative that patients relay any side effects or problems to their medical oncologist. Following are some of the most common and important ill effects:

- Low white blood counts
- Low platelet count
- Anemia
- Hair loss
- Bleeding from bladder, which is prevented by using Mesna.

Methotrexate

Methotrexate is one of the oldest chemotherapy drugs. It has been around and in use for many years. Methotrexate is a yellow powder which, when prepared for use, becomes a clear, yellow liquid, and is given by intravenous route. It is also available in tablet form. It is most commonly used in the following situations:

- Breast cancer
- Head and Neck cancer
- Lung cancer
- Acute Lymphocytic Leukemia

- Gestational Throphoblastic disease
- Bone tumors
- Lymphomas
- Treatment of arthritis

The type and extent of a cancer will determine the method and schedule of administration of this drug. This decision is made by the medical oncologist. Methotrexate is normally given intravenously or orally.

Side Effects

Methotrexate exerts its chemotherapeutic effect by its ability to counteract and compete with folic acid in cancer cells resulting in folic acid deficiency within the cells and causing their demise. Normal cells are not immune from this effect of Methotrexate either. As a result, it can cause significant side effects in the body. The degree and severity of the side effects depend on the amount and schedule of the administration of Methotrexate. It is imperative that patients relay any side effects or problems to their medical oncologist. Following are some of the most common and important ill effects:

- Low white blood counts
- Low platelet count
- Anemia
- Hair Loss
- Soreness of the mouth, difficulty swallowing
- Diarrhea
- Liver damage
- Lung damage
- Nerve damage
- Kidney damage

Most of these complications and side effects of Methotrexate can be either prevented or treated by using Leucovorin which is normally administered 24 hours after the Methotrexate is given. This will allow the Methotrexate to exert its anti-cancer effect.

Mithramycin

Mithramycin is one of the older chemotherapy drugs which has been in use for decades. This drug is used in the treatment of high calcium levels. It is given by intravenous route only.

Side Effects

The degree and severity of the side effects depend on the amount and schedule of the administration of Mithramycin. It is imperative that patients relay any side effects or problems to their medical oncologists. Following are some of the most common and important ill effects:

- Low white blood counts
- Anemia
- Low platelet count
- Loss of appetite

Mitoxantrone

Mitoxantrone is one of the newer chemotherapy drugs which has been around and in use for a few years. Mitoxantrone, when prepared for use, becomes a dark blue-colored liquid. This drug is administered intravenously. It is most commonly used in treatment of the following cancers:

- Acute Lymphocytic Leukemia
- Acute Myeloid Leukemia
- Lymphomas
- Breast cancer
- Ovarian cancer

In special situations, Mitoxantrone is injected inside the abdominal cavity for treatment of Ascites due to cancers. The type and extent of a cancer will determine the method and schedule of administration of this drug. This decision is made by the medical oncologist. Mitoxantrone is normally given daily for three days, or weekly.

Side Effects

The degree and severity of the side effects depend on the amount and schedule of the administration of Mitoxantrone. It is imperative that patients relay any side effects or problems to their medical oncologists. Following are some of the most common and significant ill effects:

- Low white blood counts
- Low platelet count
- Anemia
- Hair Loss
- Soreness of the mouth, difficulty swallowing
- Diarrhea
- Blue urine, which is due to excretion of the medicine in the urine.

Velban (Vinblastine)

Velban is one of the older chemotherapy drugs which has been around for many years. Velban, when prepared for use, becomes a clear and colorless liquid and is given by intravenous route only. It is most commonly used in treatment of the following cancers:

- Lymphomas
- Hodgkin's Disease
- Gestational Throphoblastic disease
- Testis
- Breast cancer

The type and extent of a cancer will determine the method and schedule of administration of this drug. This decision is made by the medical oncologist. Velban is normally given once every 1-2 weeks

Side Effects

The degree and severity of the side effects depend on the amount and schedule of the administration of Velban. It is imperative that patients relay any side effects or problems to their medical oncologist. Following are some of the most common and important ill effects:

- Low white blood counts
- Low platelet count
- Anemia
- Hair Loss
- Soreness of the mouth, difficulty swallowing
- Diarrhea
- Nerve damage
- Damage to the veins
- It can cause redness and irritation at the site of injection, despite proper injection.
- Severe damage to the tissues, if leaks from the injection site (Extravasation)
- Paralysis of bowels

Vincristine (Oncovin)

Vincristine is one of the older chemotherapy drugs which has been around for many years. When prepared for use, it becomes a clear and colorless liquid and is given by intravenous route only. It is most commonly used in treatment of the following cancers:

- Lymphomas
- Hodgkin's Disease
- Breast cancer
- Acute Lymphocytic Leukemia
- Soft tissue sarcomas
- Multiple Myeloma
- Neuroblastoma

The type and extent of a cancer will determine the method and schedule of administration of this drug. This decision is made by the medical oncologist. Vincristine is normally given once a week.

Side Effects

The degree and severity of the side effects depend on the amount and schedule of the administration of Vincristine. It is imperative that patients relay any side effects or problems to their medical oncologist. Following are some of the most common and important ill effects:

- Low platelet count
- Anemia
- Hair Loss
- Bowel paralysis
- Diarrhea
- Nerve damage
- Damage to the veins. It can cause redness and irritation at the site of injection, despite proper injection.
- Severe damage to the tissues, if leaks from the injection site (Extravasation)

VP-16 (Etoposide)

VP-16 is one of the newer chemotherapy drugs which has been around for many years. It is an active medicine against many cancers. VP-16 is a clear and colorless liquid, and is given by intravenous route only. Prior to administration, VP-16 has to be mixed in rather large amount of fluids. It is most commonly used in treatment of the following cancers:

- Lung
- Lymphomas

The type and extent of a cancer will determine the method and schedule of administration of this drug. This decision is made by the medical oncologist. VP-16 is normally given daily for 3 consecutive days, every 3-4 weeks.

Side Effects

The degree and severity of the side effects depend on the amount and schedule of the administration of VP-16. It is imperative that patients relay any side effects or problems to their medical oncologist. Following are some of the most common and important ill effects:

- Low white blood counts
- Low platelet count
- Anemia
- Hair Loss
- Soreness of the mouth, difficulty swallowing
- Diarrhea

Newer Drugs

Carboplatinum (Paraplatin)

Carboplatinum is one of the newer chemotherapy drugs which has been in use for over a decade. It is an active medicine against many cancers. Carboplatinum is a white powder which when prepared for use is a clear, colorless liquid. It is given by intravenous route only and is most commonly used in treatment of the following cancers:

- Ovaries
- Lung
- Head and Neck
- Leukemias
- Testis
- Endometrial

The type and extent of a cancer will determine the method and schedule of administration of this drug. This decision is made by the medical oncolooist. Carboplatinum may be given as a continuous intravenous infusion over four to five days, or given on a scheduled basis, e.g., once a week or once every three to four weeks, etc.)

Side Effects

The degree and severity of the side effects depend on the amount and schedule of the administration of Carboplatinum. It is imperative that patients relay any side effects or problems to their medical oncologist. Following are some of the most common and significant ill effects:

- Low white blood counts
- Low platelet count
- Anemia
- Hair Loss
- Nausea
- Diarrhea
- Nerve damage

Fludarabine (Fludara)

Fludarabine is one of the newer chemotherapy drugs which has been around and in use for a few years. Fludarabine is a white powder and when prepared for use, it becomes a clear and colorless liquid and is given by intravenous route only. It is most commonly used in treatment of the following cancers:

- Chronic Lymphocytic Leukemia
- Low Grade Lymphomas

The type and extent of a cancer will determine the method and schedule of administration of this drug. This decision is made by the medical oncoloaist. Fludarabine is normally given daily for 3-5 days and repeated every 4 weeks.

Side Effects

The degree and severity of the side effects depend on the amount and schedule of the administration of Fludarabine. It is imperative that patients relay any side effects or problems to their medical oncologist. Following are some of the most common and important ill effects:

- Low white blood counts
- Low platelet count
- Anemia
- Hair Loss
- Soreness of the mouth, difficulty swallowing
- Diarrhea
- Lung damage
- Tumor Lysis Syndrome

Gemcitabine (Gemzar)

Gemcitabine is among the newest cancer chemotherapy drugs which has become available in past few years. Chemically, it is very similar to Ara-C and with similar toxicities. It is an active drug in treatment of:

- Cancer of Pancreas (This drug seems to be the most effective drug in treatment of cancer of pancreas.)
- Lung cancer

Side Effects

The degree and severity of the side effects depend on the amount and schedule of the administration. It is imperative that patients relay any side effects or problems to their medical oncologist. Following are some of the most common and important ill effects:

- Low white blood counts
- Low platelet count
- Anemia
- Minimal hair loss due to Gemcitabine is seen in about 15% of patients.
- Diarrhea can be seen in up to 19% of patients receiving this medicine.
- Nausea/Vomiting
- Flu like symptoms, fever, chills, muscle ache,
- Abnormalities in Kidney and Liver function tests
- Skin rash, itching

The type and extent of a cancer will determine the method and schedule of administration of this drug. This decision is made by the medical oncologist. It is given once a week, intravenously over 30 minutes for as long as the patient responds to the drug.

Irinotecan (CPT-11)

Irinotecan is among the newest cancer chemotherapy drugs which has become available in past few years and approved by FDA in 1996 for treatment of recurrent Colon Cancer. This drug is being studied to determine its efficacy against other cancers.

Side Effects

The degree and severity of the side effects depend on the amount and schedule of the administration of this drug. It is imperative that patients relay any side effects or problems to their medical oncologist. Following are some of the most common and important ill effects of Irinotecan are:

- Severe Diarrhea, which may happen in one out of four patients.
- Low white blood counts
- Damage to the lungs

The type and extent of a cancer will determine the method and schedule of administration of this drug. This decision is made by the medical oncologis. It is given once a week or once every 3-6 weeks, intravenously, for as long as the patient responds to the drug.

Leustatin (Cladribine)

Cladribine is one of the newest chemotherapy drugs which has been around and in use for a few years. Cladribine is a white powder, when prepared for use becomes a clear, colorless liquid, and is given by intravenous route only. It is most commonly used in treatment of the following cancers:

- Hairy cell leukemia
- Low grade lymphomas
- Waldenström's macroglobulinemia

The type and extent of a cancer will determine the method and schedule of administration of this drug. This decision is made by the medical oncologist. Cladribine is normally administered daily for seven consecutive days as a continuous intravenous infusion and repeated every four weeks. A proper dosage schedule is still being studied.

Side Effects

The degree and severity of the side effects depend on the amount and schedule of the administration of Cladribine. It is imperative that patients relay any side effects or problems to their medical oncologist. Following are some of the most common and important ill effects:

- Low white blood counts
- Low platelet count
- Anemia
- Fever
- Skin rash

Navelbine (Vinorelbine)

Navelbine is one of the newest chemotherapy drugs which has been in use for a few years. Navelbine, when prepared for use, becomes a clear, colorless liquid, and is given by intravenous route only. It is most commonly used in treatment of the following cancer:

- Non small cell lung cancer

The type and extent of a cancer will determine the method and schedule of administration of the drug. This decision is made by the medical oncologist. Navelbine is normally given once a week.

Side Effects

The degree and severity of the side effects depend on the amount and schedule of the administration of Navelbine. It is imperative that patients relay any side effects or problems to their medical oncologist. Following are some of the most common and important ill effects:

- Nausea, vomiting
- Liver damage
- Nerve damage

Taxol (Paclitaxel)

Taxol is one of the newer chemotherapy drugs, and has been around, and in use for some years. It is an extract from the bark and needles of the yew tree, *Taxus brevifolia*. Taxol is a white powder and when prepared for use becomes a clear, colorless liquid which is given by intravenous route only. It is most commonly used in treatment of the following cancers:

- Ovarian
- Testis
- Metastatic breast cancer
- Head and neck cancer
- Lung cancer
- Melanoma

Taxol is most commonly used in combination with other chemotherapy drugs such as: 5-FU, Adriamycin, Vinorelbine, Cytoxan, and Cisplatinum. The type and extent of a cancer will determine the method and schedule of administration of this drug. This decision is made by the medical oncologist. Taxol is normally given once every three weeks.

Side Effects

The degree and severity of the side effects depend on the amount and schedule of the administration of Taxol. Following are some of the most common and important ill effects:

- Low white blood counts
- Low platelet count
- Anemia
- Hair loss
- Soreness of the mouth, difficulty swallowing
- Diarrhea
- Nerve damage
- Allergic reaction
- Fluid Retention

The occurrence of allergic reactions, skin reaction and fluid retention can be reduced by pretreatment of patients with steroids. It is imperative that patients relay any side effects or problems to their medical oncologists. Taxol is metabolized in the liver and excreted into bile. Dose of Taxol should be reduced in patients with liver dysfunction or massive liver metastasis.

Taxotere (Docetaxel)

This drug is prepared from the needles of European yew trees. It is from the same family of Taxol. It has shown significant activity in following cancers:

- Breast cancer. This drug was approved by FDA in May 1996 for treatment of patients with advance stage breast cancer who have failed to respond to Adriamycin.
- Non small cell lung cancer

This drug is a rather well tolerated medicine and seem to be very active in treatment of breast cancer. Over next few years we may see many more indications for it. It is administered as an intravenous infusion over 1-3 hours or over a longer period of time up to 5 day continuous infusion (24 hours a day for 5 days.) It can be combined with Cisplatinum or Carboplatinum in treatment of lung cancer.

Side Effects

It is imperative that patients relay any side effects or problems to their medical oncologist. This drug can be associated with any of the following problems;

- Low white blood counts
- Low platelet counts
- Fluid retention and weight gain

Topotecan (Hycamtin)

Topotecan is one of the newer chemotherapy drugs, and has been around, and in use for some years. It is a synthetic product, very similar to a natural compound, Camptothecin, which was derived from a Chinese tree, *Camptotheca acuminata*. Topotecan is normally given by intravenous infusion over 30 minutes, daily for five consecutive days. There is an oral product under investigation. In certain conditions, specially in treatment of leukemias, it issued as a continuos infusion for five days. The treatment cycle is repeated every 3-4 weeks. This drug is effective in treatment of the following cancers:

- Ovarian
- Small Cell Lung Cancer
- Leukemias (AML, CML)
- Non Hodgkin's Lymphomas
- Myelodysplastic Syndrome
- Selected Pediatric Cancer

Topotecan is also used in combination with other chemotherapy drugs such as: Taxol, Adriamycin, Cytoxan and Cisplatinum. The type and extent of a cancer will determine the method and schedule of administration of this drug. This decision is made by the medical oncologist. Topotecan is normally given every three weeks. Topotecan is metabolized in the liver and excreted into bile. Dose of Topotecan should be reduced in patients with kidney or liver dysfunction.

Side Effects

The degree and severity of the side effects depend on the amount and schedule of the administration of Topotecan. It is imperative that patients relay any side effects or problems to their medical oncologist. Following are some of the most common and important ill effects:

- Low white blood counts
- Low platelet count
- Fatigue
- Anemia
- Hair loss
- Nausea
- Vomiting
- Soreness of the mouth, difficulty swallowing
- Diarrhea

Chapter 66

Radiation Therapy and You

Introduction

This chapter is for patients who are receiving radiation therapy for cancer. It describes what to expect during therapy and offers suggestions for self-care during and after treatment. It explains the two most common types of radiation therapy, external radiation and internal radiation therapy. Information is included about the general effects of treatment and how to deal with specific side effects.

You may not want to read everything here at one time. Browse through it, read the sections that are of interest to you right now, and look at the others as needed. Because your doctor will plan the treatment specifically for you and the type of cancer you have, some information may not apply to you.

Radiation therapy may vary somewhat among different doctors, hospitals, and treatment centers. Therefore, your treatment or the advice of your doctor (the radiation oncologist) may be different from what you read here. Be sure to ask questions and discuss your concerns with your doctor, nurse, or radiation therapist. Ask whether they have any additional written information that might help you.

Fast Facts about Radiation Therapy

- Radiation treatments are painless.

"Radiation Therapy And You: A Guide To Self-Help During Treatment," National Cancer Institute (NCI), updated September 1999.

- External radiation treatment does not make you radioactive.

- Treatments are usually scheduled every day except Saturday and Sunday.

- You need to allow 30 minutes for each treatment session although the treatment itself takes only a few minutes.

- It's important to get plenty of rest and to eat a well-balanced diet during the course of your radiation therapy.

- Skin in the treated area may become sensitive and easily irritated.

- Side effects of radiation treatment are usually temporary and they vary depending on the area of the body that is being treated.

Radiation in Cancer Treatment

What Is Radiation Therapy?

Radiation therapy (sometimes called radiotherapy, x-ray therapy, or irradiation) is the treatment of disease using penetrating beams of high energy waves or streams of particles called radiation.

Many years ago doctors learned how to use this energy to "see" inside the body and find disease. You've probably seen a chest x-ray or x-ray pictures of your teeth or your bones. At high doses (many times those used for x-ray exams) radiation is used to treat cancer and other illnesses.

The radiation used for cancer treatment comes from special machines or from radioactive substances. Radiation therapy equipment aims specific amounts of the radiation at tumors or areas of the body where there is disease.

How Does Radiation Therapy Work?

Radiation in high doses kills cells or keeps them from growing and dividing. Because cancer cells grow and divide more rapidly than most of the normal cells around them, radiation therapy can successfully treat many kinds of cancer. Normal cells are also affected by radiation but, unlike cancer cells, most of them recover from the effects of radiation.

To protect normal cells, doctors carefully limit the doses of radiation and spread the treatment out over time. They also shield as much normal tissue as possible while they aim the radiation at the site of the cancer.

What Are the Goals and Benefits of Radiation Therapy?

The goal of radiation therapy is to kill the cancer cells with as little risk as possible to normal cells. Radiation therapy can be used to treat many kinds of cancer in almost any part of the body. In fact, more than half of all people with cancer are treated with some form of radiation. For many cancer patients, radiation is the only kind of treatment they need. Thousands of people who have had radiation therapy alone or in combination with other types of cancer treatment are free of cancer.

Radiation treatment, like surgery, is a local treatment it affects the cancer cells only in a specific area of the body. Sometimes doctors add radiation therapy to treatments that reach all parts of the body (systemic treatment) such as chemotherapy, or biological therapy to improve treatment results. You may hear your doctor use the term, adjuvant therapy, for a treatment that is added to, and given after, the primary therapy.

Radiation therapy is often used with surgery to treat cancer. Doctors may use radiation before surgery to shrink a tumor. This makes it easier to remove the cancerous tissue and may allow the surgeon to perform less radical surgery.

Radiation therapy may be used after surgery to stop the growth of cancer cells that may remain. Your doctor may choose to use radiation therapy and surgery at the same time. This procedure, known as intraoperative radiation, is explained more fully in the section "External Radiation Therapy."

In some cases, instead of surgery, doctors use radiation along with anticancer drugs (chemotherapy) to destroy the cancer. Radiation may be given before, during, or after chemotherapy. Doctors carefully tailor this combination treatment to each patient's needs depending on the type of cancer, its location, and its size. The purpose of radiation treatment before or during chemotherapy is to make the tumor smaller and thus improve the effectiveness of the anticancer drugs. Doctors sometimes recommend that a patient complete chemotherapy and then have radiation treatment to kill any cancer cells that might remain.

When curing the cancer is not possible, radiation therapy can be used to shrink tumors and reduce pressure, pain, and other symptoms of cancer. This is called palliative care or palliation. Many cancer patients find that they have a better quality of life when radiation is used for this purpose.

What Are the Risks of Radiation Therapy?

The brief high doses of radiation that damage or destroy cancer cells can also injure or kill normal cells. These effects of radiation on normal cells cause treatment side effects. Most side effects of radiation treatment are well known and, with the help of your doctor and nurse, easily treated. The side effects of radiation therapy and what to do about them are discussed the section "Managing Side Effects."

The risk of side effects is usually less than the benefit of killing cancer cells. Your doctor will not advise you to have any treatment unless the benefits control of disease and relief from symptoms are greater than the known risks.

How Is Radiation Therapy Given?

Radiation therapy can be given in one of two ways: external or internal. Some patients have both, one after the other.

Most people who receive radiation therapy for cancer have external radiation. It is usually given during outpatient visits to a hospital or treatment center. In external radiation therapy, a machine directs the high-energy rays at the cancer and a small margin of normal tissue surrounding it.

The various machines used for external radiation work in slightly different ways. Some are better for treating cancers near the skin surface; others work best on cancers deeper in the body. The most common type of machine used for radiation therapy is called a linear accelerator. Some radiation machines use a variety of radioactive substances (such as cobalt-60, for example) as the source of high-energy rays. Your doctor decides which type of radiation therapy machine is best for you. You will find more information about external radiation in the next section.

When internal radiation therapy is used, the radiation source is placed inside the body. This method of radiation treatment is called brachytherapy or implant therapy. The source of the radiation (such as radioactive iodine, for example) sealed in a small holder is called an implant. Implants may be thin wires, plastic tubes (catheters), capsules, or seeds. An implant may be placed directly into a tumor or inserted into a body cavity. Sometimes, after a tumor has been removed by surgery, the implant is placed in the 'tumor bed' (the area from which the tumor was removed) to kill any tumor cells that may remain.

Another type of internal radiation therapy uses unsealed radioactive materials which may be taken by mouth or injected into the body. If you have this type of treatment, you may need to stay in the hospital for several days.

Who Gives Radiation Treatments?

A doctor who specializes in using radiation to treat cancer. A radiation oncologist will prescribe the type and amount of treatment that is right for you. The radiation oncologist is the person referred to as "your doctor" throughout this chapter. The radiation oncologist works closely with the other doctors and health care professionals involved in your care. This highly trained health care team may include:

- The radiation physicist, who makes sure that the equipment is working properly and that the machines deliver the right dose of radiation. The physicist also works closely with your doctor to plan your treatment.

- The dosimetrist, who works under the direction of your doctor and the radiation physicist and helps carry out your treatment plan by calculating the amount of radiation to be delivered to the cancer and normal tissues that are nearby.

- The radiation therapist, who positions you for your treatments and runs the equipment that delivers the radiation.

- The radiation nurse, who will coordinate your care, help you learn about treatment, and tell you how to manage side effects. The nurse can also answer questions you or family members may have about your treatment.

Your health care team also may include a physician assistant, radiologist, dietitian, physical therapist, social worker, or other health care professional.

Is Radiation Treatment Expensive?

Treatment of cancer with radiation can be costly. It requires very complex equipment and the services of many health care professionals. The exact cost of your radiation therapy will depend on the type and number of treatments you need.

Most health insurance policies, including Part B of Medicare, cover charges for radiation therapy. It's a good idea to talk with your doctor's office staff or the hospital business office about your policy and how expected costs will be paid.

In some states, the Medicaid program may help you pay for treatments. You can find out from the office that handles social services in your city or county whether you are eligible for Medicaid and whether your radiation therapy is a covered expense.

If you need financial aid, contact the hospital social service office or the National Cancer Institute's (NCI) Cancer Information Service at 1-800-4-CANCER. They may be able to direct you to sources of help. Additional sources of cancer information are described in the resources section at the end of this chapter.

External Radiation Therapy: What To Expect

How Does the Doctor Plan My Treatment?

The high energy rays used for radiation therapy can come from a variety of sources. Your doctor may choose to use x-rays, an electron beam, or cobalt-60 gamma rays. Some cancer treatment centers have special equipment that produces beams of protons or neutrons for radiation therapy. The type of radiation your doctor decides to use depends on what kind of cancer you have and how far into your body the radiation should go. High-energy radiation is used to treat many types of cancer. Low-energy x-rays are used to treat some kinds of skin diseases.

After a physical exam and a review of your medical history, the doctor plans your treatment. In a process called simulation, you will be asked to lie very still on an examining table while the radiation therapist uses a special x-ray machine to define your treatment port or field. This is the exact place on your body where the radiation will be aimed. Depending on the location of your cancer, you may have more than one treatment port.

Simulation may also involve CT scans or other imaging studies to plan how to direct the radiation. Depending on the type of treatment you will be receiving, body molds or other devices that keep you from moving during treatment (immobilization devices) may be made at this time. They will be used each time you have treatment to be sure that you are positioned correctly. Simulation may take from a half hour to about 2 hours.

The radiation therapist often will mark the treatment port on your skin with tattoos or tiny dots of colored, permanent ink. It's important that the radiation be targeted at the same area each time. If the dots appear to be fading, tell your radiation therapist who will darken them so that they can be seen easily.

Once simulation has been done, your doctor will meet with the radiation physicist and the dosimetrist. Based on the results of your medical history, lab tests, x-rays, other treatments you may have had, and the location and kind of cancer you have, they will decide how much radiation is needed, what kind of machine to use to deliver it, and how many treatments you should have.

After you have started the treatments, your doctor and the other members of your health care team will follow your progress by checking your response to treatment and how you are feeling at least once a week. When necessary, your doctor may revise the treatment plan by changing the radiation dose or the number and length of your remaining radiation sessions.

Your nurse will be available daily to discuss your concerns and answer any questions you may have. Be sure to tell your nurse if you are having any side effects or if you notice any unusual symptoms.

How Long Does the Treatment Take?

For most types of cancer, radiation therapy usually is given 5 days a week for 6 or 7 weeks. (When radiation is used for palliative care, the course of treatment is shorter, usually 2 to 3 weeks.) The total dose of radiation and the number of treatments you need will depend on the size, location, and kind of cancer you have, your general health, and other medical treatments you may be receiving.

Using many small doses of daily radiation rather than a few large doses helps protect normal body tissues in the treatment area. Weekend rest breaks allow normal cells to recover.

It's very important that you have all of your scheduled treatments to get the most benefit from your therapy. Missing or delaying treatments can lessen the effectiveness of your radiation treatment.

What Happens during the Treatment Visits?

Before each treatment, you may need to change into a hospital gown or robe. It's best to wear clothing that is easy to take off and put on again.

In the treatment room, the radiation therapist will use the marks on your skin to locate the treatment area and to position you correctly. You may sit in a special chair or lie down on a treatment table. For each external radiation therapy session, you will be in the treatment room about 15 to 30 minutes, but you will be getting radiation for only about 1 to 5 minutes of that time. Receiving external radiation treatments is painless, just like having an x-ray taken. You will not hear, see, or smell the radiation.

The radiation therapist may put special shields (or blocks) between the machine and certain parts of your body to help protect normal tissues and organs. There might also be plastic or plaster forms that help you stay in exactly the right place. You need to remain very still during the treatment so that the radiation reaches only the area where it's needed and the same area is treated each time. You don't have to hold your breath—just breathe normally.

The radiation therapist will leave the treatment room before your treatment begins. The radiation machine is controlled from a nearby area. You will be watched on a television screen or through a window in the control room. Although you may feel alone, keep in mind that the therapist can see and hear you and even talk with you using an intercom in the treatment room. If you should feel ill or very uncomfortable during the treatment, tell your therapist at once. The machine can be stopped at any time.

The machines used for radiation treatments are very large, and they make noises as they move around your body to aim at the treatment area from different angles. Their size and motion may be frightening at first. Remember that the machines are being moved and controlled by your radiation therapist. They are checked constantly to be sure they're working right. If you have concerns about anything that happens in the treatment room, discuss these concerns with the radiation therapist.

What Is Hyperfractionated Radiation Therapy?

Radiation is usually given once daily in a dose that is based on the type and location of the tumor. In hyperfractionated radiation therapy, the daily dose is divided into smaller doses that are given more than once a day. The treatments usually are separated by 4 to 6 hours. Doctors are studying hyperfractionated therapy to learn if it is equal to, or perhaps more effective than, once-a-day therapy and whether there are fewer long-term side effects. Early results of treatment studies of some kinds of tumors are encouraging, and hyperfractionated therapy is becoming a more common way to give radiation treatments for some types of cancer.

What Is Intraoperative Radiation?

Intraoperative radiation combines surgery and radiation therapy. The surgeon first removes as much of the tumor as possible. Before the surgery is completed, a large dose of radiation is given directly to the tumor bed (the area from which the tumor has been removed) and nearby areas where cancer cells might have spread. Sometimes intraoperative radiation is used in addition to external radiation therapy. This gives the cancer cells a larger amount of radiation than would be possible using external radiation alone.

Improving Radiation Treatment

Researchers in the field of radiation therapy continue to seek ways to improve the outcome of treatment. Their challenge is to get a high dose of radiation to the tumor while the surrounding normal tissue is protected from radiation damage. New methods for using radiation to treat cancer are being investigated. Many are promising but they are not yet widely available. You may hear the following terms that describe some of these new methods of radiation treatment:

- Three-dimensional conformal radiation therapy is a radiation technique that is being used in some cancer centers. Computer simulation produces an accurate image of the tumor and surrounding organs so that multiple radiation beams can be shaped exactly to the contour of the treatment area. Because the radiation beams are precisely focused, nearby normal tissue is spared. This technique is being used to treat prostate cancer, lung cancer, and certain brain tumors.

- Stereotactic radiosurgery, which uses gamma rays or a linear accelerator, is useful for treating certain kinds of brain tumors and some malformations in the brain's blood vessels. One technique, called the 'gamma knife,' uses many powerful, precisely focused radiation beams. The patient wears a special helmet to focus the gamma rays and aim them at the target tissue from many directions. The treatment is painless and bloodless and, unlike conventional brain surgery, there is no danger of infection. Other systems use a linear accelerator to deliver the radiation in arcing paths around the patient's head.

• The cyberknife is a new, but less common, treatment that is being used to treat brain tumors. This system uses a miniature radiation machine and a robotic arm that moves around the patient's head while delivering small doses of radiation from hundreds of directions. During treatment a computer analyzes hundreds of brain images and adjusts for slight movements by the patient. This makes it possible to deliver the treatment without using a frame to hold the patient's head still. Only the tumor receives the high doses of radiation and healthy tissue is spared.

• The Peacock system is a variation of the cyberknife. It uses special machinery that delivers tiny focused beams of radiation while it rotates around the patient's head. The beams continuously change shape and size to conform to the shape and size of the tumor while avoiding vital structures in the brain. Computer software controls the intensity of the radiation.

• Precision therapy is a method of radiosurgery recently developed in Sweden. It uses high doses of radiation delivered in fewer fractions than in conventional radiation therapy. An advanced treatment planning system permits precise targeting from many angles. As with other advances in radiation treatment, it allows high doses of radiation to be delivered to tumor tissue while reducing radiation damage to healthy tissue.

What Are the Side Effects of Treatment?

External radiation therapy does not cause your body to become radioactive. There is no need to avoid being with other people because you are undergoing treatment. Even hugging, kissing, or having sexual relations with others poses no risk of radiation exposure.

Most side effects of radiation therapy are related to the area that is being treated. Many patients have no side effects at all. Your doctor and nurse will tell you about the possible side effects you might expect and how you should deal with them. You should contact your doctor or nurse if you have any unusual symptoms during your treatment, such as coughing, sweating, fever, or pain.

The side effects of radiation therapy, although unpleasant, are usually not serious and can be controlled with medication or diet. They usually go away within a few weeks after treatment ends, although some side effects can last longer. In the section "Managing Side Effects" you will find advice on how to cope with the side effects that might occur during and after your therapy. Always check with your doctor or nurse about how you should deal with side effects.

Throughout your treatment, your doctor will regularly check on the effects of the treatment. You may not be aware of changes in the cancer, but you probably will notice decreases in pain, bleeding, or other discomfort. You may continue to notice further improvement after your treatment is completed.

Your doctor may recommend periodic tests and physical exams to be sure that the radiation is causing as little damage to normal cells as possible. Depending on the area being treated, you may have routine blood tests to check the levels of red blood cells, white blood cells, and platelets; radiation treatment can cause decreases in the levels of different blood cells.

What Can I Do to Take Care of Myself during Therapy?

Each patient's body responds to radiation therapy in its own way. That's why your doctor must plan, and sometimes adjust, your treatment. In addition, your doctor or nurse will give you suggestions for caring for yourself at home that are specific for your treatment and the possible side effects.

Nearly all cancer patients receiving radiation therapy need to take special care of themselves to protect their health and to help the treatment succeed. Some guidelines to remember are given here:

- Before starting treatment, be sure your doctor knows about any medicines you are taking and if you have any allergies. Do not start taking any medicine (whether prescription or over-the-counter) during your radiation therapy without first telling your doctor or nurse.

- Fatigue is common during radiation therapy. Your body will use a lot of extra energy over the course of your treatment, and you may feel very tired. Be sure to get plenty of rest and sleep as often as you feel the need. It's common for fatigue to last for 4 to 6 weeks after your treatment has been completed.

- Good nutrition is very important. Try to eat a balanced diet that will prevent weight loss. For patients who have problems with eating or diet planning, the section, "Managing Side Effects," offers practical tips.

- Check with your doctor before taking vitamin supplements or herbal preparations during treatment.

- Avoid wearing tight clothes such as girdles or close-fitting collars over the treatment area.

Be extra kind to your skin in the treatment area:

- Ask your doctor or nurse if you may use soaps, lotions, deodorants, sun blocks, medicines, perfumes, cosmetics, talcum powder, or other substances in the treated area.

- Wear loose, soft cotton clothing over the treated area.

- Do not wear starched or stiff clothing over the treated area.

- Do not scratch, rub, or scrub treated skin.

- Do not use adhesive tape on treated skin. If bandaging is necessary, use paper tape and apply it outside of the treatment area. Your nurse can help you place dressings so that you can avoid irritating the treated area.

- Do not apply heat or cold (heating pad, ice pack, etc.) to the treated area. Use only lukewarm water for bathing the area.

- Use an electric shaver if you must shave the treated area but only after checking with your doctor or nurse. Do not use a preshave lotion or hair removal products on the treated area.

- Protect the treatment area from the sun. Do not apply sunscreens just before a radiation treatment. If possible, cover treated skin (with light clothing) before going outside. Ask your doctor if you should use a sunscreen or a sunblocking product. If so, select one with a protection factor of at least 15 and reapply it often. Ask your doctor or nurse how long after your treatments are completed you should continue to protect the treated skin from sunlight.

If you have questions, ask your doctor or nurse. They are the only ones who can properly advise you about your treatment, its side effects, home care, and any other medical concerns you may have.

Internal Radiation Therapy: What to Expect

When Is Internal Radiation Therapy Used?

Your doctor may decide that a high dose of radiation given to a small area of your body is the best way to treat your cancer. Internal radiation therapy allows the doctor to give a higher total dose of radiation in a shorter time than is possible with external treatment.

Internal radiation therapy places the radiation source as close as possible to the cancer cells. Instead of using a large radiation machine, the radioactive material, sealed in a thin wire, catheter, or tube (implant), is placed directly into the affected tissue. This method of treatment concentrates the radiation on the cancer cells and lessens radiation damage to some of the normal tissue near the cancer. Some of the radioactive substances used for internal radiation treatment include cesium, iridium, iodine, phosphorus, and palladium.

Internal radiation therapy may be used for cancers of the head and neck, breast, uterus, thyroid, cervix, and prostate. Your doctor may suggest using both internal and external radiation therapy.

In this chapter, 'internal radiation treatment' refers to implant radiation. Health professionals prefer to use the term "brachytherapy" for implant radiation therapy. You may hear your doctor or nurse use the terms, interstitial radiation or intracavitary radiation; each is a form of internal radiation therapy. Sometimes radioactive implants are called "capsules" or "seeds."

How Is the Implant Placed in the Body?

The type of implant and the method of placing it depend on the size and location of the cancer. Implants may be put right into the tumor (interstitial radiation), in special applicators inside a body cavity (intracavitary radiation) or passage (intraluminal radiation), on the surface of a tumor, or in the area from which the tumor has been removed. Implants may be removed after a short time or left in place permanently. If they are to be left in place, the radioactive substance used will lose radiation quickly and become non-radioactive in a short time.

When interstitial radiation is given, the radiation source is placed in the tumor in catheters, seeds, or capsules. When intracavitary radiation is used, a container or applicator of radioactive material is placed in a body cavity such as the uterus. In surface brachytherapy the radioactive source is sealed in a small holder and placed in or against the tumor. In intraluminal brachytherapy the radioactive source is placed in a body lumen or tube, such as the bronchus or esophagus.

Internal radiation also may be given by injecting a solution of radioactive substance into the bloodstream or a body cavity. This form of radiation therapy may be called unsealed internal radiation therapy.

679

For most types of implants, you will need to be in the hospital. You will be given general or local anesthesia so that you will not feel any pain when the doctor places the holder for the radioactive material in your body. In many hospitals, the radioactive material is placed in its holder or applicator after you return to your room so that other patients, staff, and visitors are not exposed to radiation.

How Are Other People Protected From Radiation While the Implant Is in Place?

Sometimes the radiation source in your implant sends its high energy rays outside your body. To protect others while you are having implant therapy, the hospital will have you stay in a private room. Although the nurses and other people caring for you will not be able to spend a long time in your room, they will give you all of the care you need. You should call for a nurse when you need one, but keep in mind that the nurse will work quickly and speak to you from the doorway more often than from your bedside. In most cases, your urine and stool will contain no radioactivity unless you are having unsealed internal radiation therapy.

There also will be limits on visitors while your implant is in place. Children younger than 18 or pregnant women should not visit patients who are having internal radiation therapy. Be sure to tell your visitors to ask the hospital staff for any special instructions before they come into your room. Visitors should sit at least 6 feet from your bed and the radiation oncology staff will determine how long your visitors may stay. The time can vary from 30 minutes to several hours per day. In some hospitals a rolling lead shield is placed beside the bed and kept between the patient and visitors or staff members.

What Are the Side Effects of Internal Radiation Therapy?

The side effects of implant therapy depend on the area being treated. You are not likely to have severe pain or feel ill during implant therapy. However, if an applicator is holding your implant in place, it may be somewhat uncomfortable. If you need it, the doctor will order medicine to help you relax or to relieve pain. If general anesthesia was used while your implant was put in place, you may feel drowsy, weak, or nauseated but these effects do not last long. If necessary, medications can be ordered to relieve nausea.

Be sure to tell the nurse about any symptoms that concern you. In the section "Managing Side Effects," you will find tips on how to deal with problems that might occur after implant therapy.

How Long Does the Implant Stay in Place?

Your doctor will decide the amount of time that an implant is to be left in place. It depends on the dose (amount) of radioactivity needed for effective treatment. Your treatment schedule will depend on the type of cancer, where it is located, your general health, and other cancer treatments you have had. Depending on where the implant is placed, you may have to keep it from shifting by staying in bed and lying fairly still.

Temporary implants may be either low dose-rate (LDR) or high dose-rate (HDR). Low dose-rate implants are left in place for several days; high dose-rate implants are removed after a few minutes.

For some cancer sites, the implant is left in place permanently. If your implant is permanent, you may need to stay in your hospital room away from other people for a few days while the radiation is most active. The implant becomes less radioactive each day; by the time you are ready to go home, the radiation in your body will be much weaker. Your doctor will advise you if there are any special precautions you need to use at home.

What Happens after the Implant Is Removed?

Usually, an anesthetic is not needed when the doctor removes a temporary implant. Most can be taken out right in the patient's hospital room. Once the implant is removed, there is no radioactivity in your body. The hospital staff and your visitors will no longer have to limit the time they stay with you.

Your doctor will tell you if you need to limit your activities after you leave the hospital. Most patients are allowed to do as much as they feel like doing. You may need some extra sleep or rest breaks during your days at home, but you should feel stronger quickly.

The area that has been treated with an implant may be sore or sensitive for some time. If any particular activity such as sports or sexual intercourse cause irritation in the treatment area, your doctor may suggest that you limit these activities for a while.

Remote Brachytherapy

In remote brachytherapy, a computer sends the radioactive source through a tube to a catheter that has been placed near the tumor by the patient's doctor. The procedure is directed by the brachytherapy team who watch the patient on closed-circuit television and communicate with the patient using an intercom. The radioactivity remains at the tumor for only a few minutes. In some cases, several remote treatments may be required and the catheter may stay in place between treatments.

Remote brachytherapy may be used for low dose-rate (LDR) treatments in an inpatient setting. High dose-rate (HDR) remote brachytherapy allows a person to have internal radiation therapy in an outpatient setting. High dose-rate treatments take only a few minutes. Because no radioactive material is left in the body, the patient can return home after the treatment. Remote brachytherapy has been used to treat cancers of the cervix, breast, lung, pancreas, prostate, and esophagus.

Managing Side Effects

Are Side Effects the Same for Everyone?

The side effects of radiation treatment vary from patient to patient. You may have no side effects or only a few mild ones through your course of treatment. Some people do experience serious side effects, however. The side effects that you have depend mostly on the radiation dose and the part of your body that is treated. Your general health also can affect how your body reacts to radiation therapy and whether you have side effects. Before beginning your treatment, your doctor and nurse will discuss the side effects you might experience, how long they might last, and how serious they might be.

Side effects may be acute or chronic. Acute side effects are sometimes referred to as "early side effects." They occur soon after the treatment begins and usually are gone within a few weeks of finishing therapy. Chronic side effects, sometimes called "late side effects," may take months or years to develop and usually are permanent.

The most common early side effects of radiation therapy are fatigue and skin changes. They can result from radiation to any treatment site. Other side effects are related to treatment of specific areas. For example, temporary or permanent hair loss may be a side effect of radiation treatment to the head. Appetite can be altered if treatment affects the mouth, stomach, or intestine. This section discusses common side effects first. Then the side effects that involve specific areas of the body are described.

Fortunately, most side effects will go away in time. In the meantime, there are ways to reduce discomfort. If you have a side effect that is especially severe, the doctor may prescribe a break in your treatments or change your treatment in some way.

Be sure to tell your doctor, nurse, or radiation therapist about any side effects that you notice. They can help you treat the problems and tell you how to lessen the chances that the side effects will come back. The information in this booklet can serve as a guide to handling some side effects, but it cannot take the place of talking with the members of your health care team.

Will Side Effects Limit My Activity?

Not necessarily. It will depend on which side effects you have and how severe they are. Many patients are able to work, prepare meals, and enjoy their usual leisure activities while they are having radiation therapy. Others find that they need more rest than usual and therefore cannot do as much. Try to continue doing the things you enjoy as long as you don't become too tired.

Your doctor may suggest that you limit activities that might irritate the area being treated. In most cases, you can have sexual relations if you wish. You may find that your desire for physical intimacy is lower because radiation therapy may cause you to feel more tired than usual. For most patients, these feelings are temporary. (See "Sexual Relations" later in this section.)

What Causes Fatigue?

Fatigue, feeling tired and lacking energy, is the most common symptom reported by cancer patients. The exact cause is not always known. It may be due to the disease itself or to treatment. It may also result from lowered blood counts, lack of sleep, pain, and poor appetite.

Most people begin to feel tired after a few weeks of radiation therapy. During radiation therapy, the body uses a lot of energy for healing. You also may be tired because of stress related to your illness, daily trips for treatment, and the effects of radiation on normal cells. Feelings of weakness or weariness will go away gradually after your treatment has been completed.

You can help yourself during radiation therapy by not trying to do too much. If you do feel tired, limit your activities and use your leisure time in a restful way. Save your energy for doing the things that you feel are most important. Do not feel that you have to do everything you normally do. Try to get more sleep at night, and plan your day so that you have time to rest if you need it. Several short naps or breaks may be more helpful than a long rest period.

Sometimes, light exercise such as walking may combat fatigue. Talk with your doctor or nurse about how much exercise you may do while you are having therapy. Talking with other cancer patients in a support group may also help you learn how to deal with fatigue.

If you have a full-time job, you may want to try to continue to work your normal schedule. However, some patients prefer to take time off while they're receiving radiation therapy; others work a reduced number of hours. Speak frankly with your employer about your needs and wishes during this time. A part-time schedule may be possible or perhaps you can do some work at home. Ask your doctor's office or the radiation therapy department to help by trying to schedule treatments with your workday in mind.

Whether you're going to work or not, it's a good idea to ask family members or friends to help with daily chores, shopping, child care, housework, or driving. Neighbors may be able to help by picking up groceries for you when they do their own shopping. You also could ask someone to drive you to and from your treatment visits to help conserve your energy.

How Are Skin Problems Treated?

You may notice that your skin in the treatment area is red or irritated. It may look as if it is sunburned, or tanned. After a few weeks your skin may be very dry from the therapy. Ask your doctor or nurse for advice on how to relieve itching or discomfort.

With some kinds of radiation therapy, treated skin may develop a "moist reaction," especially in areas where there are skin folds. When this happens, the skin is wet and it may become very sore. It's important to notify your doctor or nurse if your skin develops a moist reaction. They can give you suggestions on how to care for these areas and prevent them from becoming infected. Other tips on skin care can be found in the section on external radiation therapy.

During radiation therapy you will need to be very gentle with the skin in the treatment area. The following suggestions may be helpful:

- Avoid irritating treated skin.

- When you wash, use only lukewarm water and mild soap; pat dry.

- Do not wear tight clothing over the area.

- Do not rub, scrub, or scratch the skin in the treatment area.

- Avoid putting anything that is hot or cold, such as heating pads or ice packs, on your treated skin.

- Ask your doctor or nurse to recommend skin care products that will not cause skin irritation. Do not use any powders, creams, perfumes, deodorants, body oils, ointments, lotions, or home remedies in the treatment area while you're being treated and for several weeks afterward unless approved by your doctor or nurse.

- Do not apply any skin lotions within 2 hours of a treatment.

- Avoid exposing the radiated area to the sun during treatment. If you expect to be in the sun for more than a few minutes you will need to be very careful. Wear protective clothing (such as a hat with a broad brim and a shirt with long sleeves) and use a sunscreen. Ask your doctor or nurse about using sunblocking lotions. After your treatment is over, ask your doctor or nurse how long you should continue to take extra precautions in the sun.

The majority of skin reactions to radiation therapy go away a few weeks after treatment is completed. In some cases, though, the treated skin will remain slightly darker than it was before and it may continue to be more sensitive to sun exposure.

What Can Be Done about Hair Loss?

Radiation therapy can cause hair loss, also known as alopecia, but only in the area being treated. For example, if you are receiving treatment to your hip, you will not lose the hair from your head. Radiation of your head may cause you to lose some or all of the hair on your scalp. Many patients find that their hair grows back again after the treatments are finished. The amount of hair that grows back will depend on how much and what kind of radiation you receive. You may notice that your hair has a slightly different texture or color when it grows back. Other types of cancer treatment, such as chemotherapy, also can affect how your hair grows back.

Although your scalp may be tender after the hair is lost, it's a good idea to cover your head with a hat, turban, or scarf. You should wear a protective cap or scarf when you're in the sun or outdoors in cold weather. If you prefer a wig or toupee, be sure the lining does not irritate your scalp. The cost of a hairpiece that you need because of cancer treatment is a tax-deductible expense and may be covered in part by your health insurance. If you plan to buy a wig, it's a good idea to select it early in your treatment if you want to match the color and style to your own hair.

How Are Side Effects on the Blood Managed?

Radiation therapy can cause low levels of white blood cells and platelets. These blood cells normally help your body fight infection and prevent bleeding. If large areas of active bone marrow are treated, your red blood cell count may be low as well. If your blood tests show these side effects, your doctor may wait until your blood counts increase to continue treatments. Your doctor will check your blood counts regularly and change your treatment schedule if it is necessary.

Will Eating Be a Problem?

Sometimes radiation treatment causes loss of appetite and interferes with eating, digesting, and absorbing food. Try to eat enough to help damaged tissues rebuild themselves. It is not unusual to lose 1 or 2 pounds a week during radiation therapy. You will be weighed weekly to monitor your weight.

It is very important to eat a balanced diet. You may find it helpful to eat small meals often and to try to eat a variety of different foods. Your doctor or nurse can tell you whether you should eat a special diet, and a dietitian will have some ideas that will help you maintain your weight.

Coping with short-term diet problems may be easier than you expect. There are a number of diet guides and recipe booklets for patients who need help with eating problems. A National Cancer Institute booklet, "Eating Hints for Cancer Patients" [reprinted in this volume as Chapter 77] explains how to get more calories and protein without eating more food. It also has many tips that should help you enjoy eating. The recipes it contains can be used for the whole family and are marked for people with special concerns, such as low-salt diets. (To obtain this booklet, see the section at the end of this page, "Additional Resources for Cancer Information.")

If it's painful to chew and swallow, your doctor may advise you to use a powdered or liquid diet supplement. Many of these products are available at drugstores and supermarkets and come in a variety of flavors. They are tasty when used alone or combined with other foods such as pureed fruit, or added to milkshakes. Some of the companies that make these diet supplements have recipe booklets to help you increase your nutrient intake. Ask your nurse, dietitian, or pharmacist for further information.

You may lose interest in food during your treatment. Fatigue from your treatments can cause loss of appetite. Some people just don't feel like eating because of stress from their illness and treatment or because the treatment changes the way food tastes. Even if you're not very hungry, it's important to keep your protein and calorie intake high. Doctors have found that patients who eat well can better cope with having cancer and with the side effects of treatment. Medications for appetite enhancement are now available; ask your doctor or nurse about them.

The list below suggests ways to perk up your appetite when it's poor and to make the most of it when you do feel like eating.

- Eat when you are hungry, even if it is not mealtime.

- Eat several small meals during the day rather than three large ones.

- Use soft lighting, quiet music, brightly colored table settings, or whatever helps you feel good while eating.

- Vary your diet and try new recipes. If you enjoy company while eating, try to have meals with family or friends. It may be helpful to have the radio or television on while you eat.

- Ask your doctor or nurse whether you can have a glass of wine or beer with your meal to increase your appetite. Keep in mind that, in some cases, alcohol may not be allowed because it could worsen the side effects of treatment. This may be especially true if you are receiving radiation therapy for cancer of the head, neck, or upper chest area including the esophagus.

- Keep simple meals in the freezer to use when you feel hungry.

- If other people offer to cook for you, let them. Don't be shy about telling them what you'd like to eat.

- Keep healthy snacks close by for nibbling when you get the urge.

- If you live alone, you might want to arrange for "Meals on Wheels" to bring food to you. Ask your doctor, nurse, social worker, or local social service agencies about "Meals on Wheels." This service is available in most large communities.

If you are able to eat only small amounts of food, you can increase the calories per serving by:

- Adding butter or margarine.

- Mixing canned cream soups with milk or half-and-half rather than water.

- Drinking eggnog, milkshakes, or prepared liquid supplements between meals.

- Adding cream sauce or melted cheese to your favorite vegetables.

Some people find they can drink large amounts of liquids even when they don't feel like eating solid foods. If this is the case for you, try to get the most from each glassful by making drinks enriched with powdered milk, yogurt, honey, or prepared liquid supplements.

Will Radiation Therapy Affect Me Emotionally?

Nearly all patients being treated for cancer report feeling emotionally upset at different times during their therapy. It's not unusual to feel anxious, depressed, afraid, angry, frustrated, alone, or helpless. Radiation therapy may affect your emotions indirectly through fatigue or changes in hormone balance, but the treatment itself is not a direct cause of mental distress.

You may find that it's helpful to talk about your feelings with a close friend, family member, chaplain, nurse, social worker, or psychologist with whom you feel at ease. You may want to ask your doctor or nurse about meditation or relaxation exercises that might help you unwind and feel calmer.

Nationwide support programs can help cancer patients to meet others who share common problems and concerns. Some medical centers have formed peer support groups so that patients can meet to discuss their feelings and inspire each other.

There are several helpful books, tapes, and videos on dealing with the emotional effects of having cancer. You may find that the National Cancer Institute publication, "Taking Time," is a good resource for this kind of information. (To obtain this booklet, see the section at the end of this page, "Additional Resources for Cancer Information.")

The Cancer Information Service (1-800-4-CANCER) can direct you to reading matter and other resources in your area for emotional support.

What Side Effects Occur with Radiation Therapy to the Head and Neck?

Some people who receive radiation to the head and neck experience redness, irritation, and sores in the mouth; a dry mouth or thickened saliva; difficulty in swallowing; changes in taste; or nausea. Try not to let these symptoms keep you from eating.

Other problems that may occur during treatment to the head and neck are a loss of taste, which may diminish appetite and affect nutrition, and earaches (caused by hardening of ear wax). You may notice some swelling or drooping of the skin under your chin as well as changes in the skin texture. Your jaw may also feel stiff and you may be unable to open your mouth as wide as before treatment. Jaw exercises may help ease this problem. Report all side effects to your doctor or nurse and ask what you should do about them.

If you are receiving radiation therapy to the head or neck, you need to take especially good care of your teeth, gums, mouth, and throat. Side effects from treatment to these areas commonly involve the mouth, which may be sore and dry. Here are a few tips that may help you manage mouth problems:

- Avoid spices and coarse foods such as raw vegetables, dry crackers, and nuts.

- Remember that acidic foods and liquids can cause mouth and throat irritation.

- Don't smoke, chew tobacco, or drink alcohol.

- Stay away from sugary snacks because they can promote tooth decay.

- Clean your mouth and teeth often, using the method your dentist or doctor recommends.

- Use only alcohol-free mouthwash; many commercial mouthwashes contain alcohol which has a drying effect on mouth tissues.

Mouth Care

Radiation treatment for head and neck cancer can increase your chances of getting cavities in your teeth. Mouth care designed to prevent problems will be a very important part of your treatment. Before starting radiation therapy, make an appointment for a complete dental/oral checkup. Ask your dentist and radiation oncologist to consult before your radiation treatments begin.

Your dentist probably will want to see you often during your radiation therapy to help you care for your mouth and teeth. This is a good way to reduce the risk of tooth decay and help you deal with possible problems such as soreness of the tissues in your mouth. It's important that you follow the dentist's advice while you're receiving radiation therapy. Most likely, your dentist will suggest that you:

- Clean your teeth and gums thoroughly with a soft brush at least 4 times a day (after meals and at bedtime).

- Use a fluoride toothpaste that contains no abrasives.

- Floss gently between teeth daily if you flossed regularly before your illness. Use waxed, non-shredding dental floss.

- Rinse your mouth gently and frequently with a salt and baking soda solution especially after you brush. Use 1/2 teaspoon of salt and 1/2 teaspoon of baking soda in a large glass of warm water. Follow with a plain water rinse.

- Apply fluoride regularly as prescribed by your dentist.

Your dentist can explain how to mix the salt and baking soda mouthwash and how to use the fluoride treatment method that best suits your needs. You can probably get printed instructions for proper dental care at the dentist's office. If dry mouth continues after your treatment is complete, you will need to continue the mouth care recommended during treatment. Always share your dentist's instructions with your radiation nurse.

Dealing with Mouth or Throat Problems

Soreness in your mouth or throat may appear in the second or third week of external radiation therapy and it will most likely have disappeared within a month or so after your treatments have ended. You may have trouble swallowing during this time because your mouth feels dry. Your doctor or dentist can prescribe medicine for mouth discomfort and tell you about methods to relieve other mouth problems during and following your radiation therapy. If you wear dentures you may notice that they no longer fit well. This occurs if the radiation causes your gums to swell. You may need to stop wearing your dentures until your radiation therapy is over. It's important not to risk denture-induced gum sores because they may become infected and heal slowly.

Your salivary glands may produce less saliva than usual, making your mouth feel dry. Unfortunately dry mouth may continue to be a problem even after treatment is over. You may be given medication to help lessen this side effect. It's helpful to sip cool drinks throughout the day. Although many radiation therapy patients have said that drinking carbonated beverages helps relieve dry mouth, water probably is your best choice. In the morning, fill a large container with ice, add water, and carry it with you during the day so that you can take frequent sips. Keep a glass of cool water at your bedside at night, too. Sugar-free candy or gum also may help; be careful about overuse of these products as they can cause diarrhea in some people. Avoid tobacco and alcoholic drinks because they tend to dry and irritate your mouth tissues. Moisten food with gravies and sauces to make eating easier. If these measures are not enough, ask your dentist, radiation oncologist, or nurse about products that either replace or stimulate your own saliva. Artificial saliva and medication to increase saliva production are available.

Tips on Eating

You may find that it's difficult or painful to swallow. Some patients say that they feel as if something is stuck in their throat. Soreness or dryness in your mouth or throat can also make it hard to eat. The earlier section on eating problems in this booklet may be helpful. In addition, some of the following tips may help to make eating more comfortable:

- Choose foods that taste good to you and are easy to eat.

- Try changing the consistency of foods by adding fluids and using sauces and gravies to make them softer.

- Avoid highly spiced foods and textures that are dry and rough, such as crackers.

- Eat small meals, and eat more frequently than usual.

- Cut your food into small, bite-sized pieces.

- Ask your doctor for special liquid medicines to reduce the pain in your throat so that you can eat and swallow more easily.

- Ask your doctor about liquid food supplements that are easier to swallow than solids. They can help you get enough calories each day to avoid losing weight.

- If you are being treated for lung cancer, it's important to keep mucus and other secretions thin and manageable; drinking extra fluids can help.

- If familiar foods no longer taste good, try new foods and use different methods of food preparation.

Additional helpful suggestions can be found in the NCI booklet, *Eating Hints for Cancer Patients.*

What Side Effects Occur with Radiation Therapy to the Chest?

Radiation treatment to the chest may cause several changes. For example, you may find that it is hard to swallow or that swallowing hurts. You may develop a cough or a fever. You may notice that when you cough the amount and color of the mucus is different. Shortness of breath is also common. Be sure to let your treatment team know right away if you have any of these symptoms. Remember that your doctor and nurse have seen these changes in many radiation patients and they know how to help you deal with them.

Are There Side Effects with Radiation Therapy for Breast Cancer?

The most common side effects with radiation therapy for breast cancer are fatigue and skin changes. However there may be other side effects as well. If you notice that your shoulder feels stiff, ask your doctor or nurse about exercises to keep your arm moving freely. Other side effects include breast or nipple soreness, swelling from fluid buildup in the treated area, and skin reddening or tanning. Except for tanning which may take up to 6 months to fade, these side effects will most likely disappear in 4 to 6 weeks.

If you are being treated for breast cancer and you are having radiation therapy after a lumpectomy or mastectomy, it's a good idea to go without your bra whenever possible or, if this makes you more uncomfortable, wear a soft cotton bra without underwires. This will help reduce skin irritation in the treatment area.

Radiation therapy after a lumpectomy may cause additional changes in the treated breast after therapy is complete. These long-term side effects may continue for a year or longer after treatment. The skin redness will fade, leaving your skin slightly darker, just as when a sunburn fades to a sun tan. The pores in the skin of your breast may be enlarged and more noticeable. Some women report increased sensitivity of the skin on the breast; others have decreased feeling. The skin and the fatty tissue of the breast may feel thicker and firmer than it was before your radiation treatment. Sometimes the size of your breast changes—it may become larger because of fluid buildup or smaller because of the development of scar tissue. Many women have little or no change in size.

Your radiation therapy plan may include temporary implants of radioactive material in the area around your lumpectomy. A week or two after external treatment is completed, these implants are inserted during a short hospitalization. The implants may cause breast tenderness or a feeling of tightness. After they are removed, you are likely to notice some of the same effects that occur with external treatment. If so, let your doctor or nurse know about any problems that persist.

Most changes resulting from radiation therapy for breast cancer are seen within 10 to 12 months after completing therapy. Occasionally small red areas called telangiectasias appear. These are areas of dilated blood vessels and the color may fade with time. If you see new changes in breast size, shape, appearance, or texture after this time, report them to your doctor at once.

What Side Effects Occur with Radiation Therapy to the Stomach and Abdomen?

If you are having radiation treatment to the stomach or some portion of the abdomen, you may have an upset stomach, nausea, or diarrhea. Your doctor can prescribe medicines to relieve these problems. Do not take any medications for these symptoms unless you first check with your doctor or nurse.

Managing Nausea

It's not unusual to feel queasy for a few hours right after radiation treatment to the stomach or abdomen. Some patients find that they have less nausea if they have their treatment with an empty stomach. Others report that eating a light meal 1 to 2 hours before treatment lessens queasiness. You may find that nausea is less of a problem if you wait 1 to 2 hours after your treatment before you eat. If this problem persists, ask your doctor to prescribe a medicine (an antiemetic) to prevent nausea. If antiemetics are prescribed, take them within the hour before treatment or when your doctor or nurse suggests, even if you sometimes feel that they are not needed.

If your stomach feels upset just before every treatment, the queasiness or nausea may be caused by anxiety and concerns about cancer treatment. Try having a bland snack such as toast or crackers and apple juice before your appointment. It may also help to try to unwind before your treatment. Reading a book, writing a letter, or working a crossword puzzle may help you relax.

Here are some other tips to help an unsettled stomach:

- Stick to any special diet that your doctor, nurse, or dietitian gives you.

- Eat small meals.

- Eat often and try to eat and drink slowly.

- Avoid foods that are fried or are high in fat.

- Drink cool liquids between meals.

- Eat foods that have only a mild aroma and can be served cool or at room temperature.

For severe nausea and vomiting, try a clear liquid diet (broth and clear juices) or bland foods that are easy to digest, such as dry toast and gelatin.

What to Do about Diarrhea

Diarrhea may begin in the third or fourth week of radiation therapy to the abdomen or pelvis. You may be able to prevent diarrhea by eating a low fiber diet when you start therapy: avoid foods such as raw fruits and vegetables, beans, cabbage, and whole grain breads and cereals. Your doctor or nurse may suggest other changes to your diet, prescribe antidiarrhea medicine, or give you special instructions to help with the problem. Tell the doctor or nurse if these changes fail to control your diarrhea. The following changes in your diet may help:

- Try a clear liquid diet (water, weak tea, apple juice, clear broth, plain gelatin) as soon as diarrhea starts or when you feel that it's going to start.

- Ask your doctor or nurse to advise you about liquids that won't make your diarrhea worse. Weak tea and clear broth are frequent suggestions.

- Avoid foods that are high in fiber or can cause cramps or a gassy feeling such as raw fruits and vegetables, coffee and other beverages that contain caffeine, beans, cabbage, whole grain breads and cereals, sweets, and spicy foods.

- Eat frequent small meals.

- If milk and milk products irritate your digestive system, avoid them or use lactose-free dairy products.

- Continue a diet that is low in fat and fiber and lactose-free for 2 weeks after you have finished your radiation therapy. Gradually re-introduce other foods. You may want to start with small amounts of low-fiber foods such as rice, bananas, applesauce, mashed potatoes, low-fat cottage cheese, and dry toast.

- Be sure your diet includes foods that are high in potassium (bananas, potatoes, apricots), an important mineral that you may lose through diarrhea.

Diet planning is very important for patients who are having radiation treatment of the stomach and abdomen. Try to pack the highest possible food value into every meal and snack so that you will be eating enough calories and vital nutrients. Remember that nausea, vomiting, and diarrhea are likely to disappear once your treatment is over.

What Side Effects Occur with Radiation Therapy to the Pelvis?

If you are having radiation therapy to any part of the pelvis (the area between your hips), you might have some of the digestive problems already described. You also may have bladder irritation which can cause discomfort or frequent urination. Drinking a lot of fluid can help relieve some of this discomfort. Avoid caffeine and carbonated beverages. Your doctor also can prescribe some medicine to help relieve these problems.

The effects of radiation therapy on sexual and reproductive functions depend on which organs are in the radiation treatment area. Some of the more common side effects do not last long after treatment is finished. Others may be long-term or permanent. Before your treatment begins, ask your doctor about possible side effects and how long they might last.

Depending on the radiation dose, women having radiation therapy in the pelvic area may stop menstruating and have other symptoms of menopause such as vaginal itching, burning, and dryness. You should report these symptoms to your doctor or nurse, who can suggest treatment.

Effects on Fertility

Scientists are still studying how radiation treatment affects fertility. If you are a woman in your childbearing years, it's important to discuss birth control and fertility issues with your doctor. You should not become pregnant during radiation therapy because radiation treatment during pregnancy may injure the fetus, especially in the first three months. If you are pregnant before your therapy begins, be sure to tell your doctor so that the fetus can be protected from radiation, if possible.

Radiation therapy to the area that includes the testes can reduce both the number of sperm and their effectiveness. This does not mean that conception cannot occur, however. Ask your doctor or nurse about effective measures to prevent pregnancy while you are having radiation. If you have any concerns about fertility, be sure to discuss them with your doctor. For example, if you want to have children, you may be concerned about reduced fertility after your cancer treatment is completed. Your doctor can help you get information about the option of banking your sperm before treatment.

Sexual Relations

With most types of radiation therapy, neither men nor women are likely to notice any change in their ability to enjoy sex. Both sexes, however, may notice a decrease in their level of desire. This is more likely to be due to the stress of having cancer than to the effects of radiation therapy. Once the treatment ends, sexual desire is likely to return to previous levels.

During radiation treatment to the pelvis, some women are advised not to have intercourse. Others may find that intercourse is uncomfortable or painful. Within a few weeks after treatment ends, these symptoms usually disappear. If shrinking of vaginal tissues occurs as a side effect of radiation therapy, your doctor or nurse can explain how to use a dilator, a device that gently stretches the tissues of the vagina.

If you have questions or concerns about sexual activity during and after cancer treatment, discuss them with your nurse or doctor. Ask them to recommend booklets that may be helpful.

Followup Care

What Does "Followup" Mean?

Once you have completed your radiation treatments, it is important for your doctor to monitor the results of your therapy at regularly scheduled visits. These checkups are necessary to deal with radiation side effects and to detect any signs of recurrent disease. During these checkups your doctor will examine you and may order some lab tests and x-rays. The radiation oncologist also will want to see you for followup after your treatment ends and will coordinate followup care with your doctor.

Followup care might include more cancer treatment, rehabilitation, and counseling. Taking good care of yourself is also an important part of following through after radiation treatments.

Who Provides Care after Therapy?

Most patients return to the radiation oncologist for regular followup visits. Others are referred to their original doctor, to a surgeon, or to a medical oncologist. Your followup care will depend on the kind of cancer that was treated and on other treatments that you had or may need.

What Other Care Might Be Needed?

Just as every patient is different, followup care varies. Your doctor will prescribe and schedule the followup care that you need. Don't hesitate to ask about the tests or treatments that your doctor orders. Try to learn all the things you need to do to take good care of yourself.

Following are some questions that you may want to ask your doctor after you have finished your radiation therapy:

- How often do I need to return for checkups?

- Why do I need more x-rays, CT-scans, blood tests, and so on? What will these tests tell us?

- Will I need chemotherapy, surgery, or other treatments?

- How and when will you know if I'm cured of cancer?

- What are the chances that it will come back?

- How soon can I go back to my regular activities? Work? Sexual activity? Sports?

- Do I need to take any special precautions like staying out of the sun or avoiding people with infectious diseases?

- Do I need a special diet?

- Should I exercise?

- Can I wear a prosthesis?

- Can I have reconstructive surgery? How soon can I schedule it?

It's a good idea to write down the questions you want to ask your doctor. Some patients find that it's helpful to take a family member with them to help remember what the doctor says.

What if Pain Is a Problem?

Radiation therapy is not painful. However, some radiation side effects may cause discomfort. In addition, when radiation is used for palliation (see section above), some discomfort or pain may remain. Sometimes patients need help to manage cancer pain. Over-the-counter pain medicine may be enough for mild pain. Remember that you should not use a heating pad or a warm compress to relieve pain in any area treated with radiation.

If your pain is severe, ask the doctor about prescription drugs or other methods of relief. Try to be specific about your pain (how severe is it on a scale of 0-10 where 0 is no pain and 10 is the worst pain you can imagine? where is your pain? is the pain throbbing, stabbing, searing? is it continuous or intermittent? what makes it better or worse?) when you tell the doctor about it so you can get the best pain management. If you are unable to get pain relief, you may want to ask your doctor for a referral to a pain specialist.

Because fear and worry can make pain worse, you may find that relaxation exercises are helpful. Other methods such as hypnosis, biofeedback, and acupuncture may be useful for some cancer pain. Be sure to discuss these complementary or alternative treatments with your doctor or nurse. Sometimes complementary therapies can interfere with other treatment you are having. They can also be harmful when combined with other treatment.

"Questions and Answers About Pain Control: A Guide for People with Cancer and Their Families" is a free booklet that may help you understand more about controlling cancer pain. (To obtain this booklet, see the section at the end of this page, "Additional Resources for Cancer Information.")

How Can I Help Myself after Radiation Therapy?

Patients who have had radiation therapy need to continue some of the special care they used during treatment, at least for a short while. For instance, you may have skin problems for several weeks after your treatments end. Continue to be gentle with skin in the treatment area until all signs of irritation are gone. Don't try to scrub off the marks in your treatment area. If tattoos were used to mark the treatment area, they are permanent and will not wash off. Your nurse can answer questions about skin care and help you with other concerns you may have after your treatment has been completed.

You may find that you still need extra rest after your therapy is over while your healthy tissues are recovering and rebuilding. Keep taking naps as needed and try to get more sleep at night. It may take some time to get your strength back, so resume your normal schedule of activities gradually. If you feel that you need emotional or social support, ask your doctor, nurse, or a social worker for information about support groups or other ways to express your feelings and concerns.

When Should I Call the Doctor?

After treatment for cancer, you're likely to be more aware of your body and to notice even slight changes in how you feel from day to day. The doctor will want to know if you are having any unusual symptoms. Promptly tell your doctor about:

- A pain that doesn't go away, especially if it's always in the same place.
- New or unusual lumps, bumps, or swelling.
- Nausea, vomiting, diarrhea, or loss of appetite.
- Unexplained weight loss.
- A fever or cough that doesn't go away.
- Unusual rashes, bruises, or bleeding.
- Any symptoms that you are concerned about.
- Any other warning signs mentioned by your doctor or nurse.

What about Returning to Work?

Many people find that they can continue to work during radiation therapy because treatment appointments are short. If you have stopped working, you can return to your job as soon as you feel up to it. If your job requires lifting or heavy physical activity, you may need a change in your work responsibilities until you have regained your strength. Check with your employer to see if a 'return to work' release from your doctor is required.

When you are ready to return to work, it is important to learn about your rights regarding your job and health insurance. If you have any questions about employment issues, contact the Cancer Information Service (CIS). CIS staff can help you find local agencies that can help you deal with problems regarding employment and insurance rights that are sometimes faced by cancer survivors.

Additional Resources for Cancer Information

National Cancer Institute Information Resources

You may want more information for yourself, your family, and your doctor. The following National Cancer Institute (NCI) services are available to help you.

Telephone

Cancer Information Service (CIS) Provides accurate, up-to-date information on cancer to patients and their families, health professionals, and the general public. Information specialists translate the latest scientific information into understandable language and respond in English, Spanish, or on TTY equipment.

Toll-free: 1-800-4-CANCER (1-800-422-6237)
TTY: 1-800-332-8615

Internet

http://www.nci.nih.gov—NCI's primary Web site; contains information about the Institute and its programs.

http://cancertrials.nci.nih.gov—CancerTrials; NCI's comprehensive clinical trials information center for patients, health professionals, and the public. Includes information on understanding trials, deciding whether to participate in trials, finding specific trials, plus research news and other resources.

http://cancernet.nci.nih.gov—CancerNet; contains material for health professionals, patients, and the public, including information from PDQ about cancer treatment, screening, prevention, supportive care, and clinical trials, and CANCERLIT, a bibliographic database.

E-mail

CancerMail—Includes NCI information about cancer treatment, screening, prevention, and supportive care. To obtain a contents list, send e-mail to cancermail@icicc.nci.nih.gov with the word "help" in the body of the message.

Fax

CancerFax—Includes NCI information about cancer treatment, screening, prevention, and supportive care. To obtain a contents list, dial 301-402-5874 from a fax machine hand set and follow the recorded instructions.

For Further Information

Cancer patients, their families and friends, and others may find the following booklets useful. They are available free of charge by calling 1-800-4-CANCER or writing:

Office of Cancer Communications
National Cancer Institute
Building 31, Room 10A24
Bethesda, MD 20892

Booklets about Cancer Treatment

Chemotherapy and You: A Guide to Self-Help During Treatment *

Eating Hints: Recipes and Tips for Better Nutrition During Cancer Treatment *

Questions and Answers About Pain Control

What Are Clinical Trials All About?

Booklets about Living with Cancer

Taking Time: Support for People With Cancer and the People Who Care About Them

When Cancer Recurs: Meeting the Challenge Again *

Advanced Cancer: Living Each Day *

* Reprinted in this volume—see Table of Contents

Conclusion

We hope that the information in this chapter will help you understand how radiation therapy is used to treat cancer. If you know what to expect when you go for your treatments, you may not feel as anxious. Remember to talk with your nurse, doctor, or other members of your health care team whenever you have questions or feel that you need more information.

Acknowledgements

The National Cancer Institute thanks all of the many health professionals and patients who assisted with the development and review of this publication.

The National Cancer Institute (NCI) is the lead Federal agency for cancer research. Since Congress passed the National Cancer Act in 1971, NCI has continued to collaborate with top researchers and medical facilities across the country to conduct innovative research leading to progress in cancer prevention, detection, diagnosis and treatment. These efforts have resulted in a recent decrease in the overall cancer death rate, and have helped improve and extend the lives of millions of Americans.

Chapter 67

Lasers in Cancer Treatment

What Is Laser Light?

The term "laser" stands for light amplification by stimulated emission of radiation. Ordinary light, such as that from a light bulb, has many wavelengths and spreads in all directions. Laser light, on the other hand, has a specific wavelength and is focused in a narrow beam. Because of these properties, laser light can be very powerful and may be used to cut through steel or to shape diamonds. It also can be used for very precise surgical work, such as repairing a damaged retina in the eye or cutting through tissue (in place of a scalpel).

Soon after the first working laser was developed in 1960, researchers began studying the medical uses of lasers. Lasers were first used medically in 1961 to treat a type of skin discoloration and to repair detached retinas.

Types of Lasers

Although there are several different kinds of lasers, only three kinds have gained wide use in medicine:

- Carbon dioxide (CO_2)—This is mainly a surgical tool. It can cut or vaporize tissue with relatively little bleeding as the light energy changes to heat.

National Cancer Institute Fact Sheet, June 1993.

- Neodymium:yttrium-aluminum-garnet (Nd:YAG)—Light from this laser can penetrate deeper into tissue than light from the other types of lasers, and it can cause blood to coagulate quickly. It can be carried through optical fibers to less accessible parts of the body.

- Argon—This laser permits superficial penetration and is useful in dermatology and in eye surgery. It also is used with light-sensitive dyes to treat tumors in a procedure known as photodynamic therapy (PDT).

Advantages and Disadvantages of Laser Use in Medicine

Lasers have several advantages over standard surgical tools:

- Lasers are more precise than scalpels. Tissue near an incision is protected, since there is little contact with skin or other tissue.

- The heat produced by lasers sterilizes the surgery site.

- Less operating time may be needed because the precision of the laser allows for a smaller incision.

- Healing time is often shortened; since laser heat seals blood vessels, there is less bleeding, swelling, or scarring.

- Laser surgery may be less complicated. For example, with fiber optics, laser light can be directed to parts of the body without making a large incision.

- More procedures may be done on an outpatient basis.

There are disadvantages with laser surgery:

- Relatively few surgeons are trained in laser use.

- Laser equipment is expensive and bulky compared with the usual surgical tools, such as scalpels.

- Strict safety precautions must be observed in the operating room. (For example, the surgical team and the patient must wear eye protection.)

Treating Cancer with Lasers

Lasers were first used on skin tumors in 1961, and today one of the most common medical applications of lasers is in cancer treatment.

They can be used in two ways to treat cancer: by shrinking or destroying a tumor with heat, or by activating a chemical—known as a photosensitizing agent—that destroys cancer cells. In PDT, a photosensitizing agent is retained in cancer cells and can be stimulated by light to cause a reaction that kills cancer cells.

The CO_2 and Nd:YAG lasers are used to shrink or destroy tumors. They may be used with endoscopes, tubes that allow physicians to see into certain areas of the body, such as the bladder. The light from some lasers can be transmitted through a flexible endoscope fitted with fiber optics. This allows physicians to see and work in parts of the body that could not otherwise be reached except by surgery and allows very precise aiming of the laser beam. Lasers also may be used with low-power microscopes, giving the doctor a clear view of the site being treated. When used with a micromanipulator, laser systems can produce a cutting area as small as 200 microns in diameter—less than the width of a very fine thread.

Lasers are used to treat several kinds of cancer. In the digestive system, lasers are used to remove colon polyps, which may become cancerous. They are also used to remove tumors blocking the esophagus and colon. Although this procedure does not cure the cancer, it relieves some of the symptoms. The CO_2 laser is also used to treat abnormal tissue and carcinoma in situ and very early cancer of the cervix, vagina, and vulva.

Cancers of the head and neck and the respiratory system are treated (but usually cannot be cured) with lasers. Treatment with lasers for small tumors on the vocal cords may be an alternative to radiation for selected patients. As with tumors blocking the esophagus, tumors blocking the upper airway can be partially removed to make breathing easier. Blockages of the bronchi can be removed with a flexible bronchoscope and an Nd:YAG laser. Lasers can be used to shrink primary and secondary brain tumors, which may help relieve symptoms. Laser surgery for breast cancer is becoming more common and may result in a shorter hospital stay and less pain for the patient.

An argon laser is used in PDT. This treatment is based on the discovery, made over 80 years ago, that certain chemicals can kill one-celled organisms in the presence of light. Recent interest in photosensitizing agents stems from research showing that some of these substances have a tendency to collect in cancer cells.

The photosensitizing agent injected into the body is absorbed by all cells. The agent remains in or around tumor cells for a longer time than it does in normal tissue. When treated cancer cells are exposed to red light from a laser, the light is absorbed by the photosensitizing agent. This light absorption causes a chemical reaction that destroys the tumor cells. Light exposure must be carefully timed to coincide with the period when most of the agent has left healthy cells but still remains in cancer cells. There are several promising features of PDT: Cancer cells can be selectively destroyed while most normal cells are spared, the damaging effect of the photosensitizing agent occurs only when the substance is exposed to light, and the side effects are relatively mild.

A disadvantage of PDT is that argon laser light cannot pass through more than 1 centimeter of tissue (a little more than one-third of an inch). Studies are under way on the use of PDT against lung, bladder, esophageal, mesothelioma, ovarian, brain, and head and neck cancers. Researchers also are looking at different laser types and at new photosensitizers to increase effectiveness.

The Outlook for Lasers in Cancer Treatment

Doctors are trying to find new and better ways to use lasers in cancer surgery. For example, contact lasers or laser scalpels are coming into greater use. Contact lasers have artificial sapphire tips that are used directly on tissue, which gives the surgeon a "feel" for the surgery that is more like using a steel scalpel. As more cancer surgeons become trained in laser use and the technology improves, lasers may make increasing contributions to cancer treatment.

Chapter 68

Bone Marrow Transplantation and Peripheral Blood Stem Cell Transplantation

This Research Report discusses bone marrow transplantation (BMT) procedures, the diseases that can be treated with BMT or peripheral blood stem cell transplantation (PBSCT), and current research on these treatments. Less than two decades ago, BMT was strictly an investigational procedure. Today, it is recognized as an effective treatment for some types of cancer and certain other diseases.

This chapter is designed to help people better understand this method of treatment. Patients and their families who want detailed information about these procedures, health care workers, and those with a strong interest in the topic will find it helpful.

Information presented here was gathered from medical textbooks; recent articles in scientific literature; PDQ, the cancer information data base developed by the National Cancer Institute (NCI); NCI researchers; and other scientists. Knowledge about BMT and PBSCT is increasing steadily. Up-to-date information on these and other cancer-related subjects is available from the NCI-supported Cancer Information Service (CIS). The toll-free number of the CIS is 1-800-4-CANCER.

Description and Function of Bone Marrow

Bone marrow is the soft, spongy material found inside bones. The bone marrow contains a network of blood vessels and fibers surrounded

Research Report: "Bone Marrow Transplantation and Peripheral Blood Stem Cell Transplantation," U.S. Department of Health and Human Services, Public Health Service, National Institutes of Health. National Cancer Institute, NIH Publication Number 95-1178 Revised November 1994, modified April 1999.

by fat and by cells that give rise to white blood cells (WBCs), red blood cells (RBCs), and platelets. The production of blood cells is the chief function of the bone marrow. In children, the cells that give rise to blood cells can be found throughout the marrow. In adults, these cells are found mostly in the marrow of the bones of the chest, hips, back, skull, and of the upper arms and legs.

All blood cells develop from very immature cells called stem cells. Most stem cells are found in the bone marrow, although some, called peripheral blood stem cells, circulate in blood vessels throughout the body. Stem cells can divide to form more stem cells, or they can go through a series of cell divisions by which they become fully mature blood cells. Most blood cells mature in the bone marrow. However, some white blood cells (also called lymphocytes) complete their maturation in the thymus, spleen, or lymph nodes.

White Blood Cells

White blood cells (also called leukocytes) are the principal components of the immune system, the organs and cells that act together to defend the body against infection and other diseases. WBCs function by destroying "foreign" substances such as bacteria and viruses. When an infection is present, the production of WBCs increases. If the number of leukocytes is abnormally low (a condition known as leukopenia), infection is more likely to occur, and it is more difficult for the body to get rid of the infection.

There are several major types of WBCs—neutrophils, eosinophils, basophils, lymphocytes, and monocytes. Each has a different function.

- Neutrophils are a primary defense against bacterial infection. These cells can leave the bloodstream and migrate to the site of the infection. Neutrophils perform their function partially through phagocytosis, a process by which some cells "eat" other cells and foreign substances.

- Eosinophils are important in phagocytosis as well as in allergic and inflammatory reactions.

- Basophils play a special role in allergic reactions.

- Lymphocytes are found in the blood as well as in many other parts of the body. The three main types of lymphocytes—B cells, T cells, and NK cells—interact in complex ways as part of the immune response. Special B cells produce specific antibodies, proteins that help destroy foreign substances. T cells attack virus-infected cells, foreign tissue, and cancer cells. They also produce a number of substances that regulate the immune response. Among other functions, NK cells destroy cancer cells and virus-infected cells through phagocytosis and by producing substances that can kill such cells.

- Monocytes migrate into tissues and develop into macrophages when they are needed as part of the immune response. Monocytes and macrophages play a key role in phagocytosis.

As a group, neutrophils, eosinophils, and basophils may be referred to by names that describe how they look under the microscope. They are called granulocytes because of their dotted, or granular, appearance; the granules in these cells are filled with chemicals that can destroy foreign substances in the body. They also are called polymorphonuclear leukocytes (PMN's, or "polys") because of the shape of the cell nucleus. Lymphocytes and monocytes are referred to as agranulocytes or mononuclear cells.

Red Blood Cells

Red blood cells (also called erythrocytes) serve two important functions. With the help of an iron-containing protein called hemoglobin, they carry oxygen from the lungs to cells in all parts of the body. Oxygen helps cells obtain energy from the nutrients we eat. RBCs also take carbon dioxide back to the lungs from the cells; carbon dioxide is released as a waste product of cell processes. Too few RBCs or too little hemoglobin is a condition known as anemia. It can cause weakness, lack of energy, dizziness, shortness of breath, headache, and irritability.

Platelets

Platelets help prevent bleeding by causing blood clots to form at the site of an injury. An abnormally low number of platelets (a condition known as thrombocytopenia) may result in easy bruising and excessive bleeding from wounds or in mucous membranes and other tissues.

Purpose and Use of Transplantation

In bone marrow transplantation (BMT), marrow is removed from a bone with a needle. Bone marrow transplants can be divided into three groups according to where the marrow for transplantation comes from: the patient, an identical twin, or another person. In peripheral blood stem cell transplantation (PBSCT), the stem cells usually come from the patient. After treatment, the patient receives the marrow intravenously (by injection into a vein). In peripheral blood stem cell transplantation, stem cells are removed from the patient's circulating blood before treatment and then returned after treatment. The main purpose of these procedures in cancer treatment is to make it possible for patients to receive very high doses of chemotherapy and, in many cases, radiation therapy as well. To understand more about why BMT and PBSCT are used, it may be helpful to know more about how chemotherapy and radiation therapy work.

Chemotherapy and radiation therapy generally affect cells that are dividing. They are used to treat cancer because cancer cells divide more often than most other cells. Chemotherapeutic drugs and radiation are given in high doses to increase their effectiveness. However, high-dose treatment can severely damage or destroy the patient's bone marrow so that the patient is no longer able to produce needed blood cells. Destroying the marrow may be a part of treatment for diseases that affect the bone marrow (leukemias and other diseases), or it may simply be a side effect of treatment for cancers that affect other parts of the body. In any case, BMT and PBSCT allow stem cells that were damaged by treatment to be replaced with healthy stems cells that can produce the blood cells the patient needs.

BMT has been thoroughly tested in patients with certain types of cancer—among them neuroblastoma (an uncommon cancer that occurs most frequently in children) and certain types of leukemia and lymphoma. Many physicians consider it the best available treatment option for these diseases under specific circumstances. BMT also is being evaluated in the treatment of other types of cancer, including cancers of the breast, lung, ovary; germ cell tumors; multiple myeloma; certain other childhood cancers; and some primary brain tumors in both adults and children. BMT has also been used in the treatment of cancers that have spread, are not responding to other treatment, or cannot be removed by surgery (such as some that affect the head and neck). PBSCT, with or without BMT, is being studied for its usefulness in treating some of the same diseases. Patients who have cancer cells in their bone marrow or who do not have enough stem cells in their marrow may be considered for PBSCT. National Cancer Institute materials on many types of cancer are available through the Cancer Information Service (CIS) at 1-800-4-CANCER. CIS staff members also can provide information about current clinical trials (research studies) of BMT and PBSCT.

Several noncancerous disorders also are being treated with BMT. These include aplastic anemia, severe combined immunodeficiency disease (SCID), thalassemia, and myelodysplastic syndromes.

Types of Transplantation

As mentioned previously, there are three groups of bone marrow transplantation. The type of transplant a patient receives depends upon a number of factors, including the type of disease and the availability of a suitable donor.

Syngeneic Transplantation

In syngeneic transplantation, bone marrow is taken from an identical twin. Different people usually have different sets of proteins, called human leukocyte-associated (HLA) antigens, on the surface of their cells that allow white blood cells to distinguish the body's own cells from those of another person. However, because identical twins have the same genes, they also have the same set of HLA antigens (they are said to be a perfect HLA match). As a result, the patient's body usually accepts the graft (transplant). Given that identical twins represent only 0.3 percent of all births (1 birth out of every 270), syngeneic transplantation is rare.

Allogeneic Transplantation

Allogeneic transplantation, in which bone marrow comes from a person other than the patient or an identical twin, is much more common. Usually the patient's sibling or parent serves as the donor, but unrelated donors are sometimes used. (In rare cases, a child may donate marrow for a parent.)

The success of allogeneic transplantation depends largely on how closely the HLA antigens of the donor's marrow match those of the recipient's marrow, which is determined by special blood tests. (The matching of bone marrow is a much more complicated process than is the matching of blood types. Scientists look at six HLA antigens, and most institutions require a match on at least five of these proteins.) The higher the number of matches, the greater the chance that a patient's body will accept the graft. A good HLA match also reduces the chance that the transplanted bone marrow will react against the patient's body. This reaction, called graft-versus-host disease (GVHD), is a potentially serious complication of BMT; it is discussed below.

Close relatives, especially brothers and sisters, are more likely than unrelated people to have HLA-matched bone marrow. However, only 30 to 40 percent of patients have an HLA-matched sibling or parent. The odds of obtaining HLA-compatible marrow from an unrelated donor are slim. Nevertheless, recent years have seen an increase in the use of marrow from unrelated donors. In 1988 for example, unrelated donor marrow was used for just 5 percent of all allogeneic transplantations; by 1990 this number had doubled to 10 percent. This increase has been possible in part through the existence of large bone marrow registries, such as the National Marrow Donor Program (NMDP) and the American Bone Marrow Donor Registry (ABMDR) (see Resources section).

The NMDP is a federally funded program that was created in 1986 to improve a patient's chance of finding a suitable donor. The NMDP coordinates searches among donor and transplant centers throughout the United States and other countries. It receives requests for bone marrow donors from these centers, searches a central computer file (which currently contains more than 1,442,000 names) for a match, coordinates additional testing of donors, and helps with transplantation arrangements. The NMDP works in association with the American Red Cross, whose local chapters may be helpful in locating bone marrow donors.

The ABMDR is a privately funded registry of more than 500,000 potential marrow donors. Like NMDP, its function is to identify allogeneic matches by coordinating international searches among donor banks. The ABMDR also can provide information and assistance to physicians, transplant coordinators, and patients throughout the search process.

Because the likelihood of HLA matching is highest among people of similar racial and ethnic backgrounds, it is important that registries have a diverse population of potential donors so that all BMT candidates have a good chance of finding a match. Through recruitment programs for minority donors, which are in place throughout the country, NMDP and ABMDR hope to expand the donor pool for minority patients.

Autologous Transplantation

In autologous transplantation, patients receive their own marrow or peripheral stem cells. Because the patient is the donor, HLA matching is not necessary; moreover, there is virtually no risk of GVHD.

For autologous transplantation to be successful, the patient's marrow must be relatively free of disease when it is harvested (removed).

In some patients, autologous transplantation is feasible because the cancer does not involve the bone marrow. (A sample of the bone marrow, removed in a procedure called bone marrow aspiration, is checked for the presence of cancer cells.) In other patients, such as leukemia and lymphoma patients, initial treatment to induce remission (the disappearance of the signs of cancer) is necessary before bone marrow harvesting. Depending on their disease and other factors, patients may then either proceed immediately with the high-dose treatment and transplantation procedure or store their marrow and proceed with high-dose treatment and transplantation only if their disease returns.

In an effort to protect the patient from relapse caused by undetected cancer cells in the autologous marrow, the marrow often is treated before storage or transplantation. Treatment to remove or destroy cancer cells in the harvested marrow, known as purging, can be accomplished in a number of ways. These include the use of drugs to kill cancer cells or of monoclonal antibodies to kill or remove cancer cells; various methods also may be used to separate healthy cells from cancer cells. Although cancer cells may be less likely to be in the peripheral blood than in the marrow, peripheral stem cell harvests also may be purged.

Not all patients undergoing autologous BMT receive purged marrow because it is not clear whether purging truly reduces the risk of relapse after transplantation. Purging does not necessarily remove all cancer cells from the harvested marrow. Patients with solid tumors who relapse often do so at the site of the original tumor, indicating that the transplanted marrow may not be responsible for the recurrence. Moreover, purging with anticancer drugs may result in delayed recovery of bone marrow function after transplantation because stem cells in the harvested marrow may be destroyed along with cancer cells. The value of purging in BMT and PBSCT continues to be studied.

Transplantation Procedures

Transplantation of bone marrow or peripheral blood stem cells involves potentially serious risks, and patients require the care of skilled medical staff and state-of-the-art support services. For this reason, BMT and PBSCT should be performed at established transplant centers whenever possible.

The steps involved in transplantation vary from one medical center to another and with the type of transplantation done. Also, as research advances the procedures are changing. General transplantation procedures are discussed below.

Patient Selection and Consent

When considering transplantation, physicians carefully evaluate a patient's medical history to be sure this procedure is the most appropriate treatment option. The potential complications of BMT and PBSCT, which are discussed later in this Report, are given significant consideration because they can be severe and, in some cases, fatal. Patient and physician must work closely together to weigh the potential benefits against the risks.

If allogeneic BMT is determined to be an appropriate and desirable treatment, a suitable donor must be identified. As noted earlier, many resources exist for finding a donor. The number of donors is increasing constantly, and the success rate of finding a donor has increased greatly in recent years. However, there is still a very real possibility that a person without a twin will not find a donor with enough matching antigens for the treatment to proceed.

After reviewing the transplantation process, the patient is asked to sign hospital consent forms authorizing the procedure. Signing the consent forms means that the patient has been given enough information to make an informed decision about treatment and to understand what the treatment involves. Patients should be made fully aware of the risks, benefits, and costs of transplantation as well as possible treatment alternatives.

Some specific questions that patients may want to ask their physicians before signing the consent form are:

- What are the benefits of this treatment?
- What are the risks and side effects?
- How long will I be in the hospital and unable to work or go to school?
- How will I have to change my normal activities?
- How much will the treatment cost?
- Will my insurance pay for this treatment? If not, is financial help available?
- Will I have to be far from home? If so, how soon can I return home?
- How often will I need checkups?

Pretreatment Procedures

Before the actual transplantation, the patient undergoes several days of laboratory and diagnostic tests. Doctors check the patient's general medical condition, looking for signs of infection or damage to organs from previous treatment. A dental exam generally is recommended to make sure the mouth is as healthy as possible before treatment begins, because treatment will likely cause it to become sensitive and easily infected.

An intravenous catheter usually is surgically placed in one of the large veins in the chest. The catheter is used for drawing blood samples; for giving the patient blood or blood products, antibiotics, other drugs, and nutritional support; and for transplanting the new marrow. Many medical centers use Hickman or Broviac catheters, which are thin, flexible tubes similar to regular intravenous tubing. One end of the catheter remains outside the chest and must be kept very clean to prevent infection. Catheters generally can remain in place for many months. (Before they leave the hospital, patients are taught how to care for the catheter at home.) Implantable ports, in which the end of the catheter remains under the skin, are sometimes used as an alternative to Hickman or Broviac catheters. A needle is inserted through the skin and into the catheter.

Procedures for Allogeneic or Syngeneic Donors

Donors for allogeneic or syngeneic transplants need not make changes in diet, work, or social activities before bone marrow donation. Typically, the donor enters the hospital the day before or the day of the donation. Donors normally stay in the hospital for 1 or 2 nights because most receive general anesthesia, which puts them to sleep. The use of newer anesthetics has made bone marrow donation possible as an outpatient procedure at some centers. Sometimes, local anesthesia is used instead to numb the area of the body where the marrow will be removed.

Bone marrow is removed from the pelvic (hip) bones and, in rare cases, from the sternum (breastbone) as well. Generally, four to eight small incisions (not requiring stitches) are made in the pelvic area, and a large needle is inserted through these incisions 20 to 30 times to draw the marrow out of the bones. Usually, 500 to 1,000 milliliters (1 to 2 pints) of the donor's marrow is taken. This marrow contains 3 to 5 percent of all the donor's developing blood cells. Typically, the extraction process lasts about 1 hour.

Harvested bone marrow is then processed to remove blood and bone fragments. Allogeneic marrow may be treated to remove T lymphocytes in a process known as T-cell depletion (see glossary). Marrow that is to be stored may be combined with dimethyl sulfoxide (a preservative, often referred to as DMSO) and placed in a liquid nitrogen freezer to keep stem cells alive until the day of transplantation. Using this technique, known as cryopreservation, bone marrow can be preserved for 3 years or more.

Because only a small amount of marrow is removed, donating usually does not pose any significant problems for the donor. Within a few weeks, the donor's body will have replaced the donated marrow. Soreness around the incisions may linger for a few days, and donors often feel tired for some time. The time required for a donor to recover varies from person to person. Some are back to their usual routine in a day or two. Others may take several days or as long as a week, but rarely longer.

Although donor complications are uncommon and much effort is devoted to their prevention, they sometimes occur. Complications are easily treated with proper medical attention. Because incisions are made to extract the marrow, infection is a possibility. Blood loss also can occur. For this reason, allogeneic and syngeneic donors routinely store two units of their own blood beforehand to be given during and after the procedure.

Harvesting Marrow or Peripheral Blood Stem Cells for Autologous Transplantation

When autologous transplantation is planned, the procedures for harvesting marrow differ, depending on factors such as the patient's physical condition and the time between harvesting and transplantation. In general, harvesting procedures are similar to those for allogeneic and syngeneic donors. However, if purging is to be done (as discussed previously), up to 2,000 milliliters (2 quarts) may be taken so that an adequate amount of marrow remains after purging. Removal of a larger amount of marrow requires a greater number of needle punctures and a longer period of time to collect the marrow. Any problems with bleeding are treated with transfusions of blood products from a blood bank. The marrow is stored until the time of transplantation.

Peripheral stem cells are harvested in a process called apheresis or leukapheresis. In this procedure, blood is removed through an intravenous catheter or through a large vein in the arm and is run through a machine that removes stem cells. The rest of the blood is returned to the patient. Typically, apheresis takes 2 to 4 hours and is repeated an average of six times. There usually is no need for hospitalization or anesthesia. Stem cells collected by apheresis are cryopreserved in the same way as is bone marrow.

Because the concentration of stem cells circulating in blood is at least 10 times lower than that found in the marrow, researchers are exploring ways to "mobilize" the stem cells—that is, to increase the number that can be harvested. One way is to collect them during the recovery period after chemotherapy, when the number of circulating stem cells may be as much as 25 times higher than usual. Another way is to treat the patient with hematopoietic growth factors. Normally produced by the body to stimulate blood cell production, these substances also can be made in the laboratory in large quantities. The most studied hematopoietic factors are the colony-stimulating factors and interleukins, which increase the production of white blood cells and can enhance the yield of peripheral blood stem cells. The effectiveness of mobilization may be increased through a combination of approaches.

Conditioning Regimens

Conditioning—treatment with high-dose chemotherapy with or without radiation therapy—is critical to the success of the transplantation. Conditioning serves a number of functions for cancer patients. Its primary purpose is to destroy cancer cells throughout the body more effectively than may be possible through conventional treatment. In addition, cells in the marrow are destroyed, creating space for the new marrow. Conditioning serves a third purpose in patients undergoing allogeneic transplantation: Because it destroys the cells of the immune system, it reduces the risk that the recipient will reject the graft.

Conditioning regimens for transplantation vary according to the patient's disease and medical condition and according to the medical center performing the procedure. The anticancer drugs used in high-dose chemotherapy may be given over the course of 2 to 6 days. If total-body irradiation (TBI) is used, it may be given in one dose or in multiple doses over the course of several days (fractionated radiation therapy). Fractionated schedules appear to minimize the risk of side effects and are generally preferred over single doses.

Marrow or Stem Cell Infusion

Shortly after the high-dose treatment is completed, the patient receives the donated or autologous marrow through the intravenous catheter. Peripheral blood stem cells for autologous transplantation are infused in the same way. The infusion of marrow or peripheral blood stem cells is called the rescue process. The stem cells travel through the bloodstream to the bone marrow, where they begin to produce new WBCs, RBCs, and platelets. Engraftment (blood cell production from transplanted stem cells) usually occurs within about 2 to 4 weeks following transplantation. Complete recovery of immune function takes much longer, however—up to several months for autologous transplant recipients and 1 to 2 years for patients receiving allogeneic transplants. Physicians evaluate results of various blood tests to confirm that new blood cells are being produced and that the cancer has not returned. Bone marrow aspiration also can help doctors determine how well new marrow components are forming.

Supportive Care

Supportive care is an essential aspect of transplantation. The goal of supportive care is to prevent or manage the side effects of high-dose chemotherapy and/or radiation therapy. Side effects requiring supportive care include immunosuppression, anemia, and bleeding (all of which are caused by low numbers of blood cells); nausea, vomiting, and loss of appetite (caused by irritation of the gastrointestinal tract); and malfunction of the lungs, liver, kidneys, and heart (caused by damage to these organs).

One of the most serious effects of high-dose cancer treatment is immunosuppression, in which the patient's body is unable to defend itself against infection. Supportive care for immunosuppression usually includes protective isolation: Patients must stay in a hospital room, where it is easier to keep the environment free of infectious agents. Depending on the institution, medical staff and visitors entering the patient's room may be required to go through some preventive measures ranging from thorough hand washing to putting on masks and gowns. Generally, patients also may start receiving antibiotics, antiviral agents, and antifungal agents just before or soon after chemotherapy or radiation therapy in an effort to prevent infection. Intravenous immunoglobulin therapy also is used by some centers as a preventive measure against infection. In this treatment, antibodies are isolated from donor blood and administered to the patient. Protective isolation and infection-fighting substances are continued from the time the patient's own marrow is destroyed until the transplanted marrow or peripheral blood stem cells produce enough white blood cells to fight infection.

To reduce the severity of immunosuppression, many patients receive hematopoietic growth factors. Growth factors administered after BMT or PBSCT can speed engraftment, decrease the risk of infection, and reduce the likelihood of graft failure (see Graft Failure section).

Because chemotherapy and radiation therapy damage the bone marrow's ability to produce RBCs and platelets, patients usually need periodic blood transfusions to treat anemia and thrombocytopenia. To reduce the risk of GVHD, all donated blood products given to transplantation patients are treated with radiation. This destroys lymphocytes that might otherwise attack the patient's cells and cause GVHD.

Adequate nutrition is vitally important for BMT patients. Chemotherapy and radiation therapy often cause nausea, vomiting, and mouth sores, which may make eating difficult for several weeks. In addition, some treatment plans require a period of time when the patient is not permitted to eat; this allows the gastrointestinal tract to heal following chemotherapy. Patients who are unable to eat can receive all necessary nutrients through the intravenous catheter, a process called total parenteral nutrition.

Convalescence and Followup Care

Most patients stay in the hospital for 1 to 2 months after BMT. This is necessary to monitor whether engraftment has been successful and to treat any potential complications, such as infections and acute GVHD. Hospitalization time may be reduced when PBSCT is done alone or with BMT because engraftment time tends to be faster. The use of hematopoietic growth factors also can shorten the time many patients must spend in the hospital.

Generally, a patient is discharged from the hospital after the neutrophil count is greater than 500 in a standard measure of blood for at least 2 consecutive days. Other considerations are the RBC and platelet counts, the presence or absence of recurrent infections, and the patient's general physical condition. Patients may need frequent platelet and blood transfusions even after discharge; for this reason, the catheter is left in place for as long as 3 to 6 months after transplantation.

Some patients will need to return to the hospital's outpatient department daily for the first 2 weeks, while others can be seen less frequently. Followup visits to the transplant clinic continue every 1 to 2 weeks for the first several months to ensure that blood counts are normal and that the cancer has not returned. Patients are then seen every month for about 6 months. Later, the schedule of checkups is based on each patient's need. Generally, checkups are done every 2 to 6 months. Most followup includes bone marrow aspiration to determine the condition of the marrow.

Many patients need a full year to recover physically and psychologically from transplantation. Even after that period, life may not return to "normal"—the way it was before the illness: Medication may be necessary indefinitely, and the patient's lifestyle may have to be changed to help prevent fatigue, avoid infectious diseases, and cope with the long-term effects of treatment.

There are physical changes to deal with, such as dry eyes, skin sensitivity, and, for some patients, reproductive disorders. In addition, changes in liver function may require alterations in diet. Some patients also experience changes in their self-image because they have received part of their body from someone else. On the other hand, some people think of their transplantation date as a new "birthday."

Complications for the Recipient

Patients experience a number of complications after transplantation. Some are temporary and relatively minor, but others can be life threatening. The likelihood that serious complications will develop is affected by, among other factors, a patient's age and general physical condition before transplantation.

Temporary side effects that are common among patients receiving chemotherapy and/or radiation therapy include hair loss, nausea and vomiting, fatigue, loss of appetite, mouth sores, and skin reactions. Additional information about these and other side effects of cancer treatment is available in the NCI booklets *Chemotherapy and You* and *Radiation Therapy and You.*

Some patients also experience temporary side effects that are caused by drugs given to prevent or treat the more severe complications of transplantation. These side effects depend on the drugs that are used, but they include gastrointestinal problems, high blood pressure, and, in some cases, seizures and problems with vision. Hematopoietic growth factors also may produce temporary side effects such as bone pain, muscle aches, and flu-like symptoms.

Serious side effects that are related to high-dose treatment or the transplantation itself are discussed below. The seriousness of these complications is different for each person.

Infections

Patients undergoing BMT are at significant risk of developing infections for several months after transplantation. Cytomegaloviruses, Aspergillus (a type of fungus), and Pneumocystis carinii (a protozoan) are among the most important causes of life-threatening infections, including pneumonia. Many patients develop herpes zoster virus infections (shingles), and herpes simplex virus infections (cold sores and genital herpes) often become reactivated in patients who were previously infected with this virus. Mucositis, an inflammation of the mouth and gastrointestinal tract, also is common after BMT.

Some infections may be prevented by the administration of antiviral agents, antibiotics, and antifungal agents before and after transplantation. These drugs also may be used to treat infections. Patients must be watched closely just after BMT, before engraftment occurs, because this is the period in which they are at highest risk for infection. In addition, patients have routine lab work, chest x-rays, and other exams to check for signs and symptoms of infection during the entire treatment process. Because of improvements in prevention strategies, fewer patients die of infection after transplantation than did in previous years.

Infections also are a potential complication for patients undergoing PBSCT. However, because engraftment tends to occur earlier than for BMT, the period of highest risk is shortened. Often, infections that do occur are related to catheter use.

Graft-Versus-Host Disease

Graft-versus-host disease is one of the most serious potential complications of allogeneic BMT. It occurs when T cells in the donated marrow (the graft) identify the recipient's body (the host) as foreign and attack it. This situation is different from other types of organ transplantation (such as kidney or heart transplantation), in which the donated organ is rejected by the patient's immune system. Although the donated marrow can be rejected by whatever remains of the patient's original immune system, more often, it is the T lymphocytes produced by the new marrow that launch an attack against the patient. Without preventive measures, most patients undergoing allogeneic BMT would develop GVHD.

Symptoms of GVHD can develop within days or as long as 3 years after transplantation. Generally, GVHD that develops within 3 months following transplantation is known as acute GVHD; when it

721

develops later, it is called chronic GVHD. Because the time periods in which acute and chronic GVHD can develop overlap, these diseases are better identified by their symptoms, which are somewhat different for each type.

Common symptoms of acute GVHD are skin rashes, jaundice, liver disease, and diarrhea. Because recovery of immune function after BMT is delayed, patients also have persistent susceptibility to infections. Patients with mild forms of acute GVHD are likely to recover completely, but those with severe forms may die of complications of the disease. Chronic GVHD produces temporary darkening of the skin, and hardening and thickening of patches of skin and the layers of tissues under it. Occasionally, the liver, esophagus, and other parts of the gastrointestinal tract are affected. Mucous membranes may become dry, and hair loss may occur. Bacterial infections and weight loss are common. As with acute GVHD, severe cases of chronic GVHD may be fatal.

Several factors affect a patient's risk of developing GVHD. The most important is the degree of HLA matching: The more antigens that match, the lower the risk of GVHD. About 70 percent of patients who receive donor marrow with two mismatched antigens develop significant acute GVHD, versus 40 percent of patients receiving HLA-identical marrow. (Mild GVHD occasionally develops after autologous BMT or PBSCT; it usually is related to the presence of T lymphocytes in transfused blood products from another person.) Age also affects the risk of GVHD, with older patients being more susceptible to the disease than are younger ones. In addition, a recipient whose donor is of the opposite sex is more likely to develop GVHD than a recipient whose donor is of the same sex. Chronic GVHD, which affects at least one-third of allogeneic BMT patients, develops most often in those who have had acute GVHD.

To reduce the risk of GVHD after transplantation, most patients routinely receive immunosuppressive therapy with cyclosporine and/or methotrexate, drugs that help suppress T lymphocytes. Combinations of drugs appear to be most effective. Another technique for preventing GVHD is T-cell depletion, which involves eliminating T lymphocytes in the donated marrow before it is given to the patient. The T cells are removed or destroyed by means of monoclonal antibodies or other processes. Although T-cell depletion appears to reduce the chance that a patient will develop severe GVHD, this technique has other associated risks: Graft failure may be more likely when T-cell depleted marrow is used, and leukemia patients may be more likely to have a relapse.

Should GVHD occur despite efforts to prevent it, high-dose corticosteroids (such as prednisone) are given to relieve symptoms of the disease and to suppress T-cell activity. Patients may receive antithymocyte globulin, which acts against immature T cells (thymocytes), or monoclonal antibodies that are directed against T cells. Higher doses of cyclosporine also can be helpful.

Interestingly, many studies have shown that mild GVHD may be beneficial over the long term, perhaps because the activated graft cells may be better able to kill cancer cells (a so-called "graft-versus-cancer" effect). Leukemia and lymphoma patients who develop mild GVHD are less likely to have a relapse than are patients who never have the reaction. For this reason, researchers are studying ways to introduce "graft-versus-cancer" effects in autologous BMT.

Bleeding

Bleeding may be a problem, especially during the first 4 weeks after BMT, when platelet production is greatly reduced. Bleeding most often occurs in the mucous membranes of the nose and mouth; it also may develop under the skin or in the gastrointestinal tract. Platelet transfusions are given if there is any evidence of bleeding and/or to maintain the platelet count at the minimum needed to prevent bleeding. Platelets may be donated by the marrow donor or another closely HLA-matched individual.

Organ Complications

Patients may develop complications in the liver, kidneys, lungs, and/or heart. Because these vital organs are susceptible to serious damage, only patients without preexisting problems are considered for transplantation.

Several factors may contribute to the development of liver disease in patients undergoing BMT or PBSCT. Chemotherapy and radiation treatments may cause deposits of fibrous material to form in the small veins of the liver, which obstruct blood flow out of it. This obstruction is known as venocclusive disease (VOD). VOD is an important and sometimes severe complication in BMT. Symptoms of VOD include swelling of the liver, abdominal pain, weight gain, and poor liver function. Other conditions that may cause liver damage are viral hepatitis, fungal and bacterial infections, and GVHD. In addition, some drugs used to treat infection may cause liver problems. Liver disease is difficult to treat, and medical care is generally directed at controlling the patient's symptoms. Some medical centers are investigating whether certain drugs can prevent liver disease.

Chemotherapy, radiation therapy, antibiotics, and immunosuppressive agents (especially cyclosporine) also may cause kidney failure. When this happens, urine production decreases, waste products accumulate in the blood, and the patient becomes more susceptible to infection, bleeding, and drug toxicity. Should kidney problems develop, the patient's fluid balance is carefully controlled. Dietary modifications, including total parenteral nutrition, may be necessary, and drug doses may need to be changed. Some patients may need dialysis. As with liver disease, the likelihood of kidney failure may be reduced by certain drugs.

Complications also may develop in the lungs after transplantation. Often, infections are the cause of these problems. However, radiation therapy and chemotherapy also may be damaging, causing pneumonitis, an inflammation of the lungs. Some patients develop pulmonary fibrosis, a condition that may result in shortness of breath. Measures to prevent lung problems include antibiotic therapy and the use of lung shields during total-body irradiation (TBI).

Chemotherapy—in particular, doxorubicin—can damage the heart and produce a number of complications that affect its function. Certain complications can be life threatening. However, only a small percentage of patients undergoing transplantation experience heart complications.

Graft Failure

Grafting is considered a failure when bone marrow function does not return or when it is lost after a period of recovery. Unsuccessful transplantations usually result from one of two main situations. In one case, graft rejection, the recipient's body rejects the donated marrow; in the other, engraftment does not occur or doesn't continue—that is, the transplanted stem cells simply fail to grow and produce new blood cells. Graft rejection is a problem that is exclusive to allogeneic transplant recipients, whereas other types of graft failure may occur in patients receiving any type of transplant.

A number of factors may contribute to the risk of graft rejection. One of the most significant is the use of marrow with an imperfect HLA match. Graft rejection is more common among patients who have not had TBI because such patients are more likely to retain some immune activity after pretransplantation conditioning. The use of T-cell depleted donor marrow also is associated with an increased risk of graft rejection.

Engraftment is less likely to occur in patients with extensive marrow fibrosis before transplantation. Unsuccessful transplantation also may result from a viral illness or from the use of drugs that suppress the immune system (such as methotrexate). In leukemia patients graft failure often is associated with a recurrence of leukemia; the leukemic cells may inhibit the growth of the transplanted cells. In some cases the reasons for graft failure are not known.

Long-Term Effects

Long-term effects of transplantation are largely related to pretransplantation conditioning regimens. Some of these problems are discussed below.

Infertility

Chemotherapy and radiation therapy often cause temporary or permanent reproductive difficulties. The extent of these problems depends on the patient's age and sex and on the dosage and duration of treatment. Most patients who receive TBI as part of their conditioning treatment become sterile. However, sexual desire and function usually return to normal after transplantation.

Infertility is common among men who are treated with chemotherapy or radiation therapy. For this reason men are usually encouraged to consider sperm banking before treatment begins if they wish to father children after transplantation.

Menstrual irregularities often develop in women who have received high-dose chemotherapy. Although periods may return up to 2 years after transplantation in younger women, patients over the age of 25 are likely to develop early menopause. Hormone replacement therapy can help relieve the symptoms of menopause and may be recommended for other medical reasons. (However, this treatment may not be appropriate for women who have had breast cancer.) Cryopreservation of fertilized or unfertilized eggs before cancer therapy is possible for some women. Women who wish to become pregnant after they have undergone transplantation should speak with their doctor; pregnancy may not be advisable for health reasons.

Sterility can be a psychologically distressing side effect. This important issue should be addressed by the patient, partner, family, and health care team before and after transplantation.

Growth Problems

Studies have shown that some children treated with TBI may have impaired growth, particularly when single-dose TBI is given. The radiation can cause a reduction in growth hormone production and can damage children's bones. The result may be a delay in growth of about 2 years.

Cataracts

Cataracts may occur 3 to 6 years after TBI. Roughly three-quarters of patients who receive single-dose TBI develop cataracts. The number is reduced to about 20 percent in patients who receive fractionated radiation doses or in those who do not receive TBI. Patients who develop cataracts generally need corrective surgery, which often restores normal vision.

Secondary Cancers

Because BMT has been done for only a few decades, not all of the long-term effects of the procedure are known. There is some concern that high-dose chemotherapy, irradiation, immunosuppression, stem cell mobilization, or other unknown factors related to the procedure may increase the risk for secondary cancers. Studies have shown that the risk varies considerably depending on the patient's age, general health, menopausal status (for women), and previous history of radiation. The dosage and type of drug given also affect the likelihood that a second cancer may develop.

Financial Considerations

Because it is a highly technical procedure that requires extensive hospitalization, BMT is very expensive. Advances in treatment methods, including the use of PBSCT, have reduced the time many patients must spend in the hospital by speeding recovery; this shorter recovery time has brought about a reduction in cost. Still, transplantation expenses often exceed $100,000. Most centers require a guarantee of funds in advance to cover these costs. However, some health insurance plans now cover some costs of transplantation for specific diseases.

Costs are incurred not only in the hospital, but outside as well. Patients and their families may need to stay near the transplant center for several months so that the patient can receive followup care. This can involve a considerable amount of money, particularly if accommodations are far from home. After the patient returns home, other expenses may arise. No patient is able to function independently immediately after discharge from the hospital, and convalescence at home takes a significant amount of time. Family members may need to call on home helpers or visiting nurses to assist them with the care of the patient. In some cases insurers cover a portion of these costs. In other cases local service organizations may be able to help.

There are some options for relieving the financial burden associated with BMT. A hospital social worker can be a valuable resource in planning for these financial needs. Patients and their families may use an existing charitable fund from a church or service group (Kiwanis, Lions, Rotary, Masons, etc.); contributions to these funds are tax deductible.

Families can also contact the Leukemia Society of America and the American Cancer Society (listed in the white pages of the telephone directory). These organizations may be able to help with costs of transportation and other expenses.

Organizations such as the Corporate Angel Network (CAN) will sometimes help with air transportation. This organization's member companies share their scheduled executive jet flights with cancer patients needing to travel to obtain medical care.

Government programs such as Medicaid and Social Security also may provide financial assistance for health expenses and disability. Medicaid is a program for people of low income; information about coverage is available from a local public health or social services office or from a State Medicaid office. Supplemental Security Income is available to disabled people of low income and Social Security Disability to certain disabled workers. A local Social Security office (listed in the Government section of the telephone directory) can explain eligibility criteria and benefits.

Income tax deductions can be claimed for some BMT expenses. Families should check with an accountant or attorney regarding such deductions. The local Internal Revenue Service office and possibly the hospital's social services staff also can provide guidance on tax considerations.

The NCI's Cancer Information Service (1-800-4-CANCER) can provide patients and their families with additional information about financial assistance.

Psychosocial Considerations

BMT causes tremendous stress for patients and their families, who must struggle physically, emotionally, and financially with the therapy and the disruption it may bring to their lives. Families often must travel a long distance to a treatment center and arrange to live away from home for an extended period of time. (The number of treatment centers that can perform BMT has grown considerably in recent years, but they still tend to be clustered in major metropolitan areas.) For many people this means a lengthy separation from other family members. Making these adjustments can be very difficult; patients and their families may find it helpful to use support services offered through the hospital or another organization, such as the American Cancer Society.

The energy required during and after transplantation is considerable. Fatigue is a common complaint: Patients tire of the rigors of treatment, and both they and their families often feel the pressure of not knowing what will happen.

During the BMT process, medical problems are likely to take priority over psychological needs. However, the psychological stresses of BMT are considerable and should not be minimized. For many reasons, both families and patients may experience guilt, relief, fear, anger, depression, and anxiety. At any time during treatment or followup, members of the health care team may help patients and families deal with these issues. Patients and their families are encouraged to consult with a social worker, a member of the clergy, or a counselor.

The Future of Transplantation

An estimated 12,000 BMT's were performed in 1992, approximately half of which were allogeneic and half autologous. The use of autologous transplantation (including PBSCT) has grown significantly during the past several years as improvements in the procedure have been made. The number of patients who receive allogeneic transplants also is rising, in part because large donor registries have increased the number of available donors. Advances in transplantation techniques likely will further expand the use of BMT and PBSCT in the coming years.

The use of hematopoietic growth factors is one of the most promising areas of research. Other growth factors are under investigation in addition to the well-studied GM-CSF, G-CSF, and the interleukins. Erythropoietin (a red blood cell growth factor) can increase peripheral blood stem cell yield before transplantation and can reduce the need for RBC transfusions afterward. Researchers have discovered a growth factor that stimulates the production of platelets, which has been named thrombopoietin. In the future, treatment with this growth factor may be able to complement or replace transfusions with platelets. Stem cell factor, which stimulates the maturation of stem cells, may be useful for speeding engraftment. Researchers also are investigating whether growth factors can be applied to harvested stem cells in vitro (in the laboratory) to increase the number of stem cells available for transplantation.

Other biological response modifiers under investigation include interferons and monoclonal antibodies. Interferons may stop the growth of cancer cells when used before or after BMT for chronic myelogenous leukemia. Monoclonal antibodies can be bound to radioisotopes or anticancer drugs and targeted to cancer cells. In this way, drugs or radiation can be delivered directly to cancer cells without damaging healthy cells.

Because even small numbers of cancer cells can grow and cause a relapse after transplantation, researchers are exploring ways to detect cancer in patients who otherwise appear to be in remission. One technique involves the use of monoclonal antibodies linked to radioisotopes or special dyes that allow the cancer to be seen. Another technique, known as polymerase chain reaction (or PCR), magnifies the genetic abnormalities of some types of cancer so that they can be detected. Researchers also are trying to identify other factors that may indicate a high risk of relapse.

A new approach under study in allogeneic transplantation involves using umbilical cord blood, which generally contains high levels of stem cells. The feasibility of cord blood cell banking is under investigation.

Many issues surrounding BMT and PBSCT in cancer treatment are being addressed in current clinical trials; others are still under study in the laboratory. Marrow transplant technology is also being evaluated for treatment of other disorders in which the immune system's ability to function has been affected.

Clinical Trials and PDQ

To improve the outcome of treatment for patients with cancer, NCI supports clinical trials at many hospitals throughout the United States. Volunteers who take part in this research make an important contribution to medical science and may have the first chance to benefit from improved treatment methods. Physicians are encouraged to tell their patients about the option of participating in such trials. To help patients and doctors learn about current methods of treatment and clinical trials, NCI has developed PDQ, a database designed to give physicians and patients quick and easy access to:

- Descriptions of ongoing clinical trials, including information about the objectives of the studies, medical eligibility requirements, details of the treatment programs, and the names and addresses of physicians and facilities conducting the studies.

- The latest treatment information for most types of cancer.

- Names and addresses of physicians and organizations involved in cancer care.

Information specialists at the Cancer Information Service (CIS) use a variety of resources, including PDQ, to answer questions about cancer prevention, diagnosis, treatment, rehabilitation, and research. To obtain information from the PDQ data base, physicians, patients, and the public may call the CIS toll free at 1-800-4-CANCER. Staff members also can tell doctors how to obtain regular access to the data base.

In addition, PDQ statements containing up-to-date treatment information are available by fax machine through the CancerFax service. Those wanting to use this service should dial (301)-402-5874 from a fax machine telephone and follow instructions to obtain a list of the CancerFax contents and the corresponding code numbers. Users then can call the service again and enter the code numbers of the printouts they wish to receive by fax.

PDQ statements, fact sheets on various cancer topics, and citations and abstracts on selected topics from the CANCERLIT data base can be obtained through CancerNet. This service allows users to access cancer information through electronic mail. It is available through a number of different networks including BITNET and Internet.

Resources

American Cancer Society
1599 Clifton Road NE
Atlanta, GA 30329-4251
1-800-ACS-2345

The American Cancer Society (ACS) is a national voluntary organization. It offers a wide range of services to patients and their families and carries out programs of research and education. It is financed through donations from individuals and private groups. Local chapters of the ACS may be listed in the telephone directory; information is also available by dialing the toll-free number listed above.

Leukemia and Lymphoma Society
Fourth Floor
733 Third Avenue
New York, NY 10016
1-800-955-4572

The Society is a voluntary organization that offers educational materials and information to leukemia and lymphoma patients and their families. It has many local chapters whose addresses may be listed in the telephone directory. Information is also available by dialing the toll-free telephone number listed above.

National Marrow Donor Program
Suite 400
3433 Broadway Street NE
Minneapolis, MN 55413
Donor Information: 1-800-654-1247
Patient Search Information: 1-800-526-7809

The National Marrow Donor Program (NMDP) is funded by a Federal contract with the American Red Cross, the American Association of Blood Banks, and the Council of Community Blood Centers. It was created to improve the efficiency and effectiveness of the donor search so that a larger number of unrelated bone marrow transplantations can be carried out. Businesses interested in setting up corporate recruitment programs should contact NMDP at 1-800-526-7809.

American Red Cross
430 17th Street NW
Washington, DC 20006
(202) 737-8300

The American Red Cross collects and distributes blood and blood products and provides a range of services for emergency situations and people in need of social service support. It coordinates bone marrow testing and donation in association with the National Marrow Donor Program. Local chapters are listed in the white pages of the telephone directory.

American Bone Marrow Donor Registry

Search Coordinating Center
Caitlin Raymond International Registry of Bone Marrow Donor Banks
University of Massachusetts Medical Center
55 Lake Avenue North Worcester, MA 01655
Donor Information: 1-800-7-DONATE (1-800-736-6283)
Patient Search Information: 1-800-7-A-MATCH (1-800-726-2824)

The American Bone Marrow Donor Registry is a nonprofit organization that coordinates donor searches among participating donor centers in the United States and throughout the world.

International Bone Marrow Transplant Registry

Medical College of Wisconsin
P.O. Box 26509
8701 Watertown Plank Road
Milwaukee, WI 53226
414-456-8325

This research organization collects and analyzes data about allogeneic bone marrow transplantations performed at BMT centers throughout the world and autologous transplantations done in North America. (It does not make donor matches.) Staff are available to answer questions about the procedure.

Selected References

Available from Libraries

Bortin, M.M. et al. "Changing Trends in Allogeneic Bone Marrow Transplantation for Leukemia in the 1980s," *Journal of the American Medical Association*, Vol. 268(5), 1992, pp. 607-612.

Bortin, M.M. et al. "Increasing Utilization of Allogeneic Bone Marrow Transplantation: Results of the 1988-1990 Survey," *Annals of Internal Medicine*, Vol. 116(6), 1992, pp. 505-512.

Champlin, R. "T-cell Depletion To Prevent Graft-Versus-Host-Disease After Bone Marrow Transplantation," *Hematology / Oncology Clinics of North America*, Vol. 4(3), 1990, pp. 687-698.

DeVita, V.T., Jr., Hellman, S., and Rosenberg, S.A., eds. Cancer: Principles and Practices of Oncology. Philadelphia, J.B. Lippincott Company, 1993.

Ferrara, J.L.M. and Deeg, H.J. "Mechanisms of Disease: Graft-Versus-Host Disease," *The New England Journal of Medicine*, Vol. 324(10), 1991, pp. 667-674.

Holland, J.C. and Rowland, J.H. *Handbook of Psychooncology: Psychological Care of the Patient with Cancer*. New York, Oxford University Press, 1989.

Kernan, N.A. et al. "Analysis of 462 Transplantations from Unrelated Donors Facilitated by the National Marrow Donor Program," *The New England Journal of Medicine*, Vol. 328(9), 1993, pp. 593-602.

Kessinger, A. and Armitage, J. "The Use of Peripheral Stem Cell Support of High-Dose Chemotherapy," in *Important Advances in Oncology 1993*. DeVita, V.T., Jr. et al., eds. Philadelphia, J.B. Lippincott Co., 1993.

Meropol, N.J. et al. "High-Dose Chemotherapy with Autologous Stem Cell Support for Breast Cancer," *Oncology*, Vol. 6(12), 1992, pp. 53-63.

Thorne, A.C., et al. "Harvesting Bone Marrow in an Outpatient Setting Using Newer Anesthetic Agents," *Journal of Clinical Oncology*, Vol. 11(2), 1993, pp. 320-323.

Treleaven, J. and Barrett, J. *Bone Marrow Transplantation in Practice*. Edinburgh, Churchill Livingstone, 1992.

Available from the National Cancer Institute

Chemotherapy and You: A Guide to Self-Help During Treatment. Office of Cancer Communications, National Cancer Institute. NIH Publication No. 92-1136.

Radiation Therapy and You: A Guide to Self-Help During Treatment. Office of Cancer Communications, National Cancer Institute. NIH Publication No. 92-2227.

Research Report: Leukemia. Office of Cancer Communications, National Cancer Institute. NIH Publication No. 93-329.

The Immune System—How It Works. National Cancer Institute, National Institute of Allergy and Infectious Diseases. NIH Publication No. 92-3229.

What Are Clinical Trials All About? Office of Cancer Communications, National Cancer Institute. NIH Publication No. 90-2706.

Additional Information

To obtain information on this subject and to order other NCI publications, call the toll-free Cancer Information Service (CIS) at: 1-800-4-CANCER

The CIS is a nationwide telephone service that answers questions from patients and their families, the public, and health professionals. Spanish-speaking staff members are available.

This Research Report has been approved by NCI scientists. Please direct questions or comments to the Research Report Editor, Office of Cancer Communications, National Cancer Institute, Bethesda, MD 20892.

The NCI is the U.S. Government's main agency for cancer research and information about cancer. The NCI's publications are free. They may be copied or reproduced without written permission.

Chapter 69

Get a New Attitude about Cancer: A Guide for Black Americans

You could be one of the thousands of Black Americans saved over the next ten years. The fact is, Black Americans are diagnosed with cancer and die from it more often than any other group. But what most Black Americans don't know is that many more would survive cancer if it were discovered early and treated right away. By adopting a "new attitude" and making some simple lifestyle changes, you will be taking crucial steps toward maintaining your health.

Check the Facts

It is important to understand what is happening to the health of Black Americans. By understanding the facts, you also will see how important your actions are to beat cancer.

Lung Cancer

The good news is that over the past five years, the number of Black American men who smoke is decreasing. But they still get lung cancer and other smoking-related disease more than other men because they tend to smoke cigarettes with a high tar and nicotine content.

Since 1973, the number of Black American women (ages 45-54) who have died from lung cancer has increased 30 percent. Next to breast cancer, lung cancer is the leading cause of cancer death among Black American women.

"Get A New Attitude About Cancer: A Guide For Black Americans," National Cancer Institute (NCI), revised December 1992.

735

Colorectal Cancer

Since 1973, colorectal cancer in Black American men increased 30 percent; in Black American women the increase was almost 18 percent.

Breast Cancer

Since 1973, the number of Black American women of all ages who have died from breast cancer has risen 18 percent. Breast cancer is now the leading cause of cancer death for these women. Since 80 percent of women diagnosed with this form of cancer have no family history of the disease, all Black American women, particularly those age 40 and over, have a chance of getting breast cancer.

Cervical Cancer

Black American women are twice as likely to develop cervical cancer and nearly three times as likely to die from it than other women.

Prostate Cancer

For Black American men, over their lifetime, the odds of getting prostate cancer are 1 in 9, compared with 1 in 11 for all men in the United States. In fact, Black American men in the United States have the world's highest rate of prostate cancer.

Statistics

According to statistics,* the leading causes of cancer death for Black Americans are:

Black Males

1. Lung
2. Prostate
3. Colorectal

Black Females

1. Breast
2. Lung
3. Colorectal

In 1992, about 115,000 cases of cancer will be found in Black Americans.

Cancer Facts and Figures: Cancer in Minorities, 1992.

Do the Right Thing

By taking care of their health and getting checked for cancer, thousands of Black American lives can be saved.

Here some ways you can "do the right thing."

Eat Right

Scientists know that poor eating habits can increase your chances of getting cancer. Some important facts to remember are:

- Avoid eating too much fatty food. "Trimming the fat" in your diet may decrease your risk for several cancers, particularly breast, colon, and prostate cancers. Buy lean meats, and broil, boil, and bake your food. It will taste good and be good for you.

- Cut down on fats (butter, margarine, oil, fatback) when cooking food.

- Eat five servings of fruits and vegetables a day. Eating "5 A Day" is an easy way to reduce your risk of cancer. Fruits and vegetables are low in fat and rich in vitamins and fiber. One "5 A Day" serving equals either 1/2 cup of fruit or cooked vegetable, 3/4 cup of juice, 1 cup of leafy vegetable, or 1/4 cup of dried fruit. By adding five fruits and vegetables a day to your meals, you are eating your way to better health and cancer prevention.

- Eat whole grain breads and cereals daily.

- Maintain a healthy weight. Staying within your ideal weight range can lower your risk of having breast, cervical, and other cancers.

- Avoid fatty foods, eating "5 A Day," and exercising will help you maintain your healthy weight, and make you feel better, too!

Don't Smoke

Scientists also know that smoking is directly linked to cancer. The most important action to take is: Quit smoking. The chances of getting lung cancer gradually decrease once a person stops smoking. Smoking causes most deaths from lung cancer—a cancer that accounts for more than a quarter of all cancer deaths among Black Americans.

Find Cancer Early

One of the most powerful steps you can take to protect your health and your life is to find cancer early. Cancer in its earliest stage rarely has warning signs.

- Get a regular exam by your doctor and ask to be checked for cancer. For example, for women age 40 and over, getting regular mammograms can find a tumor 2 years before it can be felt as a lump. This makes it possible for doctors to catch cancer early, at its most treatable stage.

- Get a second opinion. If your exam shows that you may have cancer, a second doctor's opinion can help you make one of the most important decisions in your life. Many patients think asking for a second opinion will offend the first doctor they saw. Actually, having a second opinion is a normal medical practice and your doctor can help you with this effort.

Get Involved

Doing the right thing means more than taking care of yourself. It also means reaching back to help others take care of themselves. These messages about diet, smoking and finding cancer early as ways to fight cancer cannot reach your community without your help. Here's what you can do:

- Know how to educate yourself and others. The National Cancer Institute (NCI) has the Cancer Information Service (CIS) to help provide you with more information about cancer. The CIS provides a nationwide telephone service for cancer patients and their families and friends, the public, and health care professionals. The staff can answer questions and can send booklets about cancer. They also may know about local resources and services. One toll-free number, 1-800-4-CANCER (1-800-422-6237), connects callers with the office that serves their area.

- Take action. The NCI has a program called the National Black Leadership Initiative on Cancer (NBLIC) to help Black American communities increase their cancer awareness. The NBLIC supports community activities that can be used in churches, special groups, and service organizations to help change attitudes about cancer. Over 65 community-based groups from around the country, which include health professionals and community volunteers, hold health fairs, screening programs, educational seminars, and other programs right in your neighborhood. If you want more information about upcoming programs in your area or want to get involved with the NBLIC, call (312) 996-8046 to request the number for the NBLIC regional director for your area.

Get a New Attitude about Cancer

Take charge of your health by eating right, not smoking, seeing your doctor regularly and getting involved. By getting a new attitude about cancer, you will help not only yourself, but also help other Black Americans beat the odds in the fight against cancer.

Chapter 70

Alternative Medicine

Questions and Answers about Complementary and Alternative Medicine in Cancer Treatment

1. What is complementary and alternative medicine?

Complementary and alternative medicine (CAM)—also referred to as integrative medicine—includes a broad range of healing philosophies, approaches, and therapies. A therapy is generally called complementary when it is used in addition to conventional treatments; it is often called alternative when it is used instead of conventional treatment. (Conventional treatments are those that are widely accepted and practiced by the mainstream medical community.) Depending on how they are used, some therapies can be considered either complementary or alternative.

Complementary and alternative therapies are used in an effort to prevent illness, reduce stress, prevent or reduce side effects and symptoms, or control or cure disease. Some commonly used methods of complementary or alternative therapy include mind/body control interventions such as visualization or relaxation, manual healing including acupressure and massage, homeopathy, vitamins or herbal products, and acupuncture.

"Questions and Answers About Complementary and Alternative Medicine in Cancer Treatment," National Cancer Institute (NCI) Fact Sheet, reviewed July 1999.

2. Are complementary and alternative cancer therapies widely used?

Although there are few studies on the use of complementary and alternative therapies for cancer, one large-scale study found that the percentage of cancer patients in the United States using these therapies was nine percent overall (Lerner and Kennedy, 1992).

3. Can complementary and alternative medicine be evaluated using the same methods used in conventional medicine?

Scientific evaluation is important in understanding if and when complementary and alternative therapies work. A number of medical centers are evaluating complementary and alternative therapies by developing scientific studies to test them.

Conventional approaches to cancer treatment have generally been studied for safety and effectiveness through a rigorous scientific process, including clinical trials with large numbers of patients. Often, less is known about the safety and effectiveness of complementary and alternative methods. Some of these complementary and alternative therapies have not undergone rigorous evaluation. Others, once considered unorthodox, are finding a place in cancer treatment—not as cures, but as complementary therapies that may help patients feel better and recover faster. One example is acupuncture. According to a panel of experts at a National Institutes of Health Consensus Conference in November 1997, acupuncture has been found to be effective in the management of chemotherapy-associated nausea and vomiting and in controlling pain associated with surgery. Some approaches, such as laetrile, have been studied and found ineffective or potentially harmful.

4. What should patients do when considering complementary and alternative therapies?

Cancer patients considering complementary and alternative medicine should discuss this decision with their doctor or nurse, as they would any therapeutic approach, because some complementary and alternative therapies may interfere with their standard treatment or may be harmful when used with conventional treatment.

5. When considering complementary and alternative therapies, what questions should patients ask their health care provider?

- What benefits can be expected from this therapy?

- What are the risks associated with this therapy?
- Do the known benefits outweigh the risks?
- What side effects can be expected?
- Will the therapy interfere with conventional treatment?
- Will the therapy be covered by health insurance?

6. How can patients and their health care providers learn more about complementary and alternative therapies?

Patients and their doctor or nurse can learn about complementary and alternative therapies from the following Government agencies:

NCCAM Clearinghouse
Post Office Box 8218
Silver Spring, MD 20907-8218
Telephone: 1-888-644-6226 (toll free)
TTY/TDY (for deaf and hard of hearing callers): 1-888-644-6226 (toll free)
Web site: http://nccam.nih.gov

The NIH National Center for Complementary and Alternative Medicine (NCCAM) facilitates research and evaluation of complementary and alternative practices and has information about a variety of methods.

Food and Drug Administration
5600 Fishers Lane
Rockville, MD 20857
Telephone: 1-888-463-6332 (toll free)
Web site: http://www.fda.gov/

The Food and Drug Administration (FDA) regulates drugs and medical devices to ensure that they are safe and effective.

Federal Trade Commission
Consumer Response Center
Room 130
600 Pennsylvania Avenue, NW.
Washington, DC 20580
Telephone: 1-877-382-4357 (toll free)
TTY (for deaf and hard of hearing callers): 202-326-2502
Web site: http://www.ftc.gov/

The Federal Trade Commission (FTC) enforces consumer protection laws. Publications available from the FTC include:

- "Who Cares: Sources of Information About Health Care Products and Services"
- "Fraudulent Health Claims: Don't Be Fooled"

References

Cassileth B, Chapman C. Alternative and Complementary Cancer Therapies. *Cancer* 1996; 77(6):1026-1033.

Jacobs J. Unproven Alternative Methods of Cancer Treatment. In: DeVita, Hellman, Rosenberg, editors. Cancer: *Principles and Practice of Oncology.* 5th edition. Philadelphia: Lippincott-Raven Publishers; 1997. 2993-3001.

Lerner IJ, Kennedy BJ. The Prevalence of Questionable Methods of Cancer Treatment in the United States. *CA-A Cancer Journal* 1992; 42:181-191.

Nelson W. Alternative Cancer Treatments. *Highlights in Oncology Practice* 1998; 15(4):85-93.

Chapter 71

Marijuana Use in Supportive Care for Cancer Patients

Cancer and cancer treatment may cause a variety of problems for cancer patients. Chemotherapy-induced nausea and vomiting and anorexia and cachexia are conditions that affect many individuals with cancer.

Nausea and Vomiting

Some anticancer drugs cause nausea and vomiting because they affect parts of the brain that control vomiting and/or irritate the stomach lining. The severity of these symptoms depends on several factors, including the chemotherapeutic agent(s) used, the dose, the schedule, and the patient's reaction to the drug(s). The management of nausea and vomiting caused by chemotherapy is an important part of care for cancer patients whenever it occurs. Although patients usually receive antiemetics, drugs that help control nausea and vomiting, there is no single best approach to reducing these symptoms in all patients. Doctors must tailor antiemetic therapy to meet each individual's needs, taking into account the type of anticancer drugs being administered; the patient's general condition, age, and related factors; and, of course, the extent to which the antiemetic is helpful.

There has been much interest in the use of marijuana to treat a number of medical problems, including chemotherapy-induced nausea and vomiting in cancer patients. Two forms of marijuana have been used: compounds related to the active chemical constituent of

National Cancer Institute (NCI) Fact Sheet, modified July 1999.

marijuana taken by mouth and marijuana cigarettes. Dronabinol (Marinol), a synthetic form of the active marijuana constituent delta-9-tetrahydrocannabinol (THC), is available by prescription for use as an antiemetic. The U.S. Food and Drug Administration has approved its use for treatment of nausea and vomiting associated with cancer chemotherapy in patients who have not responded to the standard antiemetic drugs.

National Cancer Institute (NCI) scientists feel that other antiemetic drugs or combinations of antiemetic drugs have been shown to be more useful than synthetic THC as "first-line therapy" for nausea and vomiting caused by anticancer drugs. Examples include drugs called serotonin antagonists, including ondansetron (Zofran) and granisetron (Kytril), used alone or combined with dexamethasone (a steroid hormone); metoclopramide (Reglan) combined with diphenhydramine and dexamethasone; high doses of methylprednisolone (a steroid hormone) combined with droperidol (Inapsine); and prochlorperazine (Compazine). Continued research with other agents and combinations of these agents is under way to determine their usefulness in controlling chemotherapy-induced nausea and vomiting. However, NCI scientists believe that synthetic THC may be useful for some cancer patients who have chemotherapy-induced nausea and vomiting that cannot be controlled by other antiemetic agents. The expected side effects of this compound must be weighed against the possible benefits. Dronabinol often causes a "high" (loss of control or sensation of unreality), which is associated with its effectiveness; however, this sensation may be unpleasant for some individuals.

Marijuana cigarettes have been used to treat chemotherapy-induced nausea and vomiting, and research has shown that THC is more quickly absorbed from marijuana smoke than from an oral preparation. However, any antiemetic effects of smoking marijuana may not be consistent because of varying potency, depending on the source of the marijuana cigarette. To address issues surrounding the medical uses of marijuana, the National Institutes of Health convened a meeting in February 1997 to assess what is known about marijuana's therapeutic potential and to identify what future research avenues would be most productive. The group of experts concluded that more and better studies are needed to fully evaluate the potential use of marijuana as supportive care for cancer patients. One area that will be studied in the near future is a smoke-free delivery system of marijuana's active ingredient THC. Other areas to be studied are the risks associated with marijuana use, including the effects on the lungs and immune system, and the dangerous byproducts of smoked marijuana.

Anorexia and Cachexia

Anorexia, the loss of appetite or desire to eat, is the most common symptom in cancer patients that may occur early in the disease or later as the cancer grows and spreads. Cachexia is a wasting condition in which the patient has weakness and a marked and progressive loss of body weight, fat, and muscle. Anorexia and cachexia frequently occur together, but cachexia may occur in patients who are eating an adequate diet but have malabsorption of nutrients. Maintenance of body weight and adequate nutritional status can help patients feel and look better, and maintain or improve their performance status. It may also help them better tolerate cancer therapy.

There are a variety of options for supportive nutritional care of cancer patients including changes in diet and consumption of foods, enteral or parenteral feeding (delivery of nutrients by tube), and the use of drugs. Currently, an NCI-supported study is under way to evaluate the effects of THC and megestrol acetate (a synthetic female hormone) when used alone and in combination for cancer-related anorexia and cachexia. The appetite, weight, and rate of weight change among patients treated with THC will be compared with patients treated with megestrol acetate or with both therapies. In addition, researchers will evaluate the effect of the drugs alone or in combination on nausea and vomiting and assess differences in the quality of life among those patients who are treated with THC. The toxic effects related to the use of the drugs will also be assessed.

The Institute of Medicine (IOM), part of the National Academy of Sciences, has published a report assessing the scientific knowledge of health effects and possible medical uses of marijuana. The IOM project was funded by the White House Office of National Drug Control Policy. The IOM released their report on March 17, 1999.

Copies of the report, *Marijuana and Medicine: Assessing the Science Base*, are available from The National Academy Press, Lockbox 285, 2101 Constitution Avenue, NW., Washington, DC 20055; (202) 334-3313 or 1-800-624-6242. The full text of the IOM report is also available on the Internet at http://stills.nap.edu/html/marimed.

National Cancer Institute Information Resources

You may want more information for yourself, your family, and your doctor. The following National Cancer Institute (NCI) services are available to help you.

Telephone

Cancer Information Service (CIS) Provides accurate, up-to-date information on cancer to patients and their families, health professionals, and the general public. Information specialists translate the latest scientific information into understandable language and respond in English, Spanish, or on TTY equipment.

Toll-free: 1-800-4-CANCER (1-800-422-6237)
TTY: 1-800-332-8615

Internet

http://www.nci.nih.gov—NCI's primary Web site; contains information about the Institute and its programs.

http://cancertrials.nci.nih.gov—CancerTrials; NCI's comprehensive clinical trials information center for patients, health professionals, and the public. Includes information on understanding trials, deciding whether to participate in trials, finding specific trials, plus research news and other resources.

http://cancernet.nci.nih.gov—CancerNet; contains material for health professionals, patients, and the public, including information from PDQ about cancer treatment, screening, prevention, supportive care, and clinical trials, and CANCERLIT, a bibliographic database.

E-mail

CancerMail—Includes NCI information about cancer treatment, screening, prevention, and supportive care. To obtain a contents list, send e-mail to cancermail@icicc.nci.nih.gov with the word "help" in the body of the message.

Fax

CancerFax—Includes NCI information about cancer treatment, screening, prevention, and supportive care. To obtain a contents list, dial 301-402-5874 from a fax machine hand set and follow the recorded instructions.

Part Four

Cancer Prevention
and Research

Chapter 72

Taking Part in Clinical Trials: What Cancer Patients Need to Know

Purpose of This Chapter

This chapter is for people with cancer, their families, and others who care about them. It is divided into three sections. Each section answers questions many people have about clinical trials:

1. What are clinical trials?
2. What happens in a clinical trial?
3. Should I take part in a clinical trial?

The first two sections provide background information on the important role clinical trials play in improving cancer care. They also explain some of the technical terms you may hear from your doctor or nurse.

The third section of this chapter is designed to help you answer question 3 for yourself. It raises issues to think about as you decide whether a clinical trial is right for you. For example, what are the pros and cons of being in a clinical trial from the patient's point of view? This section also lists some questions to ask the doctor or nurse about any study you are considering. The resources section lists other sources of information about cancer and treatment studies.

This chapter is a part of the patient education program of the National Cancer Institute (NCI). The NCI sponsors, conducts, and

"Taking Part in Clinical Trials: What Cancer Patients Need to Know," National Cancer Institute, NIH Publication No. 98-4250 (April 1998).

oversees clinical trials and other cancer research, and provides research-based information to health professionals, patients, and the public.

What Are Clinical Trials?

Clinical trials, also called cancer treatment or research studies, test new treatments in people with cancer. The goal of this research is to find better ways to treat cancer and help cancer patients. Clinical trials test many types of treatment such as new drugs, new approaches to surgery or radiation therapy, new combinations of treatments, or new methods such as gene therapy.

A clinical trial is one of the final stages of a long and careful cancer research process. The search for new treatments begins in the laboratory, where scientists first develop and test new ideas. If an approach seems promising, the next step may be testing a treatment in animals to see how it affects cancer in a living being and whether it has harmful effects. Of course, treatments that work well in the lab or in animals do not always work well in people. Studies are done with cancer patients to find out whether promising treatments are safe and effective.

Why Are Clinical Trials Important?

Clinical trials are important in two ways.

First, cancer affects us all, whether we have it, care about someone who does, or worry about getting it in the future. Clinical trials contribute to knowledge and progress against cancer. If a new treatment proves effective in a study, it may become a new standard treatment that can help many patients. Many of today's most effective standard treatments are based on previous study results. Examples include treatments for breast, colon, rectal, and childhood cancers. Clinical trials may also answer important scientific questions and suggest future research directions. Because of progress made through clinical trials, many people treated for cancer are now living longer.

Second, the patients who take part may be helped personally by the treatment(s) they receive. They get up-to-date care from cancer experts, and they receive either a new treatment being tested or the best available standard treatment for their cancer. Of course, there is no guarantee that a new treatment being tested or a standard treatment will produce good results. New treatments also may have unknown risks. But if a new treatment proves effective or more effective than standard treatment, study patients who receive it may be among the first to benefit. Some patients receive only standard treatment and benefit from it.

In the past, clinical trials were sometimes seen as a last resort for people who had no other treatment choices. Today, patients with common cancers often choose to receive their first treatment in a clinical trial.

What Happens in a Clinical Trial?

In a clinical trial, patients receive treatment and doctors carry out research on how the treatment affects the patients. While clinical trials have risks for the people who take part, each study also takes steps to protect patients.

What Is It Like to Receive Treatment in a Study?

When you take part in a clinical trial, you receive your treatment in a cancer center, hospital, clinic, and/or doctor's office. Doctors, nurses, social workers, and other health professionals may be part of your treatment team. They will follow your progress closely. You may have more tests and doctor visits than you would if you were not taking part in a study. You will follow a treatment plan your doctor prescribes, and you may also have other responsibilities such as keeping a log or filling out forms about your health. Some studies continue to check on patients even after their treatment is over.

How Is the Research Carried Out? How Are Patients Protected?

In clinical trials, both research concerns and patient well-being are important. To help protect patients and produce sound results, research with people is carried out according to strict scientific and ethical principles. These include:

1. Each clinical trial has an action plan (protocol) that explains how it will work.

The study's investigator, usually a doctor, prepares an action plan for the study. Known as a protocol, this plan explains what will be done in the study and why. It outlines how many people will take part in the study, what medical tests they will receive and how often, and the treatment plan. The same protocol is used by each doctor that takes part.

For patient safety, each protocol must be approved by the organization that sponsors the study (such as the National Cancer Institute) and the Institutional Review Board (IRB) at each hospital or other study site. This board, which includes consumers, clergy, and health professionals, reviews the protocol to try to be sure that the research will not expose patients to extreme or unethical risks.

2. Each study enrolls people who are alike in key ways.

Each study's protocol describes the characteristics that all patients in the study must have. Called eligibility criteria, these guidelines differ from study to study, depending on the research purpose. They may include age, gender, the type and stage of cancer, and whether cancer patients who have had prior cancer treatment or who have other health problems can take part.

Using eligibility criteria is an important principle of medical research that helps produce reliable results. During a study, they help protect patient safety, so that people who are likely to be harmed by study drugs or other treatments are not exposed to the risk. After results are in, they also help doctors know which patient groups will benefit if the new treatment being studied is proven to work. For instance, a new treatment may work for one type of cancer but not for another, or it may be more effective for men than women.

3. Cancer clinical trials include research at three different phases. Each phase answers different questions about the new treatment.

Phase I trials are the first step in testing a new treatment in humans. In these studies, researchers look for the best way to give a new treatment (e.g., by mouth, IV drip, or injection? how many times a day?). They also try to find out if and how the treatment can be given safely (e.g., best dose?); and they watch for any harmful side effects. Because less is known about the possible risks and benefits in Phase I, these studies usually include only a limited number of patients who would not be helped by other known treatments.

Phase II trials focus on learning whether the new treatment has an anticancer effect (e.g., Does it shrink a tumor? improve blood test results?). As in Phase I, only a small number of people take part because of the risks and unknowns involved.

Phase III trials compare the results of people taking the new treatment with results of people taking standard treatment (e.g., Which group has better survival rates? fewer side effects?). In most cases, studies move into Phase III testing only after a treatment shows promise in Phases I and II. Phase III trials may include hundreds of people around the country.

4. In Phase III trials, people are assigned at random to receive either the new treatment or standard treatment.

Researchers assign patients by chance either to a group taking the new treatment (called the treatment group) or to a group taking standard treatment (called the control group). This method, called randomization, helps avoid bias: having the study's results affected by human choices or other factors not related to the treatments being tested.

In some studies, researchers do not tell the patient whether he or she is in the treatment or control group (called a single blind study). This approach is another way to avoid bias, because when people know what drug they are taking, it might change the way they react. For instance, patients who knew they were taking the new treatment might expect it to work better and report hopeful signs because they want to believe they are getting well. This could bias the study by making results look better than they really were.

Why Do Phase III Clinical Trials Compare Treatment Groups?

Comparing similar groups of people taking different treatments for the same type of cancer is another way to make sure that study results are real and caused by the treatment rather than by chance or other factors. Comparing treatments with each other often shows clearly which one is more effective or has fewer side effects.

Another reason Phase III trials compare the new treatment with standard treatment is so that no one in a study is left without any treatment when standard treatment is available, which would be unethical. When no standard treatment exists for a cancer, some studies compare a new treatment with a placebo (a look-alike pill that contains no active drug). However, you will be told if this is a possibility before you decide whether to take part in a study.

Your Doctor Can Tell You More

If you have any questions about how clinical trials work, ask your doctor, nurse, or other health professional. It may be helpful to bring this booklet and discuss points you want to understand better.

Should I Take Part in a Clinical Trial?

This is a question only you, those close to you, and your health professionals can answer together. Learning you have cancer and deciding what to do about it is often overwhelming. This section has information you can use in thinking about your choices and making your decision.

Clinical Trials: Weighing the Pros and Cons

While a clinical trial is a good choice for some people, this treatment option has possible benefits and drawbacks. Here are some factors to consider. You may want to discuss them with your doctor and the people close to you.

Possible Benefits

- Clinical trials offer high-quality cancer care. If you are in a study and do not receive the new treatment being tested, you will receive the best standard treatment. This may be as good as, or better than, the new approach.

- If a new treatment approach is proven to work and you are taking it, you may be among the first to benefit.

- By looking at the pros and cons of clinical trials and your other treatment choices, you are taking an active role in a decision that affects your life. You have the chance to help others and improve cancer treatment.

Possible Drawbacks

- New treatments under study are not always better than, or even as good as, standard care. They may have side effects that doctors do not expect or that are worse than those of standard treatment.

- Even if a new treatment has benefits, it may not work for you.

- Even standard treatments, proven effective for many people, do not help everyone.

- If you receive standard treatment instead of the new treatment being tested, it may not be as effective as the new approach.

- Health insurance and managed care providers do not always cover all patient care costs in a study. What they cover varies by plan and by study. To find out in advance what costs are likely to be paid in your case, talk to a doctor, nurse or social worker from the study.

Your Rights, Your Protections

- Before and during a cancer treatment study, you have a number of rights. Knowing these can help protect you from harm.

- Taking part in a treatment study is up to you. It may be only one of your treatment choices. Talk with your doctor. Together, you can make the best choice for you.

- If you do enter a study, doctors and nurses will follow your response to treatment carefully throughout the research.

- If researchers learn that a treatment harms you, you will be taken off the study right away. You may then receive other treatment from your own doctor.

- You have the right to leave a study at any time.

One of your key rights is the right to informed consent. Informed consent means that you must be given all the facts about a study before you decide whether to take part. This includes details about the treatments and tests you may receive and the possible benefits and risks they may have. The doctor or nurse will give you an informed consent form that goes over key facts. If you agree to take part in the study, you will be asked to sign this informed consent form.

The informed consent process continues throughout the study. For instance, you will be told of any new findings regarding your clinical trial, such as new risks. You may be asked to sign a new consent form if you want to stay in the study.

Signing a consent form does not mean you must stay in the study. In fact, you can leave at any time. If you choose to leave the study, you will have the chance to discuss other treatments and care with your own doctor or a doctor from the study.

Questions You Should Ask

Finding answers and making choices may be hard for people with cancer and those who care about them. It is important to discuss your treatment choices with your doctor, a cancer specialist (an oncologist) to whom your doctor may refer you, and the staff of any clinical trial you consider entering.

Ask questions about the information you receive during the informed consent process and about any other issues that concern you. Getting answers can help you work better with the doctor. You may want to take a friend or relative along when you talk to the doctor. It also may help to write down your questions and the answers you receive, or bring a tape recorder to record what is said. No question about your care is foolish. It is very important to understand your choices.

Here are some questions you may want to ask about:

The Study

- What is the purpose of the study? In what phase is this study?

- Why do researchers believe the new treatment being tested may be effective? Has it been tested before?

- Who sponsors the study, and who has reviewed and approved it?

- How are the study data and patient safety being checked?

- When and where will study results and information go?

Possible Risks and Benefits

- What are the possible short- and long-term risks, side effects, and benefits to me?

- Are there standard treatments for my type of cancer?

- How do the possible risks, side effects, and benefits in the study compare with standard treatment?

Your Care

- What kinds of treatments, medical tests, or procedures will I have during the study? Will they be painful? How do they compare with what I would receive outside the study?

- How often and for how long will I receive the treatment, and how long will I need to remain in the study? Will there be follow-up after the study?

- Where will my treatment take place? Will I have to be in the hospital? If so, how often and for how long?

- How will I know if the treatment is working?

- Will I be able to see my own doctor? Who will be in charge of my care?

Personal Issues

- How could the study affect my daily life?

- Can you put me in touch with other people who are in this study?

- What support is there for me and my family in the community?

Cost Issues

- Will I have to pay for any treatment, tests, or other charges?

- What is my health insurance likely to cover?

- Who can help answer any questions from my insurance company or managed care plan?

Others Can Help

As you make your treatment decisions, remember that you are not alone. Doctors, nurses, social workers, other people with cancer, clergy, family, and those who care about you can help and support you. The resources in the next section also can provide more information and links to other contacts in your community.

National Cancer Institute Information Resources

You may want more information for yourself, your family, and your doctor. The following National Cancer Institute (NCI) services are available to help you.

Telephone

Cancer Information Service (CIS) Provides accurate, up-to-date information on cancer to patients and their families, health professionals, and the general public. Information specialists translate the latest scientific information into understandable language and respond in English, Spanish, or on TTY equipment.

Toll-free: 1-800-4-CANCER (1-800-422-6237)
TTY: 1-800-332-8615

Internet

http://www.nci.nih.gov—NCI's primary Web site; contains information about the Institute and its programs.

http://cancertrials.nci.nih.gov—CancerTrials; NCI's comprehensive clinical trials information center for patients, health professionals, and the public. Includes information on understanding trials, deciding whether to participate in trials, finding specific trials, plus research news and other resources.

http://cancernet.nci.nih.gov—CancerNet; contains material for health professionals, patients, and the public, including information from PDQ about cancer treatment, screening, prevention, supportive care, and clinical trials, and CANCERLIT, a bibliographic database.

E-mail

CancerMail—Includes NCI information about cancer treatment, screening, prevention, and supportive care. To obtain a contents list, send e-mail to cancermail@icicc.nci.nih.gov with the word "help" in the body of the message.

Fax

CancerFax—Includes NCI information about cancer treatment, screening, prevention, and supportive care. To obtain a contents list, dial 301-402-5874 from a fax machine hand set and follow the recorded instructions.

Chapter 73

What Are
Chemoprevention Trials?

Foreword

Cancer research studies conducted with cancer patients are called clinical trials. Cancer chemoprevention (CP) trials are also research studies, but the people who participate are usually not patients with cancer; they are healthy, disease-free people or people at risk of developing cancer. Sometimes CP trials aim to prevent cancer in people with medical conditions that may lead to cancer, or aim to prevent a second cancer in people successfully treated for one cancer.

CP research is based on the belief that various CP agents may stop or reverse cancer development or prevent it from ever starting. These CP agents need to be studied scientifically over time to find out if they can indeed prevent cancer.

This chapter is part of the process of informed consent that precedes your decision to participate or not in a CP trial. The information is meant to provide a general background to understanding CP trials. It supplies answers to questions asked most often about CP trials. You may not want to read the whole chapter at one time. It is broken down into questions and answers that you can read now or later. Your doctor or nurse will provide you with additional information regarding your specific trial.

As you read this chapter, you may wish to write down questions to ask your doctor or nurse. Up-to-date information is available about cancer from the Cancer Information Service (CIS) at 1-800-4-CANCER.

National Institutes of Health (NIH) Publication 93-3459, November 1992, "What Are Chemoprevention Clinical Trials?"

We hope that this chapter will help explain how CP trials are designed and carried out. You may be interested in, or be asked to participate in a CP trial. Learn as much as you can about the trial before you make up your mind. Of course, the decision about whether or not to be in a CP trial is always up to you.

What Is a Clinical Trial?

There are many types of clinical trials. They range from studies for prevention, detection, and treatment of cancer to studies which lessen the distress of the disease and improve comfort and quality of life.

Each trial is designed to answer a scientific question and to identify new and better ways to stop cancer or to help people with cancer. CP clinical trials specifically look at ways to prevent or control cancer.

Why Are Chemoprevention Trials Important?

Advances in medicine result from new ideas and approaches developed through research. CP agents and methods must be proven safe and effective in research studies before they can be recommended for general use.

Through CP trials, researchers learn which agents are the most effective in preventing cancer. These trials also are the best way to find out how safe new agents are for healthy people. Researchers believe that CP trials will lead to findings that will help many people. But ahead of time, no one knows the answers.

Participants in CP trials are followed carefully and are monitored for early identification of any side effects. These reports are gathered and become part of the data collected from other participants across the country. By using this process, doctors and researchers combine their ideas and experience and are better able to evaluate the effectiveness of the CP agent.

How Are CP Trials Conducted?

The doctors who conduct CP trials carefully follow a treatment plan called a protocol. The trials are designed to protect the rights of the participants, to safeguard their physical and mental health, and to answer research questions.

There are regular reviews of the trial as it is being carried out. This is important because, if an agent is found to be unsafe or ineffective, it is stopped. Also, whenever there is strong evidence that a CP agent is effective, the trial is stopped and all participants and the general public are given the benefit of the new information. Participants in trials are separated into different groups by a method called randomization.

For example, some research studies compare the results of a CP agent with no drug at all. This means that some volunteers will receive the real drug and others will receive an identical looking pill called a placebo that contains no drug. Participants are selected to be in either the treatment group or the placebo group purely by chance, like the flip of a coin. In this way scientists make sure that each group contains a random mix of people. Usually, the participants are not told which group they are in. That might influence the research results. The randomization is done by other scientists in a data center and the doctors in the clinic will not know which group a participant has been assigned to. By using this method, the doctors/nurses are not influenced in any way.

Sometimes CP research studies compare different drugs. This means that participants are randomized into two or more groups. Each group takes a different CP agent, or perhaps a different dose of the same agent. In studies when more than one CP agent is being investigated, there may be no placebo group.

Why Do People Take Part in CP Trials?

People take part in CP trials for many reasons. They may hope for the benefit of a longer and healthier life. They may want to contribute to increasing the knowledge regarding the prevention of cancer. Some people enroll because they have been identified as having a "high-risk" of developing a certain type of cancer. This can be very frightening. An individual is at "high-risk" when he or she has a certain combination of lifestyle and/or hereditary factors that increase the chances (over a "normal" chance) of developing cancer. Participation in a CP trial to possibly lower one's cancer risk might be viewed as a reasonable choice.

People who participate in a CP trial and are randomized to the treatment group are among the first to benefit from the CP agent if it works. However, the effectiveness of the agent for a participant in a trial cannot be known ahead of time. Even agents which are effective for many participants may not prove to be beneficial for everyone. You should choose to take part in a study by after you understand both the possible risks and benefits.

What Are CP Agents?

CP agents generally are drugs that have shown through research some success in preventing a specific type of cancer when given in a specified dose over an extended period of time. The CP agent may be a vitamin, mineral, nutritional supplement, or medication.

How Are CP Agents Discovered?

New CP agents are identified when medical researchers observe that a substance has an anti-cancer effect. However, before a new agent is tried with people, it is studied carefully in the laboratory and in animal studies. Information from this research points out the new agents or methods most likely to succeed. These agents are then tested in CP clinical trials. As much as possible, laboratory and animal research also helps to show how to use CP agents and methods safely and effectively.

Some agents, when used to treat cancer patients, have been shown to prevent return of the original cancer and also to prevent development of new cancers. However, this research cannot predict exactly how a CP agent will work in healthy people. As with any new agent, there may be risks as well as possible benefits. There also may be some risks that are not yet known. CP trials help to find out if a new agent is safe and effective. During a trial, more and more information is found about the CP agent, its benefits, its risks, and if it works or does not work.

Are There Side Effects or Risks in CP Trials?

Yes. The agents used in CP trials sometimes can cause side effects depending upon the type of agent used and the person's response to it. Side effects vary from person to person.

Because CP trials are new areas of research, the risks may not be known ahead of time. However, every possible effort is made to identify risks assocated with the CP agents being used. Generally, the agents are not expected to cause serious side effects.

Participants need to know what is involved in a trial; what, if any, side effects or risks may be expected; and, as much as possible, what "unknowns" they may be facing. This is best accomplished by listening to the doctor's or nurse's explanation of the trial, reading a document called the informed consent form and other related materials, and asking questions.

Who Is Eligible to Enter a CP Trial?

Every CP trial is designed to answer a set of research questions. All trials have an entrance criteria. You must meet the guidelines of the criteria in order to be eligible. Each trial enrolls individuals who have certain aspects of their lives in common, such as similar lifestyles, heredity, and risk factors. This lets researchers look at them as a "group" and they can predict more accurately whether or not a CP agent is effective against a specific type of cancer.

How Do You Find Out If There Is a CP Trial Available?

By dialing 1-800-4-CANCER (1-800-422-6237), you will be connected to a CIS staff member who can answer your questions about CP trials. Spanish-speaking staff members are also available.

What Are Important Questions to Ask about a CP Trial?

If you are thinking about taking part in a CP trial, here are some important questions to ask your health care provider:

- What is the purpose of the trial?
- What part of the trial is experimental?
- What is my alternative choice if I do not choose to be in the trial?
- What kinds of tests are required?
- Whom do I contact with questions about the research and my rights?
- What are the potential risks and potential benefits?
- What are my responsibilities while on the trial?
- How long will the trial last?
- What costs may I expect?
- Will my records be confidential?
- How can the trial affect my daily life?
- What side effects could I expect from the CP agent?
- Do I have any further responsibilities after I have completed the study?

Are There Any Costs?

Each CP trial is different. Some trials are entirely cost-free to the participant. In others, participants pay for some or all of the cost of the required tests and examinations. The trials, however, are designed so that most of the tests are considered to be part of routine medical care. Insurance, if available, is billed for this part of the medical cost.

For example, the CP trial may require a mammogram, a Pap smear, or a cholesterol test, procedures that healthy people are encouraged to do regularly. These tests may be paid for by insurance. Sometimes insurance will not cover some of the required testing. These costs may be covered by the trials sponsors. Concerns about costs should be discussed with the doctor or nurse since each trial has different requirements.

What Is Informed Consent?

Informed consent, or understanding what you are agreeing to, is an important part of a trial. It is a universal requirement in all research and is required by law in the United States for any treatment. It means that you are given an explanation as well as written information so you can understand what is involved in the trial. This includes possible risks and benefits. It means you are given time to consider taking part in the trial. It means you are freely choosing to participate. It means that, if you decline to participate or later withdraw, you will continue to receive the best medical care from your health care provider.

After carefully reading the informed consent document and listening to the explanation it is your right to ask your doctor, nurse, or other health care provider any questions you may have. When you are sure you understand what will be done, and you agree to take part in the trial, you can sign the form. Of course, you may also refuse.

The informed consent process continues for the whole trial. If you enter a CP trial, you will be advised of new developments as the trial goes on and information is gathered.

After signing the consent form, you are still free to leave the trial at any time. However, you are strongly encouraged to take your participation in the trial seriously and to agree to participate only after thoughtful consideration of the risks, benefits, and responsibilities involved.

What Is It Like to Be in a CP Trial?

All trial participants are cared for in the same manner, whether they are in the CP treatment group or the placebo group. In most CP trials, even doctors and nurses in the clinic do not know which group is receiving the CP agent. participants are asked to make regular visits to the clinic during the trial. Sometimes the clinic visits are every few weeks or months at first, then less often. Most CP trials last several years.

Participants are expected to do several things. First, they should take the agent as prescribed. Second, they should visit the clinic for the scheduled appointments. They may be asked to fill out questionaires regarding how they are feeling. They may have blood samples taken or be asked to have other tests.

Participants are encouraged to keep their doctor or nurse informed about any side effects or concerns, whether expected or unexpected, while on the trial. Everything is done to assist the participants in keeping to the recommended schedules and guidelines.

Can You Leave a Trial at Any Time?

Yes. Just as you can refuse to join a trial, you can leave a trial at any time. Your rights as an individual do not change because you participate in a trial. You can always change your mind, even after you enter a trial. This will not change your relationship to your health care provider or affect the care you receive.

It is important to give serious consideration to the schedules and responsibilities of the trial as well as the possible side effects of the CP agent before agreeing to participate. The doctors who developed the trial depend upon each person's full participation to get the best possible answer to their CP question in as short a time as possible. A trial must have a specified number of participants to draw the most accurate conclusions.

What Protection Do You Have as a Participant in a CP Trial?

The ethical and legal codes that govern medical practice apply to CP trials. In addition, most clinical research is federally regulated or federally funded with built-in safeguards to protect participants. These safeguards include a regular review of the trial and its progress by researchers at other places.

For example, federally funded and federally regulated CP trials must be approved by an Institutional Review Board (IRB) located at the institution where the study is to take place. IRBs, designed to protect participants, are made up of scientists, doctors, clergy, and other people from the local community. An IRB renews a study to see that it is well designed with safeguards, for participants and that the risks are reasonable in relation to the potential benefits

Federally supported or regulated studies also go through reviews by a government agency. The National Cancer Institute sponsors and monitors many CP trials around the country.

Any well-run CP trial, whether federally supported or not, is carefully reviewed for medical ethics, participant safety, and scientific merit by the research institution. Each study should monitor the data and the safety of participants on an ongoing basis.

After participants join a CP trial and it is completed, the doctors report the trial results at scientific meetings, in medical journals whose articles are approved by experts, and to various government agencies. The names of all study participants are kept in strict confidence.

The National Cancer Program and CP Trials

A nationwide effort to conquer cancer intensified with the National Cancer Act of 1971. As a result, the National Cancer Program was created. More cancer patients are being cured today than ever before. Many others are living longer with improved quality of life.

The National Cancer Program brings together a network of researchers at many public and private institutions around the country. These include the NCI, cancer centers, universities, community hospitals, and private physicians. Groups involving hundreds of researchers are working to discover and put to use new knowledge in prevention, early detection, and diagnosis, as well as the treatment of cancer.

Today, major medical discoveries in the laboratory are leading to progress in identifying agents active in cancer prevention and treatment. CP trials continue to be one of the links between basic research and practice, where the best of research translates into directly helping people.

The Cancer Information Service (CIS)

The CIS is a nationwide telephone service that answers questions from patients and their families, the public, and health professionals. Spanish speaking staff members are available. Call 1-800-4-CANCER (1-800-422-6237)

Acknowledgments Invaluable assistance in preparing this publication was provided by: Robert M. Chamberlain, Ph.D. Oncology physicians, nurses, and patients in the Community Clinical Oncology Program.

Chapter 74

Genetic Testing for Cancer Risk

Background

Inherited genetic factors can influence cancer risk in many ways. Those that appear to have the strongest effect and are the most highly publicized are known or suspected tumor suppressor genes (e.g., BRCA1 mutations that predispose to breast and ovarian cancer).[1] Such cancer susceptibility is inherited as an autosomal dominant trait, in which one altered tumor suppressor gene is inherited from a parent and one normal-functioning tumor suppressor gene is inherited from the other parent. In individuals who develop cancer, the normal-functioning gene acquires a mutation or is lost; therefore, neither gene functions normally. In the known examples of such alterations, cancer risk is greatly increased over the risk of the general population. For example, studies of very-high-risk families suggest that lifetime breast cancer risk may be as high as 85% for women who carry a deleterious BRCA1 mutation.[2]

Defective DNA repair mechanisms may also increase cancer risk. When DNA repair systems are not functioning optimally, genes that control cell growth may have a greater chance of acquiring mutations that compromise their function. Cancer susceptibility inherited through this mechanism can be transmitted as an autosomal dominant trait (e.g., DNA mismatch repair (MSH2 gene) and nonpolyposis colon cancer risk).[3] Rare, autosomal recessive cancer predisposition syndromes,

CancerFax 208/06287 from the National Cancer Institute PDQ database, modified January 1999.

in which an altered gene is inherited from each parent, provide evidence that inadequate repair of exposure-induced DNA damage can substantially increase cancer risk (e.g., xeroderma pigmentosum, UV radiation exposure, and skin cancer).[4] Individuals who carry one copy of an altered gene, along with a normal gene, are more common in the population and may be at increased cancer risk. For example, 1%-2% of the population may be at increased breast cancer risk because they carry a single copy of an ataxia telangiectasia gene mutation.[5] Since cancer susceptibility is increased by having only one copy of the gene, susceptibility is inherited as an autosomal dominant trait. However, cancer risk in these individuals may not be as high as in individuals who carry an altered tumor suppressor gene.

Common, inherited variation in enzymes that metabolize carcinogens may also affect cancer risk. For example, glutathione S-transferase M1 deficiency, an autosomal recessive trait that nearly 50% of U.S. Caucasians have, is associated with increased lung cancer risk.[6] DNA repair proficiency and carcinogen metabolism are factors that may interact with environmental exposures to alter cancer risk. That is, certain exposures may have a lesser effect or greater effect on cancer risk in individuals, depending on each individual's ability to metabolize carcinogens or repair exposure-induced DNA damage.

References

1. Miki Y, Swensen J, Shattuck-Eidens D, et al.: A strong candidate for the breast and ovarian cancer susceptibility gene BRCA1. Science 266(5182): 66-71, 1994.

2. Easton DF, Bishop DT, Ford D, et al.: Genetic linkage analysis in familial breast and ovarian cancer: results from 214 families. American Journal of Human Genetics 52(4): 678-701, 1993.

3. Fishel R, Kolodner RD: Identification of mismatch repair genes and their role in the development of cancer. Current Opinion in Genetics and Development 5(3): 382-395, 1995.

4. Kraemer KH, Lee MM, Andrews AD, et al.: The role of sunlight and DNA repair in melanoma and nonmelanoma skin cancer. Archives of Dermatology 130: 1018-1021, 1994.

5. Athma P, Rappaport R, Swift M: Molecular genotyping shows that ataxia-telangiectasia heterozygotes are predisposed to breast cancer. Cancer Genetics and Cytogenetics 92(2): 130-134, 1996.

6. McWilliams JE, Sanderson BJ, Harris EL, et al.: Glutathione S-transferase M1 (GSTM1) deficiency and lung cancer risk. Cancer Epidemiology, Biomarkers and Prevention 4(6): 589-594, 1995.

Predictive Testing

Advances in laboratory technology and in the identification of cancer susceptibility genes (e.g., BRCA1, BRCA2, and MSH2) will soon make it possible to test large segments of the population for cancer risk. This testing will, theoretically, facilitate differentiation of individuals at increased cancer risk from those with "usual" cancer risk. However, genetic testing for cancer risk must be evaluated in the same way that other screening tests are evaluated, and many issues should be addressed before genetic testing for cancer risk is accepted and/or recommended as routine practice. Specific issues requiring further study include the following:

Good estimates are needed of the risks associated with specific mutations or types of mutations in cancer susceptibility genes. Estimates of how these risks may differ in various populations are also needed. Almost all of the currently available information is based on specific populations or families who were selected because they have a very high incidence of cancer. For example, breast and ovarian cancer risks associated with BRCA1 mutations have been estimated from families selected for having a very high incidence of breast and/or ovarian cancer.[1] The risks associated with specific mutations in these families may differ from those found outside of such families. Cancer risks may differ because, in addition to sharing genes at a specific cancer susceptibility locus, very-high-risk families also share other genes and lifestyles that affect cancer risk.[2]

In addition to estimating risks for the primary cancer(s) of interest (e.g., breast and ovarian cancer risk for BRCA1 mutation carriers), accurate risk estimates for other medical conditions (such as other cancers) are needed. For example, in addition to increased colon cancer risk, women who carry an altered MSH2 gene are at increased risk of endometrial and ovarian cancer.[3]

When testing the gene, it is necessary to identify which mutations are likely or unlikely to alter an individual's cancer risk. Some mutations will result in structurally altered proteins (e.g., mutations that produce truncated proteins) and will almost certainly increase cancer risk. Some mutations do not alter protein structure at all and will almost certainly not increase cancer risk. However, there are other mutations whose functional significance is unknown. Definitions of "normal" and "abnormal" test results are also necessary.

The cancer risk associated with a "normal" test result (no mutation detected) should be understood. The interpretation will differ according to the individual's family history of cancer and the recognized presence or absence of specific mutations in her or his family. For example, if a high-risk mutation has already been detected in a family and an individual in that family does not have that mutation, it is very unlikely that the individual has inherited genetic susceptibility to cancer—he or she is highly likely to be at average cancer risk. In contrast, if a person comes from a family that appears to represent inherited cancer susceptibility but a high-risk mutation has not been identified in that family, having a "normal" test result provides that person little new information about his or her cancer risk.

It is important to acknowledge that there are some mutations for which risk information is uncertain. It is assumed that mutations occurring with cancer in the very-high-risk cancer families confer increased cancer risk. However, additional mutations that may change protein structure have been observed outside these families. It is uncertain if such mutations confer an increased cancer risk or, if there is increased risk, what the magnitude of increase in cancer risk will be.

Intervention to reduce cancer mortality should be offered to individuals who carry a cancer susceptibility gene. Depending on the cancer site, the following interventions are currently offered: early cancer detection, prevention through prophylactic surgeries, and chemoprevention. However, the efficacy of these measures, especially among individuals in the general population, is unproved in many instances. Efficacy among individuals who carry cancer susceptibility genes is largely unknown. Also, there is a practical limit to surgical strategies for individuals at high risk for cancer in multiple organs. For example, for carriers of breast/ovarian cancer susceptibility genes, the main options are early detection and prevention through prophylactic surgical procedures. However, it is uncertain if enhanced early detection efforts will reduce mortality: it is not clear if mammography in these high-risk women younger than 50 years is beneficial; there is no proven early detection strategy for ovarian cancer. Some women are interested in prophylactic mastectomy and/or oophorectomy, but that strategy does not eliminate breast/ovarian cancer risk and it is not known to what extent, if any, it reduces cancer incidence or mortality. Tamoxifen reduces breast cancer risk in women at increased risk, but information for high-risk gene carriers is not yet available.[4] A contrasting example is chemoprevention for individuals with familial adenomatous polyposis; sulindac reduces both the size and numbers of colorectal adenomas.[5] However, the long-term risks and benefits of such therapy are unknown.

Genetic testing for cancer risk has several unusual characteristics. This is "predictive testing" in which the lifetime risk of developing cancer is less than 100%. The test result may have important health and social implications for biologic relatives, including future generations. The test result is not modifiable (although the cancer risk associated with the test result may be) and, therefore, cannot be used to measure the impact of preventive strategies on risk. These characteristics raise a host of social, legal, and ethical issues for the individuals being tested and for their relatives. These issues, which have not yet been resolved, include difficulty obtaining insurance and restricted educational and employment opportunities.

Genetic testing for cancer susceptibility must be acceptable to the public. Members of very-high-risk cancer families, as well as the general public, are interested in genetic testing for cancer risk. However, it is clear that clinicians, scientists, and the general public are only beginning to understand the limitations and social, legal, and ethical issues surrounding such testing. It is necessary to determine what conditions/situations the public considers to be acceptable for genetic testing. Current genetic testing strategies are focused on genes that confer greatly increased cancer risk, sometimes referred to as "inherited cancer" or "inherited cancer susceptibility" genes; these genes account for about 5%-10% of all breast and colon cancers.

Genetic testing protocols that are acceptable to scientists, clinicians, and the public must be available. Like genetic testing in general, genetic counseling is an integral part of the process of genetic testing for cancer susceptibility; specialists in oncology and mental health will also need to be a part of the process.[6,7] Genetic testing protocols are currently being developed and tested. Testing minors for cancer risk should be given special consideration because minors are particularly vulnerable. Testing minors should be considered only when it is clear that intervention will provide medical benefits for young people.

Genetic testing is available in academic settings and through commercial laboratories for individuals at increased risk of carrying a high-risk mutation (e.g., BRCA1 mutation testing in families with a high incidence of young-onset breast and/or ovarian cancer). Regardless of the setting, informed consent should be an essential part of the genetic counseling and testing process. Individuals who are considering genetic testing for cancer susceptibility should be given the opportunity to consider the physical, social, and legal risks balanced against the potential benefits of genetic testing for cancer risk, including the uncertainties of the state of our knowledge of cancer risk and effective interventions.

References

1. Easton DF, Bishop DT, Ford D, et al.: Genetic linkage analysis in familial breast and ovarian cancer: results from 214 families. American Journal of Human Genetics 52(4): 678-701, 1993.

2. Struewing JP, Hartge P, Wacholder S, et al.: The risk of cancer associated with specific mutations of BRCA1 and BRCA2 among Ashkenazi Jews. New England Journal of Medicine 336(20): 1401-1408, 1997.

3. Lynch HT, Smyrk TC, Watson P, et al.: Genetics, natural history, tumor spectrum, and pathology of hereditary nonpolyposis colorectal cancer: an updated review. Gastroenterology 104(5): 1535-1549, 1993.

4. Fisher B, Costantino JP, Wickerham DL, et al.: Tamoxifen for prevention of breast cancer: report of the National Surgical Adjuvant Breast and Bowel Project P-1 study. Journal of the National Cancer Institute 90(18): 1371-1388, 1998.

5. Giardiello FM, Hamilton SR, Krush AJ, et al.: Treatment of colonic and rectal adenomas with sulindac in familial adenomatous polyposis. New England Journal of Medicine 328(18): 1313-1316, 1993.

6. Anonymous: Statement of the American Society of Human Genetics on genetic testing for breast and ovarian cancer predisposition. American Journal of Human Genetics 55: i-v, 1994.

7. American Society of Clinical Oncology: Statement of the American Society of Clinical Oncology: genetic testing for cancer susceptibility, adopted February 20, 1996. Journal of Clinical Oncology 14(5): 1730-1736, 1996.

Chapter 75

Tumor Markers

Tumor markers are substances that can often be detected in higher-than-normal amounts in the blood, urine, or body tissues of some patients with certain types of cancer. Tumor markers are produced either by the tumor itself or by the body in response to the presence of cancer or certain benign (noncancerous) conditions. This text describes some tumor markers found in the blood.

Measurements of tumor marker levels can be useful—when used along with x-rays or other tests—in the detection and diagnosis of some types of cancer. However, measurements of tumor marker levels alone are not sufficient to diagnose cancer for the following reasons:

- Tumor marker levels can be elevated in people with benign conditions.

- Tumor marker levels are not elevated in every person with cancer—especially in the early stages of the disease.

- Many tumor markers are not specific to a particular type of cancer; the level of a tumor marker can be raised by more than one type of cancer.

In addition to their role in cancer diagnosis, some tumor marker levels are measured before treatment to help doctors plan appropriate

"Tumor Markers," National Cancer Institute (NCI) CancerNet, modified April 1998.

therapy. In some types of cancer, tumor marker levels reflect the extent (stage) of the disease and can be useful in predicting how well the disease will respond to treatment. Tumor marker levels may also be measured during treatment to monitor a patient's response to treatment. A decrease or return to normal in the level of a tumor marker may indicate that the cancer has responded favorably to therapy. If the tumor marker level rises, it may indicate that the cancer is growing. Finally, measurements of tumor marker levels may be used after treatment has ended as a part of followup care to check for recurrence.

Currently, the main use of tumor markers is to assess a cancer's response to treatment and to check for recurrence. Scientists continue to study these uses of tumor markers as well as their potential role in the early detection and diagnosis of cancer. The patient's doctor can explain the role of tumor markers in detection, diagnosis, or treatment for that person. Described below are some of the most commonly measured tumor markers.

Prostate-Specific Antigen

Prostate-specific antigen (PSA) is present in low concentrations in the blood of all adult males. It is produced by both normal and abnormal prostate cells. Elevated PSA levels may be found in the blood of men with benign prostate conditions, such as prostatitis (inflammation of the prostate) and benign prostatic hyperplasia (BPH), or with a malignant (cancerous) growth in the prostate. While PSA does not allow doctors to distinguish between benign prostate conditions (which are very common in older men) and cancer, an elevated PSA level may indicate that other tests are necessary to determine whether cancer is present.

PSA levels have been shown to be useful in monitoring the effectiveness of prostate cancer treatment, and in checking for recurrence after treatment has ended. In checking for recurrence, a single test may show a mildly elevated PSA level, which may not be a significant change. Doctors generally look for trends, such as steadily increasing PSA levels in multiple tests over time, rather than focusing on a single elevated result.

Researchers are studying the value of PSA in screening men for prostate cancer (checking for the disease in men who have no symptoms). At this time, it is not known whether using PSA to screen for prostate cancer actually saves lives. The National Cancer Institute-supported Prostate, Lung, Colorectal, and Ovarian Cancer Screening

Trial is designed to show whether the use of certain screening tests can reduce the number of deaths caused by those cancers. For prostate cancer, this trial is looking at the usefulness of regular screening using digital rectal exams and PSA level checks in men ages 55 to 74.

Researchers are also working on new ways to increase the accuracy of PSA tests. Improving the accuracy of PSA tests could help doctors distinguish BPH from prostate cancer, and thereby avoid unnecessary followup procedures, including biopsies.

Prostatic Acid Phosphatase

Prostatic acid phosphatase (PAP) is normally present only in small amounts in the blood, but may be found at higher levels in some patients with prostate cancer, especially if the cancer has spread beyond the prostate. However, blood levels may also be elevated in patients who have certain benign prostate conditions or early stage cancer.

Although PAP was originally found to be produced by the prostate, elevated PAP levels have since been associated with testicular cancer, leukemia, and non-Hodgkin's lymphoma, as well as noncancerous conditions such as Gaucher's disease, Paget's disease, osteoporosis, cirrhosis of the liver, pulmonary embolism, and hyperparathyroidism.

CA 125

CA 125 is produced by a variety of cells, but particularly by ovarian cancer cells. Studies have shown that many women with ovarian cancer have elevated CA 125 levels.CA 125 is used primarily in the management of treatment for ovarian cancer.

In women with ovarian cancer being treated with chemotherapy, a falling CA 125 level generally indicates that the cancer is responding to treatment. Increasing CA 125 levels during or after treatment, on the other hand, may suggest that the cancer is not responding to therapy or that some cancer cells remain in the body. Doctors may also use CA 125 levels to monitor patients for recurrence of ovarian cancer.

Not all women with elevated CA 125 levels have ovarian cancer. CA 125 levels may also be elevated by cancers of the uterus, cervix, pancreas, liver, colon, breast, lung, and digestive tract. Noncancerous conditions that can cause elevated CA 125 levels include endometriosis, pelvic inflammatory disease, peritonitis, pancreatitis, liver disease, and any condition that inflames the pleura (the tissue that surrounds the lungs and lines the chest cavity). Menstruation and pregnancy can also cause an increase in CA 125.

Carcinoembryonic Antigen

Carcinoembryonic antigen (CEA) is normally found in small amounts in the blood of most healthy people, but may become elevated in people who have cancer or some benign conditions. The primary use of CEA is in monitoring colorectal cancer, especially when the disease has spread (metastasized). CEA is also used after treatment to check for recurrence of colorectal cancer. However, a wide variety of other cancers can produce elevated levels of this tumor marker, including melanoma; lymphoma; and cancers of the breast, lung, pancreas, stomach, cervix, bladder, kidney, thyroid, liver, and ovary.

Elevated CEA levels can also occur in patients with noncancerous conditions, including inflammatory bowel disease, pancreatitis, and liver disease. Tobacco use can also contribute to higher-than-normal levels of CEA.

Alpha-Fetoprotein

Alpha-fetoprotein (AFP) is normally produced by a developing fetus. AFP levels begin to decrease soon after birth and are usually undetectable in the blood of healthy adults (except during pregnancy). An elevated level of AFP strongly suggests the presence of either primary liver cancer or germ cell cancer (cancer that begins in the cells that give rise to eggs or sperm) of the ovary or testicle. Only rarely do patients with other types of cancer (such as stomach cancer) have elevated levels of AFP. Noncancerous conditions that can cause elevated AFP levels include benign liver conditions, such as cirrhosis or hepatitis; ataxia telangiectasia; Wiscott-Aldrich syndrome; and pregnancy.

Human Chorionic Gonadotropin

Human chorionic gonadotropin (HCG) is normally produced by the placenta during pregnancy. In fact, HCG is sometimes used as a pregnancy test because it increases early within the first trimester. It is also used to screen for choriocarcinoma (a rare cancer of the uterus) in women who are at high risk for the disease, and to monitor the treatment of trophoblastic disease (a rare cancer that develops from an abnormally fertilized egg). Elevated HCG levels may also indicate the presence of cancers of the testis, ovary, liver, stomach, pancreas, and lung. Pregnancy and marijuana use can also cause elevated HCG levels.

CA 19-9

Initially found in colorectal cancer patients, CA 19-9 has also been identified in patients with pancreatic, stomach, and bile duct cancer. Researchers have discovered that, in those who have pancreatic cancer, higher levels of CA 19-9 tend to be associated with more advanced disease. Noncancerous conditions that may elevate CA 19-9 levels include gallstones, pancreatitis, cirrhosis of the liver, and cholecystitis.

CA 15-3

CA 15-3 levels are most useful in following the course of treatment in women diagnosed with breast cancer, especially advanced breast cancer. CA 15-3 levels are rarely elevated in women with early stage breast cancer.

Cancers of the ovary, lung, and prostate may also raise CA 15-3 levels. Elevated levels of CA 15-3 may be associated with noncancerous conditions, such as benign breast or ovarian disease, endometriosis, pelvic inflammatory disease, and hepatitis. Pregnancy and lactation can also cause CA 15-3 levels to rise.

CA 27-29

Similar to the CA 15-3 antigen, CA 27-29 is found in the blood of most breast cancer patients. CA 27-29 levels may be used in conjunction with other procedures (such as mammograms and measurements of other tumor marker levels) to check for recurrence in women previously treated for stage II and stage III breast cancer.

CA 27-29 levels can also be elevated by cancers of the colon, stomach, kidney, lung, ovary, pancreas, uterus, and liver. First trimester pregnancy, endometriosis, ovarian cysts, benign breast disease, kidney disease, and liver disease are noncancerous conditions that can also elevate CA 27-29 levels.

Lactate Dehydrogenase

Lactate dehydrogenase is a protein found throughout the body. Nearly every type of cancer, as well as many other diseases, can cause LDH levels to be elevated. Therefore, this marker cannot be used to diagnose a particular type of cancer.

LDH levels can be used to monitor treatment of some cancers, including testicular cancer, Ewing's sarcoma, non-Hodgkin's lymphoma, and some types of leukemia. Elevated LDH levels can be caused by a number of noncancerous conditions, including heart failure, hypothyroidism, anemia, and lung or liver disease.

Neuron-Specific Enolase

Neuron-specific enolase (NSE) has been detected in patients with neuroblastoma; small cell lung cancer; Wilms' tumor; melanoma; and cancers of the thyroid, kidney, testicle, and pancreas. However, studies of NSE as a tumor marker have concentrated primarily on patients with neuroblastoma and small cell lung cancer. Measurement of NSE level in patients with these two diseases can provide information about the extent of the disease and the patient's prognosis, as well as about the patient's response to treatment.

National Cancer Institute Information Resources

You may want more information for yourself, your family, and your doctor. The following National Cancer Institute (NCI) services are available to help you.

Telephone

Cancer Information Service (CIS) Provides accurate, up-to-date information on cancer to patients and their families, health professionals, and the general public. Information specialists translate the latest scientific information into understandable language and respond in English, Spanish, or on TTY equipment.

Toll-free: 1-800-4-CANCER (1-800-422-6237)
TTY: 1-800-332-8615

Internet

http://www.nci.nih.gov—NCI's primary Web site; contains information about the Institute and its programs.

http://cancertrials.nci.nih.gov—CancerTrials; NCI's comprehensive clinical trials information center for patients, health professionals, and the public. Includes information on understanding trials, deciding whether to participate in trials, finding specific trials, plus research news and other resources.

http://cancernet.nci.nih.gov—CancerNet; contains material for health professionals, patients, and the public, including information from PDQ about cancer treatment, screening, prevention, supportive care, and clinical trials, and CANCERLIT, a bibliographic database.

E-mail

CancerMail—Includes NCI information about cancer treatment, screening, prevention, and supportive care. To obtain a contents list, send e-mail to cancermail@icicc.nci.nih.gov with the word "help" in the body of the message.

Fax

CancerFax—Includes NCI information about cancer treatment, screening, prevention, and supportive care. To obtain a contents list, dial 301-402-5874 from a fax machine hand set and follow the recorded instructions.

Chapter 76

Cancer Tests You Should Know about: A Guide for People 65 and Over

Most people don't like to think about cancer. But think about this: the earlier cancer is found, the better the chances of beating it.

This chapter describes simple tests that can help find cancer early, long before any symptoms appear. You may have heard of some of them, such as mammograms or rectal and prostate exams. Checklists, for women and for men, will help you keep track of the tests you need.

Despite what many people think, most people who are tested will not have cancer. But if it turns out you do, this text can help you find the best care.

Why Is It Important to Find Cancer Early?

Cancers that are found early may be easier to cure. Early treatment can be simpler, making it easier to go about daily life. All in all, finding cancer early could:

- Save your life.
- Help you live life to the fullest.

Why Should You Think about Cancer?

Any one can get cancer. But you are more likely to get cancer as you get older—even if no one in your family has had it. It may surprise

National Cancer Institute, NIH Publication No. 94-3256, revised August 1993.

you to learn that more than one half of all cancers occur in people age 65 and over.

If You Did Have Cancer, Wouldn't You Know It?

Most cancers in their earliest, most treatable stages do not cause any symptoms or pain. That is why it is so important to have regular cancer tests. They can find problems early—long before you would notice anything wrong.

But What If You Do Notice Something Wrong?

Certain changes could be a sign of cancer. For example, a change in bowel habits could mean cancer of the colon or rectum. A breast lump could mean breast cancer. Don't assume these or other changes are just a normal part of growing older. See your doctor right away.

Who Should You Ask about Cancer Tests?

Perhaps you see one doctor just for your back or another doctor just for your heart. Maybe you see one doctor for checkups, but the subject of cancer has not come up. Why not bring it up yourself? Ask your family doctor, internist, or other trusted health professional about getting tested for cancer. The next section tells you about the tests to detect cancer early.

Cancer Tests

The tests in this chapter are right for most people age 65 and over. For guidelines for people under 65, call the Cancer Information Service toll-free at 1-800-4-CANCER (1-800-422-6237). But you and your doctor need to decide what is right for you. You may need certain tests more often if you have had cancer before, have some other medical conditions, or have a family member who has had cancer.

Most of the cancer tests described in this booklet take little time. Some tests may be uncomfortable, but they are not painful. Cancer tests are usually done right in your doctor's office.

Your doctor and you, together, can schedule your cancer tests. Then, as you get each test, write down the date.

You may be concerned about the cost of these cancer tests. Ask your doctor if Medicare will help or ask your own insurance company if they cover these tests. Medicare helps pay for some mammograms and Pap smears.

Cancer Tests for Women Age 65 and Over

Breasts

A woman's risk of breast cancer increases with age. Fortunately, women can take three steps to find cancer early:

Mammogram. This x-ray of the breast can reveal problems up to 2 years before a lump can be felt. To find out where to get a mammogram, ask your doctor. Or, call the National Cancer Institute's Cancer Information Service at: 1-800-4-CANCER (1-800-422-6237). Recommended: Every one to two years.

Breast Exam. Your doctor should check your breasts for problems or changes that could be a sign of breast cancer. Recommended: Every one to two years, or as part of your regular health checkup.

Breast Self-Exam. Ask your doctor or nurse for instructions. You also can call the Cancer Information Service at 1-800-4-CANCER (1-800-422-6237) for a free booklet. Recommended: Every month.

Uterus and Cervix

As women get older they have a higher risk of cancers of the female sex organs—especially cancers of the uterus and cervix. If you stopped seeing your gynecologist after menopause (change of life), it is important to ask your doctor about the following tests:

Pelvic Exam. The doctor feels the internal sex organs, bladder, and rectum for any changes in size or shape. Recommended: Every year.

Pap Smear. A Pap smear, also called a Pap test, is usually done at the same time as the pelvic exam. During this test, the doctor removes a few cells from the cervix with a swab. The cells then are checked under a microscope. After three normal annual Pap tests, your doctor may decide not to do the test for the next 1 to 3 years. Recommended: Every year.

Colon and Rectum

Cancers of the colon and rectum are more likely to occur as people get older. Three tests can help find these cancers early:

Rectal Exam. In this test, the doctor gently feels for any bumps or irregular areas on the rectum. Recommended: Every year, or as part of your regular health checkup.

Guaiac Stool Test. The guaiac (pronounced "gwyack") stool test is sometimes called a "fecal" or "stool" occult test or "hemoccult" test. This test can find unseen blood in stool samples. Your doctor can give you a simple kit to collect stool samples at home. Or, your doctor can do the test as part of a rectal exam. Recommended: Every year.

Sigmoidoscopy or "procto". The doctor looks for cancer in the colon and rectum with a thin, lighted instrument called a sigmoidoscope. Recommended: Every 3 to 5 years.

Skin

Skin cancer is the most common cancer in the United States. You can improve your chances of finding skin cancer early by doing a simple skin self-exam regularly. Check for anything new—a change in the size, texture, or color of a mole, or a sore that doesn't heal. Any changes should be reported to your doctor right away.

You should also have your doctor look at your skin during every routine physical exam.

Cancer Tests for Men Age 65 and Over

Prostate

Prostate cancer is the most common cancer in American men—especially older men. More than 80 percent of prostate cancer cases occur in men age 65 and over.

Rectal Exam. The doctor feels the prostate through the rectum. Hard or lumpy areas may mean cancer is present. Recommended: Every year.

PSA. The prostate-specific antigen test (PSA) measures the level of a specific protein in a man's blood. The protein seems to increase in cases of prostate cancer and other prostate diseases. The National Cancer Institute is studying whether screening with the PSA test along with a rectal exam may help decrease deaths from prostate cancer.

TRUS. Transrectal ultrasound (TRUS) detects cancer by using sound waves produced by an instrument inserted into the rectum. The waves bounce off the prostate, and the pattern of the echoes made by the waves is converted to a picture by computer. TRUS is not a routine test. The doctor will use this exam to help diagnose a man's problem.

Colon and Rectum

Cancers of the colon and rectum are more likely to occur as people get older. Three tests can help find these cancers early:

Rectal Exam. In this test, the doctor gently feels for any bumps or irregular areas on the rectum. Recommended: Every year, or as part of your regular health checkup.

Guaiac Stool Test. The guaiac (pronounced "gwyack") stool test is sometimes called a "fecal" or "stool" occult test or "hemoccult" test. This test can find unseen blood in stool samples. Your doctor can give you a simple kit to collect stool samples at home. Or, your doctor can do the test as part of a rectal exam. Recommended: Every year.

Sigmoidoscopy or "procto". The doctor looks for cancer in the colon and rectum with a thin, lighted instrument called a sigmoidoscope. Recommended: Every 3 to 5 years.

Skin

Skin cancer is the most common cancer in the United States. You can improve your chances of finding skin cancer early by doing a simple skin self-exam regularly. Check for anything new—a change in the size, texture, or color of a mole, or a sore that doesn't heal. Any changes should be reported to your doctor right away.

You should also have your doctor look at your skin during every routine physical exam.

What If You Find Out You Have Cancer?

Today, there are new and better ways to treat cancer. If you are told you have cancer, take these steps to get the best possible care:

- Find a doctor who is right for you and the kind of cancer you have. Oncologists are doctors specially trained to treat cancer.

- Find out what your treatment choices are and which are best for you. If you don't understand something, ask.

- Get a second opinion from another doctor before treatment begins. Doctors and most insurance companies expect their patients to do this. Many doctors will help you get a second opinion.

- Talk to your family and friends and ask for their support. Or ask your doctor to help you find other people or groups who can help. No one needs to handle cancer alone.

- Call the Cancer Information Service at 1-800-4-CANCER (1-800-422-6237) for help with all these steps. Staff members can give you information about treatment and where to get it. They also can direct you to groups that may be able to help with transportation, finances, and dealing with your problems. Spanish-speaking staff members can be reached at this toll-free number.

- Ask your doctor to check the National Cancer Institute's PDQ (Physician Data Query) system. This computer system has the most up-to-date treatment information in the United States. You or your doctor can call the Cancer Information Service (1-800-4-CANCER) to learn more about PDQ.

Want to Learn More about Cancer?

Call the Cancer Information Service toll-free at 1-800-4-CANCER (1-800-422-6237) for information and booklets about cancer. Or, write to:

Office of Cancer Communications
National Cancer Institute
Building 31, Room 10A16
Bethesda, MD 20892

For more information on aging, write to:

National Institute on Aging
P.O. Box 8057
Gaithersburg, MD 20898-8057

Why Get Tested for Cancer?

Most cancers in their earliest stages do not cause symptoms or pain. Get checked for cancer when you're feeling well... for good health and a good life.

The National Cancer Institute and the National Institute on Aging are grateful to the American Association of Retired Persons and Fox Chase Cancer Center for their ideas and guidance.

This information is part of 65+ Health, a Cancer Education Initiative for Americans 65 and over. The initiative is a partnership between the National Cancer Institute and the National Institute on Aging of the National Institutes of Health, and the National Center for Chronic Disease Prevention and Health Promotion of the Centers for Disease Control.

Mammogram and Clinical Breast Exam Every one to two years**						
Breast Self-Exam Every month	Keep track every month on your calendar					
Pelvic Exam and Pap Smear Every year***						
Rectal Exam Every year**						
Guaiac Stool Test Every year						
Sigmoidoscopy or "Procto" Every 3 to 5 years						
Skin Exam**						

Figure 76.1. Cancer Test Checklist for Women 65 and Over.* Take this checklist to your doctor. Decide together which tests are right for you and how often they should be done. Then, each time you get a test, write the date in the boxes.

*For guidelines for women under 65, call the Cancer Information Service toll-free at 1-800-4-CANCER (1-800-422-6237).

** Or as part of your regular health checkup.

*** After three normal annual Pap tests, your doctor may decide not to do the test for the next 1 to 3 years.

Rectal Exam Every year**							
Guaiac Stool Test Every year							
Sigmoidoscopy or "Procto" Every 3 to 5 years							
Skin Exam**							

Figure 76.2. *Cancer Test Checklist for Men 65 and Over* Take this checklist to your doctor. Decide together which tests are right for you and how often they should be done. Then, each time you get a test, write the date in the boxes.

*For guidelines for men under 65, call the Cancer Information Service toll-free at 1-800-4-CANCER (1-800-422-6237).

**Or as part of your regular health checkup.

Part Five

Coping Strategies

Chapter 77

Eating Hints for Cancer Patients

Your diet is an important part of your treatment for cancer. Eating the right kinds of foods during your treatment can help you feel better and stay stronger.

The National Cancer Institute (NCI) has prepared this guide to help you learn more about your diet needs and how to manage eating problems. Eating well is extra important when your body is fighting disease.

This guide is mainly for patients who are still receiving cancer treatment. However, it also may be useful after you finish treatment. Refer to it any time you find that eating well is a challenge.

Your registered dietitian, doctor, and nurse are your best sources of information about your diet. The information in here will add to their advice. Feel free to ask for their help and talk with them about changes in your diet. Ask them to explain or repeat anything that is not clear.

The Cancer Information Service (CIS) provides information about cancer, cancer treatment, research studies, and living with cancer to patients, their families, health professionals, and the public.

Eating Well During Cancer Treatment

A nutritious diet is always vital for your body to work at its best. Good nutrition is even more important for people with cancer. Why?

Excerpted from "Eating Hints for Cancer Patients," National Cancer Institute (NCI), Publication 97-2079, revised January 1997. The original booklet contains recipes that the cancer patient might find useful—see the Resources section at the end of this chapter for information on ordering a copy of this free publication from the Cancer Information Service.

- Patients who eat well during their treatment are able to cope better with the side effects of treatment. Patients who eat well may be able to handle a higher dose of certain treatments.

- A healthy diet can help keep up your strength, prevent body tissues from breaking down, and rebuild tissues that cancer treatment may harm.

- When you are unable to eat enough food or the right kind of food, your body uses stored nutrients as a source of energy. As a result, your natural defenses are weaker and your body cannot fight infection as well. Yet, this defense system is especially important to you now, because cancer patients are often at risk of getting an infection.

What Kinds of Food Do I Need?

A good rule to follow is to eat a variety of different foods every day. No one food or group of foods contains all of the nutrients you need. A diet to keep your body strong will include daily servings from these food groups:

- *Fruits and Vegetables*: Raw or cooked vegetables, fruits, and fruit juices provide certain vitamins (such as A and C) and minerals the body needs.

- *Protein Foods*: Protein helps your body heal itself and fight infection. Meat, fish, poultry, eggs, milk, yogurt, and cheese give you protein as well as many vitamins and minerals.

- *Grains*: Grains, such as bread, pasta, rice, and cereals, provide a variety of carbohydrates and B vitamins. Carbohydrates provide a good source of energy, which the body needs to function well.

- *Dairy Foods*: Milk and other dairy products provide protein and many vitamins and are the best source of calcium.

To help Americans learn how to choose a healthy diet, the U.S. Department of Agriculture (USDA) and the U.S. Department of Health and Human Services (DHHS) designed a Food Guide Pyramid. The Food Guide Pyramid gives the amounts and types of foods most Americans should try to eat each day. It emphasizes five food groups—Bread, Fruit, Vegetable, Milk, and Meat—and focuses on reducing the amount of fat in the diet. [See the section below, "Eat a Variety of Foods Each Day."]

Keep in mind that the Food Pyramid may not meet the requirements of individuals with special diet needs, such as cancer patients. In fact, the best foods for you right now may be very different from those in the Food Pyramid, depending on the type of treatment you are receiving or how you feel. You probably will need more calories and more high-protein foods, such as meats and dairy products. You may need to cut back on high-fiber foods for a while, such as vegetables, fruits, cereals, and whole grains, if your treatment causes diarrhea. Your doctor, nurse, or registered dietitian also may suggest that you add commercial nutrition supplements to your diet to make sure you get enough protein, calories, and other nutrients during treatment. (See the section, "Commercial Products To Improve Nutrition.")

Pay attention to your body. If nausea makes certain foods unappealing, then eat more of the foods you find easier to handle. For example, if you get nauseous from eating fruits but can eat protein foods, eat more protein foods and less fruit.

Sometimes changing the form of a food will make it more appetizing and help you eat better. You might try mixing canned fruit into a milkshake if eating whole, fresh fruits is a problem.

It is important to keep trying new things. Anything you eat will be a plus in getting enough calories to maintain your weight. This information describes some of the special diets that cancer patients may need to follow. (See Special Diets for Special Needs.) It also gives ideas and recipes that worked for other cancer patients when they had to change their diet or when they didn't feel like eating.

Your doctor, nurse, and registered dietitian will let you know which diet is best for you. Be sure to talk with them if you have any questions.

Can Good Nutrition Treat Cancer?

Doctors know that patients who eat well during cancer treatment are better able to cope with side effects. However, there is no evidence that any kind of diet or food can either cure cancer or stop it from coming back. In fact, some diets may be harmful, especially those that don't include a variety of foods. There is also no evidence that dietary supplements, such as vitamin or mineral pills, can cure cancer or stop it from coming back.

The NCI strongly urges you to eat nutritious foods and follow the treatment program prescribed by a doctor who uses accepted and proven methods or treatments. People who depend upon unconventional treatments may lose valuable treatment time and reduce their chances of controlling cancer and getting well.

795

The NCI also recommends that you ask your doctor, nurse, or registered dietitian before taking any vitamins or mineral supplements. Too much of some vitamins or minerals can be just as dangerous as too little. Large doses of some vitamins may even stop your cancer treatment from working the way it should. To avoid problems, don't take these products on your own. Follow your doctor's directions for safe results.

Eat a Variety of Foods Each Day

Use this list provided by the USDA, the Food Guide Pyramid, to include a variety of foods in your daily diet.

Breads, Cereals, Rice, Pasta, and Other Grain Products (Whole-Grain Enriched)

6-11 servings from entire group (include several servings of whole-grain products daily)

- 1 slice of bread
- 1/2 hamburger bun or English muffin
- 1 small roll, biscuit, or muffin
- 3 to 4 small or 2 large crackers
- 1/2 cup cooked cereal, rice, or pasta
- 1 oz. of ready-to-eat breakfast cereals

Fruits (Citrus, Melon, Berries, Other Fruits)

2-3 servings from entire group

- 1 medium apple, banana, peach, pear, etc.
- 1 grapefruit half
- 1 melon wedge
- 3/4 cup of juice
- 1/2 cup of berries
- 1/2 cup chopped, cooked, or canned fruit
- 1/4 cup dried fruit

Vegetables (Dark-green Leafy; Deep-yellow Legumes; Starchy Vegetables; Other Vegetables)

3-5 servings from entire group (include all types regularly); use dark-green leafy vegetables and legumes several times a week.

- 3/4 cup of vegetable juice
- 1 cup of leafy raw vegetables (e.g., spinach)
- 1/2 cup non-leafy vegetables (cooked or chopped raw)

Meat, Poultry, Fish, Dry Beans, Eggs, and Nuts

2-3 servings from entire group

- Amounts should total 5 to 7 oz. of cooked lean meat, poultry, or fish each day. Count 1 egg; 1/2 cup cooked dried beans, peas or seeds; and 2 tbsp. peanut butter as 1 oz. of meat

Milk, Yogurt, and Cheese

2-3 servings from entire group (3 servings for teenagers, adults under 25, and women who are pregnant or breastfeeding; 4 servings for teens who are pregnant or breastfeeding).

- 1 cup of milk
- 8 oz. of yogurt
- 1 1/2 oz. of natural cheese
- 2 oz. of processed cheese

Fats, Oils, Sweets, and Alcoholic Beverages

Use sparingly. Use unsaturated vegetable oils and margarines that list a liquid vegetable oil as the first ingredient on the label. If you drink alcoholic beverages, do so in moderation.

- 1 tbsp. mayonnaise or dressing
- 1 tsp. butter or margarine
- 2 tbsp. sour cream or cream cheese
- 1 tsp. sugar, jam, or jelly
- 1 12-oz. soda
- 1/2 cup fruit sorbet or gelatin
- 1 oz. candy
- 1 tsp. salt
- 1 oz. (about 14) potato chips
- 1 tbsp. catsup, mustard, steak sauce, or soy sauce

How Cancer Treatments Can Affect Eating

Surgery

Surgery increases the need for good nutrition because it puts stress on the body. It may slow digestion. It may lessen the ability of the mouth, throat, and stomach to work properly. It also may make the mouth, throat, and stomach sore.

- Before surgery, a high-protein, high-calorie diet may be prescribed if a patient is underweight or weak.
- After surgery, some patients may not resume normal eating at first. They may receive nutrients:
  1. Through a needle in their vein (IV or intravenous feeding)
  2. Through a tube in their nose or stomach
  3. By drinking clear liquids
  4. By following a full-liquid diet

Radiation Therapy

As it damages cancer cells, radiation therapy also may damage health cells and health parts of the body

- Treatments of head, neck, or chest may cause:
  1. Dry mouth
  2. Sore mouth
  3. Difficulty swallowing (dysphagia)
  4. Change in taste of food
  5. Dental problems
- Treatment of stomach may cause:
  1. Nausea
  2. Vomiting
  3. Diarrhea

Chemotherapy

As it destroys cancer cells, chemotherapy also may harm parts of the body needed for eating. Side effects may include:

- Nausea and vomiting
- Loss of appetite
- Diarrhea
- Constipation
- Sore mouth or throat
- Weight gain
- Change in taste of food

Biological Therapy

Biological therapy (also known as immunotherapy) side effects may include:

- Nausea and vomiting
- Diarrhea
- Sore mouth

- Severe weight loss (anorexia)
- Dry mouth
- Change in taste of food

Managing Eating Problems during Treatment

All the methods of treating cancer—surgery, radiation therapy, chemotherapy, and biological therapy (immunotherapy)—are very powerful. Although treatments target the cancer cells in your body, they sometimes can damage normal, healthy cells. This may produce unpleasant side effects that cause eating problems. (See How Cancer Treatments Can Affect Eating.)

Side effects of cancer treatment vary from patient to patient. The part of the body being treated, length of treatment, and the dose of treatment also affect whether side effects will occur. Ask your doctor about how your treatment may affect you.

The good news is that only about one-third of cancer patients have side effects during treatment, and most side effects go away when treatment ends. Your doctor will try to plan a treatment that minimizes side effects.

Cancer treatment also may affect your eating in another way. When some people are upset, worried, or afraid, they may have eating problems. Losing your appetite and nausea are two normal responses to feeling nervous or fearful. Such problems should last only a short time.

While you are in the hospital, members of the food or nutrition service, including a registered dietitian, can help you plan your diet. They also can help you solve your physical or emotional eating problems. Feel free to talk to them if problems arise during your recovery as well. Ask them what has worked for their other patients.

Don't be afraid to give food a chance. Not everyone has problems with eating during cancer treatment. Even those who have eating problems have days when eating is a pleasure.

Coping with Side Effects

The following offers practical hints for coping with treatment side effects that may affect your eating.

These suggestions have helped other patients manage eating problems that can be frustrating to handle. Try all the ideas to find what works best for you. Share your needs and concerns with your family and friends, particularly those who prepare meals for you. Let them know that you appreciate their support as you work to take control of eating problems.

Loss of Appetite

Loss of appetite or poor appetite is one of the most common problems that occurs with cancer and its treatment. Many things affect appetite, including nausea, vomiting and being upset or depressed about having cancer. A person who has these feelings, whether physical or emotional, may not be interested in eating.

The following suggestions may help make mealtimes more relaxed so that you feel more like eating.

- Stay calm, especially at mealtimes. Don't hurry your meals.

- Involve yourself in as many normal activities as possible. If you feel uneasy and do not want to take part, don't force yourself.

- Try changing the time, place, and surroundings of meals. A candlelight dinner can make mealtime more appealing. Set a colorful table. Listen to soft music while eating. Eat with others or watch your favorite TV program while you eat.

- Eat whenever you are hungry. You do not need to eat just three main meals a day. Several small meals throughout the day may be even better.

- Add variety to your menu.

- Eat food often during the day, even at bedtime. Have healthy snacks handy. Taking just a few bites of the right foods or sips of the right liquids every hour or so can help you get more protein and calories. You can find ideas for preparing snacks in Table 77.1.

Sore Mouth or Throat

Mouth sores, tender gums, and a sore throat or esophagus often result from radiation therapy, anticancer drugs, and infection. If you have a sore mouth or gums, see your doctor to be sure the soreness is a treatment side effect and not an unrelated dental problem. The doctor may be able to give you medicine that will control mouth and throat pain. Your dentist also can give you tips for care of your mouth.

Certain foods will irritate an already tender mouth and make chewing and swallowing difficult. By carefully choosing the foods you eat and by taking good care of your mouth, you can usually make eating easier. Here are some suggestions that may help:

- Try soft foods that are easy to chew and swallow, such as milkshakes; bananas, applesauce, and other soft fruits; peach, pear, and apricot nectars; watermelon; cottage cheese; mashed potatoes, macaroni and cheese; custards, puddings, and gelatin; scrambled eggs; oatmeal or other cooked cereals; pureed or mashed vegetables such as peas and carrots; pureed meats; liquids.

- Avoid foods that can irritate your mouth: citrus fruit or juice such as oranges, grapefruits, tangerines; spicy or salty foods; rough, coarse, or dry foods such as raw vegetables, granola, toast, crackers.

- Cook foods until they are soft and tender.

- Cut foods into small pieces.

- Mix food with butter, thin gravies, and sauces to make it easier to swallow.

- Use a blender or food processor to puree your food.

- Use a straw to drink liquids.

- Try foods cold or at room temperature. Hot and warm foods can irritate a tender mouth and throat.

Table 77.1. Snacks

Have these on hand for quick and easy nibbles:

Applesauce	Fruits (fresh or canned)
Bread products, including muffins and crackers	Gelatin salads and desserts
	Granola
Buttered popcorn	Hard-boiled and deviled eggs
Cakes and cookies made with whole-grains, fruits, nuts, wheat germ, or granola	Ice cream, frozen yogurt, popsicles
	Juices
Cereal	Milkshakes, instant breakfast drinks
Cheese, hard or semisoft	Nuts
Cheesecake	Peanut butter
Chocolate milk	Pizza
Cottage cheese	Puddings and custards
Cream cheese and other soft cheese	Quesadillas
Cream soups	Sandwiches
Dips made with cheese, beans, or sour cream	Vegetables (raw or cooked)
	Yogurt (regular or frozen)
Dried fruits, such as raisins, prunes, or apricots	

- If swallowing is hard, tilting your head back or moving it forward may help.

- If heartburn is a problem, try sitting up or standing for about an hour after eating.

- If your teeth and gums are sore, your dentist may be able to recommend a special product for cleaning your teeth.

- Rinse your mouth with water often to remove food and bacteria and to promote healing.

- Ask your doctor about anesthetic lozenges and sprays that can numb the mouth and throat long enough for you to eat meals.

Changed Sense of Taste or Smell

Your sense of taste or smell may change during your illness or treatment. A condition called mouth blindness or taste blindness may give foods a bitter or metallic taste, especially meat or other high-protein foods. Many foods will have less taste. Chemotherapy, radiation therapy, or the cancer itself may cause these problems. Dental problems also can change the way foods taste. For most people, changes in taste and smell go away when their treatment is finished.

There is no "foolproof" way to improve the flavor or smell of food because each person is affected differently by illness and treatments. However, the tips given below should help make your food taste better. (If you also have a sore mouth, sore gums, or a sore throat, talk to your doctor or registered dietitian. They can suggest ways to improve the taste of your food without hurting the sore areas.)

- Choose and prepare foods that look and smell good to you.

- If red meat (such as beef) tastes or smells strange, use chicken, turkey, eggs, dairy products, or fish that doesn't have a strong smell instead.

- Help the flavor of meat, chicken, or fish by marinating it in sweet fruit juices, sweet wine, Italian dressing, or sweet-and-sour sauce.

- Try using small amounts of flavorful seasonings such as basil, oregano, or rosemary.

- Try tart foods such as oranges or lemonade that may have more taste. A tart lemon custard might taste good and will also provide needed protein and calories. (Do not try this if you have a sore mouth or throat.)

- Serve foods at room temperature.
- Try using bacon, ham, or onion to add flavor to vegetables.
- Stop eating foods that cause an unpleasant taste.
- Visit your dentist to rule out dental problems that may affect the taste or smell of food.
- Ask your dentist about special mouthwashes and good mouth care.

Dry Mouth

Chemotherapy and radiation therapy in the head or neck area can reduce the flow of saliva and often cause dry mouth. When this happens, foods are harder to chew and swallow. Dry mouth also can change the way foods taste. The suggestions below may be helpful in dealing with dry mouth. Also try some of the ideas for dealing with a sore mouth or throat, which can make foods easier to swallow.

- Try very sweet or tart foods and beverages such as lemonade; these foods may help your mouth produce more saliva. (Do not try this if you also have a tender mouth or sore throat.)
- Suck on sugar-free, hard candy or popsicles or chew sugar-free gum. These can help produce more saliva.
- Use soft and pureed foods, which may be easier to swallow.
- Keep your lips moist with lip salves.
- Eat foods with sauces, gravies, and salad dressings to make them moist and easier to swallow.
- Have a sip of water every few minutes to help you swallow and talk more easily.
- If your dry mouth problem is severe, ask your doctor or dentist about products that coat and protect your mouth and throat.

Nausea

Nausea, with or without vomiting, is a common side effect of surgery, chemotherapy, radiation therapy, and biological therapy. The disease itself, or other conditions unrelated to your cancer or treatment, also may cause nausea.

Whatever the cause, nausea can keep you from getting enough food and needed nutrients. Here are some ideas that may be helpful:

- Ask your doctor about medicine to help control nausea and vomiting. These drugs are called antiemetics.

- Try toast and crackers, yogurt, sherbet, pretzels, angel food cake, oatmeal, skinned chicken (baked or broiled, not fried), fruits and vegetables that are soft or bland (such as canned peaches), clear liquids (sipped slowly), and ice chips.

- Avoid fatty, greasy, fried, spicy or hot food with strong odors; and sweets such as candy, cookies, or cake.

- Eat small amounts often and slowly.

- Avoid eating in a room that's stuffy, too warm, or has cooking odors that might disagree with you

- Drink fewer liquids with meals. Drinking liquids can cause a full, bloated feeling.

- Drink or sip liquids throughout the day, except at mealtimes. Using a straw may help.

- Drink beverages cool or chilled. Try freezing favorite beverages in ice cube trays.

- Eat foods at room temperature or cooler; hot foods may add to nausea.

- Don't force yourself to eat favorite foods when you feel nauseated. This may cause a permanent dislike of those foods.

- Rest after meals, because activity may slow digestion. It's best to rest sitting up for about an hour after meals.

- If nausea is a problem in the morning, try eating dry toast or crackers before getting up.

- Wear loose-fitting clothes.

- Avoid eating for 1 to 2 hours before treatment if nausea occurs during radiation therapy or chemotherapy.

- Try to keep track of when your nausea occurs and what causes it (specific foods, events, surroundings). If possible, make appropriate changes in your diet or schedule. Share the information with your doctor or nurse.

Vomiting

Vomiting may follow nausea and may be brought on by treatment, food odors, gas in the stomach or bowel, or motion. In some people, certain surroundings, such as the hospital, may cause vomiting.

If vomiting is severe or lasts for more than a few days, contact your doctor.

Very often, if you can control nausea, you can prevent vomiting. At times, though, you may not be able to prevent either nausea or vomiting. You may find some relief by using relaxation exercises or meditation. These usually involve deep rhythmic breathing and quiet concentration and can be done almost anywhere. If vomiting occurs, try these hints to prevent further episodes.

- Ask your doctor about medicine to control nausea and vomiting (antiemetics).

- Do not drink or eat until you have the vomiting under control.

- Once you have controlled vomiting, try small amounts of clear liquids. (See Clear Liquid Diet) Begin with 1 teaspoonful every 10 minutes, gradually increase the amount to 1 tablespoonful every 20 minutes, and finally try 2 tablespoonfuls every 30 minutes.

- When you are able to keep down clear liquids, try a full-liquid diet. (See Full Liquid Diet) Continue taking small amounts as often as you can keep them down. If you feel okay on a full-liquid diet, gradually work up to your regular diet. If you have a hard time digesting milk, you may want to try a soft diet instead of a full-liquid diet. When you feel okay on the soft diet, gradually add more foods to return to your regular diet. (You can find information about these and other diets under "Special Diets for Special Needs.")

Diarrhea

Diarrhea may have several causes, including chemotherapy, radiation therapy to the abdomen, infection, food sensitivity, and emotional upset.

Long-term or severe diarrhea may cause other problems. During diarrhea, food passes quickly through the bowel before the body absorbs enough vitamins, minerals, and water. This may cause dehydration and increase the risk of infection. Contact your doctor if the diarrhea is severe or lasts for more than a couple of days. Here are some ideas for coping with diarrhea:

- Drink plenty of liquids during the day. Drinking fluids is important because your body may not get enough water when you have diarrhea.

- Eat small amounts of food throughout the day instead of three large meals.

- Eat plenty of foods and liquids that contain sodium (salt) and potassium. These minerals are often lost during diarrhea. Good liquid choices include bouillon or fat-free broth. Foods high in potassium that don't cause diarrhea include bananas, peach and apricot nectar, and boiled or mashed potatoes.

- Try these nutritious low-fiber foods: yogurt, rice or noodles, grape juice, farina or cream of wheat, eggs (cooked until the whites are solid, not fried), ripe bananas, smooth peanut butter, white bread, skinned chicken or turkey, lean beef, or fish (boiled or baked, not fried), cottage cheese, cream cheese.

- Eliminate greasy, fatty, or fried foods, raw vegetables and fruits; high-fiber vegetables such as broccoli, corn, beans, cabbage, peas, and cauliflower; strong spices, such as hot pepper, curry, and Cajun spice mix.

- Drink liquids that are at room temperature.

- Avoid very hot or very cold foods and beverages.

- Limit foods and beverages that contain caffeine, including coffee, strong tea, some sodas, and chocolate.

- Be careful when using milk and milk products because diarrhea may be caused by lactose intolerance. (If you think you have this problem, see "Low-Lactose Diet.") Ask your doctor or registered dietitian for advice.

- After sudden, short-term attacks of diarrhea (acute diarrhea), try a clear-liquid diet during the first 12 to 14 hours. This lets the bowel rest while replacing the important body fluids lost during diarrhea. (See Clear-Liquid Diet.)

Constipation

Some anticancer drugs and other drugs, such as pain medicines, may cause constipation. This problem also may occur if your diet lacks enough fluid or bulk or if you have been bedridden.

Here are some suggestions to prevent and treat constipation:

- Drink plenty of liquids—at least eight 8-ounce glasses every day. This will help to keep your stools soft.

- Take a hot drink about one-half hour before your usual time for a bowel movement.

- Eat high-fiber foods, such as whole-grain breads, cereals, and pastas; fresh fruits and vegetables dried beans and peas; and whole-grain products such as barley or brown rice. Eat the skin on fruits and potatoes.

- Get exercise, such as walking, every day. Talk to your doctor or a physical therapist about the amount and type of exercise that is right for you.

- Add unprocessed wheat bran to foods such as cereals, casseroles, and homemade breads.

If these suggestions don't work, ask your doctor about medicine to ease constipation. Be sure to check with your doctor before taking any laxatives or stool softeners.

Weight Gain

Sometimes patients gain excess weight during treatment without eating extra calories. For example, certain anticancer drugs, such as prednisone, can cause the body to hold on to fluid, causing weight gain; this condition is known as edema. The extra weight is in the form of water and does not mean you are eating too much.

It is important not to go on a diet if you notice weight gain. Instead, tell your doctor so you can find out what may be causing this change. If anticancer drugs are causing your body to retain water, your doctor may ask you to speak with a registered dietitian. The registered dietitian can teach you how to limit the amount of salt you eat, which is important because salt causes your body to hold extra water. Drugs called diuretics also may be prescribed to get rid of extra fluid.

Tooth Decay

Cancer and cancer treatment can cause tooth decay and other problems for your teeth and gums. Changes in eating habits also may add to the problem. If you eat frequently or consume a lot of sweets, you may need to brush your teeth more often. Brushing after each meal or snack is a good idea.

Here are some ideas for preventing dental problems:

- Be sure to see your dentist regularly. Patients who are receiving treatment that affects the mouth (e.g., radiation to the head and neck) may need to see the dentist more often than usual.

- Use a soft toothbrush. Ask your doctor, nurse, or dentist to suggest a special kind of toothbrush and/or toothpaste if your gums are very sensitive.

- Rinse your mouth with warm water when your gums and mouth are sore.

- If you are not having trouble with poor appetite or weight loss, limit the amount of sugar in your diet.

- Avoid eating foods that stick to the teeth, such as caramels or chewy candy bars.

Lactose Intolerance

Lactose intolerance means that your body can't digest or absorb the milk sugar called lactose. Milk, other dairy products, and foods to which milk has been added contain lactose.

Lactose intolerance may occur after treatment with some antibiotics, radiation to the stomach, or any treatment that affects the digestive tract. The part of your intestines that breaks down lactose may not work properly during treatment. For some people, symptoms of lactose intolerance (gas, cramping, diarrhea) disappear a few weeks or months after the treatments end or when the intestine heals. For others a permanent change in eating habits may be needed.

If you have this problem, your doctor may advise you to follow a diet that is low in foods that contain lactose. (See "Low-Lactose Diet.") If milk had been a main source of protein in your diet, it will be important to get enough protein from other foods. Products such as soybean and aged cheeses are good sources of protein and other nutrients. You also may want to try low-lactose milk or liquid drops or caplets that help break down the lactose in milk and other dairy products. The recipe section of this guide can give you ideas for preparing low lactose dishes.

Saving Time and Energy

Your body needs both rest and nourishment during and after treatment for cancer. If you are usually the cook, here are some suggestions for saving time and energy in preparing meals.

- Let someone else do the cooking when possible.

- If you know that your recovery time from treatment or surgery is going to be longer than 1 or 2 days, prepare a helper list. Decide who can help you shop, cook, set the table, and clean up. Write it down, discuss it, and post it where it can easily be seen. If children help, plan a small reward for them.

- Write out menus. Choose things that you or your family can put together easily. Casseroles, TV dinners, hot dogs, hamburgers, and meals that you have prepared and frozen ahead are all good ideas. Cook larger batches to be frozen so you will have them for future use. Add instructions so that other people can help you.

- Use shopping lists. Keep them handy so that they can be used as guides either by you or other people.

- When making casseroles for freezing, only partially cook rice and macaroni products. They will cook further in the reheating process. Add 1/2 cup liquid to refrigerated or frozen casseroles when reheating because they can get dry during refrigeration. Remember that frozen casseroles take a long time to heat completely—at least 45 minutes in deep dishes in the oven.

- Don't be shy about accepting gifts of food and offers of help from family and friends. Let them know what you like and offer your recipes. If people bring food you can't use right away, freeze it. That home cooked meal can break the monotony of quickie suppers. It also can save time when you're on a tight schedule. Date the food when you put it in the refrigerator or freezer.

- Have as few dishes, pots, and pans to wash as possible. Cook in dishes and pans that can also make attractive servers. Use paper napkins and disposable dishes, especially for dessert. Paper cups are fine for kids and for medicines. Disposable pans are a great time-saver—foil containers from frozen foods make good disposable pans. Soak dirty dishes to cut down washing time.

- When you are preparing soft dishes, choose foods that the whole family can eat, such as omelets, scrambled eggs, macaroni and cheese, meatloaf, tuna salad sandwiches, or tuna casseroles. Set aside enough food to be pureed in the blender or food processor for yourself.

- Use mixes, frozen ready-to-eat main dishes, and takeout foods whenever possible. The less time spent cooking and cleaning up, the more time for relaxation and the family.

- If someone is cooking for you, share this information with them for ideas for food selection and preparation. They will also get a better sense of your special needs.

Improving Your Nutrition

There are many ways to improve your nutrition to lessen the side effects of your treatment and to keep eating as well as you can when your treatment or illness is causing side effects. Table 77.1 provides a list of snacks you may want to try. Table 77.2 offers ideas for increasing protein in your diet, and Table 77.3 shows ways of increasing calories.

When side effects of treatment occur, they usually go away after treatment ends. Long-term treatment, however, may necessitate long-term changes in your diet to help you handle side effects and keep up your strength.

The ideas and suggestions listed here have worked for other cancer patients during their treatment. Each person is different, though, and you will have to find out what works best for you.

Special Diets for Special Needs

When you have special needs because of your illness or treatment, your doctor or registered dietitian may prescribe a special diet. They also may suggest a commercial product to help you meet your nutritional needs. In the following sections, you will find guidelines for several special diets used during cancer treatment. You also will learn about products that can boost nutrition and where you can buy them. Remember that special diets and products to improve nutrition should be used only as recommended by your doctor or registered dietitian.

Special diets are an important tool for correcting nutritional problems that occur during cancer treatment. For example, a soft diet may be best if your mouth, throat, esophagus, or stomach is sore. Or, if your treatment makes it difficult for you to digest dairy products, you may need to follow a low-lactose diet. Some diets are well balanced and can be followed for long periods of time. However, some special diets should be followed for only a few days because they may not provide enough nutrients for the long term.

Table 77.2. How to Increase Protein (continued on next page)

Hard or Semisoft Cheese	■ Melt on sandwiches, bread, muffins, tortillas, hamburgers, hot dogs, other meats or fish, vegetables, eggs, or desserts, such as stewed fruit or pies. ■ Grate and add to soups, sauces, casseroles, vegetable dishes, mashed potatoes, rice, noodles, or meatloaf.
Cottage Cheese/ Ricotta Cheese	■ Mix with or use to stuff fruits and vegetables. ■ Add to casseroles, spaghetti, noodles, and egg dishes, such as omelets, scrambled eggs, and souffles. ■ Use in gelatin, pudding-type desserts, cheesecake, and pancake batter. ■ Use to stuff crepes and pasta shells or manicotti.
Milk	■ Use milk in beverages and in cooking when possible. ■ Use in preparing hot cereal, soups, cocoa, and pudding. ■ Add cream sauces to vegetable and other dishes.
Powdered Milk	■ Add to regular milk and milk drinks, such as pasteurized eggnog and milkshakes. ■ Use in casseroles, meatloaf, breads, muffins, sauces, cream soups, mashed potatoes, puddings and custards, and milk-based desserts.
Commercial Products	■ See the section on "Commercial Products To Improve Nutrition." ■ Use instant breakfast powder in milk drinks and desserts. ■ Mix with ice cream, milk, and fruit or flavorings for a high-protein milkshake.
Ice Cream, Yogurt, and Frozen Yogurt	■ Add to carbonated beverages, such as ginger ale; add to milk drinks, such as milkshakes. ■ Add to cereals, fruits, gelatin desserts, and pies; blend or whip with soft or cooked fruits. ■ Sandwich ice cream or frozen yogurt between enriched cake slices, cookies, or graham crackers.

Table 77.2. How to Increase Protein (continued from previous page)

Eggs	■ Add chopped, hard-cooked eggs to salads and dressings, vegetables, casseroles, and creamed meats.
	■ Add extra eggs or egg whites to quiches and to pancake and French toast batter. Add extra egg whites to scrambled eggs and omelets.
	■ Make a rich custard with eggs, high-protein milk, and sugar.
	■ Add extra hard-cooked yolks to deviled-egg filling and sandwich spreads.
	■ *Avoid raw eggs, which may contain harmful bacteria, because your treatment may make you susceptible to infection.* Make sure all eggs you eat are well cooked or baked; avoid eggs that are "runny."
Nuts, Seeds, and Wheat Germ	■ Add to casseroles, breads, muffins, pancakes, cookies, and waffles.
	■ Sprinkle on fruit, cereal, ice cream, yogurt, vegetables, salads, and toast as a crunchy topping; use in place of bread crumbs.
	■ Blend with parsley or spinach, herbs, and cream for a noodle, pasta, or vegetable sauce.
	■ Roll banana in chopped nuts.
Peanut Butter	■ Spread on sandwiches, toast, muffins, crackers, waffles, pancakes, and fruit slices.
	■ Use as a dip for raw vegetables such as carrots, cauliflower, and celery.
	■ Blend with milk drinks and beverages.
	■ Swirl through soft ice cream and yogurt.
Meat and Fish	■ Add chopped, cooked meat or fish to vegetables, salads, casseroles, soups, sauces, and biscuit dough.
	■ Use in omelets, souffles, quiches, sandwich fillings, and chicken and turkey stuffings.
	■ Wrap in piecrust or biscuit dough as turnovers.
	■ Add to stuffed baked potatoes.
Beans/Legumes	■ Cook and use dried peas, legumes, beans, and bean curd (tofu) in soups or add to casseroles, pastas, and grain dishes that also contain cheese or meat. Mash with cheese and milk.

Table 77.3. How to Increase Calories (continued on next page)

Butter and Margarine
- Add to soups, mashed and baked potatoes, hot cereals, grits, rice, noodles, and cooked vegetables.
- Stir into cream soups, sauces, and gravies.
- Combine with herbs and seasonings, and spread on cooked meats, hamburgers, and fish and egg dishes.
- Use melted butter or margarine as a dip for raw vegetables and seafoods, such as shrimp, scallops, crab, and lobster.

Whipped Cream
- Use sweetened on hot chocolate, desserts, gelatin, puddings, fruits, pancakes, and waffles.
- Fold unsweetened into mashed potatoes or vegetable purees.

Table Cream
- Use in cream soups, sauces, egg dishes, batters, puddings, and custards.
- Put on hot or cold cereal.
- Mix with noodles, pasta, rice, and mashed potatoes.
- Pour on chicken and fish while baking.
- Use as a binder in hamburgers, meatloaf, and croquettes.
- Add to milk in recipes.
- Make hot chocolate with cream and add marshmallows.

Cream Cheese
- Spread on breads, muffins, fruit slices, and crackers.
- Add to vegetables.
- Roll into balls and coat with chopped nuts, wheat germ, or granola.

Sour Cream
- Add to cream soups, baked potatoes, macaroni and cheese, vegetables, sauces, salad dressings, stews, baked meat, and fish.
- Use as a topping for cakes, fruit, gelatin desserts, breads, and muffins.
- Use as a dip for fresh fruits and vegetables.
- For a good dessert, scoop it on fresh fruit, add brown sugar, and let it sit in the refrigerator for a while.

Table 77.3. How to Increase Calories (continued from previous page)

Salad Dressings and Mayonnaise	▪ Spread on sandwiches and crackers. ▪ Combine with meat, fish, and egg or vegetable salads. ▪ Use as a binder in croquettes. ▪ Use in sauces and gelatin dishes.
Honey, Jam, and Sugar	▪ Add to bread, cereal, milk drinks, and fruit and yogurt desserts. ▪ Use as a glaze for meats, such as chicken.
Granola	▪ Use in cookie, muffin, and bread batters. ▪ Sprinkle on vegetables, yogurt, ice cream, pudding, custard, and fruit. ▪ Layer with fruits and bake. ▪ Mix with dry fruits and nuts for a snack. ▪ Substitute for bread or rice in pudding recipes.
Dried Fruits	▪ Cook and serve for breakfast or as a dessert or snack. ▪ Add to muffins, cookies, breads, cakes, rice and grain dishes, cereals, puddings, and stuffings. ▪ Bake in pies and turnovers. ▪ Combine with cooked vegetables, such as carrots, sweet potatoes, yams, and acorn and butternut squash. ▪ Combine with nuts or granola for snacks.
Eggs	▪ Add chopped, hard-cooked eggs to salads and dressings, vegetables, casseroles, and creamed meats. ▪ Make a rich custard with eggs, milk, and sugar. ▪ Add extra, hard-cooked yolks to deviled-egg filling and sandwich spread. ▪ Beat eggs into mashed potatoes, vegetable purees, and sauces. *(Be sure to keep cooking these dishes after adding the eggs because raw eggs may contain harmful bacteria.)* ▪ Add extra eggs or egg whites to custards, puddings, quiches, scrambled eggs, omelets, and to pancake and French toast batter before cooking.
Food Preparation	▪ Bread, meats and vegetables. ▪ Sauté and fry foods when possible, because these cooking methods add more calories than baking or broiling. ▪ Add sauces or gravies.

Only your doctor or registered dietitian should decide whether you need a special diet and for how long. If you are already following a special diet for another health problem, such as diabetes or high cholesterol, you and your doctor and registered dietitian should work together to develop your new plan.

Beginning on the next page guidelines for common special diets appear in this section, including:

- Clear-liquid diet.
- Full-liquid diet.
- Soft diet.
- Fiber-restricted diet.
- Low-lactose diet.

For each diet, you will find a brief explanation of when the diet usually is recommended, the major foods it includes, and a suggested meal pattern. This information will help you follow the diet recommended by your doctor or registered dietitian. If you think you need a special diet, talk with your doctor or registered dietitian.

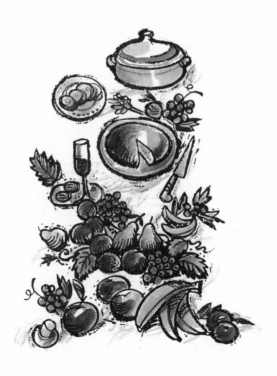

Clear-Liquid Diet

Clear-liquid diets are useful if the body can't handle the softest foods or heavy or thick liquids. Patients usually follow this type of diet after surgery or before stomach or bowel surgery. Patients with severe nausea and vomiting may also have this diet. A clear-liquid

Table 77.4. Clear-Liquid Diet (continued on next page)

Type of Food	Allowed Items	Excluded Items
Beverages	Water; carbonated beverages; cereal beverages; coffee, tea;* fruit-flavored drinks; strained lemonade, limeade, and fruit punches	Milk, milk drinks, all others**
Breads Cereals Flours	None	All
Cheeses	None	All
Desserts	Plain gelatin desserts, fruit ices without milk or pieces of fruit, popsicles	All others
Eggs	None	All
Fats	None	All

*Your doctor may recommend decaffeinated coffee or tea.
**Check with your doctor about alcohol. Alcohol cannot be used safely with some medicines.

diet of ten lasts 1 to 2 days or until you can drink or eat other beverages and foods. It cannot meet the daily servings suggested in the section "Eat a Variety of Foods Each Day" (except for fruit juices), but it helps ensure that your body doesn't lose too much fluid as you recover and become ready for a regular diet.

Table 77.4. Clear-Liquid Diet (continued from previous page)

Type of Food	Allowed Items	Excluded items
Fruits **Fruit Juices**	Apple, cranberry, and grape juice; strained citrus juices if tolerated	All others
Meat **Poultry** **Fish** **Legumes**	None	All
Milk **Milk Products**	None	All
Potatoes **Rice** **Pasta**	None	All
Soup	Bouillon, clear fat-free broths, consommé	All others
Sweets	Honey, jelly, syrups, plain sugar candy in small amounts	All others
Vegetables	Strained vegetable broth	All others
Miscellaneous	Salt	All others

Full-Liquid Diet

You may follow a full-liquid diet when your body can digest all liquids but can't handle solid food yet. Your doctor or registered dietitian may recommend this diet after surgery or when you can't chew and swallow food. All liquids served at room or body temperature are part of this diet. This diet can include most of the recommended food groups in the section, "Eat a Variety of Foods Each Day," except meat. Extra milk has been included to ensure adequate protein. When planned properly, this diet can be used for long periods. In these instances, your doctor may prescribe a commercial supplement and/or certain vitamins. However, you should only take these if your doctor or registered dietitian recommends them.

Table 77.5. Full-Liquid Diet

Type of Food	Allowed Items	Excluded Items
Beverages	Cereal beverages; coffee, tea:* fruit drinks; strained lemonade, limeade, or fruit punches; water	None**
Breads Cereals Flours	Refined or strained cooked cereal	Breads and cereals in solid form
Cheeses	Cheese soup	All others
Desserts	Plain gelatin desserts, junket, soft or baked custards, sherbets, plain cornstarch pudding, fresh or frozen yogurt, ice milk, smooth ice cream	All others, particularly those with fruits or seeds
Eggs	Pasteurized eggnog	All others
Fats	Butter, cream, oils, margarine	All others
Fruits Fruit Juices	All juices and nectars, thin fruit purees	All others

* *Your doctor may recommend decaffeinated coffee or tea.*
** *Check with your doctor before drinking alcohol. Alcohol cannot be used safely with some medicines.*

If you must follow a full-liquid diet over a long period, you can increase the protein and calorie content of the diet by:

- Adding nonfat dry milk to beverages and soups.
- Adding instant breakfast powder to milk, puddings, custards, and milkshakes.
- Adding strained meats (such as those in baby food) to broths.
- Adding butter to hot cereal and soups.
- Including sugar or syrup (glucose) in beverages.
- Using smooth ice cream in desserts and beverages.
- Using prepared breakfast mixes in milk or milkshakes.

Table 77.5. Full-Liquid Diet

Type of Food	Allowed Items	Excluded Items
Meat Poultry Fish Legumes	Small amounts of strained meat in broth or gelatin	All others
Milk Milk Products	Buttermilk and chocolate, skim, and whole milk; ice milk; milkshakes; plain yogurt	All others, yogurt with pieces of fruit
Potatoes Rice Pasta	Potatoes pureed in soup	All others
Soups	Bouillon, broth, clear cream soups, any strained or blenderized soup	All others
Sweets	Honey, jelly, syrups in small amounts	All others
Vegetables	Tomato puree for cream soups; tomato, vegetable juices	All others
Miscellaneous	Flavoring extracts, salt	All others

Soft Diet

A soft diet is useful when your body is ready for more than liquids but still unable to handle a regular solid diet. Soft food is easier to eat than regular food when the mouth, throat, esophagus, and/or stomach are sore. This soreness can occur to these parts of the body during and after radiation therapy or during chemotherapy. A soft diet can be used for long periods because it contains all needed nutrients.

Table 77.6. Soft Diet (continued on next page)

Type of Food	Allowed Items	Excluded Items
Beverages	All	None**
Breads	French, Vienna, Italian, seedless rye, white, refined whole wheat, cornbread, or any except whole-grain; if tolerated, muffins, French toast, crackers, biscuits, rolls, pancakes, waffles	Brown, cracked wheat, pumpernickel, raisin, rye with seeds, buckwheat; whole-grain crackers; rolls with coconut, raisins, nuts, or whole grains; tortillas
Cereals	Refined, cooked, or ready-to-eat, such as cream of wheat, farina, hominy grits, cornmeal, oatmeal, puffed rice	Whole-grain or bran
Flours	All except those excluded	Whole-grain, bran, or wheat
Cheeses	All except those excluded	Sharp or strongly flavored cheeses; those containing whole seeds and spices
Desserts	Ice milk, ice cream, sherbet, ices, custards, gelatins, or others with allowed fruits	Desserts made with excluded fruits, nuts, coconut
Eggs	All except those excluded	Raw, fried
Fats	Butter, cream, cream substitutes, vegetable shortening and oils, margarine, mayonnaise, sour cream, commercial French dressing	Other salad dressings; salt pork; fried foods
Fruits Fruit Juices	All juices and nectars; avocado, banana, canned or cooked apples, apricots, cherries, grapefruit and orange sections without membrane, peaches, pears, seedless grapes, tomatoes; soft melons, such as watermelon, if tolerated	All raw fruit except avocado and banana; all dried fruit; berries, crabapples, coconut, figs, grapes, pineapples, plums, rhubarb
Meat	Tender beef, lamb, veal, or liver that is baked, broiled, creamed, roasted, or stewed; roasted or stewed pork	Fried, salted, and smoked meats; chitterlings; corned beef; sausage; cold cuts

** Check with your doctor before drinking alcohol. Alcohol cannot be used safely with some medicines.

The diet consists of bland, lower fat foods that you soften by cooking, mashing, pureeing, or blending.

The table lists foods included in a soft diet as well as foods you should try to avoid. Keep in mind, however, that you may be able to eat some of the "excluded" foods without any discomfort or problems. In general, though, it is probably best to avoid fried or greasy foods and foods that may cause gas.

Table 77.6. Soft Diet (continued from previous page)

Type of Food	Allowed items	Excluded Items
Poultry	Chicken, Cornish game hen, turkey, chicken livers	Duck, goose; fried poultry
Fish	Cooked, fresh, or frozen fish without bones; tuna, salmon	Fried fish, shellfish, anchovies, caviar, herring, sardines, snails, skate
Legumes Nuts	Creamy peanut butter	All other legumes, nuts, and seed kernels
Milk Milk Products	All	None
Potatoes Rice Pasta	Baked, boiled, creamed, scalloped, mashed, au gratin; mashed sweet potatoes; dumplings; noodles; brown or white rice; spaghetti	French fries, hashbrowns, potato salad, whole sweet potatoes or yams; bread stuffing; fritters; chow mein noodles; wild rice; barley
Soups	Bouillon, broth, consommé, strained cream and vegetable	Bean, split pea, onion; bisques; gumbos; unstrained chowders
Sweets	Apple butter, butterscotch candy, caramels, chocolate, fondant, plain fudge, lollipops, marshmallows, mints, honey, jelly, syrups, sugars in small amounts	Candied fruits, nut brittle, jams, preserves, marmalade, marzipan, fruit sauces with prohibited fruits
Vegetables	Canned or cooked asparagus, carrots, beets, eggplant, mushrooms, parsley, pumpkin, spinach, squash, vegetable juice cocktail, raw lettuce if tolerated	All raw vegetables except lettuce; all canned or cooked vegetables not specifically listed as allowed
Miscellaneous	Aspic, catsup, gelatin, gravy, pretzels, soy sauce, vinegar; brown, cheese, cream, tomato, and white sauces; all finely chopped or ground leaf herbs and spices	Garlic, horseradish; olives, pickles; popcorn, potato chips; relishes; chili, a-la-king, creole, barbecue, cocktail, sweet-and-sour, Newburg, and Worcester-shire sauces; whole and seed herbs and spices

Fiber Restricted

Your doctor or registered dietitian may recommend a fiber-restricted diet if your gastrointestinal (GI) tract cannot digest fiber in foods. This type of diet is often used after GI surgery before patients return to their regular diet. A fiber-restricted diet also may be needed when treatment, such as radiation, damages the bowel or when the GI tract becomes irritated.

A fiber-restricted diet limits the amount of vegetables, fruits, cereals, and grains that you can eat. It also limits to two cups per day the amount of milk and milk products, such as cream, yogurt, and cheese, that you can eat. Milk does not contain fiber, but it leaves a residue in the GI tract that can irritate the bowel and cause diarrhea and cramping. The diet also is helpful for the many cancer patients who have a hard time digesting the milk sugar, lactose. (See the section, "Low Lactose Diet".) A fiber-restricted diet can be changed easily, depending on how you feel after eating certain foods. Use the diet in this chapter as a guide and discuss any changes with your doctor or registered dietitian.

There may be times when a low-residue diet, which is more limited than a fiber-restricted diet, is needed. On the low-residue diet, you may be able to eat most strained vegetables and fruit juices, such as white potatoes without skin, and tomato juice. All other forms of vegetables and fruits may be excluded from the diet. The low-residue diet also limits the amount of fat and dairy products you can eat. Your doctor or registered dietitian will let you know if you need to follow a low residue diet.

Your registered dietitian may gradually increase fiber and milk products in your diet according to how well you handle them.

Table 77.7 Fiber-Restricted Diet (continued on next page)

Type of Food	Allowed Items	Excluded Items
Beverages	Fruit-flavored drinks; carbonated beverages, coffee, tea;* milk drinks and milk used in cooking (2 cups milk or milk products allowed per day, if tolerated); all others except excluded items, no limitations	Prune juice, pear nectar**
Breads	French, Vienna, Italian, refined wheat, white, and rye breads without seeds; crackers; biscuits; French toast; plain hard crust; zwieback rolls	Breads, crackers, rolls, or cereals containing whole grain or graham flour; bran, seeds, nuts, or raisins; cornbread
Cereals	All refined, cooked, or dry cereals, such as cream of wheat or rice and flaked or puffed cereals	All whole-grain cereals made from prohibited flours or other foods; oatmeal; granola
Cheeses	Cottage, cream, American, Swiss, Muenster, or other mild cheese; 1 oz. may be substituted for 1 cup milk	All others
Desserts	Custards, gelatin puddings, plain cookies and cakes, sherbets; 1/2 cup ice cream (may be substituted as 1/2 cup milk allowance), pastries made with allowed ingredients	All desserts containing seeds, nuts, coconut, or raisins; tough-skinned fruits
Eggs	All except raw	Raw
Fats	Butter, oils, cream, dry cream substitutes, margarine, mayonnaise, shortenings, smooth salad dressings, sour cream	Salad dressing made with excluded foods; tartar sauce
Fruits	Canned or cooked fruits without seeds, skins, or membranes — apples, applesauce, cherries, grapefruit, oranges, tangerine, peaches, pineapple, pears, fruit cocktail; raw — ripe bananas, melon, grapefruit, oranges, tangerine; juice — all except prune juice and pear nectar (2 servings allowed per day)	All other fruits; dried fruits; berries; figs; grapes with seeds; stewed prunes, prune purée; plums; pear nectar

Your doctor may recommend decaffeinated coffee or tea.
**Check with your doctor before drinking alcohol. Alcohol cannot be used safely with some medicines.*

Table 77.7 Fiber-Restricted Diet (continued from previous page)

Type of Food	Allowed Items	Excluded Items
Meat **Poultry**	Tender beef, ham, lamb, liver, poultry, or veal that is baked, broiled, or stewed; lean or low-fat cold cuts and frankfurters	Fried meats and poultry, smoked or cured meats, cold cuts, corned beef, frankfurters, pastrami, sausage
Fish	Fresh or frozen fish without bones, canned tuna or salmon, cooked shellfish	All fried or smoked fish, sardines, herring
Legumes **Nuts**	None	All dried legumes, lima beans, peas, nuts
Milk **Milk Products**	Buttermilk and chocolate, skim, low-fat, and whole milk, if tolerated; yogurt, plain, custard-style, with allowed fruits and without nuts (2 cups, including that used in cooking, allowed per day)	Yogurt containing fruits
Potatoes **Rice** **Pasta**	Boiled, creamed, mashed, and scalloped potatoes without skin; macaroni, noodles, white rice, spaghetti (1 serving potato allowed per day; all others, no limitation)	Potato skin, potato cakes, french fries, hash browns, potato salad, sweet potato, brown and wild rice, barley, hominy
Soups	Cream and broth-based soups made with allowed foods	All others
Sweets	Honey, jelly, syrup, plain hard candy, molasses, marshmallows, gumdrops	Jams, preserves, candies with fruits, coconut, raisins, nuts, candied fruits
Vegetables	Canned or cooked asparagus tips, green or wax beans, mushrooms, peas, pumpkin, raw lettuce, if tolerated (no limitation on vegetable juices; 1 serving whole vegetables allowed per day)	All raw vegetables except lettuce; canned or cooked vegetables not specifically allowed, such as the high-fiber vegetables: beans, carrots, peas, spinach and other greens, beets
Miscellaneous	Ground or finely chopped herbs and spices, salt, flavoring extracts, catsup, chocolate, mild gravy, white sauce, soy sauce, vinegar	All other spices and condiments, olives, pickles, potato chips, popcorn

Low-Lactose Diet

All milk products contain lactose (or milk sugar). The doctor or registered dietitian may recommend a low-lactose diet after radiation therapy to the intestines, which often makes lactose hard to digest for a time. Fermented milk products, such as buttermilk, acidophilus

Table 77.8. Low-Lactose Diet (continued on next page)

Type of Food	Allowed Items	Excluded Items
Beverages	Water, lactose-free carbonated beverages, fruit-flavored drinks, fruit punches, lemonade, limeade, nondairy product drinks, low-lactose milk, acidophilus milk, coffee, and tea*	Artificial fruit drinks containing lactose, all beverages and nutritional supplements made with milk and milk products with the exception of buttermilk, low-lactose milk, and yogurt**
Bread	All	None
Cereals	Any cooked or dry cereal not containing lactose	Instant hot cereals, high-protein cereals, all cereals with added milk or lactose
Flours	All	None
Cheeses	Fermented cheeses (cheddar and any cheese aged with bacteria)	All others
Desserts	Fruit ices; gelatins; angel food cake; desserts made with nondairy products, buttermilk, or sour cream	Ice cream, puddings, and other desserts containing milk or milk products
Eggs	All except raw eggs and eggs prepared with milk or milk products	Creamed, scrambled, omelets, or other eggs prepared with milk; raw eggs
Fats	Margarine not containing milk solids, vegetable oils, mayonnaise, shortening	All others: cream, half-and-half, table and whipping cream, butter
Fruits Fruit Juices	All fresh, canned, or frozen fruit juices; fruits not processed with lactose	Any canned or frozen fruits and fruit juices processed with lactose
Meat Poultry Fish Legumes Nuts	Any except those specifically excluded	Creamed or breaded fish, poultry, meat; cold cuts, hot dogs, liver, sausage, or other processed meats containing milk or lactose; gravies made with milk

* Your doctor may recommend decaffeinated coffee or tea.
** Check with your doctor before drinking alcohol. Alcohol cannot be used safely with some medicines.

825

milk, sour cream, and yogurt, usually are easier to handle than whole milk. You also can buy low-lactose milk or use liquid drops or caplets that help break down the lactose in milk and other dairy products. Lactose is often used as a filler in many products such as instant coffee and some medicines. Carefully read labels on commercial foods to see if they contain lactose or any milk products or milk solids.

Lactose tolerance varies from person to person. Ask your doctor or registered dietitian about choosing allowed foods and about low-lactose dairy products that you can buy at the grocery store.

Table 77.8. Low-Lactose Diet (continued from previous page)

Type of Food	Allowed Items	Excluded Items
Milk **Milk Products**	Fermented milk products such as acidophilus milk, buttermilk, yogurt, and sour cream; low-lactose products; "lactose-digesting" pills or caplets	All milk, milk products except those allowed
Potatoes **Rice** **Pasta**	White or sweet potatoes, macaroni, noodles, spaghetti or other pasta, rice	Any prepared with milk, such as commercially prepared creamed or scalloped potato products containing dried milk
Soups	Broth-based soups.	Cream soups, chowders, commercially prepared soups that contain milk or milk products
Sweets	Honey, jams, preserves, syrups, molasses	Candy containing lactose, milk, or cocoa; butterscotch candies; caramels; chocolates (Read all labels carefully.)
Vegetables	All vegetables except those prepared with milk	Any prepared with milk, such as creamed, scalloped, or any processed vegetables containing lactose
Miscellaneous	Catsup, chili sauce, horseradish, olives, pickles, vinegar, gravies prepared without milk, mustard, all herbs and spices, peanut butter, unbuttered popcorn	Chocolate, cocoa, milk gravies, cream sauces, chewing gum, instant coffee, powdered soft drinks, artificial juices containing milk or lactose

Commercial Products to Improve Nutrition

If you cannot get enough calories and protein from your diet, commercial nutrition supplements, such as formulas and instant breakfast powders, may be helpful. There also are products that can be added to any food or beverage to boost calorie content. These supplements are high in protein and calories and have extra vitamins and minerals. They come in liquid, pudding, and powder forms. Prepackaged blenderized diets made from whole foods also are available. These are a convenient and inexpensive alternative to homemade preparations. Most commercial nutrition supplements contain little or no lactose. However, it is important to check the label if you are sensitive to lactose. (See the section, "Low Lactose Diet.")

These products need no refrigeration until you open them. Thus, you can carry nutrition supplements with you and take them whenever you feel hungry or thirsty. They are good chilled as between-meal and bedtime snacks. You may want to take a can or two with you when you go for treatments or other times when long waits may tire you. Ask your registered dietitian which supplements would be best for you.

Many supermarkets and drugstores carry a variety of commercial nutrition supplements. If you don't see these products on the shelf, ask the store manager if they can be ordered. You also may want to ask your doctor or registered dietitian for information about products for special patients. Be sure to ask for manufacturers' names, and, as mentioned above, be sure to read the label to see if any of the products contains lactose.

Resources

Information about cancer is available from many sources, including the ones listed below. For additional information you may wish to check the local library, bookstores or support groups in your community.

Cancer Information Service

The Cancer Information Service (CIS), a program of the National Cancer Institute NCI), is a nationwide telephone service for cancer patients and their families and friends, the public, and health care professionals. The staff can answer questions (in English or Spanish) and can send free National Cancer Institute materials about cancer. They also know about support groups and other resources and services.

One toll-free number, 1-800-4-CANCER (1-800-422-6237), connects callers with the office that serves their area

American Cancer Society

The American Cancer Society (ACS) is a voluntary organization with local units all over the country. This organization supports research, conducts educational programs, and offers support groups and many other services to patients and their families. The American Cancer Society also provides free booklets. To obtain booklets or for information about services and activities in local areas, call the toll-free number 1-800-ACS-2345 (1-800-227-2345), or the number listed under American Cancer Society in the white pages of the telephone book.

Chapter 78

Management of Cancer Pain

Facts about Cancer Pain Treatment

If you are being treated for cancer pain, you may have concerns about your medicine or other treatments. Here are some common concerns people have and the facts about them.

Concern: I can only take medicine or other treatments when I have pain.

Fact: You should not wait until the pain becomes severe to take your medicine. Pain is easier to control when it is mild than when it is severe. You should take your pain medicine regularly and as your doctor or nurse tells you. This may mean taking it on a regular schedule and around-the-clock. You can also use the other treatments, such as relaxation and breathing exercises, hot and cold packs, as often as you want to.

Concern: I will become "hooked" or "addicted" to pain medicine.

Fact: Studies show that getting "hooked" or "addicted" to pain medicine is very rare. Remember, it is important to take pain medicine regularly to keep the pain under control.

Concern: If I take too much medicine, it will stop working.

Managing Cancer Pain, Clinical Practice Guideline Number 9, March 1994. U.S. Department of Health and Human Services, Agency for Health Care Policy and Research.

Fact: The medicine will not stop working. But sometimes your body will get used to the medicine. This is called tolerance. Tolerance is not usually a problem with cancer pain treatment because the amount of medicine can be changed or other medicines can be added. Cancer pain can be relieved, so don't deny yourself pain relief now.

Concern: If I complain too much, I am not being a good patient.

Fact: Controlling your pain is an important part of your care. Tell your doctors and nurses if you have pain, if your pain is getting worse, or if you are taking pain medicine and it is not working. They can help you to get relief from your pain.

You may have concerns about your treatment that were not discussed here. Talk to your doctor or nurse about your concerns.

Purpose of This Chapter

This chapter is about cancer pain and how it can be controlled. Not everyone with cancer has pain. But those who do can feel better with proper pain treatment.

Reading this chapter should help you to:

- Learn why pain control is important to you.

- Work with your doctors and nurses to find the best method to control your pain.

- Talk to your doctors and nurses about your pain and how well the treatment is working for you.

Why Pain Should Be Treated

Pain can affect you in many ways. It can keep you from being active, from sleeping well, from enjoying family and friends, and from eating. Pain can also make you feel afraid or depressed.

When you are in pain or uncomfortable, your family and friends may worry about you.

With treatment, most cancer pain can be controlled. When there is less pain, you will probably feel more active and interested in doing things you enjoy.

If you have cancer and you are feeling pain, you need to tell your doctor or nurse right away. Getting help for your pain early on can make pain treatment more effective.

What Causes Cancer Pain?

There are many causes of cancer pain. Most of the pain of cancer comes when a tumor presses on bone, nerves, or body organs. Cancer treatment can cause pain, too.

You may also have pain that has nothing to do with your illness or its treatment. Like everyone else, you can get headaches, muscle strains, and other aches and pains. Because you may be taking medicine for cancer treatment or pain, check with your doctor or nurse on what to take for these everyday aches and pains.

Other conditions, such as arthritis, can cause pain, too. Pain from these other conditions can be treated along with cancer pain. Again, talk to your doctors and nurses about your medical history. They will be able to tell you how each condition can be treated and what is best for you.

Treating Cancer Pain

Cancer pain is usually treated with medicine. But surgery, radiation therapy, and other treatments can be used along with medicine to give even more pain relief. Ask your doctor or nurse how the other treatments can help you.

Choosing the Right Medicine

Pain treatments work differently for different people. Even when a doctor or nurse uses the right medicines and treatments in the right way, you may not get the pain relief you need. While you are being treated for your pain, tell your doctors and nurses how you feel and if the treatments help. The information you give them will help them to help you get the best pain relief.

Your doctors and nurses will work to find the right pain medicine and treatments for you. You can help by talking with them about:

- Pain medicines you have taken in the past and how well they have worked for you.

- Medicines and other treatments (including health foods, vitamins, and other "nonmedical" treatments) you are taking now. Your doctor or nurse needs to know about other treatments you are trying and other medicines you take. This is important because some treatments and medicines do not work well together. Your doctors and nurses can find medicines that can be taken together.

831

- Allergies that you have, including allergies to medicines.

- Fears and concerns that you have about the medicine or the treatment.Talk to your doctors and nurses about your fears and concerns. They can answer your questions and help you to understand your pain treatment.

Types of Pain Medicine

Many medicines are used to treat cancer pain, and your doctor may give you one or more of them to take. The list below describes the different types of medicine that you may be taking and the kind of pain they work on. Ask your doctor or nurse to tell you more about the medicine you are taking. Do not start to take a new medicine without checking with your doctor or nurse first. Even aspirin can be a problem in some people who are taking other medicines or having cancer treatment.

For Mild to Moderate Pain

- Nonopioids: Acetaminophen and nonsteroidal anti-inflammatory drugs (NSAIDs), such as aspirin and ibuprofen. You can buy many of these over-the-counter (without a prescription). Others need a prescription.

For Moderate to Severe Pain

- Opioids: Morphine, hydromorphone, oxycodone, and codeine. A prescription is needed for these medicines. Nonopioids may also used along with opioids for moderate to severe pain.

For Tingling and Burning Pain

- Antidepressants: Amitriptyline, imipramine, doxepin, trazodone. A prescription is needed for these medicines. Taking an antidepressant does not mean that you are depressed or have a mental illness.

- Anticonvulsants: Carbamazepine and phenytoin. A prescription is needed for these medicines. Taking an anticonvulsant does not mean that you are going to have convulsions.

For Pain Caused by Swelling

- Steroids: Prednisone, dexamethasone. A prescription is needed for these medicines.

About Side Effects

All medicines can have some side effects, but not all people get them. Some people have different side effects than others. Most side effects happen in the first few hours of treatment and gradually go away. Some of the most common side effects of pain medicines are:

- *Constipation* (not being able to have a bowel movement). The best way to prevent constipation is to drink lots of water, juice, and other liquids, and to eat more fruits and vegetables. Exercise also helps to prevent constipation. Your doctor or nurse may also be able to give you a stool softener or a laxative.

- *Nausea and vomiting.* When this happens, it usually only lasts for the first day or two after starting a medicine. Tell your doctors and nurses about any nausea or vomiting. They can give you medicine to stop these side effects.

- *Sleepiness.* Some people who take opioids feel drowsy or sleepy when they first take the medicine. This usually does not last too long. Talk to your doctor or nurse if this is a problem for you.

- *Slowed breathing.* This sometimes happens when the dose of medicine is increased. Your doctor or nurse can tell you what to watch for and when to report slowed breathing.

More serious side effects of pain medicines are rare. As with the more common side effects, they usually happen in the first few hours of treatment. They include trouble breathing, dizziness, and rashes. If you have any of these side effects, you should call your doctor or nurse right away.

How Pain Medicine Is Taken

Most pain medicine is taken by mouth (orally). Oral medicines are easy to take and usually cost less than other kinds of medicine. Most oral medicines are in tablet form, but sometimes they are liquids that you drink. If it is hard for you to swallow and you cannot take a tablet or liquid for some other reason, there are other ways to get these medicines. These include:

- *Rectal suppositories* (medicine that dissolves in the rectum and is absorbed by the body).

- *Patches* that are filled with medicine and placed on the skin (transdermal patches).

- *Injections.* There are many kinds of injections to give pain relief. Most injections use a tube or needle to place medicine directly into the body. These include:

  Subcutaneous injection—medicine is placed just under the skin using a small needle.

  Intravenous injection—medicine is placed directly into the vein through a needle that stays in the vein.

  Epidural or intrathecal injections—medicine is placed directly into the back using a small tube. Most of these injections give pain relief that lasts for many hours.

  Subdermal and intramuscular injections—commonly known as "shots," are injections that are placed more deeply into the skin or muscle using a needle. These injections are not recommended for long-term cancer pain treatment. Constantly having shots into the skin and muscle can be painful. Also, shots take longer to work, and you have to wait for them.

When to Take Your Pain Medicine

To help your pain medicine work best:

- Take your medicine on a regular schedule (by the clock). Taking medicine regularly and as your doctor tells you will help to keep pain under control. Do not skip a dose of medicine or wait for the pain to get worse before taking your medicine.

- Ask your doctor or nurse how and when to take extra medicine. If some activities make your pain worse (for example, riding in a car), you may need to take extra doses of pain medicines before these activities. The goal is to PREVENT the pain. Once you feel the pain, it is harder to get it under control.

- Treating pain is important, and there are many medicines and treatments that can be used. If one medicine or treatment does not work, there is another one that can be tried. Also, if a schedule or way that you are taking the medicine does not work for you, changes can be made. Talk to your doctors and nurses because they can work with you to find the pain medicine that will help you the most.

- It may be helpful for you to keep a record of how the medicine is working. Keeping a record and sharing it with your doctor or nurse will help to make your treatment more effective.

Other Treatments

Your doctor or nurse may recommend that you try other treatments along with your medicine to give you even more pain relief. Relaxation exercises help reduce pain. Many people find that cold packs, heating pads, massage, and rest help to relieve pain. Music or television may distract you from the pain. Your family members may want to help you to use these treatments. These treatments will help to make your medicines work better and relieve other symptoms, but they should not be used instead of your medicine.

Nondrug Treatments of Pain

Here are a few examples of treatments that can help to relieve your pain. You may use these treatments along with your regular medicine:

- Biofeedback
- Breathing and relaxation
- Imagery
- Massage, pressure, vibration
- Transcutaneous electrical nerve stimulation (TENS)
- Distraction
- Hot or cold packs
- Rest

Talk to your doctors and nurses about these treatments. They will be able to give you more information. Also, counseling and support groups may be able to tell you more.

When Medicine Is Not Enough

Some patients have pain that is not relieved by medicine. In these cases other treatments can be used to reduce pain:

- *Radiation therapy.* This treatment reduces pain by shrinking a tumor. A single dose of radiation may be effective for some people.

- *Nerve blocks.* Pain medicine is injected directly around a nerve or into the spine to block the pain.

- *Neurosurgery.* In this treatment pain nerves (usually in the spinal cord) are cut to relieve the pain.

- *Surgery.* When a tumor is pressing on nerves or other body parts, operations to remove all or part of the tumor can relieve pain.

Talk to your doctor about other pain treatments that will work for you.

The First Step

The key to getting the best pain relief is talking with your doctors and nurses about your pain. They will want to know how much pain you feel, where it is, and what it feels like. Answering the questions below may help you describe your pain.

- Where is the pain? You may have pain in more than one place. Be sure to list all of the painful areas.

- What does the pain feel like? Does it Ache? Throb? Burn? Tingle? You may wish to use other words to describe your pain.

- How bad is the pain?You can also use a number scale and rate your pain from 0 to 10: 0 means no pain and 10 means the worst pain. You can also describe your pain with words like none, mild, moderate, severe, or worst possible pain.

- What makes the pain better or worse? You may have already found ways to make your pain feel better. For example, using heat or cold, or taking certain medicines.

You may have also found that sitting or lying in certain positions or doing some activities affects the pain.

If you are being treated for pain now, how well is the treatment working? You may want to describe how well the treatment is working by saying how much of the pain is relieved all, almost all, none, etc.

Has the pain changed? You may notice that your pain changes over time. It may get better or worse or it can feel different. For example, the pain may have been a dull ache at first and has changed to a tingle. It is important to report changes in your pain. Changes in pain do not always mean that the cancer has come back or grown. Describe how the pain was before and how it is now.

After talking with you about your pain, your doctor or nurse may want to examine you or order x-rays or other tests.

These tests will help the doctor or nurse find the cause of your pain.

Having a Plan

You can work with your doctor or nurse to write a pain control plan to meet your needs. In a pain control plan, you and your doctor or nurse plan your pain control activities. This will include when to take your medicine, how and when to take extra medicine, and other things you can do to ease and prevent your pain. Your doctor or nurse may also list the medicines and other treatments you can use to help you with any side effects or other aches and pains, such as headaches.

Making the Plan Work

Some people find that the first pain control plan does not work for them. You and your doctor or nurse can change your pain control plan at any time. Here are some questions to ask yourself about the pain plan:

- Is the pain plan hard to follow?
- Is there any part of the plan that is hard to understand?
- Are you pleased with the pain control?
- Are you having trouble getting the medicine?
- Are you having trouble taking the medicine?
- Are you having side effects from the medicine?
- Is the medicine or the treatment causing a problem for you or your family?
- Are the nondrug treatments working for you?

Write down any other questions you have for your doctor or nurse.

Benefits and Risks of Treatment

This chapter talks about many different treatments for cancer pain. It also talks about side effects of medicines. Information about benefits and risks (side effects) of medicines may also be important to you. The list below describes the benefits and risks of the different types of medicines.

Nonopioids

Benefits: Control mild to moderate pain. Some can be bought without a prescription.

Risks: Some of these medicines can cause stomach upset. They can also cause bleeding in the stomach, slow blood clotting, and cause kidney problems. Acetaminophen does not cause these side effects, but high doses of it can hurt the liver.

Opioids

Benefits: These medicines control moderate to severe pain and do not cause bleeding.

Risks: May cause constipation, sleepiness, nausea and vomiting. Opioids sometimes cause problems with urination or itching. They may also slow breathing, especially when they are first given, but this is unusual in people who take opioids on a regular basis for pain.

Antidepressants

Benefits: Antidepressants help to control tingling or burning pain from damaged nerves. They also improve sleep.

Risks: These medicines may cause dry mouth, sleepiness, and constipation. Some cause dizziness and lightheadedness when standing up suddenly.

Anticonvulsants

Benefits: Help to control tingling or burning from nerve injury.

Risks: May hurt the liver and lower the number of red and white cells in the blood. It is important to have regular blood tests to check for these effects.

Steroids

Benefits: Help relieve bone pain, pain caused by spinal cord and brain tumors, and pain caused by inflammation. Steroids also increase appetite.

Risks: May cause fluid to build up in the body. May also cause bleeding and irritation to the stomach. Confusion is a problem for some patients when taking steroids.

Counseling and Peer Support

Pain can make you feel many emotions. You may feel sad, helpless, vulnerable, angry, depressed, lonely, isolated, or other emotions.

Lots of people feel these things when they are in pain. Often, when the pain is successfully treated, these feelings lift. Many people who have had cancer feel that counseling, religious, and other support groups have helped them to get back a sense of control and well being.

To find out more about support groups and to receive books and pamphlets about cancer pain, call or write to:

National Cancer Institute
Cancer Information Service
1-800-4-CANCER

Ask for the booklet *Questions and Answers About Pain Control.*

American Cancer Society
1-800-ACS-2345

The booklet *Questions and Answers About Pain Control* is also available from this group:

Wisconsin Cancer Pain Initiative
Medical Science Center, Room 3675
University of Wisconsin Medical School
1300 University Avenue
Madison, WI 53706
608-262-0978

For adults, ask for *Cancer Pain Can Be Relieved*. For children with cancer pain, ask for *Children's Cancer Pain Can Be Relieved*. For adolescents with cancer pain, ask for *Jeff Asks About Cancer Pain*.

Some Other Suggestions

Write down a list of nondrug pain control methods, along with additional instructions that may be required.

Write down important phone numbers, such as your doctor, your nurse, your pharmacy, and emergency telephone numbers.

Call your doctor or nurse immediately if your pain increases or if you have new pain. Also call your doctor early for a refill of pain medicines. Do not let your medicines get below 3 or 4 days' supply.

Slow Rhythmic Breathing For Relaxation

Deep breathing exercises can help relax you. These exercises may work along with your medicine to lessen or relieve your pain.

- Breathe in slowly and deeply.

- As you breathe out slowly, feel yourself beginning to relax; feel the tension leaving your body.

- Now breathe in and out slowly and regularly, at whatever rate is comfortable for you.

- To help you focus on your breathing and breathe slowly and rhythmically: (a) breathe in as you say silently to yourself, "in, two, three"; (b) breathe out as you say silently to yourself, "out, two, three." or Each time you breathe out, say silently to yourself a word such as "peace" or "relax." Do steps 1 through 4 only once or repeat steps 3 and 4 for up to 20 minutes.

- End with a slow deep breath. As you breathe out say to yourself "I feel alert and relaxed."

Relaxation Breathing Source: McCaffery and Beebe, *Pain: Clinical manual for nursing practice*, 1989. Adapted and reprinted with permission.

Pain Control Record

You can create a chart to rate your pain and to keep a record of how well the medicine is working. Write the information in the chart. Use the pain intensity scale to rate your pain before and after you take the medicine (see Figure 78.1).

Constipation

Constipation is a very common problem when taking opioid medications. When this happens, do the following:

- Increase fluid intake (8 to 10 glasses of fluid per day).

- Exercise regularly.

- Increase fiber in the diet (bran, fresh fruits, vegetables).

- Use a mild laxative, such as milk of magnesia, if no bowel movement in 3 days.

- Take (fill in medication) every day at (time) with a full glass of water.

- Use a glycerin suppository every morning (this may help make a bowel movement less painful).

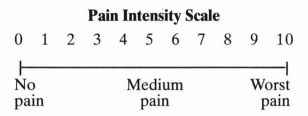

Pain Intensity Scale

0   1   2   3   4   5   6   7   8   9   10

| No | Medium | Worst |
| pain | pain | pain |

Figure 78.1. Pain Intensity Scale

For Further Information

The information in this chapter was taken from the Clinical Practice Guideline on Management of Cancer Pain. The guideline was written by a panel of private-sector experts sponsored by the Agency for Health Care Policy and Research. Other guidelines on common health problems are being developed.

To order a single copy of this booklet call the National Cancer Institute, Cancer Information Service at: 800-4-CANCER or write to:

Cancer Pain Guideline
AHCPR Publications Clearinghouse
P.O. Box 8547
Silver Spring, MD 20907

Chapter 79

Behavioral Therapy for Cancer Pain

Panel Endorses Behavioral Therapy for Cancer Pain

Behavioral therapies for chronic cancer pain should be accepted as part of cancer treatment and reimbursed as fully as surgery and chemotherapy, according to the recent recommendation of a National Institutes of Health technology assessment panel.

Despite the traditional bias of many insurance companies against behavioral therapies such as meditation, biofeedback, and hypnosis, said panel chairman Julius Richmond, M.D., professor of health policy emeritus at Harvard Medical School, Boston, available data support their effectiveness in relieving chronic pain. The panel of outside experts found that behavioral and relaxation techniques can help reduce pain arousal, while hypnosis reduces the perception of pain for a variety of conditions, including cancer. Richmond said that increasingly creative approaches have been used to relieve pain because traditional therapies such as surgery and drugs haven't worked. However, he emphasized that the panel doesn't view behavioral painrelief therapies as competitive with traditional medical treatment, but rather as an option in a comprehensive treatment plan.

Francis J. Keefe, Ph.D., a professor of medical psychology at Duke University Medical Center, Durham, N.C., noted that behavioral painrelief methods are especially important in oncology because 60% to

"Panel Endorses Behavioral Therapy for Cancer Pain," *Journal of the National Cancer Institute*, Vol. 87, No. 22, November 15, 1995.

80% of patients with advanced cancer have pain. Even today, he said, cancer patients often fear addiction and won't take enough medication to relieve their pain. According to Philip R. Lee, M.D., assistant secretary for health in the Department of Health and Human Services, cancer pain is widely undertreated even though it can be controlled in 90% of all cancer patients.

Early Introduction

The key to behavioral therapies is to introduce them early in the cancer patient's treatment and to use them along with—not as a substitute for—opioid drugs, said Ada Jacox, R.N., Ph.D., a professor in Johns Hopkins University's School of Nursing, Baltimore. Jacox said this early use of behavioral therapies is especially important because cancer patients often have pain from multiple sources (including treatments), which may last for years.

The panel stressed that behavioral therapies can be cost-effective. "These techniques are often as effective as medical therapy and often cheaper," said Alan F. Schatzberg, M.D., professor and chairman of the Department of Psychiatry at Stanford University School of Medicine, Palo Alto, Calif. While the panel found no scientific evidence that surgical debulking of a tumor to relieve pain is effective, Schatzberg said, hypnosis—in part because of its capacity for evoking intense relaxation—can be an effective noninvasive and inexpensive way of helping relieve cancer pain.

Helen J. Crawford, Ph.D., a researcher at the Department of Psychology at Virginia Polytechnic Institute and State University, Blacksburg, told the panel that hypnosis for chronic pain is equal to or more effective than bio-feedback—which uses monitoring instruments to help a patient influence physiological responses—and cognitive behavioral training, which strives to change a patient's negative thought patterns about pain.

Crawford said hypnosis appears to activate some of the descending inhibitory control systems that come from higher cognitive control centers in the brain's cerebral cortex. But, she said, "Still not fully understood is how hypnosis techniques can, even within minutes, dramatically reduce or eliminate what appear to be strongly developed neurosignatures of pain."

The NIH panel found that despite growing acceptance, many barriers to the use of behavioral pain-relief strategies remain. But, panelists said, "all are potentially surmountable," including attitudinal, bureaucratic, and financial obstacles.

No "Soft" Science

John D. Loeser, M.D., director of the University of Washington School of Medicine's Multidisciplinary Pain Center, Seattle, said that medical students are not trained to focus on what they perceive to be a "soft" science such as behavior. With this orientation, he said, physicians find it easier to write a prescription for a painkiller than to explore behavioral approaches.

But that attitude is changing, according to a recent survey, said panelist Brian M. Berman, M.D., director of the Division of Complementary Medicine at the University of Maryland School of Medicine, Baltimore. And ultimately, panelists said, physicians may not be the best health professionals to deliver behavioral therapies, "Physicians have so much to do, that this is just another skill for them to learn," said Stanley Krippner, Ph.D., a psychology professor at Saybrook Institute Graduate School and Research Center in San Francisco. He said master's level psychologists as well as nurse practitioners and social workers can help patients learn behavioral pain-control therapies.

As to the attitudes of patients themselves, panel member Bonnie B. O'Connor, Ph.D., assistant professor in the Department of Community and Preventive Medicine at the Medical College of Pennsylvania in Hershey, said that by the time patients come to behavioral pain-control therapies, "they've been from pillar to post and suffered greatly," and are often willing to try anything that might give them relief.

Panel member John P. Docherty, M.D., vice chairman of the Department of Psychiatry at Cornell University Medical College, said that managed care poses a threat to the delivery of behavioral therapies for the reduction of chronic pain because of "carve-outs" for mental health services—typically about 3% of plan revenues. If behavioral therapies for pain reduction are included in the carve-out, they could be seen as a potential drain on the plan's scarce resources, limiting their use.

Outside of managed care plans, insurance companies have their own ways of shutting out behavioral therapies. Loeser said that, in general, insurance companies fund only standard therapy and that "one way you control costs is you don't let anything new in." But, noted chairman Richmond, "When communities begin to demand something, things begin to happen." He predicted that patients themselves will force broader reimbursement of behavioral therapies for chronic pain because they will start demanding them.

—by Peggy Eastman

Chapter 80

Cancer Fatigue

While everyone knows what it feels like to be occasionally exhausted, cancer patients who suffer from fatigue—resulting from the disease itself or its treatment—often suffer from a debilitating exhaustion that can last days, weeks or months.

Cancer fatigue, often described by patients as a total lack of energy, is a near universal problem among cancer patients. It is the most common side effect of cancer and its treatment, affecting 76 percent of patients undergoing therapy. Unfortunately, while medical science has been making steady progress in treating cancer itself, cancer-related fatigue is frequently over-looked, under-recognized and under-treated.

"For many patients, fatigue is the constant reminder that they have cancer. Yet despite its prevalence and distressing consequences, it is one of the least understood symptoms of cancer," said Russell Portenoy, M.D., Department of Pain Medicine and Palliative Care, Beth Israel Medical Center, New York City, and chairman of The Fatigue Coalition, a multi-disciplinary group of medical practitioners, researchers and patient advocates that authored a recent survey about fatigue.

The causes and effects of fatigue are complex, and there is no established method to assess it. Patients may not report it and clinicians are usually focused on other indicators. Indeed, it is often dismissed by medical professionals with such comments as, "Of course you're tired—you have cancer," rather than viewed as a medical condition that can and should be addressed. While thousands of cancer

"About Cancer Fatigue," from the Oncology Nursing Society, www.cancerfatigue.org, 1999. Reprinted with permission.

studies have been conducted, researchers are only now beginning to study cancer fatigue.

Symptoms of Cancer Fatigue

Patients treated by either surgery, radiation or chemotherapy experience such side effects as pain, nausea, and fatigue as a consequence of the treatment. Some treatments, the cancer itself or other disorders can also lead to anemia (an abnormally low level of red blood cells), a frequent source of fatigue for cancer patients. The symptoms of cancer fatigue include not only feeling tired—weak, worn out, drained, "wiped out"—but also leg pain, difficulty climbing stairs or walking short distances, shortness of breath after light activity, and difficulty performing ordinary tasks such as cooking, cleaning, taking a shower or making the bed.

Cancer fatigue can have mental and emotional effects as well. Patients may have difficulty concentrating while reading or watching television, or have trouble thinking clearly and making decisions.

Fatigue also may underlie patients' feelings of low self-esteem and frustration, often resulting in feelings of helplessness or despair. Changes in sleep, daily activity or eating patterns can cause fatigue, as can anxiety, depression or stress.

Consequences of Fatigue

Aside from the discomfort of feeling exhausted, fatigue can pose a number of obstacles to coping with cancer and reaping the full benefits of available treatments. Fatigue can significantly interfere with a patient's quality of life and may limit the number of chemotherapy cycles that could be administered, which may limit the effectiveness of treatment altogether.

"It's not acceptable to tell patients that fatigue is just something they must live with," said Dr. Portenoy. "We need to create greater awareness about cancer-related fatigue and develop approaches for assessing and treating it. For some patients, treating fatigue may be as important as treating the disease."

Treating Cancer Fatigue

In many cases, the known causes of cancer-related fatigue can be treated and possibly relieved, at least to some degree. Proper nutrition, vitamin and mineral supplements, anti-depressant and anti-anxiety medications, lifestyle modifications and even psychological counseling can help alleviate fatigue.

To treat the anemia that contributes to fatigue, oncologists have traditionally relied on blood transfusions to raise red blood cell levels and help restore energy, if only temporarily. Although transfusions can bring quick but temporary results, many physicians try to avoid them because of potential risks. Today, medication for chemotherapy-related anemia can increase red blood cells, reduce the need for transfusion, and may improve a patient's ability to engage in everyday activities and cope with the disease.

Focusing Attention on Cancer Fatigue

Fatigue, like pain, is not easily measured. Caregivers need to realize that unrecognized fatigue may be a major factor when patients can't perform their jobs properly, keep up their daily activities or maintain social contacts.

In the early 1970s, medical authorities began to call attention to the prevalence and costs of under-treating pain. And, last year, the American Pain Society Quality of Care Committee issued a consensus statement calling for guidelines to improve patient well-being and to recognize potential obstacles to adequate pain management.

"Management of fatigue deserves the same attention as management of cancer pain," said David Cella, Ph.D., Director, Center on Outcomes, Research and Education, Evanston Northwestern Health Care, Northwestern University in Chicago, and a member of The Fatigue Coalition.

The Fatigue Coalition was formed in 1996 and will implement a series of educational and research initiatives during the next several years to elevate the importance of diagnosing and treating fatigue in cancer patients. The Coalition's first undertaking was a national survey of oncologists, cancer patients and caregivers to determine the incidence and impact of cancer fatigue.

"It is The Coalition's mission to promote greater understanding of cancer fatigue in the hope of improving the everyday life of cancer patients and their families," Dr. Cella said.

Cancer and Chemotherapy-Induced Anemia and Fatigue

Anemia, an abnormally low level of red blood cells, is a common complication of cancer and treatments such as chemotherapy and radiation therapy. Both cancer and its treatment can interfere with the supply of red blood cells—by inhibiting the production of bone marrow, or as a result of chronic blood loss during surgery. Although it is seldom life-threatening, cancer-related anemia can cause debilitating fatigue, and may have a severe impact on quality of life.

Prevalence. Although there is no accurate estimate of its prevalence among cancer patients, evidence suggests that most patients with cancer will develop anemia at some point during the course of their disease.

Symptoms. Fatigue affects up to 76% of cancer patients and is the most frequently reported symptom of anemia. Other clinical symptoms of anemia include dizziness, loss of appetite, inability to concentrate, shortness of breath, and cardiovascular problems such as chest pain and elevated heart rate.

Quality of life. Anemia and its chief symptom, fatigue, can affect quality of life in many ways. Loss of energy associated with anemia can limit a patient's ability to perform everyday activities, including work, social, and leisure activities. Fatigue also may result in emotional problems such as loss of self-esteem and depression. For some, severe fatigue may diminish a patient's ability to cope with the disease and its treatment.

Diagnosis. Cancer-related anemia can be diagnosed with a blood test which measures the volume of red blood cells in whole blood.

Treatment. Severe, chronic cancer-related anemia traditionally has been treated with blood transfusions as needed. However, transfusions may result in complications such as fever, allergic disorders, infections, and suppression of the immune system in about 20 percent of cases. Medications to stimulate red blood cell production are an alternative to blood-transfusion therapy. Proper nutrition, vitamin and mineral supplements, antidepressant and anti-anxiety medication, lifestyle modifications, and even psychological counseling also may help alleviate the fatigue associated with cancer and anemia.

Quick Tips for Coping with Cancer Fatigue

Though everyone experiences cancer fatigue differently, the following tips may help you manage your symptoms:

- Plan your day so that you have time to rest

- Take short naps or breaks rather than one, long rest period

- Eat as well as you can, and drink plenty of fluids

- Take short walks or do light exercise if possible

- Try easier or shorter versions of activities you enjoy

- Try activities that are less strenuous, like listening to music or reading

- Keep a diary of how you feel each day to help you plan your daily activities

- Join a support group

- Save your energy for the activities that are most important to you

- Become comfortable allowing others to take care of some of the things you normally do

- See what helps you feel less tired, and make those activities a priority for you

- Talk to your nurse or doctor about fatigue, there may be treatment available for your condition

Understanding Cancer Treatment-Related Fatigue: Facts You Should Know

- Fatigue is the most common side effect of cancer treatment.

- The fatigue experienced by a person with cancer is different from fatigue of everyday life. Cancer treatment-related fatigue can appear suddenly. It can be overwhelming. It is not always relieved by rest. It can last after treatment ends.

- Cancer treatment-related fatigue can affect many aspects of a person's life. It may affect an individual's mood or emotions. It may also affect a person's ability to do usual activities. Fatigue can make it hard to concentrate.

- Fatigue can have many causes; cancer treatment, loss of appetite, lack of exercise, and the cancer itself are all examples of causes of fatigue.

- Lack of understanding within a family about cancer fatigue can lead to communication problems, resentment, and feelings of guilt.

- For some people, careful planning of activities, exercise, and managing symptoms and side effects may help to alleviate fatigue.

- Cancer fatigue is real. It should not be ignored. Talk to your oncology nurse about what can be done to preserve quality in your life.

Managing Your Cancer Treatment-Related Fatigue

Fatigue is a feeling of tiredness that can keep you from doing the things you normally do or want to do. Fatigue is very common among people receiving cancer treatments. Factors such as cancer itself, low blood counts, nutritional problems, and sleep problems contribute to fatigue, but the exact cause is not known.

Signs of Fatigue

- You feel weary or exhausted. It may be physical, emotional, and/or mental exhaustion.

- Your body, especially your arms and legs, may feel heavy.

- You have less desire to do normal activities like eating or shopping.

- You may find it hard to concentrate or think clearly.

What You Can Do to Manage Your Fatigue

Rest. Rest and sleep are important, but don't overdo it. Too much rest can decrease your energy level. In other words, the more you rest, the more tired you will feel. If you have trouble sleeping, talk to your doctor or nurse.

Activity. Stay as active as you can. Regular exercise like walking several times each week may help.

Nutrition. Drink plenty of liquids. Eat as well as you can, and eat nutritious foods.

Energy Conservation. You can do more by spreading your activities throughout the day. Take rest breaks between activities. Rest breaks save energy for the things you want to do. Let others help you with meals, housework, or errands. Do not force yourself to do more than you can manage.

Energy Restoration. Do activities that you enjoy and make you feel good. Many people enjoy nature activities such as bird watching or gardening. Try listening to music, or visiting with friends and family, or looking at pleasant pictures. Try to do these activities at least three times per week.

Talk to Your Nurse

- If you have been too tired to get out of bed for the past 24 hours.

- If you feel confused or cannot think clearly.

- If your fatigue becomes worse.

Self-Care for the Caregiver: Managing Your Own Fatigue

Caregiver fatigue can be brought on by the physical and emotional demands placed on you because of the cancer diagnosis and treatment.

Below is a list of Fatigue Fighting Tips. It is important to maintain your own health and well being so that you can provide the best possible care to your loved one.

- Take time for yourself and your own needs.

- Watch for signs of stress such as impatience, loss of appetite, or difficulty sleeping.

- Eat a well-balanced diet. Drink plenty of water or juice every day.

- Exercise by taking short walks daily, or at least three times a week.

- Listen to relaxation tapes or music to help reduce stress.

- Space your activities with short rest periods. Get a good night's sleep.

- Don't overload your daily list of "things to do." Be realistic.

- Let family members and friends help. Delegate household chores, meals, baby sitting, or shopping.

- Share your feelings with family members or other caregivers, or join a support group.

- Keep the lines of communication open between your loved one, your family and friends, and the oncology nurse.

- Give yourself credit—the care you give does make a difference.

Chapter 81

Depression in Cancer Patients

Facts on Depression and Cancer

This year, an estimated 1.2 million Americans will be diagnosed with cancer. Receiving such a diagnosis is often traumatic, causing emotional upset, sadness, anxiety, poor concentration, and withdrawal. Often, this turmoil begins to abate within two weeks, with a return to usual functioning in about a month. When that doesn't happen, the patient must be evaluated for clinical depression, which occurs in about 10% of the general population and in about 25% of persons with cancer. Early diagnosis and treatment are important because depression adds to a patient's suffering and interferes with his or her motivation to engage in cancer treatment.

The symptoms of depression include:

- Persistent sad or "empty" mood

- Loss of interest or pleasure in ordinary activities, including sex

- Decreased energy, fatigue, being "slowed down"

- Sleep disturbances (insomnia, early-morning waking or oversleeping)

- Eating disturbances (loss of appetite and weight, or weight gain)

- Difficulty concentrating, remembering, making decisions

"Co-Occurrence of Depression with Cancer," National Institutes of Mental Health (NIMH) Fact Sheet.

- Feelings of guilt, worthlessness, helplessness
- Thoughts of death or suicide; suicide attempts
- Irritability
- Excessive crying
- Chronic aches and pains that don't respond to treatment

When five or more of these symptoms lasts for more than two weeks, are not caused by other illness or medication, or disrupt usual functioning, an evaluation for depression is indicated. While it may be difficult to say whether fatigue or appetite loss are due to depression or to cancer, their presence along with other depressive symptoms strongly indicates a diagnosis of clinical depression.

Depression Is Often Undiagnosed and Untreated

Depression in cancer patients goes unrecognized for several reasons. Sometimes, depression is misinterpreted to be a reaction to the diagnosis. Or the depressive symptoms are attributed to the cancer itself, which can also cause appetite loss, weight loss, insomnia, and loss of energy. Finally, depression may be viewed as just the side effect of cancer treatments such as corticosteroids or chemotherapy. These diagnostic hurdles can all be overcome by careful evaluation, which is important because regardless of the cause, when depression is present it must be treated.

Treating Depression Has Many Benefits

Research shows that, compared to patients without depression, depressed cancer patients experience greater distress, more impaired functioning and less ability to follow medical regimens. Studies also show that treating depression in these patents not only improves the psychological condition but reduces suffering and enhances quality of life. Therefore. professionals, patients, and families must be alert for depressive symptoms in cancer patients, and seek evaluation for depression when indicated.

Risk Factors

Studies also indicate that the more severe the medical condition, the more likely it is that a person will experience clinical depression.

Other factors which increase the risk of depression in persons with cancer are: history of depressive illness each year, alcohol or other substance abuse, poorly controlled pain, advanced disease, disability or disfigurement, medications such as steroids and chemotherapy agents, the presence of other physical illness, social isolation, and socio-economic pressures.

Effective Treatment for Depression

With treatment, up to 80% of all depressed people can improve, usually within weeks. Treatment includes medication, psychotherapy or a combination of both. The severity of the depression, the other conditions present, and the medical treatments being used must be considered to determine the appropriate treatment. Altering the cancer treatment may also help diminish depressive symptoms.

Antidepressant Medications

Several types of antidepressant medication are effective, none of them habit-forming. Most side-effects can be eliminated or minimized by adjustment in dosage or type of medication, so it is important for patients to discuss all effects with the doctor. Also, because responses differ, several trials of medicine may be needed before an effective treatment is found. In severe depression, medication is usually required and is often enhanced by psychotherapy.

In special circumstances, low doses of psychostimulant can be used to treat depression in cancer patients. These may be used when standard antidepressants produce side effects that, due to the patients physical condition are either intolerable or medically dangerous. Also psychostimulants may help alleviate post-surgical pain and their rapid effect (1-2 days) can aid medical recovery.

Psychotherapy

Interpersonal Therapy and Cognitive/Behavioral Therapy have also been shown to be effective in treating depression. These short-term (10-20 weeks) treatments involve talking with a therapist to recognize and change behaviors, thoughts, or relationships that cause or maintain depression and to develop more healthful and rewarding habits.

Psychological treatment of patients with cancer, even those without depression, has been shown to be beneficial in a number of ways.

These include: improving self-concept and sense of control, and reducing distress, anxiety, pain, fatigue, nausea, and sexual problems. In addition, there is some indication that psychological intervention may increase survival time in some cancer patients.

Electroconvulsive Therapy

Electroconvulsive therapy (ECT) is a safe and often effective treatment for severe depression. Because it is fast-acting, it may be of particular use for depression in cancer patients who experience severe weight loss or debilitation, or who cannot take or do not respond to antidepressant medications.

Medical Management

The benefits from the standard treatments described above are maximized by the effective management of pain and other medical conditions in depressed cancer patients.

The Path to Healing

Depression can be overcome through recognition of symptoms, and evaluation and treatment by a qualified professional. Family and friends can help by encouraging the depressed person to seek or remain in treatment. Participating in a support group may be a helpful addition to treatment. For additional information about depression, write to:

DEPRESSION
National Institute of Mental Health (NIMH)
6001 Executive Boulevard
Rm. 8184, MSC 9663
Bethesda, MD 20892-9663

For free brochures on depression and its treatment, call: 1-800-421-4211

Chapter 82

Facing Forward: A Guide for Cancer Survivors

Introduction

Who Should Read "Facing Forward"?

If you are an adult who is getting on with your life after a diagnosis for cancer, this guide is for you. Whether your treatment took place in childhood, 5 years ago, or last week, you may share common concerns with other cancer survivors. The purpose of this guide is to present a concise overview of some of the most important survivor issues and practical ideas to help you look ahead. If you are just finishing cancer treatment, the information may prepare you for situations you have not yet experienced. As you read about handling possible problems, keep in mind that not everyone will have all these concerns. If you are a long term cancer survivor, many of these issues will not be new to you. But some of the ideas and resources may add to your own experience.

Facing Forward should also be shared with your family or friends—the people who care about you. In some cases, they can use this guide to understand issues you may face so that they can support you with real understanding of your needs. In other cases, they will use the ideas and resources in this guide when acting on your behalf—for example, in processing your bills and dealing with your insurance company and your medical care providers. Finally, it is

Facing Forward: A Guide for Cancer Survivors, National Cancer Institute, NIH Publication 93-2424, October 1992.

important for your family to know about how your concerns may affect them, and the options they have for getting help.

How to Use the Materials

The key to using *Facing Forward* is to let it meet your needs. Each section can stand alone, so if you are interested only in one issue right now, that section is all you need to read. Or you may want to read it from beginning to end to get the big picture.

Facing Forward is divided into four major sections:

- Continuing to Care for Your Health
- Taking Care of Your Feelings
- Managing Insurance Issues
- Earning a Living

Each section follows the same format:

- *What You Can Expect* relates the experiences of other cancer survivors. The situations presented in these sections represent a combination of documented experiences. Some of the accounts were suggested by cancer survivors who reviewed the materials.
- *Briefs* present quick facts or statistics about cancer issues.
- *Tips* offers practical suggestions for handling problems.
- *Options* offers alternative approaches for taking control of your situation.
- *Resources* lists materials and organizations that can give you more detailed information and help.

Each section can be used in four main ways:

- To bring up some key issues that you may find interesting.
- To suggest topics and questions you may want to discuss with professionals who can help, such as your doctors and nurses, social workers, and clergy.
- To serve as a long-term resource you can use over time as problems arise.
- To help you organize your cancer information.

Take notes and write down the answers to the questions you ask professionals. Write in names and telephone numbers for your doctors, nurses, and social works; local cancer support resources; and insurance inquiries. Record helpful options you've found—you may want to pass the information to friends or coworkers who become cancer survivors. Keep track of your medical history: the tests, treatments, and medications you have received and when you received them.

How "Facing Forward" Was Developed

The National Cancer Institute's Office of Cancer Communications and the National Coalition for Cancer Survivorship worked together on the project. Our first step was to ask cancer survivors which issues were most important to them and what kinds of information they needed to take charge of their lives. Next, we looked at the growing body of research (and personal histories) on the issues important to survivors. We pulled together some of the key facts and recommendations from the experts and put the information in a style we hoped would be easy to use. Finally, we tested the materials with cancer survivors to be sure it was clear, appropriate, and relevant to "real life" situations.

We hope this guide helps you find the options that work best for you, family members, and friends as you begin facing forward after cancer.

Continuing to Care for Your Health

What You Can Expect

After you have been treated for cancer, you will have two ongoing health needs. First, you'll want to take the health steps that doctors suggest for anyone your age. Second, you'll have special needs for caring for your body based on your type of cancer, treatment, and current state of health. (See "Briefs.")

Other long-term health needs for cancer survivors differ from person to person. In addition to regular checkups, you may need rehabilitation or home care. Some survivors may need help in dealing with emotional or sexual problems, while others may seek pain control therapy. And more cancer treatment sometimes occurs. To get a good picture of your individual needs, ask your doctor. He or she can let you know what you need to do this year—and in the future—to take care of your health. The following stories highlight some of the most common issues for cancer survivors.

861

"I had expected that leaving the hospital after cancer treatment would be the happiest day of my life. When that time came, though, I was actually more afraid than happy. I felt very alone, and I missed the support of being watched over and cared for by the medical team. My social worker said that this was a common reaction, but I remember that my family had a hard time understanding it." —Jack C.

"In the first couple of years after my recovery, the thing I hated most was going in for my checkups. Just seeing the hospital again reminded me of a part of my life I'd rather have forgotten. I had an almost physical reaction to the sounds and smells of the place. But more than that, those visits reminded me that I'd been sick and that my cancer might recur. In my daily life, I'd kept those thoughts out of my mind. Fortunately, it's better now. Maybe I've just gotten used to the routine, and I also understand how important these checkups are to my health." —Janet V.

"I find I walk a fine line between watching for signs of recurrence or long-term effects of my radiation therapy and going overboard. I never used to be like this, but it's hard not to be scared by changes that might mean problems. My first doctor was not very sympathetic about my concerns, so I found another doctor who is. She understands, and she doesn't tell me 'it's all in your head.'" —Louise F.

"I'm in a support group for cancer survivors, and we have people with all kinds of cancers who've made all kinds of adjustments: living with artificial limbs, ostomies, breast changes, energy loss, chronic pain. But we all have one thing in common. At one time or another we each have been so angry that this happened to us. Before I joined the group, my anger was having as much of a negative effect on my life as my disability. Talking about it, and seeing how others cope, helped me put things in perspective." —Sacha R.

"When I think about my cancer treatment, I almost feel like it began when I left the hospital after surgery. Much of my care took place at home—for a while my room looked like a hospital. Now I'm back to the hospital some times for radiation therapy to control my pain. I'm getting used to the fact that my cancer is more like a lifelong, chronic disease that I need to manage than something the doctors can 'cure' once and for all." —Irene L.

"My family wonders if it's a waste of time and money for me to get yearly checkups for the colon cancer I had 15 years ago. But I feel that I'm doing something important for my health." —Rhea S.

Briefs

Basics of Health Care for Cancer Survivors

- Get regular checkups. In general, people who have been treated for cancer return regularly to the doctor every 3-4 months at first, and once or twice a year later on. Ask your doctor how often you should be rechecked.

- Be alert to signs of a possible return of cancer and long-term effects of treatment. Ask your doctor to explain what symptoms should be watched.

- Get tested as needed for other cancers. Your doctor can tell you how often you should have tests to detect breast cancer and colon cancer. With early detection, these cancers often can be controlled.

- Have good health habits: Eating right and getting enough sleep and exercise will help you feel better.

Tips for Managing Your Care

- Keep accurate, up-to-date records of all the medical care you receive for cancer and other conditions. Future decisions about your care may depend on how you have been treated in the past. If you move or go to several different doctors, no one but you will have your complete history.

- Do things you enjoy, even if you don't feel perfect. Pleasure can be a powerful tool for health.

- Work as a partner with your doctors and other health professionals in your continuing care. When you first were treated for cancer, you may have taken an active part in making decisions about your care. The same active role can help you take control of your long term health needs. The two main steps are to ask questions and give information to your caregivers.

Ask questions. You need information to carry out your role in managing your care. These facts are as important to quality of care as any other aspect of treatment. With this in mind, no question you have about your care is "dumb." Many people bring a tape recorder, take notes, or ask a friend along to help them remember everything that's said. It is also a good idea to bring a list of questions when you visit your doctor. The following are some questions you may want to ask:

- How often should I have a checkup?

- What are the signs of cancer's return or of long-term effects?

- How likely are they to occur?

- What changes might I see that are not danger signs?

- What kind of diet should I have?

- What are my treatment options for handling chronic pain, the return of cancer, the long-term effects of therapy?

- What is the best way to talk to you about my concerns? (By phone? At a special appointment? At a regular visit scheduled in advance to run longer?)

- Who else is available to talk with me about specific problems (e.g. sexual concerns, care instructions, general fitness)?

Give information. Doctors need to know key facts about you to pre-scribe the best treatments and help keep you involved in your care. Tell them:

- What medicines you now are taking for all conditions (including over-the-counter medicines such as aspirin or laxatives). Doctors need this information to avoid problems when they give you a new medicine.

- About fears or concerns you have, especially those that might be keeping you from following treatment. Talking openly may help solve the problem.

- About changes in your lifestyle. Even changes that seem minor could affect your treatment. For example, if you quit smoking you may need a different dose of some medicines.

- How you are feeling. Include danger signs you may have noticed as well as any other changes that may be worrying you.

- About problems you may have and how much the doctor tells you about your cancer. You have a right to hear as much or as little information as you wish.

Options for Coping with Body Changes

Get help if you need it. Ask your nurse or the social worker at your hospital about homemaker services, home health services, seminars and classes, rides to the hospital, and other community aid.

Find out how to use special tools to over come disability or discomfort. Mechanical aids can replace many lost functions. Talk to your rehabilitation professional.

Learn from others who have the same problem. Ask your local cancer support organization, social worker, or doctor's office staff to put you in touch with other survivors. They can give you practical tips to make your new situation easier.

Find ways to meet your needs for intimacy.

- Most survivors of any cancer can still enjoy sexual touching and sexual closeness.

- Talk to your doctor, nurse, or therapist to learn proven ideas for solving problems.

Focus on your best features. Make the most of them with makeup, clothes, or accessories. Feel good about yourself.

Find new shopping sources for products that help you look better. Ask your local cancer support organization, your social worker, and other survivors for ideas and addresses (see Resources).

Resources

Additional Reading

Cancer patients, their families and friends, and others may find the following booklets useful. They are available free of charge by calling the Cancer Information Service (1-800-4-CANCER).

- * *Chemotherapy and You: A Guide to Self-Help During Treatment.* Explains chemotherapy and addresses problems and concerns of patients undergoing this treatment.

- *Datos sobre el tratamiento de quimioterapia contra el cancer.* Introduces chemotherapy to Spanish-speaking persons.

- *Eating Hints for Cancer Patients*. Provides recipes and tips that help patients meet their needs for good nutrition during treatment.

- *El tratamiento de radioterapia: guia para el paciente durante el tratamiento*. Provides an explanation of radiation therapy for Spanish-speaking persons.

- * *Radiation Therapy and You: A Guide to Self-Help During Treatment*. Explains radiation therapy and addresses concerns of patients receiving radiation treatment.

- *Taking Time: Support for People With Cancer and the People Who Care About Them*. Discusses the emotional side of cancer— how to deal with the disease and to learn to talk with friends, family members, and others about cancer.

- *What Are Clinical Trials All About?* Explains clinical trials (studies of new cancer treatments) to help patients decide if they want to take part in a trial.

- *What You Need To Know About...* This is a series of booklets. Each provides information about a specific type of cancer. These booklets discuss symptoms, diagnosis, treatment, emotional is-sues, and questions to ask the doctor about a number of cancer types. Some are available in Spanish.

- * *When Cancer Recurs: Meeting the Challenge Again*. Explains the ways that cancer may recur and discusses types of treat-ment and methods of coping with recurrence.

[* Publications marked with an asterisk are reprinted in this volume: See Table of Contents]

Magazines and Journals

Hundreds of articles on cancer are published each year. You can locate those that appear in popular magazines and journals in the Reader's Guide to Periodical Literature, which is available in most public libraries. If you need help using the guide or finding an article, ask a librarian.

You can find articles published in over 3,000 health-science jour-nals by looking in *Index Medicus*. Medical libraries, most colleges and universities, and some public libraries carry this resource.

You also can locate cancer-related articles published in technical jour-nals by using or having access to the National Library of Medicine's (NLM) MEDLARS program. MEDLARS, in turn, provides access to

CANCERLIT, a computerized database system which contains almost 1 million citations and abstracts of articles on cancer from technical literature published since 1963.

Librarians in medical libraries and in libraries at nursing schools can retrieve information stored in MEDLARS. However, if you or your doctor want to get information using your own computer system, you can contact NLM at the following address or telephone number:

MEDLARS MANAGEMENT SECTION
National Library of Medicine
8600 Rockville Pike
Bethesda, MD 20894
(301) 496-6193
(800) 638-8480

Your local library also may be able to do a computer information search. If it belongs to the Federal Library System, you may be able to borrow government publications.

Additional Resources

Looking Good

Some people who've had cancer treatment must adjust to a new body image. Cosmetic aids, such as artificial limbs or wigs, may help boost self-confidence as well as provide physical comfort. After a mastectomy, for example, a woman may wear a breast form to give shape and weight to where her breast was removed. Patients who lose hair due to chemotherapy may wear wigs.

If you are a woman interested in making the most of your appearance, contact the Look Good, Feel Better program through local American Cancer Society offices or at 1-800-395-LOOK.

If you are over 65, have had a mastectomy and want reconstructive surgery or a prosthesis, you may want to contact your local Medicare office. Medicare covers either of these if necessary due to a mastectomy. The coverage is the same in all states.

If you plan to buy a cosmetic aid, you may want to contact your local American Cancer Society unit, which may have a list of stores that sell them. The unit also may maintain a "wig bank," a collection of wigs that are given free of charge to cancer patients. Or call the Cancer Information Service at 1-800-4-CANCER, which may have a list of local stores that sell the product you need. And check with your insurance company. Some policies cover some cosmetic aids.

These books on cosmetic aids also may be useful:

- *Looking Up: The Complete Guide to Looking and Feeling Good for the Recovering Cancer Patient*, Suzy Kalter. McGraw-Hill: 1987. Provides tips (with photos) on hair care, wigs, makeup, and exercise. (Out of print; check your local library to find a copy.)

- *Buyer's Guide to Wigs and Hairpieces*. This 2-page summary is available, as well as additional literature as needed. Contact Ruth L. Weintraub Co. Inc., 420 Madison Avenue, Suite 406, New York, NY 10017, (212)838-1333.

- A full-color catalogue of wigs for medical purposes is available nationwide. Contact Jacques Darcel, 50 West 57th Street, New York, NY 10019, (212)753-7576.

Sexual Concerns

Cancer and cancer treatment may affect sexual relationships. Although treatment for cancer sometimes causes sexual problems, often a patient's or partner's feelings about cancer and sex can make a difference. Your doctor, nurse, or social worker may be able to help. They also may be able to help you find a sex therapist who helps couples understand their sexual problems and suggests ways to deal with them. The following association can provide names of sex therapists in your area:

American Association of Sex Educators, Counselors, and Therapists (ASECT)
Suite 1717
435 North Michigan Avenue
Chicago, IL 60611
(312) 644-0828

If you write ASECT, be sure to include a self-addressed, stamped envelope and a $3.00 handling fee.

The American Cancer Society has two publications on sexuality that may be helpful:

- *Sexuality and Cancer: For the Woman Who Has Cancer and Her Partner*

- *Sexuality and Cancer: For the Man Who Has Cancer and His Partner*

Contact your local unit or the national office at 1-800-ACS-2345 to get copies.

Taking Care of Your Feelings

What You Can Expect

What kinds of feelings are "normal"? There is no "right" way to feel; the important thing is to handle your emotions in a way that works for you. Many survivors find that the key for them is talking their feelings out—with family and friends, health professionals, other patients, and counselors such as clergy and psychotherapists.

The following stories show the range of feelings that many cancer survivors have. Each of them is a normal reaction that is often part of the cancer survivor's life.

"In the first 6 months after my cancer treatment, I saw my cancer more as a threat to my life plans for marriage and a career than I did as a threat to my life. I felt the most depressed and anxious during the first 3 months, but then I started to get back to normal. I say started, because I'm not sure I'm there yet. It's getting better, but I still feel a little off balance." —Marcia B.

"I don't intend to focus on cancer for the rest of my life. I follow my care plan but I don't dwell on the disease or talk about it to others. Some (I suppose) well-meaning people at the office said that my reaction is called denial, and that it is bad for me. I talked about it with the doctor, and he said denial can be positive when it helps you get on with your life. I have my ups and downs like every one else, but I feel good about the way I'm handling my disease." —Joe K.

"I have to say that there's been one positive result of my having had cancer. It made me look at the real possibility of my own death, something I had never thought much about before. That made me take a hard look at my life and decide what really mattered to me. As a survivor, I now see every day as a precious gift." —Vicki W.

"My cancer treatment ended 10 years ago, but I still get anxious every time I go in for a checkup. The nurse told me that's a common reaction." —Dave L.

"I was very surprised at how few of my friends really made the effort to 'be there' for me. I talked to the nurse about this during my last checkup. She said that people often want to help but they don't know how—and they may be embarrassed to ask. So I decided to make the first move with some of the people I cared about most. It was hard, but I think I broke down a wall when I spoke openly about my feelings and my needs. I feel much more in touch and supported now" —Rhonda L.

"My cancer has led to some difficult family situations. The hardest thing was learning to adjust to different family roles. My wife went back to work during my recovery, and my teenage daughter had to take care of the house. As I got better, none of us was sure what roles were 'normal' and my daughter especially didn't want any changes that limited her independence. At that point the doctor suggested family therapy. I had my doubts, but seeing the real problems behind the obvious problems made a difference. After we worked through solutions together, I think we're closer now than ever before." —Ralph Y.

"The most important source of hope and support for me has been my faith in God. When I face my fears and uncertainties, I know I'm not alone." —Frances C.

"Surviving cancer has been not one condition but many. It was such happiness at the birth of a daughter in the midst of concerns about the future. It was the joy of eating Chinese food for the first time after radiation burns in my esophagus had healed. It has been the anxiety of waiting for test results and the fear that the cancer would recur. It has been having a positive attitude and wanting to strangle the people who told me that was all it would take." —Frank T.

"People have recovered from every type of cancer, no matter how gloomy the first reports. Yes, we're all going to die someday of something. But I plan to push that day back as far as I can, and to go out fighting whenever the time comes." —Betty R.

Briefs

Surviving Cancer: Hopeful Trends

- There are over 8 million cancer survivors in America today.

- If lung cancer deaths were excluded, cancer mortality would have declined 14 percent between 1950 and 1990.

- The number of people who have survived cancer for 5 or more years has increased significantly since 1973 for cancers of the colon, stomach, testis, and bladder, and for Hodgkin's disease and leukemia.

- Studies show that for most patients the emotional upset after cancer diagnosis and treatment decreases over time.

Tips for Coping With Survivor Stress

The following tips come from the experiences of survivors in the American Cancer Society's "I Can Cope" program. They are adapted from ideas appearing in a book, *I Can Cope—Staying Healthy With Cancer*, coauthored by the program's cofounder, Judi Johnson.

- Be kind to yourself. Instead of telling yourself you can't do something you should do, focus on what you can do and what you want to do. Instead of telling yourself you look awful, think of ways to make the most of your best features.

- Help others. Reaching out to someone else can reduce the stress caused by brooding.

- Don't be afraid to say no. Polite but firm refusals help you stay in control of your life.

- Talk about your concerns. It's the best way to release them.

- Learn to pace yourself. Stop before you get tired.

- Give in sometimes. Not every argument is worth winning.

- Get enough exercise. It's a great way to get rid of tension and aggression in a positive way.

- Take time for activities you enjoy, whether it's a hobby, club, or special project.

- Take one thing at a time. If you're feeling overwhelmed, divide your list into manageable parts.

- Set priorities. Don't try to be Superman or Superwoman.

- Solve problems like an expert. First, identify the problem and write it down, so it's clear in your mind. Second, list your options with the pros and cons of each. Third, choose a plan.

Fourth, list the steps to accomplish it. Then give yourself a deadline and act. Sometimes just having a plan can reduce the stress of the problem.

- Eat properly.
- Get enough sleep.
- Laugh at least once a day.

Is a Survivors' Group Right?

If you answer "yes" to most of the following questions, joining a cancer survivors' group may be a positive step for you.

- Are you comfortable sharing your feelings with others in a similar situation?
- Are you interested in hearing others' feelings about their experiences?
- Could you benefit from the advice of others who have gone through cancer treatment?
- Do you enjoy being part of a group?
- Do you have helpful information or hints to share with others?
- Would reaching out to support other cancer survivors give you satisfaction?
- Would you feel comfortable working with survivors who have different ways of facing forward?
- Are you interested in learning more about cancer and survivor issues?
- Focus on the positive. If you have a setback, think about all of the good things you've done.

Options for Getting Emotional Support

- Join a cancer survivors' group. Ask your doctor, nurse, or social worker about programs available at local hospitals. Call your local cancer support organizations, including the American Cancer Society, which may sponsor groups in your area. Check the telephone book for contact information.
- Talk to your family and friends. Help them understand how they can help you. Talk about their needs for support.

- Talk to your clergyman or clergywoman. Consider professional mental health assistance. Consult a psychologist, nurse therapist, clinical social worker, or psychiatrist. For marital or family issues, consult a licensed or family therapist.

- Work with someone on the medical team to solve problems. Get help in dealing with your hospital, clinic, or health maintenance organization. Ask about health concerns that cause you stress.

- Support yourself. Draw on your own strength. Read about how others cope. Ask at your local bookstore for accounts by cancer survivors.

- Reach out to others. Helping others can help you feel stronger and more in control. For some people, helping other cancer survivors is a satisfying way to reach out.

Resources

Additional Reading

Taking Time: Support for People With Cancer and the People Who Care About Them. Discusses the emotional side of cancer: how to deal with the disease and learn to talk with friends, family members, and others about cancer. Available free of charge by calling the National Cancer Institute's Cancer Information Service at 1-800-4 CANCER.

Newsletters

The Networker National Coalition for Cancer Survivorship
1010 Wayne Avenue
5th Floor
Silver Spring, MD 20910
(301) 650-8868

Surviving
Pat Fobair
Stanford University Medical Center
Department of Radiation Oncology
Division of Radiation Therapy, Room H013
300 Pasteur Drive
Stanford, CA 94305
(415) 723-7881

Additional Resources

- Cancer Survivor Groups. To find out about groups in your area, contact:

    Your local Cancer Information Service at 1-800-4-CANCER.

    Your local office of the American Cancer Society at 1-800-ACS-2345.

    Your hospital social services department.

Family Concerns

To help alleviate or resolve tensions that cancer may cause in families and other close relationships, the following associations can provide referrals to marriage and family counselors:

- Your local Cancer Information Service at 1-800-4-CANCER.

- Your local religious and community social service agencies (check the yellow pages for the telephone numbers).

- Your local senior centers.

- Your local community mental health centers.

- American Association for Marriage and Family Therapy, 1100 17th Street, NW Washington, DC 20036 (202) 452-0109

- American Association of Sex Educators, Counselors, and Therapists (ASECT) Suite 1717, 435 North Michigan Avenue Chicago, IL 60611 (312) 644-0828

- American Family Therapy Association 2020 Pennsylvania Avenue Suite 273 Washington, DC 20006 (202) 944-2776

- National Association of Social Workers 750 First Street, NE Suite 700 Washington, DC 20020 (202) 408-8600

Managing Insurance Issues

What You Can Expect

If you are like most cancer survivors, the costs of initial treatment and continuing care are a major concern. What happens to insurance coverage and costs after you've had treatment for cancer?

In general, people who had life and health insurance before treatment are able to keep it, although costs and benefits may changes.

Those who change jobs or apply for new policies, however, often face problems.

The stories of the following cancer survivors show common post-treatment insurance experiences.

"I'm grateful my insurance benefits are safe at my company. I only wish my job had more going for it. I'm working hard to find something that pays better and offers more growth. But along with finding the right job, I'm also looking for a good benefits package that is fully open to a cancer survivor. So far, the two haven't come together." —Ron L.

"I never even thought about life insurance before I got cancer. My wife and I are young, and we had enough expenses. But after my diagnosis, I felt like I should get some insurance for my wife's sake. It turned out to be harder than I'd expected. Several companies refused to accept me at all. I have coverage now, but the policy has an 'exclusion' for cancer, and it pays nothing if cancer is the cause of death. My doctor says it's very unlikely that my cancer will recur. But I'm still looking for another policy where having had cancer doesn't hurt me." —Burt W.

"I knew I had health insurance, but I had no idea what it covered. And when I went into the hospital, the last thing on my mind was the cost of the treatment. When the bills started coming in, I was shocked that my company's insurance policy didn't cover everything. At first, I felt like everything about my health had gone out of my control, but I started to take charge again by learning about the claims process and pleading my own case." —Bill G.

"My insurance company paid for all of my cancer care, but my radiation treatment made me unable to father a child. When my wife and I looked into artificial insemination, we found that insurance would not cover the cost of donor sperm. We decided to adopt a child instead." —Brian K.

"When my health insurance company canceled my individual policy after my cancer treatment, I started checking into other options. My best bet turned out to be joining my new company's group policy, even though employees have to pay all their own premiums. The benefits are pretty good, and they accepted me despite the cancer history. But I had to fill out a health history and have a physical exam that none of my coworkers had to complete. There was also a 5-year 'waiting period' before I could submit any bills for cancer care. Luckily, I got through 5 years with no major expenses." —Jean T.

"I had been covered under my husband's health insurance policy, and we had no problems until he changed jobs. When the new company saw my cancer history, they denied him family coverage. I was finally able to get insurance through my state health insurance pool." —Laura S.

"Health insurance after cancer treatment worked pretty much like my car insurance: After I had an accident, my rates went up." —Barbara K.

Briefs

States That Provide Health Insurance Coverage for the Hard-to-Insure

A number of states currently sell comprehensive health insurance to state residents with serious medical conditions who can't find a company to insure them. Listed below are states and the companies that run their programs. (Several other states have programs planned that are not yet operational.) If your state isn't listed, you may want to contact the State Department of Insurance to find out if such programs are available in your state. Call directory assistance in your state capital for contact information.

Arizona
Arizona Department of Insurance
2910 North 44th Street
Suite 210
Emil Barberich (Hotline Monitor)
Phoenix, AZ 85018
(800) 544-9208
(602) 912-8450

California
California Major Risk Medical
Insurance Program c/o Blue Cross of California
P.O. Box 9044
Oxnard, CA 93031-9044
(800) 289-6574

Colorado
Colorado Uninsurable Health Insurance Plan
Philadelphia American Life Insurance
3121 Buffalo Speedway
Houston, TX 77098
(303) 863-1960
(800) 67-CUHIP

Connecticut
Health Reinsurance Association of Connecticut
Travelers' Insurance Company
One Tower Square
9MS
Hartford, CT 06183-2937
(800) 842-0004

Florida
Florida Comprehensive Health Association
971 E. Tennessee Street
Tallahassee, FL 32308
(800) 766-3242

Georgia
Georgia Insurance Department
#2 Martin Luther King Drive, SE
Atlanta, GA 30334
(404) 656-6054

Hawaii
State Health Insurance Program
1000 Bishop Street, Room 908
Honolulu, HI 96813
(808) 586-4141

Illinois
Illinois Comprehensive Health Insurance Plan
Blue Cross and Blue Shield of Illinois
P.O. Box 2401
ICHIP Administrative Unit
18th Floor
Chicago, IL 60690
(800) 367-6410

Indiana
Indiana Comprehensive Health
Insurance Association
9525 Delegates Row
P.O. Box 40438
Indianapolis, IN 46240-0438
(800) 552-7921
(317) 581-1005

Iowa
Iowa Comprehensive Health Association
P.O. Box 40699
Indianapolis, IN 46240-0699
(800) 877-5156

Kansas
Kansas Health Insurance Association
c/o LaHood and Associates
P.O. Box 12170
Overland Park, KS 66282-2170
(913) 362-0040
(800) 255-6065

Louisiana
Louisiana Health Insurance Association
7904 Wrenwood
Suite D
Baton Rouge, LA 70809
(504) 926-6245

Maine
Maine Bureau of Insurance
State House Station 34
Augusta, ME 04333
(207) 582-8707

Minnesota
Minnesota Comprehensive Health Association
P.O. Box 64560
St. Paul, MN 55164
(800) 382-2000

Mississippi
Mississippi Comprehensive Health Insurance
Risk Pool Association
P.O. Box 13748
Jackson, MS 39236
(601) 362-0799

Missouri
Missouri Health Insurance Pool
1831 Chestnut Street
St. Louis, MO 63103
(800) 843-6447

Montana
Montana Comprehensive Health Association
404 Fuller Avenue
Helena, MT 59601
(800) 447-7828
(406) 444-8200

Nebraska
Nebraska Comprehensive Health Insurance Pool
Blue Cross and Blue Shield of Nebraska
P.O. Box 3248
Main Post Office Station
Omaha, NE 68180-0001
(800) 356-3485

New Mexico
New Mexico Comprehensive Health Insurance Pool
Blue Cross and Blue Shield of New Mexico
P.O. Box 27630
Albuquerque, NM 87125-7630
(800) 432-0750

North Dakota
Comprehensive Health Association of North Dakota
4510 13th Avenue, SW
Fargo, ND 58121
(701) 282-1100
(800) 737-0016

Oregon
Oregon Medical Insurance Pool
796 Winter Street, NE
Salem, OR 97310
(800) 848-7280

South Carolina
South Carolina Health Insurance Pool
P.O. Box 61153
Columbia, SC 29260
(800) 868-2500
(803) 736-0043

Tennessee
Tennessee Comprehensive Health Insurance Pool
P.O. Box 6249
Chattanooga, TN 37401-6249
(800) 533-9892
(615) 755-5918

Utah
Utah Comprehensive Health Insurance Pool
P.O. Box 27797
Salt Lake City, UT 84127
(800) 624-6519 (in Utah)
(800) 662-0876 (out of state)
(801)481-6063

Washington
Washington State Health Insurance Pool
P.O. Box 31726
Omaha, NE 68131
(800) 228-4044

Wisconsin
Wisconsin Health Insurance Risk Sharing Plan
Blue Cross Blue Shield United of Wisconsin
1515 North River Center Drive
Milwaukee, Wl 53212
(800) 828-4777

Wyoming
Wyoming Health Insurance Pool

P.O. Box 2419
Cheyenne, WY 82003
(800) 438-5768

The following states have Blue Cross and Blue Shield plans that offer some policy year-round or at a designated time period for the hard-to-insure. Many states have restrictions/waiting periods based on the individual's medical history.

Alaska
Short-term program that provides six-month coverage.
Blue Cross of Washington and Alaska
2550 Denali Street
Suite 600
Anchorage, AK 99503
(907) 258-5065

District of Columbia
Plan available to residents of the Washington, DC metropolitan area: the District of Columbia (DC), Montgomery and Prince George's County in Maryland (MD), and most of Northern Virginia (VA), Enrollment is available in spring and fall for MD/DC residents, year-round for VA residents.
Blue Cross and Blue Shield of the National Capital Area
550 12th Street, SW
Washington, DC 20065
(202) 484-9100

Maryland
Enrollment available in the spring and fall each year.
Blue Cross and Blue Shield Open Enrollment Policy
10455 Mill Run Circle
Owings Mills, MD 21117
(800) 544-8703

Massachusetts
Year-round enrollment available.
Blue Cross and Blue Shield of Massachusetts Non-Group Coverage
P.O. Box 9140
North Quincy, MA 02171-9140
(800) 822-2700
(617) 956-3934

Michigan
Year-round enrollment available.
Blue Cross and Blue Shield of Michigan
600 East Lafayette
Department B613
Detroit, Ml 48226
(800) 637-2227
(517) 322-9470

New Hampshire
Year-round enrollment available.
Blue Cross and Blue Shield of New Hampshire
2 Pillsbury Street
Concord, NH 03306
(800) 225-2666

New Jersey
Year-round enrollment available.
Blue Cross and Blue Shield of New Jersey
3 Penn Plaza
Newark, NJ 07105
(201) 491-2729

New York
Year-round enrollment available.
Empire Blue Cross and Blue Shield Tradition Plus
622 Third Avenue
New York, NY 10017
(212) 476-7111

North Carolina
Year-round enrollment available.
Blue Cross and Blue Shield of North Carolina Access Plan
P.O. Box 2291
Durham, NC 27707
(919) 490-3829

Pennsylvania
Year-round enrollment available.
Independence Blue Cross and Pennsylvania Blue Shield
1901 Market Street
Philadelphia, PA 19103-1480

(800) 453-2566
(215) 568-8204

Rhode Island
Enrollment available one month of the year.
Blue Cross and Blue Shield of Rhode Island
444 Westminister Street
Providence, RI 02903
(800) 527-7290
(401) 831-7300

Vermont
Year-round enrollment available.
Blue Cross and Blue Shield of Vermont
P.O. Box 186
Montpelier, VT 05601
(800) 247-2583 (existing insured)
(800) 272-3674 (newcomers)
(802) 223-6131

Virginia
Year-round enrollment available.
Blue Cross and Blue Shield of Virginia
P.O. Box 13047
Roanoke, VA 24045
(800) 334-7676

The following states have coverage only for employees eligible under Small Employer Group Health Reform.

Alabama
Alabama Insurance Department
P.O. Box 303351
Montgomery, Al 36130-3351
(205) 269-3550

Delaware
Delaware Insurance Department
841 Silver Lake Boulevard
Dover, DE 19901
(302) 739-4251

Idaho
Idaho Insurance Department
700 W. State Street
Boise, ID 83720
(208) 334-2250

Ohio
Ohio Insurance Department
2100 Stella Court
Columbus, OH 43266-0566
(614) 644-2651

Texas
Texas Insurance Department
Mail Code 106-A
P.O. Box 149104
Austin, TX 78714-9104
(512) 322-3415

Tips for Making the Most of Your Insurance

Get all the benefits your policy provides.

- Get a copy of your insurance policies and find out exactly what your coverage includes.

- Keep careful records of all your covered expenses and claims.

- File claims for all covered costs. Surprisingly, many cancer survivors don't take full advantage of their insurance, either because they don't know about a benefit or are confused or put off by the paperwork.

- Get help in filing a claim if you need it. If friends or family can't assist, ask a social worker for help. Private companies and some community organizations also offer insurance filing aid.

- If your claim is turned down, file again. Ask your doctor to explain to the company why the services meet the requirements for coverage under your policy. If you are turned down again, find out if the company has an appeals process.

Keep insurance needs in mind when you are changing job status.

- Don't leave a job with insurance benefits until you have a new job with good coverage or you have made other plans for insurance.

This is also an important thing for your spouse to keep in mind if you are covered under his or her policy.

- Look at the differences in insurance coverage and other benefits offered by various employers. You may be better off taking a new job with a lower salary that has better insurance coverage.

- Consider continuing to take part in your current company's group plan after you leave. If a new job does not work out, you could be left with no coverage. Federal law (Public Law 99-272), the Consolidated Omnibus Budget Reconciliation Act (COBRA), requires many employers to allow employees who quit, are let go, or whose hours are reduced to pay their own premiums for the company's group plan. This protection lasts 18 months for employees (up to 29 months if they lose their jobs due to disability and are eligible for Social Security disability benefits at the time they leave the job) and 36 months for their dependents. If an employee leaves a company and takes a new job, continuation coverage by the former company can be kept for up to 18 months if the new company's coverage is limited or excludes a pre-existing condition, such as cancer. (COBRA applies to employers with 20 or more workers who already offer group health insurance.) Contact your personnel department to enroll. In addition, you can contact your state insurance commissioner to learn if your state has continuation-of-benefits laws. They may help you receive additional insurance rights protection.

- Take advantage of your right in some company group policies to convert to an individual policy when you leave the company or retire. Typically, a cancer survivor can obtain coverage for about a year under a converted policy. Premiums for individual policies, however, may be considerably higher and less comprehensive. You may want to check around with different companies for the best coverage at the lowest rates because each may have a different system for assessing premiums.

- Look for work in a large company, whose group insurance plans rarely exclude employees with a history of illness.

Work with your doctors to get maximum coverage of clinical trials' costs.

Many clinical trials (treatment studies) offer some part of care free of charge. But some insurers will not cover certain costs when a new treatment is under study. If you are taking part in or considering a clinical trial:

- Ask your doctor about the experience of other patients in the trial. Have their insurers paid for their care? Have there been any consistent problems?

- Talk to your doctor about the paperwork he or she submits to your insurer. Often the way the doctor describes a treatment can help or hurt your chances of insurance coverage.

- Be sure you know what's in your policy. Check it to see if there's a specific exclusion for "experimental treatment."

Many companies handle new treatments on a case-by-case basis, rather than having a blanket policy. You always can ask about their coverage of specific therapies. However, some patients say that their questions may have hurt their chances for coverage by raising a red flag.

Find ways to supplement your insurance.

Take all the Federal income tax deductions for health care costs that you are allowed. Examples include gas mileage for trips to and from medical appointments, out-of-pocket costs for prescription drugs and equipment, and meals during lengthy medical visits.

What Your Health Insurance Coverage Should Include

When looking into a new health insurance plan, it's a good idea to make sure that the coverage provided suits your health care needs. Health insurance for the cancer survivor should provide, at the very least, the following:

- *Benefits.* Inpatient hospital care, physician services, laboratory and x-ray services, prenatal care, inpatient psychiatric care, outpatient services, and nursing home care. Prescription drug coverage may be important if you will be taking a medicine for a long time.

- *Financial protection.* The insurer should pay at least 80 percent of the covered services, except for inpatient psychiatric care, which may require that the policyholder pay more than 20 percent of expenses. In addition, the insurer should pay at least $250,000 for catastrophic illness coverage, with the patient paying no more than 30 percent of his or her income toward these expenses.

Confirm conversations with insurance representatives in writing. If you think the representative is wrong, ask to speak with his/her supervisor. Consider filing an insurance complaint if you feel you have been treated unfairly.

- If your insurer is a private company (e.g., Blue Cross, Prudential), it is regulated by your state department of Insurance.

- If your insurer is a licensed health care service plan (e.g., Kaiser and other HMOs), it is regulated by your state department of insurance.

- If your insurer is a federal qualified Health Maintenance Organization, it is regulated by the U.S. Health Care Financing Administration, Office of Prepaid Health Care Operations and Oversight.

- If your insurer is a private employer or union self-insurance or a self-financed plan, it is regulated by the U.S. Department of Labor, Pension & Welfare Benefits Administration.

- If your insurer is Medicaid (sometimes called other names; e.g., in California it's known as MediCal), it is regulated by your state department of social services or medical assistance services.

- If your insurer is Medicare, it is regulated by the U.S. Social Security Administration.

- If your insurer is Supplemental Security Income, it is regulated by the U.S. Social Security Administration.

- If your insurer is Veterans Benefits, it is regulated by the Department of Veterans Affairs, Veterans Assistance Service.

- If your insurer is CHAMPUS, it is regulated by the Department of Veterans Affairs, Veterans Assistance Service.

Options for Getting Insurance after Cancer Treatment

- Obtain dependent coverage under your spouse's insurance plan.

- Join your current company plan.

- Join a health maintenance organization. Look for open enrollment periods when you may be accepted regardless of your health history.

- Request group insurance through a professional, fraternal, membership, or political organization to which you belong.

- Use Medicare. It covers most people age 65 or older and those who are permanently disabled.

- Use Medicaid or other state or local benefits. Coverage and eligibility criteria differ from state to state; check with your local office.

- Get coverage through an independent broker.

- Join a state "high risk" health insurance pool for people who cannot get conventional coverage (see "Briefs.").

Resources

Additional Reading

With so many issues involved, cancer survivors may not be aware of their needs for specific insurance coverage and benefits. Materials that can help include:

Comprehensive Health Insurance for High Risk Individuals: A State-by-State Analysis

Communicating for Agriculture
2626 East 82nd Street, Suite 325
Bloomington MN 55425
(800) 445-1525
There is a $24 charge for this product which includes shipping and handling; prepayment is required.

National Insurance Consumer Organization (NICO)
P.O. Box 15492
Alexandria, VA 22309
(703) 549-8050
Offers general information only. For a list of NICO publications, send a self-addressed, stamped envelope.

Health Insurance: Risk Pools
Pub.#HRD-88-66BR
U.S. General Accounting Office
P.O. Box 6015
Gaithersburg, MD 20884
(202) 512-6000 FAX
(301) 258-4066

Additional Resources

Many people need help paying for medical costs that aren't covered by their insurance. For financial assistance, you may want to contact:

- Local Groups
  - Local cancer support organizations, which may provide referrals to community sources for financial aid.
  - Your local office on aging, if you are an older adult.
  - The county board of assistance or welfare office.
- United States Government. The U. S. Government has a number of programs designed to help people with low incomes or disabilities pay their bills. For information, call your local office of:
  - Aid to Families With Dependent Children (AFDC) and Food Stamps Programs. Look for the numbers under the Local Government, Social Services, section of your telephone book.
  - Medicare/Medicaid Information. Call your local Social Security Administration office to receive an explanation of the medical costs covered by these Federal health insurance programs. Note: For people under age 65, Medicare coverage does not begin until 2 years from the date they are declared disabled.
  - Social Security Administration. Call 1-800-772-1213 for general information on Social Security benefits you may be eligible to receive.
  - The Department of Veterans Affairs. Request information about medical benefits for veterans and their dependents.
  - The Cancer Information Service of the National Cancer Institute. Call 1-800-4 CANCER to request information about drug companies with assistance programs for cancer patients with low incomes.
- Your Hospital. Financial help may also be available within hospitals. To find out about setting up monthly payment plans for hospital bills, contact your:
  - Hospital patient advocate.
  - Hospital financial aid counselor.
  - Hospital social worker.
  - Patient representative in the hospital business office.

Earning a Living

What You Can Expect

Many cancer survivors wonder whether having a cancer history will make a difference in their job prospects. Common questions include: Will I be able to return to work? Take time off for more treatment if I need it? Work as hard as I once did? Advance in my career?

There is no one answer to these questions. Some people choose not to go back to their jobs while others are not physically able to return. But most work-able cancer survivors do return to work. Sometimes it takes a year or more before survivors are ready to return full-time, but once they go back, they almost always are back to stay. Cancer survivors have included professional and Olympic athletes, business executives, artists and musicians, film stars, and world leaders.

When cancer survivors return to work, some have highly supportive employers who help ease the change from patient back to employee. Others get back to the routine without much help from their company or organization. And at some workplaces, wrong ideas and false fears about cancer cause job-related problems that survivors must overcome.

The following stories reflect the workplace experiences of cancer survivors.

"After I had my colostomy, my employer asked me to quit my job because the cancer was upsetting my fellow workers. He said a demotion or transfer was possible if I didn't agree. Except for my wife, that job was my whole world. So rather than quit, I decided to fight for it."—Jon H.

"My employer denies that my treatment last year for cancer had anything to do with my not getting a promotion and raise. My boss said I was being defensive when I suggested that I was being discriminated against because of my illness. He said he just didn't feel I was ready for the responsibility at this time. I don't know what to believe, but I'm looking into my options." —Betty C.

"When I went back to work, my boss was honest with me. She said that my situation had been discussed at a managers' meeting. Some people had questioned what impact my coming back would have on the company's insurance rates. Her boss asked how she planned to get the job done with an employee she could no longer count on to stay healthy. Fortunately she did some research and found out that the turnover rate, absenteeism records, and work performance of people with a cancer history are very much the same as unaffected workers. Her facts helped correct management's wrong ideas." —Roy P.

"I wasn't happy with my job before my cancer was diagnosed, and I'm no happier with it now that I'm finished treatment and back to work. At first I was just grateful that they took me back. I stopped job hunting for fear that my cancer history would lock me out of better chances. But a friend convinced me that I shouldn't give up before I started. I haven't found the job I want yet, but I have found employers who've given me fair consideration." —Jean D.

Briefs

Cancer Survivors as Employees

- 80 percent of people with cancer return to work after diagnosis.

- Research shows that cancer survivors are as productive on the job as other workers and that they aren't absent from work any more often.

- About 1 in 4 cancer survivors experience some form of employment discrimination.

Tips for Dealing with Coworkers after Cancer Treatment

When your coworkers hear about your illness, many of them will want to help, but they won't know how. Others may be frightened by your situation, especially when they don't know much about cancer and today's potential for treatment and cure. Here are some ideas for helping them—and you—to resume a good working relationship.

Plan how you will deal publicly with your cancer when you are back on the job. There is no "right" way to interact with others about your illness. Once they are back at work, some cancer survivors don't want to focus on their cancer or to be associated with the disease in people's minds. Others are very open with coworkers about their experiences. They may have a frank discussion with their manager or close coworkers to air concerns, correct wrong ideas, and decide how to work together. The best approach is the one that feels comfortable for you.

891

Keep up contacts during your treatment and recovery. Your coworkers will be concerned about you. If they have information about your treatment and progress, they will be less anxious and frightened.

It is also important to stay "connected" to the people with whom you work. Talk by phone. When you are able, have lunch with friends or stop in for an office party. Plan to rest before and after if necessary. Your return to work will be easier for you and your coworkers if you have stayed involved.

Ask your employer to educate company employees about cancer. Research has found that people believe three major myths about cancer that sometimes affect their attitudes towards cancer survivors:

Myth #1—Cancer is a death sentence.

Myth #2—Cancer is contagious.

Myth #3—Cancer makes workers less productive.

When coworkers learn the facts about cancer, they realize that these myths are untrue. Open discussion calms concerns and resolves fears. You may want to invite a speaker to discuss the issues such as an expert from a local cancer support organization, or a doctor, nurse, or social worker who specializes in cancer.

Your company medical department, personnel office, union, or employee assistance program are possible sponsors for an educational program. Information efforts might include making written materials available, holding a brown bag lunch discussion, or correcting wrong ideas at staff or union meetings.

Join (or form) a workplace support group for cancer survivors. Such groups may include only cancer survivors or both people with and without cancer. Depending on what members want, support groups can be anonymous or open. They can provide mutual emotional support for members, or they can make active efforts to stand up for the rights of cancer survivors.

Consider talking to other coworkers who learn they have cancer. Share your experiences and insights. Let people who have just found out they have cancer know that they are not alone. Offer to do something for them that you wish someone had done for you.

Get help if you need it. If coworkers attitudes about cancer are making it hard to do your job, your first step may be trying to resolve the situation informally with the people involved. Correcting others' wrong ideas, without being defensive, can be difficult. But a direct approach may help things change for the better.

When your own efforts don't work, you may want to get help. Your manager, shop steward, employee assistance counselor, or personnel office may be able to change coworkers' ideas, procedures, or the way your job fits in with others' to lessen problems. It is a good idea to have a workable solution to suggest when you raise a problem. (See "Ask your employer to adjust to your needs.")

Most survivors understandably hesitate to "rock the boat," calling company attention to personal problems. When hurtful remarks or actions get you down, talking to a friend or counselor may help you put things in perspective. When coworker attitudes get in the way of doing your job, however, it becomes an issue that management needs to address. (See "Ask your employer to adjust to your needs.")

Your Protection Under Law

On July 26, 1992, the employment provisions of the Americans with Disabilities Act (ADA) went into effect. The ADA bans discrimination by both private and public employers against qualified workers who have disabilities or histories of disability. While the ADA does not specifically include cancer survivors, it is expected that survivors will be included based on past legal rulings.

For two years, the ADA will cover private employers with 25 or more workers. Thereafter, it will cover employers with 15 or more workers. Under this law employers:

- Cannot require you to take pre-employment exams designed to screen out people with disabilities such as histories of cancer.

- Can ask you medical questions only after you are offered employment and only if the questions relate specifically to the job.

- Complaints filed under this law are handled by the field offices of the Equal Employment Opportunities Commission (EEOC). These offices can be located by calling 1-800-669-4000.

Other protection will continue to be provided by the Federal Rehabilitation Act of 1973, which states that federal employers or companies receiving federal funds cannot discriminate against handicapped workers, including cancer survivors. This law protects cancer survivors in hiring practices, promotions, transfers, and layoffs at the federal level.

In addition to federal protection, you may be eligible for employment protection under state laws. To learn more about your legal rights, check with:

- Your local American Cancer Society office. They have state-specific information pamphlets about cancer and employment discrimination.

- Your social worker, who may know about laws in your state. He or she also can tell you which state agency is responsible for protecting your rights.

- The National Coalition for Cancer Survivorship (see "Resources"). This group offers information and some legal referrals.

- Your Congressional representative or senator. Staff working for these officials can give you information about federal and state laws. If you aren't sure who represents your district, call the library or local chapter of the League of Women Voters.

Tips for Changing Jobs after Cancer Treatment

When you look for a new job after cancer treatment, it is important to anticipate the concerns that your cancer history may raise. Here are some ideas to help you prepare for the job search.

- Don't discriminate against yourself. First, take an honest look at your current skills and capabilities. Then, apply for jobs you know you can do. Don't try to do more—or settle for less—than you are able to handle.

- Organize your resume to your best advantage. For example, a chronological resume may raise questions if cancer treatment or recovery interrupted your career. To avoid pointing up those gaps, you might organize your resume by skills or achievements instead of by dates of employment.

- Get a letter from your doctor (on office or hospital stationery) that explains your health situation for employers. Have the doctor talk specifically about your physical ability to perform the type of work you are seeking. If you are in good health now, ask the doctor to verify your good health in the letter. The doctor also may include statements about the documented work ability of cancer survivors nationwide.

- Don't lie about your cancer history if an employer or an application asks you directly.

- Always qualify your "yes" with positive statements about your current health (including the doctor's letter noted above).

- Don't volunteer health information if no one asks. You have no legal responsibility to mention your cancer unless it directly relates to the job you seek.

- Practice answering possible questions about your health history before an interview. Be confident and avoid sounding defensive.

- Consider working with a job counselor who can help you prepare fully for your job search.

Options for Handling Job Problems

Decide what you want to do about an employment problem.

- Do you still want to work there?

- Are you willing to take action to correct a problem?

- Would you rather try to find a different job?

Educate your employer.

- Give management the facts about cancer survivors' dependability on the job (See "Briefs.")

- Have your doctor explain how, if at all, your personal cancer history may affect your work or your schedule.

Ask your employer to adjust to your needs.

- Start by talking informally to your supervisor, the personnel office, employee assistance program, shop steward, or union representative.

- Ask for a specific change that would make it easier for you to keep your job (e.g., flextime, working at home, special equipment at the office).

- Document your requests and the outcome for your records.

The Federal Government and many private companies are now required to make "reasonable accommodations" to meet the needs of "disabled" employees if this does not cause the employer "undue hardship." Although cancer survivors may not feel "disabled," they may be legally protected under this umbrella term. Simple changes employers are required to make include:

- Making facilities accessible (e.g., having desks, aisles, and restrooms that accommodate a wheelchair).

- Allowing an employee to work a flexible schedule to adjust for treatment-related absences.

- Changing the way a job works (e.g., letting an employee work part-time or share a job).

The Job Accommodation Network can help you and your employer find out about accommodations that have worked for other companies. This hotline is a project of the President's Committee on the Employment of People with Disabilities. Call 1-800-526-7234 for more information.

Get help working with your employer if you need it.

- People that can support you include: your doctor or nurse; medical social workers, state rehabilitation workers; staff and volunteers at your local American Cancer Society; advocacy groups for disabled workers; your family and friends.

Talk about your legal rights with the agencies that enforce anti-discrimination laws.

- State commissions on discrimination

- State affirmative action offices

- U.S. Department of Health and Human Services, Office for Civil Rights in your region

- U.S. Department of Labor, Office of Federal Contract Compliance programs in your region

A medical social worker or your local American Cancer Society can help you find out whom to contact.

Talk to an attorney with experience in solving on-the-job discrimination problems.

- Talk to your local bar association or cancer support organization to find a qualified lawyer.

- The National Coalition for Cancer Survivorship offers limited referrals to attorneys with expertise in this area (see "Resources").

- Discuss any formal procedures your company may have for settling disputes.

- Consider filing a discrimination complaint under state or federal law.

Resources

Information about cancer is available from the sources listed below. You may wish to check for additional information at your local library or bookstore and from support groups in your community

Additional Reading

Many cancer survivors have concerns related to their jobs. They may worry, for example, about job discrimination. The following publications can help you understand your legal rights as a person with a history of cancer.

Cancer: Your Job, Insurance, and the Law. American Cancer Society. Answers job and insurance-related questions often asked by cancer survivors. Booklet is free. Call 1-800-ACS-2345.

Charting the Journey: An Almanac of Practical Resources for Cancer Survivors. National Coalition for Cancer Survivorship (NCCS) Guides cancer survivors to resources for legal concerns, medical treatment, emotional support, self-help, and family issues. Call 301-650-8868. For NCCS members, cost is $12.00; nonmembers can order from Consumer Reports Books, 9180 Le Saint Drive, Fairfield, OH 45014, cost is $14.95.

Additional Resources

National Rehabilitation Information Center (NARIC)
8455 Colesville Road, Suite 935
Silver Spring, MD 20910
(800) 34-NARIC(voice/TDD)

The National Rehabilitation Information Center provides information regarding job rehabilitation.

National Coalition for Cancer Survivorship (NCCS)
1010 Wayne Avenue, 5th Floor
Silver Spring, MD 20910
(301) 650-8868

The National Coalition for Cancer Survivorship is a network of independent groups and individuals concerned with survivorship and support of cancer survivors and their loved ones. NCCS's primary goal is to promote a national awareness of issues affecting cancer survivors. Its objectives are to:

- Serve as a clearing house for information on services and materials for survivors.

- Advocate the rights and interests of cancer survivors.

- Encourage the study of survivorship.

- Promote the development of cancer support activities.

Cancer Information Service. The Cancer Information Service, a program of the National Cancer Institute, is a nationwide telephone service for cancer patients and their families and friends, the public, and health care professionals. The staff can answer questions (in English or Spanish) and send free National Cancer Institute booklets about cancer. They also know about local resources and services. One toll-free number 1-800-4-CANCER (1-800-422-6237), connects callers all over the country with the office that serves their area.

American Cancer Society (ACS). The American Cancer Society is a voluntary organization with a national office and local units all over the country. This organization supports research, conducts educational programs, and offers many services to patients and their families. The American Cancer Society also provides free booklets on cancer. To obtain booklets, or for information about services and activities in local areas, call the Society's toll-free number, 1-800-ACS-2345 (1-800 227-2345), or the number listed under American Cancer Society in the white pages of the telephone book.

Moving Ahead

The National Cancer Institute hopes that this guide has given you ideas and information you can use—now and in the future. We encourage you to write to us about your own ideas and experiences. We plan to update Facing Forward as needed to include new advice, research findings, and relevant changes in laws or social policies.

In compiling this guide, we have heard from cancer survivors with many points of view. A common thread was respect for their fellow survivors and a recognition that some of the changes in their lives have been positive ones.

One survivor, Bill, described it like this:

"Cancer survivorship can be a catalyst for spiritual awakening, providing life with depth and poignancy. Survivors themselves are often gutsy and assertive, and they dare to take chances. They are often optimistic, independent-minded, and compassionate and have elevated self-esteem and pride...New attitudes towards work, pleasure, and relationships develop with utmost clarity, while superficial distractions and frivolous people are filtered out... [Survivors] share a new understanding of time, a sense of needing to make every minute count."

National Coalition for Cancer Survivorship President (1989-90) Fitzhugh Mullan has compared cancer survivorship to crossing a river and starting a new life on the other bank—with no maps or trails to show the way. We hope that Facing Forward offers some useful signposts for your unique journey and helps you, in Mullan's words, " [civilize the new land] to make life there tolerable, and even good."

Chapter 83

Advanced Cancer: Living Each Day

Introduction

This chapter was written to help persons who have gone through the struggles of diagnosis, treatment, and, perhaps, recurrence of cancer, persons for whom a cure or longterm remission is no longer likely. Terms that doctors use for this stage of illness are advanced, terminal, or endstage disease. Although these terms can have different meanings, they are used interchangeably in this chapter.

"Advanced Cancer" is meant to help people who are facing death from cancer live their remaining days as well as they can. It is based on the most current information available and on interviews with patients, their families, and their caregivers.

Throughout the chapter, several themes are stressed:

- Many of your concerns can be eased with medical skill, support from caregivers, and knowledge about your illness.

- Talking with others about your anxieties, frustrations, concerns, and problems may be one of the best things you can do for yourself.

- Loss of control over your illness does not mean loss of control over the days ahead. You can choose the way you wish to face each day.

"Advanced Cancer: Living Each Day," National Institutes of Health (NIH) Publication 94-856, February 1994.

Some of the information in this chapter may not be suitable for all readers. As you read this chapter, select the parts that are right for you. Please keep in mind that "Advanced Cancer" was written primarily for adult patients and their families. If you are a parent, relative, or friend of a child or young person who has terminal cancer, you may wish to call the National Cancer Institute's Cancer Information Service or the American Cancer Society for more information.

We hope that this chapter will help ease your concerns. Perhaps it will show you that each day can be meaningful and offer comfort, sometimes in a new or unexpected way. Even at this difficult time, there are many things that can be done to help you lead a dignified, satisfying life.

Living One Day at a Time

Few people like to think about dying. We all know that death will come, but most of us spend little time thinking about it. Approaching death often brings a change in how we look at life and what we value. For many people, having a serious illness leads them to live one day at a time rather than to put off until tomorrow, next week, or next year what could be done or said today. One patient expressed his philosophy this way:

> "The death rate for any generation is 100 percent. We all die. However, I know what probably will kill me, while most people don't. We have no guarantee of how long we will live. But I believe it is truly the quality of life, not the quantity, that is most important."

There is no right or wrong way to face the end of life. Do what is most comfortable and useful for you. Many people with a serious illness are able to find peace of mind by coming to terms with their emotions and beliefs about life and death. You may be able to find meaning for yourself, in your own way and at your own pace.

The Will to Survive

We are all born with the will to survive. Exactly what influence this has on diseases—especially cancer—has been debated for a long time. But there is little argument that a strong desire to live can enhance the quality of life.

Many people with terminal cancer have lived far longer than expected. They often share a positive attitude about the value of life.

They also seem to have a combination of hope, endurance, willpower, and courage. When asked to explain how they have managed, they often give answers such as, "I'm needed too much at work," or "I can't die until my grandchild is born." They do not want to give up or retreat from living. A keen interest in daily events helps to get them through uncomfortable treatments or disease-related problems.

This does not mean that a positive attitude alone necessarily will lengthen your life. Nor does it mean that you are doing something wrong if you are sick and not getting better. But emphasizing the positive aspects of your life can add meaning, purpose, and comfort to your remaining time.

How You May Feel when Time Is Limited

Each of us is unique, and we each find our own way to live and die. Still, many patients with advanced cancer have many feelings in common and may approach this time in their lives in similar ways. You may not experience all the emotions discussed in this chapter or in the exact way they are described. Your feelings may come, go away, and then come again. Information is presented to reassure you and those close to you that your reactions are not unusual; they are a part of the way we, as humans, make peace with ourselves. When patients are first told or first realize that their cancer can no longer be treated effectively, they often react by denying that this could be happening to them. They believe they will find a way to beat the odds. This is a way of coping with an overwhelming situation, and it may be helpful at first. With time, however, patients and their loved ones are often able to face reality. One patient explained it this way:

"The reality of death does not go away by denying it. When you do this, you can miss the comfort you get from sharing fears and concerns. You miss the sense of well-being you get knowing you have taken care of your loved ones."

The feeling of "No, not me!" often changes to "Why me?" This question may result from feelings of anger and rage. You may be angry with the doctor, family members, neighbors, your disease, and even yourself without good cause. This is a normal reaction, and with some time, if you can accept and understand your anger, hopefully it will pass. It may help to talk about your feelings with your family, a close friend, or a social worker. It also may help to keep in mind that you are not responsible for your disease.

Next you may begin to realize that there is no answer to the question, "Why me?" Your anger is not the solution, and you may find yourself "bargaining" for a longer life. People make all kinds of promises in hopes of a longer life. A promise might be "If I can live just one more month, I'll go to church every day," or "If I just can see my son married, I won't ask for more."

It is not unusual to bargain. In fact, taking notice of what you ask for and then working to accomplish your wishes may help relieve some anxieties about things left undone and words left unsaid.

At times you may feel depressed because you have lost control of some aspects of your life or your independence. It may help to focus on what you value most in life—family, friends, or other things that you cherish—rather than on what you cannot change.

As your illness progresses, depression from losses that already have occurred may give way to grief over the people and life you are going to lose. This grieving should not be discouraged; it must be worked through to gain peace of mind and acceptance. Frequently, talking through these feelings with a loved one, clergy, social worker, counselor, or support group can ease the grieving process.

During this time, you may find yourself wanting to have fewer people around. It may help you and your family and friends to understand that this type of withdrawal often occurs toward the end of life. Conversation may not be needed as long as someone who cares for you is nearby. A smile or a gentle touch sometimes can say much more than words. Not all people who face the end of life are able to find peace and accept death; however, with time and support from those around you, acceptance is often possible. You need to know that everything that can be done for your peace and comfort will be done. Don't be afraid to ask for such support and assurances.

Your Inner Strength

Most people are overwhelmed emotionally when they first learn that their cancer no longer can be controlled. They may not be able to cope as well as they did in the past. Sometimes they may temporarily lose their will to live, but their reactions often change with time. Your feelings of hopelessness may change because of physical and emotional reserves you didn't know you had. Calling on your inner strength can help revive your spirits and your drive to enjoy each experience and each day. Concentrating on the present instead of the future can be helpful. For many patients, the future becomes the end of each day. As one person explained:

"Before this happened I had a 5 year plan, a 10 year plan, even a 20 year plan. No more. What I realized was that I could only die in the future, but I was alive right now, and I always would be alive in the here and now."

Others prefer to plan ahead—days, months, even a year or so. This reaffirms to themselves and others that they are not finished with living and accomplishing goals. With places to go and things to do, life stretches before them.

Your plans may involve doing things that you enjoy each day. You may want to plan a few "special days" with family members or friends—a day outing, a concert, or an afternoon together. Or you may want to focus on fulfilling a lifelong dream, such as taking a trip. Without a plan, whether it is general or very specific, you may find that your time consists only of routine daily activities. But try not to do too many activities. Becoming tired may weaken your defense against depression and despair and may make coping with your illness more difficult.

Some people view their illness as a challenge to be met or a battle to be fought. They think of each day they survive as a victory. One woman expressed her outlook this way:

"I get satisfaction by being engaged in the fight. It's me and my doctors against the cancer, and we know we might not win in the end. But by God, we're going to give it a run for its money."

Others cope by rethinking what is important in their lives and what is not. As one person said:

"Disease rearranges your values, and you cast off things. You reduce the trivia to a minimum; you simplify life."

It may be helpful to put together a "living legacy" —a book, cassette, video, piece of artwork, or poem that reflects who you are—to share with your family and other loved ones. However you choose to cope, your inner strength can help you live each day as fully as possible.

What You Can Do for Yourself

Living with a serious illness can be discouraging. You will have good days and bad days, just as you did before, and your ability to deal with these changes may vary. In the morning you may feel down, but by afternoon your outlook may improve. On one day, you may have little energy, but on another, your mood and spirit may rebound. During the bad times, try to remember the good moments and remind yourself there can be more good times ahead.

Taking charge of your life is one way to help yourself. Take an active role in the kind of care you receive. Participate in daily activities with your family and friends.

Do things for yourself that make you feel good, such as attending religious services or encouraging visits from friends. Let others help you. Let them know what they can do for you and what you can do for yourself. They will be grateful for specific suggestions. Your caregivers may recommend things that don't seem as important to you now, such as exercise, medications, and food. But these measures will help you keep your strength and independence for as long as possible. Working with your caregivers and family helps you maintain a sense of control, purpose, and hope.

Set the tone for those around you. Making those around you feel comfortable now will help them to be comfortable around you throughout your illness. As one patient said:

> "You have to do this because no one knows how you want to be treated, and they may be waiting for a cue. No one else will talk about it unless you do."

At the same time, remember that you don't have to be noble and heroic if you don't feel that way. Sometimes loved ones may want you to try to keep your feelings of sadness or anger inside because they can't face their own painful emotions; however, your feelings are important and need to be shared.

Facing the Challenge

It may be very hard to accept that your body is no longer as strong and reliable as it once was. As cancer progresses, you will not be as independent as you once were. This new dependence on others may affect your self-respect. Your role in the family and at work will change as well. When this happens, remember that the qualities that made you a good friend, loving parent, caring mate or responsible worker haven't changed. One woman had this to say about her feelings about herself:

> "It shouldn't take a fatal diagnosis to find self-awareness, self-concern, and self-love. But, I'm afraid, for most of us, it does. I

think I've straightened myself out in these areas. In fact, I've discovered that I'm a stronger person than I might have anticipated. I am just a bit gutsier than I thought, and I'm delighted to know that about myself."

You may be able to continue many of your regular activities, such as playing sports, doing volunteer work, or traveling. Advances in the ability to control pain and to administer needed medications and treatments outside the hospital can give those in the later stages of cancer more independence while receiving medical care.

Arranging family albums, scrapbooks, or hobby collections; working on a computer; or keeping a daily journal of your feelings and experiences are activities you can do if you are less active. Just remember to conserve your strength for the activities you really want to pursue.

Keep in mind that you can have control over many aspects of your life whether you are bedridden or not. You can make decisions about your care, your activities, food preferences, and what you need to make yourself comfortable. In the hospital, for example, you can wear your own clothes or use your own blanket and pillow. In some cases, you also may be able to participate in decisions about your schedule for resting, bathing, and so on.

Maintaining independence makes many patients feel better about themselves. However, well-meaning family and friends may try to make decisions for you, and sometimes you must rely on others for your care. When you face situations such as these, just remember: You know better than anyone what you need to make the most of each day.

Handling Your Emotions

As mentioned earlier, people who are dying from cancer may be sad, depressed, angry, scared, or all of these. These feelings are very human and natural. You already may be grieving for the loss of the person you were before you had cancer. As your friends will grieve for you, you now may be grieving for your loss of them.

You may be wondering what experiences you will miss in life, what the moment of death will be like, and whether you will continue to "be" after death. You may think about what will become of your family and friends and how these people will react to your death.

Don't bottle up your emotions. Letting feelings out will help relatives, friends, and caregivers understand your needs; may relieve some of your sadness, depression, or anger; and even may reduce physical discomfort. For some people, writing about emotions can help, and occasionally you may want to punch a pillow, scream, or have a good, long cry. Go ahead and express your feelings.

If you are feeling angry, it will help both you and others to understand that your anger may not be meant for them. You might even think of ways to make your anger work for you. For example, perhaps you can focus your energy on changing some aspect of your care that displeases you.

Many people with a terminal illness develop an interest in expressing or trying to resolve spiritual or religious issues. Even if you don't consider yourself a "religious person" or haven't taken part in religious services, you may find comfort in exploring spiritual matters with a friend, family member, or member of the clergy. For some, prayer and/or meditation can be a positive spiritual boost.

Talking It Over

Honest and open communication about your illness can help you in several ways. It can help those close to you understand how you want to be treated, and the weight of your problems may be lightened just by talking them over with a family member, a friend, or other cancer patients who may think of ideas to help comfort you. Sharing your feelings also may reduce stress.

You may find this kind of communication difficult, and it may be hard for others. Still, talking over your worries and concerns and knowing how your loved ones feel can give you strength and reassurance. To discuss these issues, try to choose people who are comfortable with your illness.

Let your friends and relatives know that they can offer comfort simply by being themselves, by listening without trying to solve problems, and by being at ease with you.

But keep in mind, not everyone can handle your suffering and loss. Friendships and family relationships may change—not because of you but because others may not be able to cope with their own emotional pain about your illness. If this is the case, you might want to talk to a member of your medical team or to someone trained in counseling. such as a nurse, social worker, psychologist, member of the clergy, or, if you are receiving care at home, a professional home health care worker. Also, you may find support by attending self-help groups where people meet to share common concerns. Your caregivers, hospital, hospice, or local unit of the American Cancer Society can help find the right person or group for you.

Making the Unknown Known

Some say it is not death people fear but the days, weeks, or months that precede it. Many are afraid that there will be pain during this time and wonder if they will become a burden. Patients with a serious illness fear the unknown, isolation, abandonment, and loss of physical and emotional control. They worry about the future of those who will outlive them.

Understanding your condition can help you and your family resolve these fears. The more you learn about your condition and treatment, the more your fears of the unknown are reduced. Don't hesitate to ask your doctors, nurses, and other caregivers if there is something you want to know. Remember: It is your right to receive answers, even to the most direct questions about your future.

Sometimes your health care providers will seem hesitant to offer information. They may not be able to explain exactly what to expect. Or they may wait until you seem ready for the information. You can signal your readiness by asking specific questions—about your life, your illness, and about dying.

Try to include one or more relatives, friends, or others who are supportive in talks with your health care providers. If they explain directly to your caregivers, your caregivers gain a clearer understanding of how they can help you, and their concerns can be eased.

Relieving Your Pain and Discomfort

Many people with cancer fear physical pain. However, not everyone with cancer has pain. And those who do have pain are not in pain all the time. If you have pain, it can be treated. Talk to your doctor or nurse about pain control. Don't wait until your pain is severe. Pain almost always can be lessened.

Cancer patients may have pain for a variety of reasons. Pain may be due to the cancer itself, or it could result from treatment methods. For example, after surgery, a person feels pain as a result of the operation itself. Sometimes, the pain is unrelated to the cancer, such as a muscle sprain, a toothache, or a headache. Whatever the cause, pain can be relieved.

The best way to manage pain is to treat its cause. Whenever possible, the cause of the pain is treated by removing the tumor or decreasing its size. To do this, your doctor may suggest surgery, radiation therapy, or chemotherapy. However, your doctor may be more likely to recommend pain relief methods to control your pain. These methods include pain medicines, operations on nerves, nerve blocks, physical therapy, and techniques such as relaxation, distraction, and imagery.

Many people are reluctant to use pain medications for fear of becoming addicted. But taking medication to relieve pain will not make you an "addict." In fact, studies show that medically supervised use of narcotics (also known as analgesics) to control cancer pain does not cause addiction. Also, research shows that patients who take medication to prevent rather than reduce pain, tend to use less medication. And if the cause of your pain can be corrected, you will be able to stop taking your medications.

Physical therapy, biofeedback, relaxation techniques, self-hypnosis, and imagery also may help relieve pain. Other types of pain control include skin stimulation, pressure, vibration, massage, cold or warm compresses, menthol applied to the skin, and transcutaneous electric nerve stimulation. Some of these methods cause nerve endings to become numb in a specific area of the body, providing pain relief without the drowsiness caused by some pain medications. Special procedures that use anesthetics are available for the 10 to 15 percent of patients whose pain therapy is ineffective or causes severe side effects.

You know the most about your pain, such as where it is, how bad it is, what eases it, or what makes it feel worse. Your doctors and nurses rely on you to tell them about your pain. Together, you can decide which methods of relief might be best for you.

Don't hesitate to talk about your pain to your doctor or nurse. You have a right to the best pain control you can get. Relieving your pain means you can continue to do the everyday things that are important to you.

A booklet about handling pain, "Questions and Answers About Pain Control: A Guide for People With Cancer and Their Families," is available from the Cancer Information Service and the American Cancer Society.

Feelings of Isolation

As cancer progresses, your life is disrupted. Social activities with family, friends, or coworkers become less frequent. Routines change because of treatments, visits to the doctor, or your need to rest.

These changes can lead to feelings of loneliness and isolation, even when you are surrounded by family and friends. One way to lessen these feelings is to live as normally as possible. Continue to do the things you always have done, such as hobbies, reading, walking the dog, or enjoying the company of children. Let your family and friends know that you want to continue with life as it was before. Encourage them, as much as you can, to carry on with their regular routines.

Don't hesitate to ask friends and relatives to visit if you are feeling up to it. They may want to stop by but may be afraid to contact you because they don't know what to say or how to act.

In spite of all your efforts, there will be days when you feel alone because you realize others cannot fully understand or share your experience. Some days you may simply want to be left alone, and that is okay too.

People who live alone or those who do not have family and friends close by may find an illness especially difficult. In these situations, some have found it easier to cope by having volunteers or caregivers visit. For others, the company of a pet often helps.

Talking with other people who have terminal cancer might provide the understanding and companionship you need. Joining a support group, where you can talk with other cancer patients, is another way to ease feelings of isolation.

At times you may need to rely on yourself for encouragement. If this happens, try to focus on the pleasures you can give yourself, such as a leisurely walk, a beautiful bouquet of flowers, or a good book. Draw on your own strength and try to be your own best friend.

The People in Your Life

For many people, family and close friends are the most important sources of emotional support. As one man said:

> "My wife and friends who love me are like a circle. They form a protective shield around me. I don't know what I'd do without them."

Those who are close to you need understanding as much as you do. It may be helpful to try to consider how they feel and what they can and can't do. Your loved ones may need time, just as you do, to adjust to your illness and to their feelings of confusion, shock, helplessness, or anger. Letting family and friends know that you want them close and that you need their support will help them cope with these difficult emotions. For many patients and their families, sharing feelings and taking the time to say goodbye provide reassurance and comfort. Don't hesitate to ask your nurse, social worker, clergy, or counselor to help bring together family members to talk and listen.

How Young and Teenage Children May React

Children whose parent, grandparent, brother, or sister has cancer almost always are aware of a change in their lives. Even very young children sense when something is wrong. They may be frightened by the changes in their daily routine or become angry when someone they depend on is seriously ill. They may worry that they might have caused the illness. It is important to reassure children that nothing they said, did, or thought caused the cancer and that someone will be there to take care of them.

Because of these possible reactions, it is best to be honest and encourage communication. Let your children or grandchildren know that it's okay to ask questions and that you will answer them as honestly and as thoroughly as you can. Tell children as much as you think they can understand.

Keep in mind that many young people understand more than we can imagine. In fact, children who are not told the truth about an illness in the family often depend on their imagination and fears to explain the changes around them. For example, they may believe that the family member's cancer is punishment for something they have said or done. As a result, they may feel unnecessary anxiety and guilt. Health professionals generally agree that telling children the truth about an illness reduces stress and guilt. If you find it difficult to talk with your children or explain your illness, you might want to ask a close friend, relative, or health care provider for help.

Children need to know that they are still loved and important and that they will continue to be cared for as before. Perhaps a friend can give some time and attention to a child who needs comforting, affection, and guidance. Choose someone the child likes and suggest that he or she help with a special project or attend an important school event if you cannot; ask a friend or family member to videotape your child's performance and then view it with your child when you can enjoy the time together.

Taking the time to listen to a child's triumphs, problems, and fears is important. This holds true for adolescents as well as for younger children. Teenagers are sometimes expected to assume responsibilities beyond their maturity. Try to give them the independence they need, but also be sure to include them as valued family members.

Your doctor or social worker can guide you to an appropriate counselor if you think outside assistance would be helpful. Local hospice counselors also are a good source for helping family members cope.

How Adult Children May React

The potential loss of a parent may change how adult children feel about themselves, may raise questions and fears concerning their own mortality, and may affect their views of what is important in life. Adult children also may be torn by the multiple demands in their lives: roles as parents, children, and professionals. They can experience feelings of guilt about the limited time they are able to spend with you.

Throughout your illness, you and your children may have some of the same emotional reactions. Some of these reactions are shock and depression at the diagnosis; hope that treatment will work; disappointment, frustration, anger, and fear when treatment does not work; and grief associated with the changes and losses that have occurred as a result of the cancer.

As your illness progresses, it will be helpful to share decision-making tasks with your children. Try to involve them in issues that are important to you, such as what type of treatment, if any, you prefer or what types of activities you would like to continue. Sharing these tasks with your children can minimize conflict and fears that may arise between siblings when other important decisions need to be made.

Your ability to reach out to your children and openly share your feelings, goals, and wishes will help them through this time. It also will allow them to feel that they have contributed positively to making this part of your lives together the best possible. It may help to remember that just as parents want the best for their children, children want the best for their parents. Children want to see that their parents' needs are met in the most compassionate and effective way possible; no child wants to see a parent suffer.

Partners

Communication is a two-way street between you and your partner. Being honest about your emotions can help you draw support from each other. Loving words, hugs, and kisses can bring a sense of comfort and closeness.

Be realistic about demands on your partner, who also may be having a difficult time. Your partner may feel guilty about your illness and any time spent away from you. Another source of stress for a partner is their changing role in the family. For example, your partner may need to tackle new duties, such as paying bills or providing childcare.

Talking things over is especially important if you have been separated by hospitalization for long periods of time. Sometimes in the absence of their partners, patients begin to draw support from, and relate more personally to, members of their health care team. Partners may have a hard time adjusting to this if they sense they no longer are participating in your care.

Your partner also must take time to meet his or her own needs. If these needs are neglected, your partner will have less energy, cheer, and support to give. Try to have other relatives or friends stay with you while your partner attends to the details of daily life. Some time away from each other will refresh both of you. You must remember that you didn't spend 24 hours a day together before your illness. Try, as much as possible, to maintain your relationship in the same way that you did before.

Intimacy

You may find yourself unable to express yourself sexually as you did before because of physical changes and emotional concerns. However, this does not mean that you must deny needs and desires for intimacy. There are many ways to show love and find satisfaction.

Open, honest communication is the key. Re-examining your attitudes about intimacy will help you and your partner maintain the closeness, warmth, and sense of belonging fostered in a loving relationship. Physical satisfaction can be found in a variety of ways, such as touching, kissing, stroking, and holding.

Sexual problems may stem from feelings about your medical condition or treatment as well as from the condition or treatment itself. With patience and communication between partners, many of these problems can be solved. Understanding why sexual activity may not be the same as before can prevent unrealistic expectations and relieve feelings of selfconsciousness or anxiety.

Don't be afraid to seek help or advice. You are entitled to all the information you need or want. You may wish to seek counseling from a professional who specializes in addressing sexuality issues. Your doctor, social worker, or other caregivers also may be able to offer some guidance. Or they may be able to suggest books that deal with sexuality or that offer cancer patients specific information on this subject.

Choices for Care

Special machines and treatments that can save or extend lives are frequently such an accepted part of treating illness that many persons with terminal cancer choose to be hospitalized. They want to know that every resource to extend the length of their life is available. But, more and more, cancer patients and their families are choosing care at home or in a homelike setting, such as a hospice facility.

Home Care

Home care is a practical and comfortable alternative to hospital care for many patients. Home health care professionals can provide cancer drugs, pain medications, nutritional supplements, physical therapy, and many complex nursing and medical care procedures. They also can help you understand and work through some of the difficult emotional issues that you and your family may be experiencing. Another advantage to home care is that family members and friends can be with you and help with your care. Some people prefer to be treated at home because hospital care can seem impersonal. For many, home care helps ease some of the emotional difficulties that families may experience when a loved one has a terminal illness. As one nurse who cared for her mother at home said:

> "The times we all were together with Mom, the rest of the family usually sat and talked with her, while I attended to her personal care or coaxed her to eat. During those times, we quietly seemed to draw strength from each other just by being together."

Home care involves bringing members of the health care team into your home, or possibly into the home of your son, daughter, other relative, or friend. Depending on the needs and concerns of you and your family, the home health team may include all or many of the following professionals: nurses or nurse practitioners, social workers, dietitians, physical therapists, pharmacists, oncologists, radiation therapists, clergy, and a psychologist or psychiatrist. In addition, many patients find that they need a home health aide to help with bathing, personal care, or preparation of light meals. In many cases, respite care workers, usually specially trained volunteers, also are available to provide limited, temporary care to the patient, allowing the caregiver several hours away from the home. Your primary care physician will remain in close contact with the team and monitor your care but probably will not make daily or regular visits to your home, as many of the other team members do.

The home health care team works closely with you and your family to provide the support that you and those around you need. For example, if 24-hour care is needed, members of the team will work different shifts to accommodate that need. Or, if a family caregiver needs to leave the house for a few hours to run errands, a respite care worker may stop by just to make sure everything is okay.

Home care is provided through various for-profit and not-for-profit private agencies, public and private hospitals, and public health departments. You may wish to discuss home health care further with your nurse, physician, oncologist, or clergy. You may also wish to consider hospice care, another alternative to standard hospital care, described briefly below.

Hospice Care

Hospice programs provide specialized care for patients and their families, either at home or away from home, in freestanding facilities, within hospitals, or in nursing homes. The primary concern of hospice caregivers is the quality of life and control of pain. Hospice care is based on a team approach, similar to the one described in the previous section on home care.

Hospice caregivers try to provide the most effective ways to relieve pain and other symptoms. Emotional, social, and spiritual health also are important considerations in hospice care. Support is available to help family members care for patients.

Approximately 1,800 hospice programs across the country currently offer comprehensive hospice care. The National Hospice Organization promotes and monitors the quality of hospice care. For information about hospice concepts and practices, call the Cancer Information Service. Your doctor, nurse, or social worker also can provide information on hospice care.

Making Treatment Decisions

It is your right to make decisions about your treatment. It is also important for you and those around you to realize that these decisions may change over time. Family, friends, and caregivers may find it hard to accept, but for some patients, continuing to live with their illness is no longer a top priority. Other patients may want to try every available drug or treatment in the hope that something will work. Either way, it is not up to family members, friends, or caregivers to decide how much or how little treatment you should have. It is up to you. Frequently, patients will establish durable powers of attorney and living wills so that their wishes are known by family members and the health care team.

Refusal of treatment does not necessarily mean certain death; however, refusing treatment should be based on your feelings about life, death, and the benefits and side effects of treatment. Should you decide to stop treatment, you still can receive pain medication and treatments to reduce the symptoms of your disease. This will help you remain as comfortable as possible. Remember, however, that you can change your mind and ask to resume your cancer therapy.

Your doctors will, almost certainly, offer information and advice about your decision to stop treatment. Many religious groups have issued statements about the decision to end treatment. You may want to explore the position that your religious group or church takes on this issue. Contact a member of the clergy or other counselor if you would like more information.

Patients' Rights

You have other rights, too. You are entitled to complete information about your illness and what the future might bring, and you have the right to share or withhold that information from others. You also should be informed about any procedures and treatments that are planned, the benefits and risks, and any alternative treatments that may be available. You may be asked to sign an "informed consent" form, which includes this information. Before you sign such a form, be sure to ask your doctor any questions you might have.

The Patient Self-Determination Act

A new Federal law, the Patient Self-Determination Act (PSDA), requires that all medical care facilities receiving Medicare and Medicaid payments inform patients of their rights and choices in making decisions about the type and extent of their medical care. The PSDA also requires that medical care facilities give patients information about living wills and power of attorney (described below). For more information about the PSDA, contact any hospital or medical care facility in your area.

The Living Will/Durable Power of Attorney for Health Care

A living will is a legal document that allows you to state, in writing, that you do not wish to be kept alive by artificial means or heroic measures. It is a recognized statement of your right to refuse treatment and has been upheld in court.

If you decide to prepare a living will, be sure to talk with your doctor, nurse, or lawyer to identify and define terms that may be important to your future medical care, such as "artificial means," "heroic measures," and "code status." You also may want to consider appointing someone who can make decisions for you about your medical care in the event you can no longer do so. This is referred to as "durable power of attorney." Choose a person who knows how you feel about specific treatments and who is familiar with any religious considerations that need to be taken into account. Just make sure that the term "durable" appears on the power of attorney document you prepare.

If you sign a living will and a durable power of attorney, tell everyone close to you that you have these documents and give them copies. Your health care team and lawyer also should be informed and given copies. This will ensure that your wishes are carried out.

Each state has its own laws concerning living wills and power of attorney. Call the Cancer Information Service for information on how to obtain a copy of the living will used in your state and for more information on durable power of attorney. You also may contact any hospital or medical care facility in your area for this information.

Planning for Your Family

Careful planning reduces the financial, legal, and emotional difficulties your family and friends face after your death. Though it is difficult, discussing practical matters now, such as wills and debts, can eliminate many problems later. Your early decisions also help relieve unspoken family worries. Advice from professional advisers, including lawyers, clergy, social workers, and insurance company representatives, can help you make these important decisions.

You may want to help your family plan a funeral or memorial service that has your personal and special touch. Talk with your family and clergy about how you would like to be honored and remembered. Your choice of music, readings, and participants will speak your personal message to those gathered to remember you.

You can help your family by organizing records, documents, and instructions they will need. If you cannot gather all of these items, make a list of where they are located. The papers should be kept in a fireproof box or with your lawyer. If they are kept in your safety deposit box, be sure a family member or friend has access to the box so that papers can be removed when needed. Although the original documents must be used for any legal purposes, you may want to make copies for family members.

Conclusion

We hope this chapter has been helpful to you and those close to you. Our intention has been to give you some practical information and to encourage discussion with family and friends. Open communication offers a chance to learn one of life's most important lessons. As one cancer patient said:

> "We can choose to wait for death, or we can choose to live until we die. Knowing that death is in the near future is no reason to give up on the life we have today."

We hope that this chapter will help you face this time in your life. Try to remember that even when there seems to be little hope, there are ways to fight feelings of hopelessness and to acknowledge the good things around you.

Try to keep in mind that survival statistics are just numbers. They are no guarantee that you will die at a certain time. In fact, the numbers that should mean the most to you—and perhaps to all of us at any time of life—are those that measure the good days, the comfortable nights, and the hours of happiness and joy, however you find them.

Resources

Information about cancer is available from many sources, including the ones listed below. You may wish to check for additional information at your local library or bookstore and from support groups in your community.

Cancer Information Service (CIS). The Cancer Information Service, a program of the National Cancer Institute, is a nationwide telephone service for cancer patients and their families and friends, the public, and health care professionals. The staff can answer questions (in English or Spanish) and can send free National Cancer Institute booklets about cancer. They also know about local resources and services. One toll-free telephone number, 1-800-4-CANCER (1-800-422-6237), connects callers with the office that serves their area.

American Cancer Society (ACS). The American Cancer Society is a voluntary organization with a national office and local units all over the country. This organization supports research, conducts educational programs, and offers many services to patients and their families. The American Cancer Society also provides free booklets on cancer. To obtain booklets, or for information about services and activities in local areas, call the Society's toll-free number, 1-800-ACS-2345, or the number listed under American Cancer Society in the white pages of the telephone book.

Chapter 84

When Cancer Recurs: Meeting the Challenge Again

In the back of every cancer patient's mind is the possibility that the disease may return. And yet when it does, most patients think, "How can this be happening to me again?"

The shock is back. The fears are back—of telling your family and friends, of more treatment, and possibly of death. The anger is there too—after all you've been through, it should have been enough. And the unanswered question is, "Will the treatment work this time?"

Even though you may feel some of the same things you felt when you were first diagnosed, now there's a difference. You've been through this before. You've faced cancer and its treatment and the changes that came to your life. You know that medical and emotional support is available to you. Facing cancer again is difficult, but it is a challenge you can handle.

This chapter is about cancer that has returned—its diagnosis and treatment, suggestions for coping, and where to get help.

As you read this chapter, remember that there are more than 100 different types of cancer. Each is different, and each person responds to treatment differently. No publication can cover every situation for every person. For this reason, the information given here is general, and some of it may not apply to you. Still, a lot of people have found ways to handle recurring cancer in similar ways, and their experiences may help you.

"When Cancer Recurs: Meeting the Challenge Again," National Cancer Institute (NCI). NIH publication 93-2709, revised November 1997.

921

Many people who have faced the return of cancer say that learning more about your illness and its treatment helps you to take part in your care. Having a positive attitude toward treatment may help you control some of your emotional and physical reactions to it. Drawing on your own strengths and the support from the people and resources around you can help you meet this challenge again. You can call the Cancer Information Service (CIS) at 1-800-4-CANCER to get the most up-to-date information about treatment for your type of cancer and to talk with someone who can offer suggestions on how to cope.

Why Cancer Can Recur

"Recur" means to "happen again." When cancer recurs, it means that the disease that was thought to be cured, or at least to be inactive (in remission), has become active again. Cancer may recur after several months, a few years, or many years.

Cancer that has recurred is very much like the first cancer in the way that it starts: Abnormal cells begin to grow and multiply quickly. If not stopped, cancer cells can destroy normal tissues and organs.

Recurrent cancer starts from cells that were not killed by the original therapy. Your previous treatment was meant to destroy the original cancer and the cells that may have broken away from it. However, a small number of cancer cells may have survived and only now have grown into large enough tumors to be detected.

The cancer that recurs is the same type as the original cancer, no matter where it is found. For example, if colon cancer recurs in the liver, it is not liver cancer; it is colon cancer that has spread to the liver.

Where Cancers Can Recur

Not every cancer cell that breaks away from a tumor is able to grow elsewhere. Most are stopped by the body's natural defenses or destroyed by treatment. Cancers differ in their ability to recur and in the places where they may recur. For this reason, recurrent cancers are classified by location: local, regional, or metastatic.

Local recurrence means that the cancer has come back in the same place as the original cancer. The term "local" also means that there is no sign of cancer in nearby lymph nodes or other tissues. For instance, a woman who has had a mastectomy could later have a local recurrence of breast cancer in or around the area of the surgery.

A regional recurrence involves growth of a new tumor in lymph nodes or tissues near the original site but with no evidence of cancer at distant places in the body. A man who has had a melanoma removed from his arm, for instance, might have a regional recurrence in the lymph nodes under his arm.

In metastatic recurrence, cancer has spread to organs or other tissues far from the original site. For example, a man with prostate cancer could have metastasis to his bones.

Diagnosing Recurrent Cancer

Over the past several months or years, you may have had a number of tests and checkups. Most likely, your doctor told you to watch for changes in your body and to report any unusual symptoms.

You may have noticed a weight change, bleeding, or constant pain, or your doctor may have found signs of further illness while examining you. In either case, tests are used to find the exact cause of the problem and decide on the best treatment.

Specific procedures and tests help your doctor answer these questions:

- Are the signs and symptoms caused by cancer or by some other medical problem?

- If cancer is present, is it a recurrence or is it a different type?

- Has the cancer spread to more than one place?

Because certain types of cancer tend to recur in certain parts of the body, your doctor is likely to check those places first. Information from physical exams and tests helps the doctor make an accurate diagnosis and choose the treatment that is best for you.

In addition to the routine physical exam (feeling for lumps, swelling, and so on), your doctor may need to look at your colon, stomach, bladder, breathing passages, or other organs. A number of instruments are used for viewing different parts of the body. The names of most of the instruments end in "scope" For example, a bronchoscope is used to view the air passages of a lung. In some cases, the doctor may even take a tissue sample (biopsy) through the scope and look at the sample under a microscope.

A number of lab tests are used to help diagnose recurrent cancer. For example, blood samples can be tested to check the levels of certain proteins or enzymes that may change when cancer recurs. The carcinoembryonic antigen (CEA) assay is a blood test that detects changes in the body that often accompany some cancers.

Other tests, such as the examination of a stool smear, can detect internal bleeding that may be too slight for you to notice. If blood is found, a series of x-rays or another type of test is done to learn if the bleeding is caused by cancer or by some other problem.

These are only a few examples of lab tests used to diagnose cancer and other health problems. Your doctor will select those that may be helpful in your case.

X-Rays and Scans

To learn the location and size of suspected cancer, the doctor can use x-rays, computed tomography (CT) scans, nuclear scanning, ultrasound, or magnetic resonance imaging (MRI).

These tests use radiation, computers, magnets, and other sophisticated equipment. If you have questions about how they are used, their risks or benefits, or what you should expect during the procedure, be sure to talk with your doctor, nurse, or technician about your concerns.

X-Rays

Tumors that cause a change in density of a normal structure can often be seen with the standard x-ray; for example, decreased bone density from breast cancer that has spread or increased density of lung cancer that has grown into the air spaces of the lung. Other tests combine x-rays with a barium solution, dye, or air to give sharp pictures of organs such as the stomach, kidney, and colon that cannot be seen clearly with x-rays alone. An example of this kind of study is the "lower GI (gastrointestinal) series" (barium enema followed by an x-ray).

CT Scan

In a CT scan, a series of x-rays are taken from many directions and combined into one cross-sectional picture with the aid of a computer. The CT scan gives more detailed pictures than standard x-rays for certain body parts and is often used for tissues such as the liver and brain.

Nuclear Scanning

Nuclear scans are often used to see many parts of the body. A substance that is very slightly radioactive is swallowed or injected into the bloodstream. A machine called a scanner then takes pictures of the areas of the body where the substance is taken up. A cancer can show up in the pictures as an area of more or less radioactivity than the tissue around it.

Ultrasound

An ultrasound test uses a microphone-like device that sends sound waves that bounce off internal organs. The sound echoes to form a picture of the organ.

MRI

Instead of x-rays, MRI uses radio waves and a powerful magnet to create images of internal organs. Like a CT scan, MRI uses a computer to combine many images into a single picture. That picture may include organs, muscles, blood vessels, and other parts of the body that are hard to see with other kinds of scanners.

Biopsy

A biopsy is often the best way to tell if cancer is present. While an abnormal area may be seen through scopes or on x-ray films, a biopsy shows whether it is made of cancer cells.

For some cancers, the doctor uses a needle to withdraw fluid (aspirate) or remove small tissue samples (needle biopsy). A surgical biopsy, done under local or general anesthesia, removes the entire tumor or a piece of it. The sample of cells or tissues that is removed is examined under a microscope.

If your cancer has recurred, an accurate diagnosis is the first step in determining the best course of treatment and getting the disease under control again.

Treatment Methods

In planning your treatment for recurrent cancer, many of the same factors that affected treatment decisions for the original cancer will be taken into account. How your cancer is treated depends on the type of cancer, its size and location, your general health, and other treatments you've had.

Your doctor may recommend surgery, radiation, anticancer drugs (chemotherapy), or a combination of these treatments. For certain cancers, such as those in the reproductive organs, the doctor may suggest hormone therapy. In other cases, biological therapy may be considered.

It is important that you take an active part in your treatment by asking questions and expressing your feelings. Talk to your doctor about treatment goals, methods, and side effects to help determine which treatment will be best for you.

The following paragraphs describe the most common treatments, some of the newer methods now under study, and "unproven" treatments that you may have heard about. You will also find a list of questions that patients often ask about the various treatments.

Surgery

Surgery is often used to treat cancer when it is first diagnosed, but it is used less often in recurrent disease. Your doctor may recommend an operation to remove a recurrence if it seems to be limited to a single spot on the skin or in the lung, liver, bone, brain, or lymph nodes. For many sites of recurrence, other methods such as radiation, chemotherapy, or biological therapy have been shown to be more effective.

When cancer recurs in a weight-bearing bone (such as in the leg), there may be a threat of fracture caused by the growing tumor. In such a case, the doctor may suggest an operation to support the bone and prevent a break. This procedure can help relieve pain and keep the patient active while waiting for other forms of treatment to take effect and control the cancer.

Radiation Therapy

Radiation treatment directs high levels of radiation (tens of thousands of times the amount used, for instance, to produce a chest x-ray) at a cancerous tumor to destroy the cancer cells. Both normal and cancer cells are affected by radiation, but many normal cells replace themselves quickly while cancer cells do not.

Doctors use radiation to treat cancer in almost every part of the body. Sometimes radiation therapy is used before surgery to shrink a cancerous tumor. After surgery, it may be used to stop the growth of any cancer cells that remain in a certain part of the body. In some cases, doctors use radiation and anticancer drugs, rather than surgery, to destroy a cancer and prevent it from returning.

The type of cancer, location, stage (extent of disease), and other factors will determine whether radiation therapy is right for a patient.

Sites that may be treated with radiation include the brain, lung, and bone.

Although radiation treatment can cause side effects, most are not serious. They usually disappear within a few weeks after treatment ends, although some last longer. The type of side effects will often depend on the part of the body that is being treated and the amount of radiation received. Fatigue and skin irritation are common side effects among patients receiving radiation therapy. Many patients have no side effects at all. If radiation therapy is prescribed for you, ask your doctor to explain the side effects that might occur and how you can best manage them. *Radiation Therapy and You* [reprinted in this volume as Chapter 66], a booklet available from the National Cancer Institute (NCI), answers many questions about this type of treatment.

Chemotherapy

Chemotherapy is the use of drugs to treat cancer. These drugs may be used alone or in combination with radiation therapy, surgery, or biological therapy.

Chemotherapy may be given by mouth or by injection into the veins or muscles. The drugs reach and destroy cancer cells in nearly every part of the body. Treatment may consist of a single drug or a combination of drugs.

Because anticancer drugs can reach sites that are far away from the original cancer and can destroy cancer cells throughout the body, chemotherapy is the primary treatment for many kinds of recurrent cancers that have spread beyond a single site or region.

Chemotherapy can affect any rapidly growing cells in the body, normal as well as cancer cells. The normal cells most likely to be affected are the blood-producing cells in the bone, cells lining the digestive tract and reproductive organs, and hair follicles. Again, the normal cells are able to replace themselves while the cancer cells cannot.

Every person reacts differently to chemotherapy. Some people have few or no side effects; others say their side effects are less severe than they expected; still others have a more difficult time. Ask your doctor, nurse, or pharmacist about side effects that could occur with the specific anticancer drugs prescribed for you. They can give you suggestions to help manage problems that may occur during treatment. Most side effects gradually begin to stop after treatment ends. However, the fatigue that some patients experience during chemotherapy sometimes lingers for a while.

927

The NCI's booklet *Chemotherapy and You* [reprinted in this volume as Chapter 63] provides further information about this type of cancer treatment.

Hormone Therapy

Some cancers are sensitive to changes in hormone levels. By adding, removing, or limiting the activity of a certain hormone, doctors can slow the growth or therapy is often used to treat cancers of the breast and prostate.

Sometimes surgery or radiation treatment is used to stop the body from producing hormones that cancer cells need to grow. Hormone therapy can cause a number of side effects, depending on the type of drug or surgical procedures. Patients may have nausea, swelling, or weight gain. In some cases, the treatment interferes with the body's production or use of hormones. For example, breast cancer patients taking tamoxifen may have some symptoms of menopause, such as hot flashes.

Biological Therapy

Biological therapy—sometimes called immunotherapy—is a promising new area of cancer treatment. It uses both natural and manmade substances to boost the body's own immune (defense) system against cancer. Called "biological response modifiers" or BRMs, they help the body's immune system fight the growth of cancer cells. Researchers are studying biological therapies in clinical trials to learn how BRMs work best and against which cancers.

Supportive Therapy

When you were first treated for cancer, you may have had physical therapy or used the services of a psychological counselor or social worker. You may want to consider seeking those kinds of help again. Two other types of supportive therapy that could also be important to you are nutritional support and pain management.

Nutrition

Eating well during cancer therapy is very important. Studies have shown that patients who eat well may be able to cope better with the cancer and its treatment.

Eating well means choosing foods that have the protein, calories, and other elements needed to keep the body working normally. Dieting during treatment is not advised because it deprives the body of needed calories and nutrients.

You could have problems with eating and digesting food because of treatment side effects. There are ways to ease some of these side effects, however. The NCI publication *Eating Hints* [reprinted in this volume as Chapter 77] has many suggestions for healthy eating habits during treatment, as do the booklets *Chemotherapy and You* and *Radiation Therapy and You*, which discuss specific nutrition problems associated with those treatments.

If eating enough to stay at your normal weight continues to be a problem in spite of your efforts, ask a dietitian at the hospital where you had your treatment to help plan a diet for you. For severe nutrition problems, special treatments can be given at home or in the hospital.

Pain Control

Although many people with cancer do not have serious problems with pain, others need help managing their pain. Pain from cancer or its treatment may need only a light medication—such as Tylenol (acetaminophen) or another medication with acetaminophen—to relieve it. If the pain is not helped by light pain relievers, ask your doctor about prescription medicines or other methods of pain relief. Some individuals can use intravenous medications received through a catheter where they can control the amount and rate of medication. These and other methods are being studied to see if they can help cancer patients.

Many patients try to avoid using pain medicine on a regular basis. Bear in mind, though, that the medicine works best if taken before the pain becomes severe. Talk with your doctor if you are concerned about how often to take the medicine or if it doesn't seem to be working. If you're having radiation therapy or chemotherapy, be sure to check with your doctor before taking any medicines.

When describing a pain to your doctor, be as specific as you can. To recommend the best pain treatment for you, your doctor will want to know the following things:

- Where exactly is your pain? Does it ever move from one spot to another?

- How does the pain feel (dull, sharp, burning, etc.)?

- How often does it occur?

- How long does the pain last?

- Does it start at a specific time (before or after meals, after certain activities, etc.)?

- Does anything (lying down, sitting, eating, etc.) seem to relieve the pain?

Because pain can be worse when you are frightened or worried, you may find some relief by using relaxation exercises or meditation. These activities, which usually involve deep, rhythmic breathing and quiet concentration, can be done almost anywhere.

A number of nonmedical ways to reduce pain have been gaining attention in recent years. Hypnosis and biofeedback have been helpful for some people with serious illness. If you want to learn about them, ask your doctor or nurse to refer you to a health professional who is trained to teach these methods. The NCI publication *Questions & Answers About Pain Control* provides many suggestions for managing pain.

Investigational and Unproven Treatments

The words "investigational" and "unproven" may be similar in meaning, but there are important differences when they are used to describe cancer treatments. Understanding the difference can help you when discussing and choosing among your treatment options.

Investigational Treatments

Investigational treatments are new methods of treating disease that are given under strict scientific controls. These methods have been tested on animals and have shown promise for treating humans. Doctors test the value of new treatments with the help of cancer patients who take part in studies called clinical trials.

Patients who take part in clinical trials may be the first to benefit from improved treatment methods. They also can make an important contribution to medical care because the results of the studies may help many people. Patients participate in clinical trials only if they choose to and are free to leave the trial at any time. More information about these studies is provided in NCI's booklet *What Are Clinical Trials All About?*

Examples of investigational treatments of cancer being studied in clinical trials at this time include new combinations of drugs, biological therapies, and bone marrow transplants. If proven effective, the investigational treatments of today could become standard treatments in the future.

Unproven Methods

A treatment method described as "unproven" is one for which the substance used (a vitamin, food, etc.) or the way it is given has not been shown, by accepted scientific methods, to be effective. Unproven methods you may have heard about use various diets, vitamins, and herb mixtures.

The American Cancer Society (ACS) has developed a list of clues to help you know whether a new treatment is "investigational" or "unproven." One way is to look at how results of the treatment are reported. Findings from clinical trials are usually first reported in medical and scientific journals and may later be reported in newspapers and magazines directed to the general public. Unproven methods are usually reported only in newspapers and magazines. They generally rely on first-person accounts by patients and do not discuss scientific data. Using these unproven treatments may actually be harmful because they may cause dangerous reactions or may delay or interfere with treatments proven to be effective.

Call the CIS if you want to learn more about unproven methods. The booklet *Unproven Methods of Cancer Management*, available from ACS, provides information about many of these treatments. Be sure to carefully consider the list of suggested questions below as you think about your treatment options.

Questions to Ask the Doctor

Before you and your doctor agree on a treatment plan, you should understand why one treatment is recommended over others. Compare the possible benefits, risks, side effects, and effect on the quality of your life of the recommended treatment with other treatments.

The questions listed below are examples of what patients often want to know about their treatment. You may want to add your own questions to the list to discuss with your doctor, nurse, or social worker. Family members or others close to you may have questions, too.

Questions to Ask about Any Recommended Treatment

- What is the goal of this treatment? Is it a cure, will it shrink the tumor and relieve the symptoms, or is it for comfort only?

- Why do you think this treatment is the best one for me?

- Is this the standard treatment for my type of cancer?

- Are there other treatments? What are they?

- Am I eligible for any clinical trials?

- What benefits can I expect from the treatment?

- Are there side effects with this treatment? Are they temporary or permanent?

- Is there any way to prevent or relieve the side effects?

- How safe is this treatment? What are the risks?

- How will I know if the treatment is working?

- Will I need to be in the hospital?

- What will happen if I don't have the treatment?

- What does my family need to know about the treatment? Can they help?

- How long will I be on this treatment?

- How much will the treatment cost?

Questions about Radiation Therapy

- What benefits can I expect from this therapy?

- What type of radiation treatment will I be getting?

- How long do the treatments take? How many will I need? How often?

- Can I schedule treatments at a certain time of day?

- What if I have to miss a treatment?

- What risks are involved?

- What side effects should I expect? What can I do about them?

- Who will give me the treatments? Where are they given?

- Will I need a special diet?

- Will my activities be limited?

Questions about Chemotherapy and Hormone Therapy

- What do you expect the drugs to do for me?

- Which drugs will I be getting? How is each one given?

- Where are the treatments given?

- How long do the treatments take? How many will I need?

- What happens if I miss a dose?

- What risks are involved?

- What side effects should I expect?

- What can I do about them?

- Will I need a special diet or other restrictions?

- Can I take other medicines during treatment?

- Can I drink alcoholic beverages during treatment?

Questions about Biological Therapy

- Exactly what kind of therapy will I receive?

- How is it given? Has this type of therapy already been shown to work against my kind of cancer?

- What side effects should I expect?

- What can be done about them? Where will I have to go for treatment?

- Who will be the doctor responsible for my care?

- How long will the treatment last, and how long will I be in the hospital?

- How much will the treatment cost? Will my insurance pay for it?

Questions about Investigational Treatments or Unproven Methods

- What benefits can I expect from the treatment?

- What can you learn from it?

- Is there scientific evidence that the treatment can help?

- What are the known or potential risks? Possible side effects?

- Will I have to get the new treatment from a different doctor?

- Will my insurance cover the costs of treatment?

- Will I have to travel to get the treatment? How often?

Helping Yourself

Gathering Information

You may remember that much of the fear and anxiety that you felt the first time cancer appeared in your life was "fear of the unknown." You can help yourself again by gathering information, taking part in your treatment as actively as possible, and finding the support you need to deal with your feelings about the recurrence of your cancer.

If you know how your illness can affect your body and if you stay informed about the progress of your treatment, you have a better chance to take part in your care.

Learn as much as you can about what is happening to you. If you have questions, ask your doctor and other members of your treatment team. Your pharmacist is a good person to talk to if you have questions about your medicines. If you don't understand the answer to a question, ask it again.

Some patients hesitate to ask their doctors about their treatment options. They may think that doctors do not like to have their recommendations questioned. Most doctors, however, believe that the best patient is an informed patient. They understand that coping with treatment is easier when patients understand as much as possible, and they encourage patients to discuss their concerns.

When you see your doctor to talk about possible treatments or to get help for problems that come up during treatment, take your list of questions and ask a friend or relative to go with you. You'll get the most useful advice if you and your companion speak openly with the doctor about your needs, expectations, wishes, and concerns.

Taking Part in Your Treatment

Taking an active part in your care can help you have a sense of control and well-being. You can be involved in many ways. One is to follow your doctor's recommendations about caring for yourself such as staying on a special diet or avoiding alcohol.

Another way you can help is to keep your doctor informed. Report honestly how you feel, and if problems arise, be as specific as possible when describing them. Don't ever hesitate to report symptoms to your doctor or to ask advice about what to do about them. Although many health-related signs and symptoms may not seem important to you, they could provide valuable information to your doctor. Know what signs you should look for, and if any of them appear, tell your doctor as soon as possible.

Remember the difference between "doing" and "overdoing." Rest is very important to you now—both physically and emotionally. Some things you can do to keep up your strength are to:

- *Eat well.* This may be one of the most important things you can do to improve your body's response to treatment.

- *Get extra rest.* Your body will use a lot of extra energy during treatment. Get more sleep at night, and take naps whenever you feel the need.

- *Adjust activities.* Try not to demand too much of yourself. Ask other people to take over some of your tasks if necessary. If your energy level is low, do the things that are most important to you and cut back on the others.

Managing Your Emotions

The diagnosis of cancer, whether for the first time or when it recurs, can threaten anyone's sense of well-being. Some people, when they first find out that cancer has returned, feel shock and denial. Many had put their experiences with cancer completely behind them, and the new diagnosis hits them as hard as—or even harder than—it did the first time. Others are not surprised, as if they had been expecting it all along.

There may be times when you'll feel overcome by fear, anxiety, depression, or anger. These emotions are natural. They are common ways to cope with a difficult situation, and many people with recurrent cancer experience them. Feel free to express these feelings if they occur. None of these is a "wrong" reaction, and letting them out will help you deal with them.

Starting cancer treatments again can place demands on your spirits as well as your body. Your attitudes and actions really can make a difference. Remember that you have coped with this situation before. Keeping your treatment goals in mind may help you keep your spirits up during therapy and see you through "down" spells that may occur.

As you go through treatment, you're bound to feel better about yourself on some days than on others. The uncertainty of living with recurrent cancer can sometimes contribute to ups and downs. When a bad day comes along, try to remember that there have been good days, and there will be more. Feeling low today does not mean you will feel that way tomorrow or that you are giving up. At these times, try distracting yourself with a book, a hobby, or plans for a new garden.

Many people say it helps to have something to look forward to—even simple things like a drive, a visit from a friend, or a telephone call. Sometimes, however, you may just want to cry, and that's okay, too.

You may need to rely more on the people closest to you to help during your treatment, but this may be difficult at first. You may not want to accept help, and some people may have trouble giving it. Many people do not understand cancer, and they may avoid you because they're afraid of your illness. Others may worry that they will upset you by saying the wrong thing.

At a time when you might expect others to rush to your aid, you may have to make the first move. Try to be open in talking with others about your illness, your treatment, your needs, and your feelings. Once people know that you can discuss these things, they may be more willing to open up and help.

By sharing your feelings, you and your loved ones will be better able to help each other through a difficult time. Another booklet from NCI, *Taking Time*, offers useful advice for cancer patients and their families.

Sometimes it is easier to talk to someone outside your family or your friends. Try talking to health professionals such as your doctor, nurse, psychologist, social worker, or a clergyman with whom you feel comfortable. These professionals care about your emotional as well as physical well-being. When they know about your personal concerns, how your home life or lifestyle has been affected, and what changes in your situation you'd like to see, they will be better able to support you emotionally.

At times you are likely to feel stressed by the continuing changes in your life. Some stress can help because it may push you to take action. Too much stress, though, can harm your health and make you feel like you are losing control. You may not be able to remove all the stress around you, but you can try to limit it. Relaxation techniques can be used to reduce stress and help you cope better with your illness. Rhythmic breathing, imagery, and distraction are among the techniques that are easy to learn and use whenever you need them. If you are interested, ask your doctor or nurse to refer you to someone trained to teach these techniques. The local library also has useful books on relieving stress.

There are many reasons for cancer patients to feel sad, worried, or depressed. You can probably manage some of these problems on your own or with the help of family, friends, or clergy, but for others you may want professional help. A counselor trained to help cancer patients deal with their feelings can offer the support you may need.

These counselors understand the special problems that go along with serious illness as well as the various ways of coping that others have found useful. If you think this kind of professional support could help you, ask your doctor or nurse for the name of an appropriate counselor.

Employment and Insurance Issues

If you have a job, you may want to return to work as soon as you can. You may even find it possible to continue to work during the time you are receiving treatment. This depends on the kind of treatment you are getting, what side effects you have, and how you feel about working.

Sometimes cancer patients find that they are treated differently on the job because of their medical condition. If this happens to you, be aware of your rights. Your employer may be violating laws that protect people against such unfair practices.

Although as many as 1 million cancer patients in the United States experience some form of employment discrimination, this practice is illegal. Find out the legal facts on equal opportunity by contacting your local department of employment services.

You need to fully understand your insurance rights, not only as a cancer patient but also as an employee of your company. Carefully read the health insurance policy provided by your employer. If you have any questions, contact your state insurance commission or department. This agency determines what types of insurance policies must be offered and when rates may be raised.

If you have trouble learning what your rights are, or if you have any questions about employment issues, contact the Cancer Information Service, the American Cancer Society, or the National Coalition for Cancer Survivorship (NCCS). They can help you find local agencies that respond to problems cancer survivors face regarding their rights. The addresses and telephone numbers of these groups are listed in the next section.

Resources for Patients and Families

General information about cancer is widely available. Some of the resources and publications listed below might be helpful to you. You may also wish to see what the local library has to offer and contact support groups in your community. You don't have to be an active member of these groups to use their information services.

Cancer Information Service
1-800-4-CANCER

The National Cancer Institute-supported Cancer Information Service (CIS) is a nationwide telephone service that responds to inquiries from cancer patients and their families, health care professionals, and the public. Information specialists can provide information and publications on all aspects of cancer. They also may know about cancer-related services in local areas. By dialing 1-800-4-CANCER (1-800-422-6237), you will be connected to a CIS serving your area, where a trained staff member can answer your questions and listen to your concerns. Spanish-speaking CIS staff members are available.

People who have cancer, those who care about them, and doctors need up-to-date and accurate information about cancer treatment. To help these people, NCI has developed Physician Data Query (PDQ). This computer system gives quick and easy access to:

- Cancer treatment information for both patients and doctors.

- Information about research studies, called clinical trials, that test new and promising cancer treatments and are open to patients.

- Names of organizations and doctors involved in caring for people with cancer.

To get information from PDQ, doctors may use an office computer, the services of a medical library, or call the CIS. Patients can also get PDQ information from the CIS.

Publications

You may also want to read some other NCI booklets and fact sheets that discuss various aspects of cancer, cancer treatment, and patient concerns. Available free of charge, the publications may be ordered by calling the Cancer Information Service at 1-800-4-CANCER or by writing to the National Cancer Institute, Building 31, Room 10A24, Bethesda, Maryland 20892. The following booklets might be especially helpful:

- *Answers to Your Questions About Metastatic Cancer.* This fact sheet presents information on detection, treatment methods, and common areas of recurrence.

- *Chemotherapy and You: A Guide to Self-Help During Treatment.* * This is a detailed guide about anticancer drugs and how they act.

- *Eating Hints.* * This is a collection of helpful, practical information to help make mealtime more pleasant for people with cancer.

- *Questions & Answers About Pain Control.* This booklet discusses pain control using both medical and nonmedical methods. It is also available from ACS.

- *Radiation Therapy and You: A Guide to Self-Help During Treatment.* * Radiation therapy, its goals and side effects, and suggestions to help patients manage are discussed in this booklet.

- Research Reports. These in-depth reports cover current knowledge of various types of cancer. When requesting a report, specify a primary cancer site (such as lung or breast).

- *Taking Time: Support for People With Cancer and the People Who Care About Them.* This booklet discusses the special emotional and personal problems that people with cancer face.

- *What Are Clinical Trials All About?* This booklet describes what types of trials are available, who is eligible, what is involved if you are in a clinical trial, and what are important questions to ask before enrolling in a clinical trial.

- *What You Need To Know About...* This is a series of booklets about different types of cancer. Specify a primary cancer site in your request.

* Reprinted in this volume—see Table of Contents

Support Programs and Organizations

Health professionals and patients alike have learned the value of mutual support among patients. When someone with a serious illness feels frightened or depressed, it often helps to discuss those feelings with another person who has been through the same experience. This can help patients get practical information, understand their feelings, and develop their own ways of handling their problems. The following programs and organizations provide support for patients, family members, and others who are close to someone with a serious illness.

American Cancer Society. The American Cancer Society (ACS) is a nonprofit organization that offers a variety of services to patients and their families. Through ACS's CanSurmount Program, people who have recovered from cancer are available to talk with newly diagnosed and recurrent cancer patients about cancer-related problems and treatments. The ACS also offers the I Can Cope Program, which is a course designed to address the educational and psychological needs of people with cancer. To find an ACS chapter near you, check your local telephone book or contact the national office at the following address and telephone number:

American Cancer Society
National Headquarters
599 Clifton Road, N.E.
Atlanta, Georgia 30329
(404) 320-3333

Leukemia and Lymphoma Society. The Society offers supplemental financial assistance and consultation services to cancer patients with leukemia and related disorders.

Leukemia and Lymphoma Society
733 Third Avenue
New York, New York 10017
(212) 573-8484

Make Today Count. This program brings together patients with cancer or other life-threatening illnesses and their families to help them cope with their illness and the changes in lifestyle that it often requires. Support is provided through group meetings, home visit programs, and newsletters. To receive information about this program, contact Make Today Count at the following address and telephone number:

Make Today Count, American Cancer Society
11311 Amherst Avenue
Silver Spring, MD 20902
(888) 227-6333

National Coalition for Cancer Survivorship. The National Coalition for Cancer Survivorship (NCCS) is a network of cancer survivors and related organizations across the country. It provides cancer survivors and their families with local support groups; a national clearinghouse of resources on support and on life after a cancer diagnosis; advocacy to reduce cancer-based discrimination; and a unified voice of cancer survivors. To find a local group of NCCS, contact the national office at the following address and telephone number:

National Coalition for Cancer Survivorship
323 Eighth Street, S.W.
Albuquerque, New Mexico 87102
(505) 764-9956

United Ostomy Association. The United Ostomy Association is a network of local chapters that offers emotional support, aid, and education to those who have had colostomy, ileostomy, or urostomy surgery.

United Ostomy Association
36 Executive Park, Suite 120
Irvine, California 92714
(714) 660-8624
(local chapters listed under "Ostomy")

Home Health Care Services. Some patients will need help caring for themselves during or after their cancer treatments. Many state and county health departments have programs that provide instruction in caring for the cancer patient at home. Such knowledge may be very useful after surgery or during bouts of illness. Commercial services, such as visiting nurses, may be listed under "home health agencies" in your telephone book.

American Red Cross. The American Red Cross (ARC) provides instruction in first aid and home nursing. Your local chapter may be able to help you locate someone to assist with activities such as personal care, housework, and shopping, if you need this type of help. To receive information about ARC, contact the national office at the following address and telephone number:

American Red Cross
National Headquarters
17th and D Streets, N.W.
Washington, D.C. 20006
(202) 737-8300

Chapter 85

Restoring Sexuality after Cancer

Sex and cancer are two seemingly incompatible subjects: One is a life-affirming, physically driven pleasurable event; the other represents a menacing physical and emotional battle. When it comes to cancer, an immediate reordering of priorities occurs, and all too often, sexuality becomes a casualty. But being able to enjoy sex after cancer treatment is a significant and necessary part of the recovery process. Never before has there been such a need to discuss quality-of-life issues as they relate to cancer survivors. An estimated 8 million Americans are living with cancer; 5 million of them have survived five or more years since their diagnosis and are now cancer-free.

But many doctors, while out to save lives, neglect their patients' sex lives. They often fail to recognize when a patient's sexuality has been sacrificed to cancer and its treatment. These doctors rarely discuss sexual performance with their patients, before or after treatment. "Often, discussing sex depends on a doctor's age, and how well adjusted they are to their own sexuality," says Dr. Fredrick J. Moritz, director of gynecologic oncology at Johns Hopkins.

Avoiding the issue all too often creates additional problems for people with cancer. It ends up shortchanging them physically and emotionally at a time when they most need to reaffirm and identify with with that has normally been a comforting part of their life. Truly informed healthcare decisions cannot be made until patients fully

"Restoring Sexuality After Cancer," *The Johns Hopkins Medical Letter*, page 7, April 1998. Reprinted with permission

understand the effect that cancer therapies may have on their sexual health.

What part sex plays in a person's life needs to be factored into the decision process when choosing a more-or-less aggressive therapy. For example, in some cases of prostate cancer, a man should choose between pelvic radiation and radical prostatectomy not just on the basis of statistical success, but also with an understanding of the degree to which each procedure may affect his ability to function sexually. In addition to surgery's impact, drug and radiation therapies may strike a powerful blow to the hormones and trigger menopause prematurely.

Still, while sexual expression may temporarily be put on hold by cancer, the need for intimacy and human warmth only increases. The eventual restoration of sex life can be a key part of feeling alive, whole, and healthy again. "Living is the main goal in cancer treatment,: says Dr. Moritz, "and this means traveling, dancing, spending time with your loved ones, and having sex." Dr. Montz recommends a comprehensive approach to cancer treatment, with nutritionists, clerics, and sexual therapists getting involved as needed.

Knowing What to Expect

"Being able to enjoy sex is a significant part of quality of life after cancer treatement," says Leslie R. Schover, Ph.D., a clinical psychologist and sex therapist at the Cleveland Clinic Foundation, and a leading authority on cancer and sexuality. Her book, *Sexuality and Fertility After Cancer* (John Wiley & Sons, 1997) details all the options cancer patients have, and how to take advantage of them. Dr. Schover writes that a frank discussion on the subject should touch upon:

- The physical side effects of radiation therapy and chemotherapy on sexual desire and performance;

- Tips on lovemaking after therapy;

- How women and men might feel when they see their partner's surgically altered body for the first time.

Chapter 86

Frequently Asked Questions about Hospice

1. When should a decision about entering a hospice program be made—and who should make it?

At any time during a life limiting illness, it is appropriate to discuss all of a patients care options, including hospice. By law the decision belongs to the patient.

Understandably, most people are uncomfortable with the idea of stopping an all-out effort to beat the disease. Hospice staff members are highly sensitive to these concerns and always available to discuss them with the patient and family.

2. Should I wait for our physician to raise the possibility of hospice, or should I raise it first?

The patient and family should feel free to discuss hospice care at any time with their physician, other health care professionals, clergy or friends.

3. What if our physician doesn't know about hospice?

Most physicians know about hospice. If your physician wants more information about hospice, it is available from the Academy of Hospice Physicians, medical societies, state hospice organizations, or the National Hospice Helpline, 1-800-658-8898.

Reprinted with permission from the National Hospice Organization. http://www.teleport.com/~hospice/faq.htm

4. Can a hospice patient who shows signs of recovery be returned to regular treatment?

Certainly. If the patient's condition improves and the disease seems to be in remission, patients can be discharged from hospice and return to aggressive therapy or go on about their daily life.

If a discharged patient should later need to return to hospice care, Medicare and most private insurance will allow additional coverage for this purpose.

5. What does the hospice admission process involve?

One of the first things hospice will do is contact the patient's physician to make sure he or she agrees that hospice care is appropriate for this patient at this time. (Hospices have medical staff available to help patients who have no physician.)

The patient will also be asked to sign consent and insurance forms. These are similar to the forms patients sign when they enter a hospital.

The so-called hospice election form says that the patient understands that the care is palliative (that is, aimed at pain relief and symptom control) rather than curative. It also outlines the services available. The form Medicare patients sign also tells how electing the Medicare hospice benefit affects other Medicare coverage for a terminal illness.

6. Is there any special equipment or changes I have to make in my home before hospice care begins?

Your hospice provider will assess your needs, recommend any equipment, and help make arrangements to obtain any necessary equipment. Often the need for equipment is minimal at first and increases as the disease gets worse. In general, hospice will assist in any way it can to make home care as convenient, clean, and safe as possible.

7. How many family members or friends does it take to care for a patient at home?

There is no set number. One of the first things a hospice team will do is to prepare an individualized care plan that will, among other things, address the amount of caregiving needed in your situation. Hospice staff members visit regularly and are always accessible to answer medical questions and provide support.

8. Must someone be with the patient at all times?

In the early weeks of care, its usually not necessary for someone to be with the patient all the time. Later, however, since one of the most common fears of patients is the fear of dying alone, hospice generally recommends someone be there continuously.

9. How difficult is caring for a dying loved one at home?

Its never easy and sometimes can be quite hard. At the end of a long, progressive illness, nights especially can be very long, lonely, and scary. So, hospices have staff available around the clock to consult with the family and make night visits if the need arises.

To repeat: Hospice can also provide trained volunteers to provide respite care, or to give family members a break.

10. What specific assistance does hospice provide home-based patients?

Hospice patients are cared for by a team of doctors, nurses, social workers, counselors, home health aides, clergy, therapists, and volunteers—and each provides assistance based on his or her area of expertise. In addition, hospices help provide medications, supplies, equipment, hospital services, and additional helpers in the home, if and when needed.

11. Does hospice do anything to make death come sooner?

Hospices do nothing either to speed up or to slow down the dying process. Just as doctors and midwives lend support and expertise during the time of child birth, so hospice provides its presence and specialized knowledge during the dying process.

12. Is caring for the patients at home the only place hospice care can be delivered?

No. Although 90% of hospice patient time is spent in a personal residence, some patients live in nursing homes or hospice centers.

13. How does hospice manage pain?

Hospice believes that emotional and spiritual pain are just as real and in need of attention as physical pain, as it addresses each.

Hospice nurses and doctors are up to date on the latest medications and devices for pain and symptom relief. In addition, physical

947

and occupational therapists assist patients to be as mobile and self-sufficient as possible, and they are often joined by specialists schooled in music therapy, art therapy, massage and diet counseling.

14. What is hospice's success rate in battling pain?

Very high. Using some combination of medications, counseling and therapies, most patients can be kept pain free and comfortable.

15. Will medications prevent the patient from being able to talk or know what's happening?

Usually not. It is the goal of hospice to allow the patient to be pain free but alert. By constantly consulting with the patient, hospices have been very successful in reaching this goal.

16. Is hospice affiliated with any religious organizations?

Hospice is not an off-shoot of any religion. While some churches and religions have started hospices (sometimes in connection with their hospitals), these hospices serve a broad community and do not require patients to adhere to any particular set of beliefs.

17. Is hospice care covered by insurance?

Hospice coverage is available widely. It is provided by Medicare nationwide, by Medicaid in over 30 states, and by most private health insurance policies. To be sure of coverage, families should, of course, check with their employer or health insurance provider.

18. If the patient is eligible for Medicare, will there be any additional expenses to be paid?

Medicare covers all services and supplies for the hospice patient. In some hospices, the patient may be required to pay a 5% or $5 co-payment on medication and respite care. You should find out about any co-payment when finding a hospice.

19. If the patient is not covered by Medicare or any other health insurance, will hospice still provide care?

The first thing hospice will do is assist families in finding out whether the patient is eligible for any coverage they may not be aware of. Barring this, most hospices will provide for anyone who cannot pay using money raised for the community or from memorial or foundation gifts.

20. Does the hospice provide any help to the family after the patient dies?

Hospice provides continuing contact and support for family and friends for at least a year following the death of a loved one. Most hospices also sponsor bereavement groups and support for anyone in the community who experienced a death of a family member, a school friend, and the like.

Part Six

Additional Help and Information

Chapter 87

Glossary of Cancer Terms

A

Abdomen (AB-do-men): The part of the body that contains the pancreas, stomach, intestines, liver, gallbladder, and other organs.

Accelerated phase (ak-SEL-er-ay-ted): Refers to chronic myelogenous leukemia that is progressing. The number of immature, abnormal white blood cells in the bone marrow and blood is higher than in the chronic phase, but not as high as in the blast phase.

Achlorhydria (a-klor-HY-dree-a): A lack of hydrochloric acid in the digestive juices in the stomach. Hydrochloric acid helps digest food.

Acoustic (ah-KOOS-tik): Related to sound or hearing.

Actinic keratosis (ak-TIN-ik ker-a-TO-sis): A precancerous condition of thick, scaly patches of skin; also called solar or senile keratosis.

Acute leukemia: Leukemia that progresses rapidly.

Adenocarcinoma (AD-in-o-kar-sin-O-ma): Cancer that begins in cells that line certain internal organs.

Adenoma (AD-in-o-ma): A noncancerous tumor.

Adjuvant therapy (AD-joo-vant): Treatment given in addition to the primary treatment to enhance the effectiveness of the primary treatment.

Excerpted from the comprehensive glossary of the National Cancer Institute web page at: http://rex.nci.nih.gov/info_cancer/cancer_defs/

Adrenal glands (a-DREE-nal): A pair of small glands, one located on top of each kidney. The adrenal glands produce hormones that help control heart rate, blood pressure, the way the body uses food, and other vital functions.

Aflatoxin (AF-la-TOK-sin): A substance made by a mold that is often found on poorly stored grains and nuts. Aflatoxins are known to cause cancer in animals.

Agranulocyte (A-gran-yoo-lo-SITE): A type of white blood cell; monocytes and lymphocytes are agranulocytes.

Allogeneic bone marrow transplantation (AL-o-jen-AY-ik): A procedure in which a patient receives bone marrow from a compatible, though not genetically identical, donor.

Alpha-fetoprotein (AL-fa FEE-to-PRO-teen): A protein often found in abnormal amounts in the blood of patients with liver cancer.

Alveoli (al-VEE-o-lye): Tiny air sacs at the end of the bronchioles.

Amputation (am-pyoo-TAY-shun): Surgery to remove all or some of a body part.

Amylase (AM-il-aze): An enzyme that helps the body digest starches.

Anaplastic (an-ah-PLAS-tik): A term used to describe cancer cells that divide rapidly and bear little or no resemblance to normal cells.

Anastamosis (an-AS-ta-MO-sis): A procedure to connect healthy sections of the colon or rectum after the diseased portion has been surgically removed.

Androgen (AN-dro-jenz): A hormone that promotes the development and maintenance of male sex characteristics.

Anemia (a-NEE-mee-a): A decrease in the normal amounts of red blood cells.

Anesthesia (an-es-THEE-zha): Loss of feeling or awareness. A local anesthetic causes loss of feeling in a part of the body. A general anesthetic puts the person to sleep.

Anesthetic (an-es-THET-ik): A substance that causes loss of feeling or awareness. A local anesthetic causes loss of feeling in a part of the body. A general anesthetic puts the person to sleep.

Angiogenesis (an-gee-o-GEN-e-sis): Blood vessel formation, which usually accompanies the growth of malignant tissue.

Angiogram (AN-jee-o-gram): An x-ray of blood vessels; the patient receives an injection of dye to outline the vessels on the x-ray.

Angiography (an-jee-O-gra-fee): A procedure to x-ray blood vessels. The blood vessels can be seen because of an injection of a dye that shows up in the x-ray pictures.

Angiosarcoma (AN-jee-o-sar-KO-ma): A type of cancer that begins in the lining of blood vessels.

Antiandrogen (an-tee-AN-dro-jen): A drug that blocks the action of male sex hormones.

Antibiotics (an-ti-by-AH-tiks): Drugs used to treat infection.

Antibody (AN-ti-BOD-ee): A protein produced by certain white blood cells in response to a foreign substance (antigen). Each antibody can bind only to a specific antigen. The purpose of this binding is to help destroy the antigen. Antibodies can work in several ways, depending on the nature of the antigen. Some antibodies disable antigens directly. Others make the antigen more vulnerable to destruction by white blood cells.

Anticonvulsant (an-ti-kon-VUL-sant): Medicine to stop, prevent, or control seizures (convulsions).

Antigen: Any foreign or "non-self" substance that, when introduced into the body, causes the immune system to create an antibody.

Antithymocyte globulin (anti-THIGH-moe-site GLA-bu-lin): A protein preparation used to prevent and treat graft-versus-host disease.

Anus (AY-nus): The opening of the rectum to the outside of the body.

Aplastic anemia: A deficiency of certain parts of the blood caused by a failure of the bone marrow's ability to generate cells.

Apoptosis (ay-paw-TOE-sis): A normal cellular process involving a genetically programmed series of events leading to the death of a cell.

Areola (a-REE-oe-la): The area of dark-colored skin that surrounds the nipple.

Arterial embolization (ar-TEE-ree-al EM-bo-lih-ZAY-shun): Blocking an artery so that blood cannot flow to the tumor.

Arteriogram (ar-TEER-ee-o-gram): An x-ray of blood vessels, which can be seen after an injection of a dye that shows up in the x-ray pictures.

Asbestos (as-BES-tus): A natural material that is made up of tiny fibers. If the fibers are inhaled, they can lodge in the lungs and lead to cancer.

Ascites (a-SYE-teez): Abnormal buildup of fluid in the abdomen.

Aspiration (as-per-AY-shun): Removal of fluid from a lump, often a cyst, with a needle and a syringe.

Astrocytoma (as-tro-sye-TOE-ma): A type of brain tumor that begins in the brain or spinal chord in small, star-shaped cells called astrocytes.

Asymptomatic: Presenting no signs or symptoms of disease.

Ataxic gait (ah-TAK-sik): Awkward, uncoordinated walking.

Atypical hyperplasia (hy-per-PLAY-zha): A benign (noncancerous) condition in which tissue has certain abnormal features.

Autologous bone marrow transplantation (aw-TAHL-o-gus): A procedure in which bone marrow is removed from a patient and then is given back to the patient following intensive treatment.

Axilla (ak-SIL-a): The underarm.

Axillary (AK-sil-air-ee): Pertaining to the lymph nodes under the arm.

Axillary dissection (AK-sil-air-ee): Surgery to remove lymph nodes under the arm.

B

B cells: White blood cells that develop in the bone marrow and are the source of antibodies. Also known as B lymphocytes.

Barium enema: A series of x-rays of the lower intestine. The x-rays are taken after the patient is given an enema with a white, chalky solution that contains barium. The barium outlines the intestines on the x-rays.

Barium solution: A liquid containing barium sulfate that is used in x-rays to highlight parts of the digestive system.

Barrett's esophagus: A change in the cells of the tissue that lines the bottom of the esophagus. The esophagus may become irritated when the contents of the stomach back up (reflux). Reflux that happens often over a long period of time can lead to Barrett's esophagus.

Basal cell carcinoma (BAY-sal sel kar-sin-O-ma): A type of skin cancer that arises from the basal cells.

Basal cells: Small, round cells found in the lower part, or base, of the epidermis, the outer layer of the skin.

Basophil: A type of white blood cell. Basophils are granulocytes.

BCG (Bacillus Calmette-Guerin): A substance that activates the immune system. Filling the bladder with a solution of BCG is a form of biological therapy for superficial bladder cancer.

Benign (beh-NINE): Not cancerous; does not invade nearby tissue or spread to other parts of the body.

Benign prostatic hyperplasia (hy-per-PLAY-zha): A noncancerous condition in which an overgrowth of prostate tissue pushes against the urethra and the bladder, blocking the flow of urine. Also called benign prostatic hypertrophy or BPH.

Benign tumor (beh-NINE): A noncancerous growth that does not spread to other parts of the body.

Beta-carotene: A substance from which vitamin A is formed; a precursor of vitamin A.

Bilateral: Affecting the right and left side of body.

Bile: A yellow or orange fluid made by the liver. Bile is stored in the gallbladder. It passes through the common bile duct into the duodenum, where it helps digest fat.

Biological response modifiers (by-o-LOJ-i-kal): Substances that stimulate the body's response to infection and disease. The body naturally produces small amounts of these substances. Scientists can produce some of them in the laboratory in large amounts and use them in cancer treatment. Also called BRMs.

Biological therapy (by-o-LOJ-i-kul): The use of the body's immune system, either directly or indirectly, to fight cancer or to lessen side effects that may be caused by some cancer treatments. Also known as immunotherapy, biotherapy, or biological response modifier therapy.

Biopsy (BYE-ahp-see): The removal of a sample of tissue, which is then examined under a microscope to check for cancer cells.

Bladder: The hollow organ that stores urine.

Blast phase: Refers to advanced chronic myelogenous leukemia. In this phase, the number of immature, abnormal white blood cells in the bone marrow and blood is extremely high. Also called blast crisis.

Blasts: Immature blood cells.

Blood-brain barrier: A network of blood vessels with closely spaced cells that makes it difficult for potentially toxic substances (such as anti-cancer drugs) to penetrate the blood vessel walls and to enter the brain.

Bone marrow: The soft, spongy tissue in the center of large bones that produces white blood cells, red blood cells, and platelets.

Bone marrow aspiration (as-per-AY-shun) or biopsy (BY-op-see): The removal of a small sample of bone marrow (usually from the hip) through a needle for examination under a microscope to see whether cancer cells are present.

Bone marrow biopsy (BYE-ahp-see): The removal of a sample of tissue from the bone marrow with a large needle. The cells are checked to see whether they are cancerous. If cancerous plasma cells are found, the pathologist estimates how much of the bone marrow is affected. Bone marrow biopsy is usually done at the same time as bone marrow aspiration.

Bone marrow transplantation (trans-plan-TAY-shun): A procedure in which doctors replace marrow destroyed by treatment with high doses of anticancer drugs or radiation. The replacement marrow may be taken from the patient before treatment or may be donated by another person.

Bone scan: A technique to create images of bones on a computer screen or on film. A small amount of radioactive material is injected and travels through the bloodstream. It collects in the bones, especially in abnormal areas of the bones, and is detected by a scanner.

Bowel: Another name for the intestine. There is both a small and a large bowel.

Brachytherapy (BRAK-i-THER-a-pee): Internal radiation therapy using an implant of radioactive material placed directly into or near the tumor.

Brain stem: The stemlike part of the brain that is connected to the spinal cord.

Brain stem glioma (glee-O-ma): A type of brain tumor that occurs in the lowest, stemlike part of the brain.

BRCA1: A gene located on chromosome 17 that normally helps to restrain cell growth. Inheriting an altered version of BRCA1 predisposes an individual to breast, ovary, and prostate cancer.

Breast reconstruction: Surgery to rebuild a breast's shape after a mastectomy.

Bronchi (BRONK-eye): Air passage that leads from the windpipe to the lungs.

Bronchioles (BRON-kee-ols): The tiny branches of air tubes in the lungs.

Bronchitis (BRON-KYE-tis): Inflamation (swelling and reddening) of the bronchi.

Bronchoscope (BRON-ko-skope): A flexible, lighted instrument used to examine the trachea and bronchi, the air passages that lead into the lungs.

Bronchoscopy (bron-KOS-ko-pee): A test that permits the doctor to see the breathing passages through a lighted tube.

Buccal mucosa (BUK-ul myoo-KO-sa): The inner lining of the cheeks and lips.

Burkitt's lymphoma: A type of non-Hodgkin's lymphoma that most often occurs in young people between the ages of 12 and 30. The disease usually causes a rapidly growing tumor in the abdomen.

Bypass: A surgical procedure in which the doctor creates a new pathway for the flow of body fluids.

C

Calcium (KAL-see-um): A mineral found mainly in the hard part of bones.

Cancer: A term for diseases in which abnormal cells divide without control. Cancer cells can invade nearby tissues and can spread through the bloodstream and lymphatic system to other parts of the body.

Carcinogen (kar-SIN-o-jin): Any substance that is known to cause cancer.

Carcinogenesis: The process by which normal cells are transformed into cancer cells.

Carcinoma (kar-sin-O-ma): Cancer that begins in the lining or covering of an organ.

Carcinoma in situ (kar-sin-O-ma in SY-too): Cancer that involves only the cells in which it began and has not spread to other tissues.

Cartilage (KAR-ti-lij): Firm, rubbery tissue that cushions bones at joints. A more flexible kind of cartilage connects muscles with bones and makes up other parts of the body, such as the larynx and the outside of the ears.

Catheter (KATH-et-er): A tube that is placed in a blood vessel to provide a pathway for drug or nutrients.

Cauterization (KAW-ter-i-ZAY-shun): The use of heat to destroy abnormal cells.

CEA assay: A laboratory test to measure the level of carcinoembryonic antigen (CEA), a substance that is sometimes found in an increased amount in the blood of patients with certain cancers.

Cell: The basic unit of any living organism.

Cell differentiation: The process during which young, immature (unspecialized) cells take on individual characteristics and reach their mature (specialized) form and function.

Cell motility: The ability of a cell to move.

Cell proliferation: An increase in the number of cells as a result of cell growth and cell division.

Cellular adhesion: The close adherence (bonding) to adjoining cell surfaces.

Central nervous system: The brain and spinal cord. Also called CNS.

Cerebellum (sair-uh-BELL-um): The portion of the brain in the back of the head between the cerebrum and the brain stem.

Cerebral hemispheres (seh-REE-bral HEM-iss-feerz): The two halves of the cerebrum.

Cerebrospinal fluid (seh-REE-bro-spy-nal): The watery fluid flowing around the brain and spinal cord. Also called CSF.

Cerebrum (seh-REE-brum): The largest part of the brain. It is divided into two hemispheres, or halves.

Cervical intraepithelial neoplasia (SER-vih-kul in-tra-eh-pih-THEEL-ee-ul NEE-o-play-zha): A general term for the growth of abnormal cells on the surface of the cervix. Numbers from 1 to 3 may be used to describe how much of the cervix contains abnormal cells. Also called CIN.

Cervix (SER-viks): The lower, narrow end of the uterus that forms a canal between the uterus and vagina.

Chemoprevention (KEE-mo-pre-VEN-shun): The use of natural or laboratory made substances to prevent cancer.

Chemotherapy (kee-mo-THER-a-pee): Treatment with anticancer drugs.

Cholangiosarcoma (ko-LAN-jee-o-sar-KO-ma): A type of cancer that begins in the bile ducts.

Chondrosarcoma (KON-dro-sar-KO-ma): A cancer that forms in cartilage.

Chordoma (kor-DO-ma): A form of bone cancer that usually starts in the lower spinal column.

Chromosome (KRO-mo-soam): Part of a cell that contains genetic information. Normally, human cells contain 46 chromosomes that appear as a long thread inside the cell.

Chronic leukemia (KRON-ik): Leukemia that progresses slowly.

Chronic phase (KRON-ik): Refers to the early stages of chronic myelogenous leukemia or chronic lymphocytic leukemia. The number of immature, abnormal white blood cells in the bone marrow and blood is higher than normal, but lower than in the accelerated or blast phase.

Clinical trials: Research studies that involve patients. Each study is designed to find better ways to prevent, detect, diagnose, or treat cancer and to answer scientific questions.

CNS (central nervous system): The brain and the spinal cord.

CNS prophylaxis (pro-fi-LAK-sis): Chemotherapy or radiation therapy to the central nervous system (CNS). This is preventive treatment. It is given to kill cancer cells that may be in the brain and spinal cord, even though no cancer has been detected there.

Colectomy (ko-LEK-to-mee): An operation to remove all or part of the colon. In a partial colectomy, the surgeon removes only the cancerous part of the colon and a small amount (called a margin) of surrounding healthy tissue.

Colon (KO-lun): The long, coiled, tubelike organ that removes water from digested food. The remaining material, solid waste called stool, moves through the colon to the rectum and leaves the body through the anus.

Colonoscope (ko-LON-o-skope): A flexible, lighted instrument used to view the inside of the colon.

Colonoscopy (ko-lon-OS-ko-pee): An examination in which the doctor looks at the colon through a flexible, lighted instrument called a colonoscope.

Colony-stimulating factors: Substances that stimulate the production of blood cells. Treatment with colony-stimulating factors (CSF) can help the blood-forming tissue recover from the effects of chemotherapy and radiation therapy.

Colorectal (ko-lo-REK-tul): Related to the colon and/or rectum.

Colostomy (ko-LOS-to-mee): An opening created by a surgeon into the colon from the outside of the body. A colostomy provides a new path for waste material to leave the body after part of the colon has been removed.

Colposcopy (kul-POSS-ko-pee): A procedure in which a lighted magnifying instrument (called a colposcope) is used to examine the vagina and cervix.

Combination chemotherapy: Treatment in which two or more chemicals are used to obtain more effective results.

Common bile duct: Bile ducts are passageways that carry bile. Two major bile ducts come together into a "trunk"-the common bile duct which empties into the upper part of the small intestine (the part next to the stomach).

Computed tomography (tom-OG-rah-fee): An x-ray procedure that uses a computer to produce a detailed picture of a cross section of the body; also called CAT or CT scan.

Condylomata acuminata (kon-di-LOW-ma-ta a-kyoo-mi-NA-ta): Genital warts caused by certain human papillomaviruses.

Conization (ko-ni-ZAY-shun): Surgery to remove a cone-shaped piece of tissue from the cervix and cervical canal. Conization may be used to diagnose or treat a cervical condition. Also called cone biopsy.

Continent reservoir (KAHN-tih-nent RES-er-vwar): A pouch formed from a piece of small intestine to hold urine after the bladder has been removed.

Corpus: The body of the uterus.

Craniopharyngioma (KRAY-nee-o-fah-rin-jee-O-ma): A type of brain tumor that develops in the region of the pituitary gland near the hypothalamus, the area of the brain that controls body temperature, hunger, and thirst. These tumors are usually benign, but are sometimes considered malignant because they can press on or damage the hypothalamus and affect vital functions.

Craniotomy (kray-nee-OT-o-mee): An operation in which an opening is made in the skull so the doctor can reach the brain.

Cryosurgery (KRY-o-SER-jer-ee): Treatment performed with an instrument that freezes and destroys abnormal tissues.

Cryptorchidsm (kript-OR-kid-izm): A condition in which one or both testicles fail to move from the abdomen, where they develop before birth, into the scrotum; also called undescended testicles.

CT (or CAT) scan: A series of detailed pictures of areas inside the body; the pictures are created by a computer linked to an x-ray machine. Also called computed tomography scan or computed axial tomography scan.

Curettage (kyoo-re-TAHZH): Removal of tissue with a curette.

Curette (kyoo-RET): A spoon-shaped instrument with a sharp edge.

Cutaneous (kyoo-TAY-nee-us): Related to the skin.

Cyst (sist): A sac or capsule filled with fluid.

Cystectomy (sis-TEK-to-mee): Surgery to remove the bladder.

Cystoscope (SIS-to-skope): An instrument that allows the doctor to see inside the bladder and remove tissue samples or small tumors.

Cystoscopy (sist-OSS-ko-pee): A procedure in which the doctor inserts a lighted instrument into the urethra (the tube leading from the bladder to the outside of the body) to look at the bladder.

D

Dermatologist (der-ma-TOL-o-jist): A doctor who specializes in the diagnosis and treatment of skin problems.

Dermis (DER-mis): The lower or inner layer of the two main layers of cells that make up the skin.

Diabetes (dye-a-BEE-teez): A disease in which the body does not use sugar properly. (Many foods are converted into sugar, a source of energy for cells.) As a result, the level of sugar in the blood is too high. This disease occurs when the body does not produce enough insulin or does not use it properly.

Diagnosis: The process of indentifying a disease by the signs and symptoms.

Dialysis (dy-AL-i-sis): The process of cleansing the blood by passing it through a special machine. Dialysis is necessary when the kidneys are not able to filter the blood.

Diaphanography (DY-a-fan-OG-ra-fee): An exam that involves shining a bright light through the breast to reveal features of the tissues inside. This technique is under study; its value in detecting breast cancer has not been proven. Also called transillumination.

Diaphragm (DY-a-fram): The thin muscle below the lungs and heart that separates the chest from the abdomen.

Diathermy (DIE-a-ther-mee): The use of heat to destroy abnormal cells. Also cauterization or electrodiathermy.

Diethylstilbestrol (die-ETH-ul-stil-BES-trol): A drug that was once widely prescribed to prevent miscarriage. Also called DES.

Differentiation: In cancer, refers to how mature (developed) the cancer cells are in a tumor. Differentiated tumor cells resemble normal cells and grow at a slower rate than undifferentiated tumor cells, which lack the structure and function of normal cells and grow uncontrollably.

Digestive system: The organs that take in food and turn it into products that the body can use to stay healthy. Waste products the body cannot use leave the body through bowel movements. The digestive system includes the salivary glands, mouth, esophagus, stomach, liver, pancreas, gallbladder, intestines, and rectum.

Digestive tract (dye-JES-tiv): The organs through which food passes when we eat. These are the mouth, esophagus, stomach, small and large intestines, and rectum.

Digital rectal exam: An exam to detect cancer. The doctor inserts a lubricated, gloved finger into the rectum and feels for abnormal areas. Also called DRE.

Dilation and Curettage (di-LAY-shun and KYOO-re-tahzh): A minor operation in which the cervix is expanded enough (dilation) to permit the cervical canal and uterine lining to be scraped with a spoon-shaped instrument called a curette (curettage). This procedure also is called D and C.

Dilator (DIE-lay-tor): A device used to stretch or enlarge an opening.

DNA: The substance of heredity; a large molecule that carries the genetic information that cells need to replicate and to produce proteins.

Douching (DOO-shing): Using water or a medicated solution to clean the vagina and cervix.

Dry orgasm: Sexual climax without the release of semen.

Duct (dukt): A tube through which body fluids pass.

Ductal carcinoma in situ (DUK-tal kar-sin-O-ma in SY-too): Abnormal cells that involve only the lining of a duct. The cells have not spread outside the duct to other tissues in the breast. Also called DCIS or intraductal carcinoma.

Dumping syndrome: A group of symptoms that occur when food or liquid enters the small intestine too rapidly. These symptoms include cramps, nausea, diarrhea, and dizziness.

Duodenum (doo-o-DEE-num): The first part of the small intestine.

Dysplasia (dis-PLAY-zha): Abnormal cells that are not cancer.

Dysplastic nevi: (dis-PLAS-tik NEE-vye): Atypical moles; moles whose appearance is different from that of common moles. Dysplastic nevi are generally larger than ordinary moles and have irregular and indistinct borders. Their color often is not uniform, and ranges from pink or even white to dark brown or black; they usually are flat, but parts may be raised above the skin surface.

E

Edema (eh-DEE-ma); Swelling; an abnormal buildup of fluid.

Ejaculation: The release of semen through the penis during orgasm.

Electrodesiccation (e-LEK-tro-des-i-KAY-shun): Use of an electric current to destroy cancerous tissue and control bleeding.

Electrolarynx (e-LEK-tro-LAR-inks): A battery-operated instrument that makes a humming sound to help laryngectomees talk.

Embolization (EM-bo-li-ZAY-shun): Blocking an artery so that blood cannot flow to the tumor.

Encapsulated (en-KAP-soo-lay-ted): Confined to a specific area; the tumor remains in a compact form.

Endocervical curettage (en-do-SER-vi-kul kyoo-re-TAZH): The removal of tissue from the inside of the cervix using a spoon-shaped instrument called a curette.

Endocrinologist (en-do-kri-NOL-o-jist): A doctor that specializes in diagnosing and treating hormone disorders.

Endometriosis (en-do-mee-tree-O-sis): A benign condition in which tissue that looks like endometrial tissue grows in abnormal places in the abdomen.

Endometrium (en-do-MEE-tree-um): The layer of tissue that lines the uterus.

Endoscope (EN-do-skope): A thin, lighted tube through which a doctor can look at tissues inside the body.

Endoscopic retrograde cholangiopancreatography (en-do-SKAH-pik RET-ro-grade ko-LAN-jee-o-PAN-kree-a-TAW-gra-fee): A procedure to x-ray the common bile duct. Also called ERCP.

Endoscopy (en-DOS-ko-pee): An examination of the esophagus and stomach using a thin, lighted instrument called an endoscope.

Ependymoma (eh-PEN-dih-MO-ma): A type of brain tumor that usually develops in the lining of the ventricles, but may also occur in the spinal chord.

Enterostomal therapist (en-ter-o-STO-mul): A health professional trained in the care of urostomies and other stomas.

Environmental tobacco smoke: Smoke that comes from the burning end of a cigarette and smoke that is exhaled by smokers. Also called ETS or second-hand smoke. Inhaling ETS is called involuntary or passive smoking.

Enzyme: A substance that affects the rate at which chemical changes take place in the body.

Ependymoma (eh-PEN-di-MO-ma): A type of brain tumor.

Epidermis (ep-i-DER-mis): The upper or outer layer of the two main layers of cells that make up the skin.

Epidermoid carcinoma (ep-i-DER-moyd): A type of lung cancer in which the cells are flat and look like fish scales. Also called squamous cell carcinoma.

Epiglottis (ep-i-GLOT-is): The flap that covers the trachea during swallowing so that food does not enter the lungs.

Epithelial carcinoma (ep-i-THEE-lee-ul kar-si-NO-ma): Cancer that begins in the cells that line an organ.

Epithelium (EP-i-THEE-lee-um): A thin layer of tissue that covers organs, glands, and other structures in the body.

ERCP (endoscopic retrograde cholangiopancreatography) (en-do-SKOP-ik RET-ro-grade ko-LAN-gee-o-PAN-kree-a-TOG-ra-fee): A procedure to x-ray the common bile duct.

Erythrocytes (e-RITH-ro-sites): Cells that carry oxygen to all parts of the body. Also called red blood cells (RBCs).

Erythroleukemia (e-RITH-ro-loo-KEE-mee-a): Leukemia that develops in erythrocytes. In this rare disease, the body produces large numbers of abnormal red blood cells.

Erythroplakia (eh-RITH-ro-PLAY-kee-a): A reddened patch with a velvety surface found in the mouth.

Esophageal (e-soff-a-JEE-al): Related to the esophagus.

Esophageal speech (e-SOF-a-JEE-al): Speech produced with air trapped in the esophagus and forced out again.

Esophagectomy (e-soff-a-JEK-to-mee): An operation to remove a portion of the esophagus.

Esophagoscopy (e-soff-a-GOSS-ko-pee): Examination of the esophagus using a thin, lighted instrument.

Esophagram (e-SOFF-a-gram): A series of x-rays of the esophagus. The x-ray pictures are taken after the patient drinks a solution that coats and outlines the walls of the esophagus. Also called a barium swallow.

Esophagus (e-SOF-a-gus): The muscular tube through which food passes from the throat to the stomach.

Estrogen (ES-tro-jin): A female hormone.

Etiology: The study of the causes of abnormal condition or disease.

Ewing's sarcoma (YOO-ingz sar-KO-ma): A bone cancer that forms in the middle (shaft) of large bones. It most often affects the hipbones and the bones of the upper arm and thigh.

External radiation: Radiation therapy that uses a machine to aim high-energy rays at the cancer.

F

Fallopian tubes (fa-LO-pee-in): Tubes on each side of the uterus through which an egg moves from the ovaries to the uterus.

Familial polyposis (pol-i-PO-sis): An inherited condition in which several hundred polyps develop in the colon and rectum.

Fecal occult blood test (FEE-kul o-KULT): A test to check for hidden blood in stool. (Fecal refers to stool. Occult means hidden.)

Fertility (fer-TIL-i-tee): The ability to produce children.

Fetus (FEET-us): The unborn child developing in the uterus.

Fiber: The parts of fruits and vegetables that cannot be digested. Also called bulk or roughage.

Fibroid (FY-broid): A benign uterine tumor made up of fibrous and muscular tissue.

Fibrosarcoma: A type of soft tissue sarcoma that begins in fibrous tissue, which holds bones, muscles, and other organs in place.

Fluoroscope (FLOOR-o-skope): An x-ray machine that makes it possible to see internal organs in motion.

Fluoroscopy (Floor-OS-ko-pee): An x-ray procedure that makes it possible to see internal organs in motion

Fluorouracil (floo-ro-YOOR-a-sil): An anticancer drug. Its chemical name is 5-fluorouracil, commonly called 5-FU.

Follicles (FAHL-ih-kuls): Shafts through which hair grows.

Fractionation: Dividing the total dose of radiation therapy into several smaller, equal doses delivered over a period of several days.

Fulguration (ful-gyoor-AY-shun): Destroying tissue using an electric current.

G

Gallbladder (GAWL-blad-er): The pear-shaped organ that sits below the liver. Bile is stored in the gallbladder.

Gamma knife: Radiation therapy in which high-energy rays are aimed at a tumor from many angles in a single treatment session.

Gastrectomy (gas-TREK-to-mee): An operation to remove all or part of the stomach.

Gastric (GAS-trik): Having to do with the stomach.

Gastric atrophy (GAS-trik AT-ro-fee): A condition in which the stomach muscles shrink and become weak. It results in a lack of digestive juices.

Gastroenterologist (GAS-tro-en-ter-OL-o-jist): A doctor who specializes in diagnosing and treating disorders of the digestive system.

Gastrointestinal tract (GAS-tro-in-TES-ti-nul): The part of the digestive tract where the body processes food and eliminates waste. It includes the esophagus, stomach, liver, small and large intestines, and rectum.

Gastroscope (GAS-tro-skope): A thin, lighted instrument to view the inside of the stomach.

Gastroscopy (gas-TROS-ko-pee): An examination of the stomach with a gastroscope, an instrument to view the inside of the stomach.

Gene: The biological or basic unit of heredity found in all cells in the body.

Gene deletion: The total loss or absence of a gene.

Gene therapy: Treatment that alters genes (the basic units of heredity found in all cells in the body). In studies of gene therapy for cancer, researchers are trying to improve the body's natural ability to fight the disease or to make the tumor more sensitive to other kinds of therapy.

Genetic: Inherited; having to do with information that is passed from parents to children through DNA in the genes.

Genitourinary system (GEN-i-toe-YOO-rin-air-ee): The parts of the body that play a role in reproduction, in getting rid of waste products in the form of urine, or in both.

Germ cells: The reproductive cells of the body specifically, either egg or sperm cells.

Germ cell tumors: A type of brain tumor that arises from primitive (developing) sex cells, or germ cells.

Germinoma (jer-mih-NO-ma): The most frequent type of germ cell tumor in the brain.

Germline mutation: See hereditary mutation.

Gland: An organ that produces and releases one or more substances for use in the body. Some glands produce fluids that affect tissues or organs. Others produce hormones or participate in blood production.

Glioblastoma multiforme (glee-o-blast-TO-ma mul-tih-FOR-may): A type of brain tumor that forms in the nervous (glial) tissue of the brain.

Glioma (glee-O-ma): A name for brain tumors that begin in the glial cells, or supportive cells, in the brain. "Glia" is the Greek word for glue.

Glottis (GLOT-is): The middle part of the larynx; the area where the vocal cords are located.

Grade: Describes how closely a cancer resembles normal tissue of its same type, and the cancer's probable rate of growth

Grading: A system for classifying cancer cells in terms of how malignant or aggressive they appear microscopically. The grading of a tumor indicates how quickly cancer cells are likely to spread and plays a role in treatment decisions.

Graft: Healthy skin, bone, or other tissue taken from one part of the body to replace diseased or injured tissue removed from another part of the body.

Graft-versus-host disease: A reaction of donated bone marrow against a patient's own tissue. Also called GVHD.

Granulocyte (GRAN-yoo-lo-site): A type of white blood cell. Neutrophils, eosinophils, and basophils are granulocytes.

Groin: The area where the thigh meets the hip.

GVHD (graft-versus-host disease): A reaction of donated bone marrow against a patient's own tissue.

Gynecologic oncologists (guy-ne-ko-LA-jik on-KOL-o-jists): Doctors who specialize in treating cancers of the female reproductive organs.

Gynecologist (guy-ne-KOL-o-jist): A doctor who specializes in treating diseases of the female reproductive organs.

H

Hair follicles (FOL-i-kuls): The sacs in the scalp from which hair grows.

Hairy cell leukemia: A rare type of chronic leukemia in which the abnormal white blood cells appear to be covered with tiny hairs.

Helicobacter pylori (HEEL-i-ko-BAK-ter pie-LOR-ee): Bacteria that cause inflammation and ulcers in the stomach.

Hematogenous: Orginating in the blood, or disseminated by the circulation or through the bloodstream.

Hematologist (hee-ma-TOL-o-jist): A doctor who specializes in treating diseases of the blood.

Hepatitis (hep-a-TYE-tis): Inflammation of the liver.

Hepatitis B: A type of hepatitis that is carried and passed on through the blood. It can be passed on through sexual contact or through the use of "dirty" (bloody) needles.

Hepatoblastoma (HEP-a-to-blas-TO-ma): A type of liver tumor that occurs in infants and children.

Hepatocellular carcinoma (HEP-a-to-SEL-yoo-ler kar-si-NO-ma): The most common type of primary liver cancer.

Hepatocyte (HEP-a-to-site): A liver cell.

Hepatoma (HEP-a-TO-ma): A liver tumor.

Hereditary mutation: A gene change in the body's reproductive cells (egg or sperm) that becomes incorporated into the DNA of every cell in the body of offspring; hereditary mutations are passed on from parents to offspring.

Herpes virus (HER-peez-VY-rus): A member of the herpes family of viruses. One type of herpesvirus is sexually transmitted and causes sores on the genitals.

HER-2/neu: Oncogene found in some breast and ovarian cancer patients that is associated with a poor prognosis.

Hormonal therapy: Treatment of cancer by removing, blocking, or adding hormones.

Hormone receptor test: A test to measure the amount of certain proteins, called hormone recptors, in breast cancer tissue. Hormones can attach to these proteins. A high level of hormone receptors means hormones probably help the cancer grow.

Hormone therapy: Treatment that prevents certain cancer cells form getting the hormones they need to grow.

Hormones: Chemicals produced by glands in the body and circulate in the bloodstream. Hormones control the actions of certain cells or organs.

Human papillomaviruses (pap-i-LOW-ma VY-rus-ez): Viruses that generally cause warts. Some papillomaviruses are sexually transmitted. Some of these sexually transmitted viruses cause wartlike growths on the genitals, and some are thought to cause abnormal changes in cells of the cervix.

Humidifier (hyoo-MID-ih-fye-er): A machine that puts moisture in the air.

Hydrocephalus (hy-dro-SEF-uh-lus): The abnormal buildup of cerebrospinal fluid in the ventricles of the brain.

Hypercalcemia (hy-per-kal-SEE-mee-a): A higher-than-normal level of calcium in the blood. This condition can cause a number of symptoms, including loss of appetite, nausea, thirst, fatigue, muscle weakness, restlessness, and confusion.

Hyperfractionation: A way of giving radiation therapy in smaller-than-usual doses two or three times a day.

Hyperplasia (hye-per-PLAY-zha): A precancerous condition in which there is an increase in the number of normal cells lining the uterus.

Hyperthermia (hy-per-THER-mee-a): Treatment that involves heating a tumor.

Hypothalamus (hy-po-THAL-uh-mus): The area of the brain that controls body temperature, hunger, and thirst.

Hysterectomy (hiss-ter-EK-to-mee): An operation in which the uterus and cervix are removed.

I

Ileostomy (il-ee-OS-to-mee): An opening created by a surgeon into the ileum, part of the small intestine, from the outside of the body. An ileostomy provides a new path for waste material to leave the body after part of the intestine has been removed.

Imaging: Tests that produce pictures of areas inside the body.

Immune system (im-YOON): The complex group of organs and cells that defends the body against infection or disease.

Immunodeficiency: A lowering of the body's ability to fight off infection and disease.

Immunology: A science that deals with the study of the body's immune system.

Immunosuppression: The use of drugs or techniques to suppress or interfere with the body's immune system and its ability to fight infections or disease. Immunosuppression may be deliberate, such as in preparation for bone marrow or other organ transplantation to prevent rejection by the host of the donor tissue, or incidental, such as often results from chemotherapy for the treatment of cancer.

Immunotherapy (IM-yoo-no-THER-a-pee): Treatment that uses the body's natural defenses to fight cancer. Also called biological therapy.

973

Implant (or internal) radiation: Internal radiation therapy that places radioactive materials in or close to the cancer.

Impotent (IM-po-tent): Inability to have an erection and/or ejaculate semen.

Incidence: The number of new cases of a disease diagnosed each year.

Incision (in-SI-zhun): A cut made in the body during surgery.

Incontinence (in-kON-ti-nens): Inability to control the flow of urine from the bladder.

Infertility: The inability to produce children.

Infiltrating cancer: See invasive cancer.

Inflammatory breast cancer: A rare type of breast cancer in which cancer cells block the lymph vessels in the skin of the breast. The breast becomes red, swollen, and warm, and the skin of the breast may appear pitted or have ridges.

Inguinal orchiectomy (IN-gwin-al or-kee-EK-to-mee): Surgery to remove the testicle through the groin.

Insulin (IN-su-lin): A hormone made by the islet cells of the pancreas. Insulin controls the amount of sugar in the blood.

Interferon (in-ter-FEER-on): A type of biological response modifier (a substance that can improve the body's natural response to disease). It stimulates the growth of certain disease-fighting blood cells in the immune system.

Interleukin (in-ter-LOO-kin): A substance used in biological therapy. Interleukins stimulate the growth and activities of certain kinds of white blood cells.

Interleukin-2 (in-ter-LOO-kin): A type of biological response modifier (a substance that can improve the body's natural response to disease). It stimulates the growth of certain blood cells in the immune system that can fight cancer. Also called IL-2.

Internal radiation (ray-dee-AY-shun): Radiation therapy that uses radioactive materials placed in or near the tumor.

Intestine (in-TES-tin): The long, tube-shaped organ in the abdomen that completes the process of digestion. It consists of the small and large intestines.

Intraepithelial (in-tra-eh-pih-THEEL-ee-ul): Within the layer of cells that forms the surface or lining of an organ.

Intrahepatic (in-tra-hep-AT-ik): Within the liver.

Intrahepatic bile duct (in-tra-hep-AT-ik): The bile duct that passes through and drains bile from the liver.

Intraoperative radiation therapy: Radiation treatment given during surgery. Also called IORT.

Intraperitoneal chemotherapy (IN-tra-per-i-to-NEE-al): Treatment in which anticancer drugs are put directly into the abdomen through a thin tube.

Intrathecal chemotherapy (in-tra-THEE-cal KEE-mo-THER-a-pee): Chemotherapy drugs infused into the thin space between the lining of the spinal cord and brain to treat or prevent cancers in the brain and spinal cord.

Intravenous (in-tra-VEE-nus): Injected in a vein. Also called IV.

Intravenous pyelogram (in-tra-VEE-nus PIE-el-o-gram): A series of x-rays of the kidneys and bladder. The x-rays are taken after a dye that shows up on x-ray film in injected into a vein. Also called IVP.

Intravenous pyelography (om-tra-VEE-nus py-LOG-ra-fee): X-ray study of the kidneys and urinary tract. Structures are made visible by the injection of a substance that blocks x-rays. Also called IVP.

Intravesical (in-tra-VES-ih-kal): Within the bladder.

Invasion: As related to cancer, the spread of cancer cells into healthy tissue adjacent to the tumor.

Invasive cancer: Cancer that has spread beyond the layer of tissue in which it developed. Invasive breast cancer is also called infiltrating cancer or infiltrating carcinoma.

Invasive cervical cancer: Cancer that has spread from the surface of the cervix to tissue deeper in the cervix or to other parts of the body.

IORT (intraoperative radiation therapy): Radiation treatment given during surgery.

Islet cell cancer (EYE-let): Cancer arising from cells in the islets of Langerhans.

Islets of Langerhans (EYE-lets of LANG-er-hanz): Hormone-producing cells in the pancreas.

IV (intravenous) (in-tra-VEE-nus): Injected in a vein.

IVP (intravenous pyelogram) (in-tra-VEE-nus PYE-el-o-gram): X-ray study of the kidneys, uterus, and urinary tract. Structures are made visible by the injection of a substance that blocks x-rays.

J

Jaundice (JAWN-dis): A condition in which the skin and the whites of the eyes become yellow and the urine darkens. Jaundice occurs when the liver is not working properly or when a bile duct is blocked.

K

Kaposi's sarcoma (KAP-o-seez-sar-KO-ma): A relatively rare type of cancer that develops on the skin of some elderly persons or those with a weak immune system, including those with acquired immune deficiency syndrome (AIDS).

Kidneys (KID-neez): A pair or organs in the abdomen that remove waste from the blood. The waste leaves the blood as urine.

Krukenberg tumor (KROO-ken-berg): A tumor of the ovary caused by the spread of stomach cancer.

L

Laparoscopy (lap-a-ROS-ko-pee): A surgical procedure in which a lighted instrument shaped like a thin tube is inserted through a small incision in the abdomen. The doctor can look through the instrument and see inside the abdomen.

Laparotomy (lap-a-ROT-o-mee): An operation that allows the doctor to inspect the organs in the abdomen.

Large cell carcinomas: A group of lung cancers in which the cells are large and look abnormal.

Laryngeal (lair-IN-jee-al): Having to do with the larynx.

Laryngectomee (lair-in-JEK-toe-mee): A person who has had his or her voice box removed.

Laryngectomy (lair-in-JEK-toe-mee): An operation to remove all or part of the larynx.

Laryngoscope (lair-IN-jo-skope): A flexible lighted tube used to examine the larynx.

Laryngoscopy (lair-in-GOS-ko-pee): Examination of the larynx with a mirror (indirect laryngoscopy) or with a laryngoscope (direct laryngoscopy).

Larynx (LAIR-inks): An organ in the throat used in breathing, swallowing, and talking. It is made of cartilage and is line by a mucous membrane similar to the lining of the mouth. Also called the "voice box."

Laser (LAY-zer): A powerful beam of light used in some types of surgery to cut or destroy tissue.

Lesion (LEE-zhun): An area of abnormal tissue change.

Leukemia (loo-KEE-mee-a): Cancer of the blood cells.

Leukocytes (LOO-ko-sites): Cells that help the body fight infections and other diseases. Also called white blood cells (WBCs).

Leukoplakia (loo-ko-PLAY-kee-a): A white spot or patch in the mouth

Li-Fraumeni Syndrome: A rare family predisposition to multiple cancers, caused by an alteration in the p53 tumor suppressor gene.

Ligation (lye-GAY-shun): The process of tying off blood vessels so that blood cannot flow to a part of the body or to a tumor.

Limb perfusion (per-FYOO-zhun): A chemotherapy technique that may be used when melanoma occurs on an arm or leg. The flow of blood to and from the limb is stopped for a while with a tourniquet, and anticancer drugs are put directly into the blood of the limb. This allows the patient to receive a high dose of drugs in the area where the melanoma occurred.

Liver: A large, glandular organ, located in the upper abdomen, that cleanses the blood and aids in digestion by secreting bile.

Liver scan: An image of the liver created on a computer screen or on film. For a liver scan, a radioactive substance is injected into a vein and travels through the bloodstream. It collects in the liver, especially in abnormal areas, and can be detected by the scanner.

Lobe: A portion of the liver, lung, breast, or brain.

Lobectomy (lo-BEK-to-mee): The removal of a lobe.

Lobular carcinoma in situ (LOB-yoo-lar-sin-O-ma in SY-too): Abnormal cells in the lobules of the breast. This condition seldom becomes invasive cancer. However, having lobular carcinoma in situ is a sign that the woman has an increased risk of developing breast cancer. Also called LCIS.

Lobule (LOB-yule): A small lobe.

Local: Reaching and affecting only the cells in a specific area.

Local therapy: Treatment that affects cells in the tumor and the area close to it.

Lower GI series: A series of x-rays of the colon and rectum that is taken after the patient is given a barium enema. (Barium is a white, chalky substance that outlines the colon and rectum on the x-ray.)

Lubricant (LOO-brih-kant): An oily or slippery substance. A vaginal lubricant may be helpful for women who feels pain during intercourse because of vaginal dryness.

Lumbar puncture: The insertion of a needle into the lower part of the spinal column to collect cerebrospinal fluid or to give intrathecal chemotherapy. Also called a spinal tap.

Lumpectomy (lump-EK-toe-mee): Surgery to remove only the cancerous breast lump; usually followed by radiation therapy.

Luteinizing hormone-releasing hormone (LHRH) agonist (LOO-tin-eye-zing...AG-o-nist): A substance that closely resembles LHRH, which controls the production of sex hormones. However, LHRH agonists affect the body differently than does LHRH. LHRH agonists keep the testicles from producing hormones.

Lymph (limf): The almost colorless fluid that travels through the lymphatic system and carries cells that help fight infection and disease.

Lymph nodes: Small, bean-shaped organs located along the channels of the lymphatic system. The lymph nodes store special cells that can trap bacteria or cancer cells traveling through the body in lymph. Clusters of lymph nodes are found in the underarms, groin, neck, chest, and abdomen. Also called lymph glands.

Lymphangiogram (lim-FAN-jee-o-gram): An x-ray of the lymphatic system. A dye is injected to outline the lymphatic vessels and organs.

Lymphangiography (imf-an-jee-OG-ra-fee): X-ray study of lymph nodes and lymph vessels made visible by the injection of a special dye.

Lymphatic system (lim-FAT-ik): The tissues and organs that produce, store, and carry white blood cells that fight infection and disease. This system includes the bone marrow, spleen, thymus, and lymph nodes and a network of thin tubes that carry lymph and white blood cells. These tubes branch, like blood vessels, into all the tissues of the body.

Lymphedema (LIMF-eh-DEE-ma): A condition in which excess fluid collects in tissue and causes swelling. It may occur in the arm or leg after lymph vessels or lymph nodes in the underarm or groin are removed.

Lymphoma: Cancer that arises in cells of the lymphatic system.

Lymphocytes (LIMF-o-sites): White blood cells that fight infection and disease.

Lymphocytic (lim-fo-SIT-ik): Referring to lymphocytes, a type of white blood cell.

Lymphoid (LIM-foyd): Referring to lymphocytes, a type of white blood cell. Also refers to tissue in which lymphocytes develop.

M

M proteins: Antibodies or parts of antibodies found in unusually large amounts in the blood or urine of multiple myeloma patients.

Magnetic resonance imaging (mag-NET-ik REZ-o-nan IM-a-jing): A procedure in which a magnet linked to a computer is used to create detailed pictures of areas inside the body. Also called MRI.

Maintenance therapy: Chemotherapy that is given to leukemia patients in remission to prevent a relapse.

Malignant (ma-LIG-nant): Cancerous; can invade nearby tissue and spread to other parts of the body.

Mammogram (MAM-o-gram): An x-ray of the breast.

Mammography (mam-OG-ra-fee): The use of x-rays to create a picture of the breast.

Mastectomy (mas-TEK-to-mee): Surgery to remove the breast (or as much of the breast as possible).

Mediastinoscopy (MEE-dee-a-stin-AHS-ko-pee): A procedure in which the doctor inserts a tube into the chest to view the organs in the mediastinum. The tube is inserted through an incision above the breastbone.

Mediastinotomy (MEE-dee-a-stin-AH-toe-mee): A procedure in which the doctor inserts a tube into the chest to view the organs in the mediastinum. The tube is inserted through an incision next to the breastbone.

Mediastinum (mee-dee-a-STY-num): The area between the lungs. The organs in this area include the heart and its large veins and arteries, the trachea, the esophagus, the bronchi, and lymph nodes.

Medical oncologist (on-KOL-o-jist): A doctor who specializes in treating cancer. Some oncologists specialize in a particular type of cancer treatment. For example, a radiation oncologist specializes in treating cancer with radiation.

Medulloblastoma (MED-yoo-lo-blas-TOE-ma): A type of brain tumor that recent research suggests develops from primitive (developing) nerve cells that normally do not remain in the body after birth. Medulloblastomas are sometimes called primitive neuroectodermal tumors.

Melanin (MEL-a-nin): A skin pigment (substance that gives the skin its color). Dark-skinned people have more melanin than light-skinned people.

Melanocytes (mel-AN-o-sites): Cells in the skin that produce and contain the pigment called melanin.

Melanoma: Cancer of the cells that produce pigment in the skin. Melanoma usually begins in a mole.

Membrane: A very thin layer of tissue that covers a surface.

Meninges (meh-NIN-jeez): The three membranes that cover the brain and spinal cord.

Meningioma (meh-nin-jee-O-ma): A type of brain tumor that develops in the meninges. Because these tumors grow very slowly, the brain may be able to adjust to their presence; meningiomas often grow quite large before they cause symptoms.

Menopause (MEN-o-pawz): The time of a woman's life when menstrual periods permanently stop. Also called "change of life."

Menstrual cycle (MEN-stroo-al): The hormone changes that lead up to a woman's having a period. For most women, one cycle takes 28 days.

Metastasize (meh-TAS-ta-size): To spread from one part of the body to another. When cancer cells metastasize and form secondary tumors, the cells in the metastatic tumor are like those in the original (primary) tumor.

Microcalcifications (MY-krow-kal-si-fi-KA-shunz): Tiny deposits of calcium in the breast that cannot be felt but can be detected on a mammogram. A cluster of these very small specks of calcium may indicate that cancer is present.

Mole: An area on the skin (usually dark in color) that contains a cluster of melanocytes.

Monoclonal antibodies (MON-o-KLO-nul AN-ti-BOD-eez): Substances that can locate and bind to cancer cells wherever they are in the body. They can be used alone, or they can be used to deliver drugs, toxins, or radioactive material directly to tumor cells.

Monocyte: A type of white blood cell.

Morphology: The science of the form and structure of organisms (plants, animals, and other forms of life).

MRI (magnetic resonance imaging): A procedure in which a magnet linked to a computer is used to create detailed pictures of areas inside the body.

Mucus: A thick fluid produced by the lining of some organs of the body.

Multiple myeloma (mye-eh-LO-ma): Cancer that affects plasma cells. The disease causes the growth of tumors in many bones, which can lead to bone pain and fractures. In addition, the disease often causes kidney problems and lowered resistance to infection.

Mutations: Changes in the way cells function or develop, caused by an inherited genetic defect or an environmental exposure. Such changes may lead to cancer.

Mycosis fungoides (my-KO-sis fun-GOY-deez): A type of non-Hodgkin's lymphoma that first appears on the skin. Also called cutaneous T-cell lymphoma.

Myelin (MYE-eh-lin): The fatty substance that covers and protects nerves.

Myelodysplastic syndrome (MYE-eh-lo-dis-PLAS-tik SIN-drome): See Preleukemia.

Myelogenous (mye-eh-LAH-jen-us): Referring to myelocytes, a type of white blood cell. Also called myeloid.

Myelogram (MYE-eh-lo-gram): An x-ray of the spinal cord and the bones of the spine.

Myeloid (MYE-eh-loyd): Referring to myelocytes, a type of white blood cell. Also called myelogenous.

Myometrium (my-o-MEE-tree-um): The muscular outer layer of the uterus.

N

Neck dissection (dye-SEK-shun): Surgery to remove lymph nodes and other tissues in the neck.

Neoplasia (NEE-o-play-zha): Abnormal new growth of cells.

Neoplasm: A new growth of tissue. Can be referred to as benign or malignant.

Nephrectomy (nef-REK-to-mee): Surgery to remove the kidney. Radical nephrectomy removes the kidney, the adrenal gland, nearby lymph nodes, and other surrounding tissue. Simple nephrectomy removes just the affected kidney. Partial nephrectomy removes the tumor, but not the entire kidney.

Nephrotomogram (nef-ro-TOE-mo-gram): A series of special x-rays of the kidneys. The x- rays are taken from different angles. They show the kidneys clearly, without the shadows of the organs around them.

Neurologist (noo-ROL-o-jist): A doctor who specializes in the diagnosis and treatment of disorders of the nervous system.

Neuroma (noo-RO-ma): A tumor that arises in nerve cells.

Neurosurgeon (NOO-ro-SER-jun): A doctor who specializes in surgery on the brain and other parts of the nervous system.

Neutrophil (NOO-tro-fil): A type of white blood cell.

Nevus (NEE-vus): The medical term for a spot on the skin, such as a mole. A mole is a cluster of melanocytes that usually appears as a dark spot on the skin. The plural of nevus is nevi (NEE-vye).

Nitrosoureas (nye-TRO-so-yoo-REE-ahz): A group of anticancer drugs that can cross the blood-brain barrier. Carmustine (BCNU) and lomustine (CCNU) are nitrosoureas.

Nonmelanoma skin cancer: Skin cancer that does not involve melanocytes. Basal cell cancer and squamous cell cancer are nonmelanoma skin cancers.

Nonseminoma (non-sem-i-NO-ma): A classification of testicular cancers that arise in specialized sex cells called germ cells. Nonseminomas include embryonal carcinoma, teratoma, choriocarcinoma, and yolk sac tumor.

Nonsmall cell lung cancer: A form of lung cancer associated with smoking, exposure to environmental tobacco smoke, or exposure to radon. Nonsmall cell lung cancer is classified as squamous cell carcinoma, adenocarcinoma, and large cell carcinoma depending on what type of cells are in the cancer.

O

Oat cell cancer: A type of lung cancer in which the cells look like oats. Also called small cell lung cancer.

Oligodendroglioma (OL-ih-go-den-dro-glee-O-ma): A rare, slow growing type of brain tumor that occurs in the cells that produce myelin, the fatty covering that protects nerves.

Ommaya reservoir (o-MYE-a REZ-er-vwahr): A device implanted under the scalp and used to deliver anticancer drugs to the fluid surrounding the brain and spinal cord.

Oncogene: The part of the cell that normally directs cell growth, but which can also promote or allow the uncontrolled growth of cancer if damaged (mutated) by an environmental exposure to carcinogens, or damaged or missing because of an inherited defect.

Oncologist (on-KOL-o-jist): A doctor who specializes in treating cancer. Some oncologists specialize in a particular type of cancer treatment. For example, a radiation oncologist specializes in treating cancer with radiation.

Oncology: The study of tumors encompassing the physical, chemical, and biologic properties.

Oophorectomy (oo-for-EK-to-mee): The removal of one or both ovaries.

Ophthalmoscope (off-THAL-mo-skope): A lighted instrument used to examine the inside of the eye, including the retina and the optic nerve.

Optic nerve: The nerve that carries messages from the retina to the brain.

Oral surgeon: A dentist with special training in surgery of the mouth and jaw.

Orchiectomy (or-kee-EK-to-mee): Surgery to remove the testicles.

Organisms: Plants, animals, and other forms of life that are made up of complex and interconnected systems of cells and tissue.

Oropharynx (or-o-FAIR-inks): The area of the throat at the back of the mouth.

Osteosarcoma (OSS-tee-o-sar-KO-ma): A cancer of the bone that is most common in children. Also called osteogenic sarcoma.

Ostomy (AHS-toe-mee): An operation to create an opening from an area inside the body to the outside. See Colostomy.

Otolaryngologist (AH-toe-lar-in-GOL-o-jist): A doctor who specializes in treating diseases of the ear, nose, and throat.

Ovaries (O-var-eez): The pair of female reproductive glands in which the ova, or eggs, are formed. The ovaries are located in the lower abdomen, one on each side of the uterus.

P

p53: A gene in the cell that normally inhibits the growth of tumors, which can prevent or slow the spread of cancer.

Palate (PAL-et): The roof of the mouth. The front portion is bony (hard palate), and the back portion is muscular (soft palate).

Palliative treatment: Treatment that does not alter the course of a disease, but improves the quality of life.

Palpation (pal-PAY-shun): A technique in which a doctor presses on the surface of the body to feel the organs or tissues underneath.

Pancreas: A gland located in the abdomen. It makes pancreatic juices, and it produces several hormones, including insulin. The pancreas is surrounded by the stomach, intestines, and other organs.

Pancreatectomy (pan-kree-a-TEK-to-mee): Surgery to remove the pancreas. In a total pancreatectomy, the duodenum, common bile duct, gallbladder, spleen, and nearby lymph nodes also are removed.

Pancreatic juices: Fluids made by the pancreas. Pancreatic juices contain proteins called enzymes that aid in digestion.

Papillary tumor (PAP-i-lar-ee): A tumor shaped like a small mushroom with its stem attached to the inner lining of the bladder.

Papilledema (pap-il-eh-DEE-ma): Swelling around the optic nerve, usually due to pressure on the nerve by a tumor.

Pap test: Microscopic examination of cells collected from the cervix. It is used to detect changes that may be cancer or may lead to cancer, and it can show noncancerous conditions, such as infection or inflammation. Also called Pap smear.

Paralysis (pa-RAL-ih-sis): Loss of ability to move all or part of the body.

Paraneoplastic syndrome (pair-a-nee-o-PLAS-tik): A group of symptoms that may develop when substances released by some cancer cells disrupt the normal function of surrounding cells and tissue. Such symptoms do not necessarily mean that the cancer has spread beyond the original site.

Pathologist (pa-THOL-o-jist): A doctor who identifies diseases by studying cells and tissues under a microscope.

Pediatric (pee-dee-AT-rik): Pertaining to children.

Pelvis: The lower part of the abdomen, located between the hip bones.

Percutaneous transhepatic cholangiography (per-kyoo-TAN-ee-us trans-heh-PAT-ik ko-LAN-jee-AH-gra-fee): A test sometimes used to help diagnose cancer of the pancreas. During this test, a thin needle is put into the liver. Dye is injected into the bile ducts in the liver so that blockages can be seen on x-rays.

Perfusion: The process of flooding fluid through the artery to saturate the surrounding tissue. In regional perfusion, a specific area of the body (usually an arm or a leg) is targeted and high doses of anticancer drugs are flooded through the artery to reach the surrounding tissue and kill as many cancer cells as possible. Such a procedure is performed in cases where the cancer is not thought to have spread past a localized area.

Perineal prostatectomy (pe-ri-NEE-al): Surgery to remove the prostate through an incision made between the scrotum and the anus.

Peripheral blood stem cell transplantation (per-IF-er-al): A procedure that is similar to bone marrow transplantation. Doctors remove healthy immature cells (stem cells) from a patient's blood and store them before the patient receives high-dose chemotherapy and possibly radiation therapy to destroy the leukemia cells. The stem cells are then returned to the patient, where they can produce new blood cells to replace cells destroyed by the treatment.

Peripheral stem cell support (per-IF-er-ul): A method of replacing blood-forming cells destroyed by cancer treatment. Certain cells (stem cells) in the blood that are similar to those in the bone marrow are removed from the patient's blood before treatment. The cells are given back to the patient after treatment.

Peristalsis (pair-ih-STAL-sis): The rippling motion of muscles in the digestive tract. In the stomach, this motion mixes food with gastric juices, turning it into a thin liquid.

Peritoneal cavity: The lower part of the abdomen that contains the intestines (the last part of the digestive tract), the stomach, and the liver. It is bound by thin membranes.

Peritoneum (PAIR-i-to-NEE-um): The large membrane that lines the abdominal cavity.

Pernicious anemia (per-NISH-us a-NEE-mee-a): A blood disorder caused by a lack of vitamin B12. Patients who have this disorder do not produce the substance in the stomach that allows the body to absorb vitamin B12.

Petechiae (peh-TEE-kee-a): Tiny red spots under the skin; often a symptom of leukemia.

Pharynx (FAIR-inks): The hollow tube about 5 inches long that starts behind the nose and ends at the top of the trachea (windpipe) and esophagus (the tube that goes to the stomach).

Photodynamic therapy (fo-to-dy-NAM-ik): Treatment that destroys cancer cells with lasers and drugs that become active when exposed to light.

Pigment: A substance that gives color to tissue. Pigments are responsible for the color of skin, eyes, and hair.

Pineal gland (PIN-ee-al): A small gland located in the cerebrum.

Pineal region tumors: Types of brain tumors that occur in or around the pineal gland, a tiny organ near the center of the brain. The pineal region is very difficult to reach, therefore these tumors often cannot be removed.

Pineoblastoma (PIN-ee-o-blas-TOE-ma): A fast growing type of brain tumor that occurs in or around the pineal gland, a tiny organ near the center of the brain.

Pineocytoma (PIN-ee-o-sye-TOE-ma): A slow growing type of brain tumor that occurs in or around the pineal gland, a tiny organ near the center of the brain.

Pituitary gland (pih-TOO-ih-tair-ee): The main endocrine gland; it produces hormones that control other glands and many body functions, especially growth.

Plasma: The liquid part of the blood.

Plasma cells: Special white blood cells that produce antibodies.

Plasmacytoma: A tumor that is made up of cancerous plasma cells.

Plasmapheresis (plas-ma-fer-EE-sis): The process of removing certain proteins from the blood. Plasmapheresis can be used to remove excess antibodies from the blood of multiple myeloma patients.

Plastic surgeon: A surgeon who specializes in reducing scarring or disfigurement that may occur as a result of accidents, birth defects, or treatment for diseases (such as melanoma).

Platelets (PLAYT-lets): Blood cells that help clots form to help control bleeding. Also called thrombocytes.

Pleura (PLOOR-a): The thin covering that protects and cushions the lungs. The pleura is made up of two layers of tissue that are separated by a small amount of fluid.

Pleural cavity: A space enclosed by the pleura, thin tissue covering the lungs and lining the interior wall of the chest cavity. It is bound by serous membranes.

Pneumatic larynx (noo-MAT-ik): A device that uses air to produce sound to help a laryngectomee talk.

Pneumonectomy (noo-mo-NEK-to-mee): An operation to remove an entire lung.

Pneumonia (noo-MONE-ya): An infection that occurs when fluid and cells collect in the lung.

Polyp (POL-ip): A mass of tissue that projects into the colon.

Positron emission tomography scan: For this type of scan, a person is given a substance that reacts with tissues in the body to release protons (parts of an atom). Through measuring the different amounts of protons released by healthy and cancerous tissues, a computer creates a picture of the inside of the body. Also called PET scan.

Postremission therapy: Chemotherapy to kill leukemia cells that survive after remission induction therapy.

Precancerous (pre-KAN-ser-us): A term used to describe a condition that may or is likely to become cancer.

Precancerous polyps: Growths in the colon that often become cancerous.

Prednisone: A drug often given to multiple myeloma patients along with one or more anticancer drugs. Prednisone appears to act together with anticancer drugs in helping to control the effects of the disease on the body.

Preleukemia (PREE-loo-KEE-mee-a): A condition in which the bone marrow does not function normally. It does not produce enough blood cells. This condition may progress and become acute leukemia. Preleukemia also is called myelodysplastic syndrome or smoldering leukemia.

Primitive neuroectodermal tumors (NOO-ro-ek-toe-DER-mul): A type of brain tumor that recent research suggests develops from primitive (developing) nerve cells that normally do not remain in the body after birth. Primitive neuroectodermal tumors are often called medulloblastomas.

Proctoscopy (prok-TOS-ko-pee): An examination of the rectum and the lower end of the colon using a thin lighted instrument called a sigmoidoscope.

Proctosigmoidoscopy (PROK-toe-sig-moid-OSS-ko-pee): An examination of the rectum and the lower part of the colon using a thin, lighted instrument called a sigmoidoscope.

Progesterone (pro-JES-ter-own): A female hormone.

Prognosis (prog-NO-sis): The probable outcome or course of a disease; the chance of recovery.

Prophylactic cranial irradiation (pro-fi-LAK-tik KRAY-nee-ul ir-ray-dee-AY-shun): Radiation therapy to the head to prevent cancer from spreading to the brain.

Prostatectomy (pros-ta-TEK-to-mee): An operation to remove part or all of the prostate.

Prostate gland (PROS-tate): A gland in the male reproductive system just below the bladder. It surrounds part of the urethra, the canal that empties the bladder. It produces a fluid that forms part of semen.

Prostate-specific antigen: A protein whose level in the blood goes up in some men who have prostate cancer or benign prostatic hyperplasia. Also called PSA.

Prostatic acid phosphatase (FOS-fa-tase): An enzyme produced by the prostate. Its level in the blood goes up in some men who have prostate cancer. Also called PAP.

Prosthesis (pros-THEE-sis): An artificial replacement for a body part.

Prosthodontist (pros-tho-DON-tist): A dentist with special training in making replacements for missing teeth or other structures of the oral cavity to restore the patient's appearance, comfort, and/or health.

Proteins (PRO-teenz): Substances that are essential to the body's structure and proper functioning.

PTC (percutaneous transhepatic cholangiography) (per-kyoo-TAN-ee-us trans-heh-PAT-ik ko-LAN-jee-AH-gra-fee): A test sometimes used to help diagnose cancer of the pancreas. During this test, a thin needle is put into the liver. Dye is injected into the bile ducts in the liver so that blockages can be seen on x-rays.

R

Radiation fibrosis (ray-dee-AY-shun-fye-BRO-sis): The formation of scar tissue as a result of radiation therapy to the lung.

Radiation oncologist (ray-dee-AY-shun on-KOL-o-jist): A doctor who specializes in using radiation to treat cancer.

Radiation therapy (ray-dee-AY-shun): Treatment with high-energy rays (such as x-rays) to kill cancer cells. The radiation may come from outside the body (external radiation) or from radioactive materials placed directly in the tumor (implant radiation). Also called radiotherapy.

Radical cystectomy (RAD-i-kal sis-TEK-to-mee): Surgery to remove the bladder as well as nearby tissues and organs.

Radical prostatectomy: Surgery to remove the entire prostate. The two types of radical prostatectomy are retropubic prostatectomy and perineal prostatectomy.

Radioactive (RAY-dee-o-AK-tiv): Giving off radiatiion.

Radiologist: A doctor who specializes in creating and interpreting pictures of areas inside the body. The pictures are produced with x-rays, sound waves, or other types of energy.

Radionuclide scanning: An exam that produces pictures (scans) of internal parts of the body. The patient is given an injection or swallows a small amount of radioactive material. A machine called a scanner then measures the radioactivity in certain organs.

Radiosensitizers: Drugs that make cells more sensitive to radiation.

Radon (RAY-don): A radioactive gas that is released by uranium, a substance found in soil and rock. When too much radon is breathed in, it can damage lung cells and lead to lung cancer.

Rectum: The last 8 to 10 inches of the large intestine. The rectum stores solid waste until it leaves the body through the anus.

Recur: To occur again. Recurrence is the reappearance of cancer cells at the same site or in another location.

Red blood cells: Cells that carry oxygen to all parts of the body. Also called erythrocytes.

Reed-Sternberg cell: A type of cell that appears in patients with Hodgkin's disease. The number of these cells increases as the disease advances.

Reflux: The term used when liquid backs up into the esophagus from the stomach.

Regional chemotherapy: Treatment with anticancer drugs that affects mainly the cells in the treated area.

Relapse: The return of signs and symptoms of a disease after a period of improvement.

Remission: Disappearance of the signs and symptoms of cancer. When this happens, the disease is said to be "in remission." A remission can be temporary or permanent.

Remission induction therapy: The initial chemotherapy a patient with acute leukemia receives to bring about a remission.

Renal capsule: The fibrous connective tissue that surrounds each kidney.

Renal cell cancer: Cancer that develops in the lining of the renal tubules, which filter the blood and produce urine.

Renal pelvis: The area at the center of the kidney. Urine collects here and is funneled into the ureter.

Reproductive cells: Egg and sperm cells. Each mature reproductive cell carries a single set of 23 chromosomes.

Reproductive system: The group of organs and glands involved with having a child. In women, these are the uterus (womb), the fallopian tubes, the ovaries, and the vagina (birth canal). The reproductive system in men includes the testes, the prostate, and the penis.

Resection (ree-SEK-shun): Surgical removal of part of an organ.

Respiratory system (RES-pi-ra-tor-ee): The organs that are involved in breathing. These include the nose, throat, larynx, trachea, bronchi, and lungs.

Respiratory therapy (RES-pi-ra-tor-ee): Exercises and treatments that help patients recover lung function after surgery.

Retinoblastoma: An eye cancer caused by the loss of both gene copies of the tumor- suppressor gene RB; the inherited form typically occurs in childhood, because one gene is missing from the time of birth.

Retropubic prostatectomy (re-tro-PYOO-bik): Surgical removal of the prostate through an incision in the abdomen.

Risk factor: Something that increases the chance of developing a disease.

RNA (ribonucleic acid): One of the two nucleic acids found in all cells. The other is DNA (deoxyribonucleic acid). RNA transfers genetic information from DNA to proteins produced by the cell.

S

Salivary glands (SAL-i-vair-ee): Glands in the mouth that produce saliva.

Salpingo-oophorectomy (sal-PING-o-OO-for-EK-to-mee): Surgical removal of the fallopian tubes and ovaries.

Sarcoma (sar-KO-ma): A malignant tumor that begins in connective and supportive tissue.

Scans: Pictures of organs in the body. Scans often used in diagnosing, staging, and monitoring patients include liver scans, bone scans, and computed tomography (CT) or computed axial tomography (CAT) scans. In liver scanning and bone scanning, radioactive substances that are injected into the bloodstream collect in these organs. A scanner that detects the radiation is used to create pictures. In CT scanning, an x-ray machine linked to a computer is used to produce detailed pictures of organs inside the body.

Schiller test (SHIL-er): A test in which iodine is applied to the cervix. The iodine colors healthy cells brown; abnormal cells remain unstained, usually appearing white or yellow.

Schwannoma (shwah-NO-ma): A type of benign brain tumor that begins in the Schwann cells, which produce the myelin that protects the acoustic nerve; the nerve of hearing.

Screening: Checking for disease when there are no symptoms.

Scrotum (SKRO-tum): The external pouch of skin that contains the testicles.

Sebum (SEE-bum): An oily substance produced by certain glands in the skin.

Seizures (SEE-zhurz): Convulsions; sudden, involuntary movements of the muscles.

Semen: The fluid that is released through the penis during orgasm. Semen is made up of sperm from the testicles and fluid from the prostate and other sex glands.

Seminal vesicles (SEM-in-al VES-i-kulz): Glands that help produce semen.

Seminoma (sem-in-O-ma): A type of testicular cancer that arises from sex cells, or germ cells, at a very early stage in their development.

Shunt: A catheter (tube) that carries cerebrospinal fluid from a ventricle in the brain to another area of the body.

Side effects: Problems that occur when treatment affects healthy cells. Common side effects of cancer treatment are fatigue, nausea, vomiting, decreased blood cell counts, hair loss, and mouth sores.

Sigmoidoscope (sig-MOY-da-skope): An instrument used to view the inside of the colon.

Sigmoidoscopy (sig-moid-OSS-ko-pee): A procedure in which the doctor looks inside the rectum and the lower part of the colon (sigmoid colon) through a lighted tube. The doctor may collect samples of tissue or cells for closer examination. Also called proctosigmoidoscopy.

Skin graft: Skin that is moved from one part of the body to another.

Small cell lung cancer: A type of lung cancer in which the cells are small and round. Also called oat cell lung cancer.

Small intestine: The part of the digestive tract that is located between the stomach and the large intestine.

Smoldering leukemia: See Preleukemia.

Soft tissue sarcoma: A sarcoma that begins in the muscle, fat, fibrous tissue, blood vessels, or other supporting tissue of the body.

Somatic cells: All the body cells except the reproductive cells.

Somatic mutations: See mutation.

Speech pathologist: A specialist who evaluates and treats people with communication and swallowing problems. Also called a speech therapist.

Speculum (SPEK-yoo-lum): An instrument used to widen the opening of the vagina so that the cervix is more easily visible.

Sperm banking: Freezing sperm before cancer treatment for use in the future. This procedure can allow men to father children after loss of fertility.

SPF (Sun protection factor): A scale for rating sunscreens. Sunscreens with an SPF of 15 or higher provide the best protection from the sun's harmful rays. SPF stands for sun protection factor.

Spinal tap: A test in which a fluid sample is removed from the spinal column with a thin needle. Also called a lumbar puncture.

Spleen: An organ that produces lymphocytes, filters the blood, stores blood cells, and destroys those that are aging. It is located on the left side of the abdomen near the stomach.

Splenectomy (splen-EK-toe-mee): An operation to remove the spleen.

Sputum (SPYOO-tum): Mucus from the lungs.

Squamous cell carcinoma (SKWAY-mus): Cancer that begins in squamous cells, which are thin, flat cells resembling fish scales. Squamous cells are found in the tissue that forms the surface of the skin, the lining of the hollow organs of the body, and the passages of the respiratory and digestive tracts.

Squamous cells (SKWAY-mus): Flat cells that look like fish scales; they make up most of the epidermis, the outer layer of the skin.

Squamous intraepithelial lesion (SKWAY-mus in-tra-eh-pih-THEEL-ee-ul LEE-zhun): A general term for the abnormal growth of squamous cells on the surface of the cervix. The changes in the cells are described as low grade or high grade, depending on how much of the cervix is affected and how abnormal the cells are. Also called SIL.

Stage: The extent of a cancer, especially whether the disease has spread from the original site to other parts of the body.

Staging: Doing exams and tests to learn the extent of the cancer, especially whether it has spread from its original site to other parts of the body.

Stem cells: The cells from which all blood cells develop.

Stereotaxis (stair-ee-o-TAK-sis): Use of a computer and scanning devices to create three- dimensional pictures. This method can be used to direct a biopsy, external radiation, or the insertion of radiation implants.

Sterile: The inability to produce children.

Steroids (STEH-roidz): Drugs used to relieve swelling and inflammation.

Stoma: An opening in the abdominal wall; also called an ostomy or urostomy.

Stool: The waste matter discharged in a bowel movement; feces.

Stool test: A test to check for hidden blood in the bowel movement.

Subglottis (SUB-glot-is): The lowest part of the larynx; the area from just below the vocal cords down to the top of the trachea.

Sun Protection Factor (SPF): A scale for rating sunscreens. Sunscreens with an SPF of 15 or higher provide the best protection from the sun's harmful rays.

Sunscreen: A substance that blocks the effect of the sun's harmful rays. Using lotions or creams that contain sunscreens can protect the skin from damage that may lead to cancer.

Supportive care: Treatment given to prevent, control, or relieve complications and side effects and to improve the patient's comfort and quality of life.

Supraglottis (SOOP-ra-GLOT-is): The upper part of the larynx, including the epiglottis; the area above the vocal cords.

Surgery: A procedure to remove or repair a part of the body or to find out if disese is present.

Systemic (sis-TEM-ik): Reaching and affecting cells all over the body.

Systemic therapy (sis-TEM-ik): Treatment that uses substances that travel through the bloodstream, reaching and affecting cancer cells all over the body.

T

T-cell lymphoma (lim-FO-ma): A cancer of the immune system that appears in the skin; also called mycosis fungoides.

Testicles (TES-ti-kuls): The two egg-shaped glands that produce sperm and male hormones.

Testosterone (tes-TOS-ter-own): A male sex hormone.

Thermography (ther-MOG-ra-fee): A test to measure and display heat patterns of tissues near the surface of the breast. Abnormal tissue generally is warmer than healthy tissue. This technique is under study; its value in detecting breast cancer has not been proven.

Thoracentesis (thor-a-sen-TEE-sis): Removal of fluid in the pleura through a needle.

Thoracic (thor-ASS-ik): Pertaining to the chest.

Thoracotomy (thor-a-KOT-o-mee): An operation to open the chest.

Thrombocytes (THROM-bo-sites): See Platelets.

Thrombophlebitis (throm-bo-fleh-BYE-tis): Inflammation of a vein that occurs when a blood clot forms.

Thymus: An organ in which lymphocytes mature and multiply. It lies behind the breastbone.

Tissue (TISH-oo): A group or layer of cells that together perform specific functions.

Tonsils: Small masses of lymphatic tissue on either side of the throat.

Topical chemotherapy (kee-mo-THER-a-pee): Treatment with anticancer drugs in a lotion or cream.

Total pancreatectomy (pan-cree-a-TEK-to-mee): Surgery to remove the entire pancreas.

Toxins: Poisons produced by certain animals, plants, or bacteria.

Trachea (TRAY-kee-a): The airway that leads from the larynx to the lungs. Also called the windpipe.

Tracheoesophageal puncture (TRAY-kee-o-eh-SOF-a-JEE-al PUNK-chur): A small opening made by a surgeon between the esophagus and the trachea. A valve keeps food out of the trachea but lets air into the esophagus for esophageal speech.

Tracheostomy (TRAY-kee-AHS-toe-mee): Surgery to create an opening (stoma) into the windpipe. The opening itself may also be called a tracheostomy.

Tracheostomy button (TRAY-kee-AHS-toe-mee): A 1- to 1-1/2-inch-long plastic tube placed in the stoma to keep it open.

Tracheostomy tube (TRAY-kee-AHS-toe-mee): A 2- to 3-inch-long metal or plastic tube that keeps the stoma and trachea open. Also called a trach ("trake") tube.

Transformation: The change that a normal cell undergoes as it becomes malignant.

Transfusion (trans-FYOO-zhun): The transfer of blood or blood products from one person to another.

Transitional cell carcinoma: Cancer that develops in the lining of the renal pelvis. This type of cancer also occurs in the ureter and the bladder.

Transitional cells: Cells lining some organs.

Transplantation (trans-plan-TAY-shun): The replacement of an organ with one from another person.

Transrectal ultrasound: The use of sound waves to detect cancer. An instrument is inserted into the rectum. Waves bounce off the prostate and the pattern of the echoes produced is converted into a picture by a computer.

Transurethral resection (TRANZ-yoo-REE-thral ree-SEK-shun): Surgery performed with a special instrument inserted through the urethra. Also called TUR.

Transurethral resection of the prostate (TRANZ-yoo-REE-thral): The use of an instrument inserted through the penis to remove tissue from the prostate. Also called TUR or TURP.

Transvaginal ultrasound: Sound waves sent out by a probe inserted in the vagina. The waves bounce off the ovaries, and a computer uses the echoes to create a picture called a sonogram. Also called TVS.

Tumor (TOO-mer): An abnormal mass of tissue that results from excessive cell division. Tumors perform no useful body function. They may either be benign (not cancerous) or malignant (cancerous).

Tumor debulking: Surgically removing as much of the tumor as possible.

Tumor marker: A substance in blood or other body fluids that may suggest that a person has cancer.

Tumor necrosis factor (ne-KRO-sis): A type of biological response modifier (a substance that can improve the body's natural response to disease). Scientists are still learning how this substance causes cancer cells to die.

Tumor-suppressor gene: Genes in the body that can suppress or block the development of cancer.

U

Ulcerative colitis: A disease that causes long-term inflammation of the lining of the colon.

Ultrasonography: A test in which sound waves (called ultrasound) are bounced off tissues and the echoes are converted into a picture (sonogram).

Ultrasound: A test that bounces sound waves off tissues and internal organs and changes the echoes into pictures (sonograms). Tissues of different densities reflect sound waves differently.

Ultraviolet (UV) radiation (ul-tra-VYE-o-let ray-dee-AY-shun): Invisible rays that are part of the energy that comes from the sun. UV radiation can burn the skin and cause melanoma and other types of skin cancer. UV radiation that reaches the earth's surface is made up of two types of rays, called UVA and UVB rays. UVB rays are more likely than UVA rays to cause sunburn, but UVA rays pass further into the skin. Scientists have long thought that UVB radiation can cause melanoma and other types of skin cancer. They now think that UVA radiation also may add to skin damage that can lead to cancer. For this reason, skin specialists recommend that people use sunscreens that block or absorb both kinds of UV radiation.

Upper GI series: A series of x-rays of the upper digestive system that are taken after a person drinks a barium solution, which outlines the digestive organs on the x-rays.

Ureter (yoo-REE-ter): The tube that carries urine from the kidney to the bladder.

Urethra (yoo-REE-thra): The tube that empties urine from the bladder.

Urinalysis: A test that determines the content of the urine.

Urinary tract (YUR-in-air-ee): The organs of the body that produce and discharge urine. These include the kidneys, ureters, bladder, and urethra.

Urine (YUR-in): Fluid containing water and waste products. Urine is made by the kidneys, stored in the bladder, and leaves the body through the urethra.

Urologist (yoo-RAHL-o-jist): A doctor who specializes in diseases of the urinary organs in females and the urinary and sex organs in males.

Urostomy (yoo-RAHS-toe-mee): An operation to create an opening from inside the body to the outside, making a new way to pass urine.

Uterus (YOO-ter-us): The small, hollow, pear-shaped organ in a woman's pelvis. This is the organ in which an unborn child develops. Also called the womb.

V

Vagina (vah-JYE-na): The muscular canal extending from the uterus to the exterior of the body.

Vasectomy (vas-EK-to-mee): An operation to cut or tie off the two tubes that carry sperm out of the testicles.

Ventricles (VEN-trih-kulz): Four connected cavities (hollow spaces) in the brain.

Vinyl chloride (VYE-nil KLO-ride): A substance used in manufacturing plastics. It is linked to liver cancer.

Viruses (VYE-rus-ez): Small living particles that can infect cells and change how the cells function. Infection with a virus can cause a person to develop symptoms. The disease and symptoms that are caused depend on the type of virus and the type of cells that are infected.

Vital: Necessary to maintain life. Breathing is a vital function.

Vocal cords: Two small bands of muscle within the larynx. They close to prevent food from getting into the lungs, and they vibrate to produce the voice.

W

Wart: A raised growth on the surface of the skin or other organ.

Whipple procedure: A type of surgery used to treat pancreatic cancer. The surgeon removes the head of the pancreas, the duodenum, a portion of the stomach, and other nearby tissues.

White blood cells: Cells that help the body fight infection and disease. These cells begin their development in the bone marrow and then travel to other parts of the body.

Wilms' tumor: A kidney cancer that occurs in children, usually before the age of five.

X

Xerogram: An x-ray of soft tissue.

Xeroradiography (ZEE-roe-ray-dee-OG-ra-fee): A type of mammography in which a picture of the breast is recorded on paper rather than on film.

X-ray: High-energy radiation used in low doses to diagnose diseases and in high doses to treat cancer.

Chapter 88

Directory of Cancer Organizations

People with cancer and their families sometimes need assistance coping with the emotional as well as the practical aspects of their disease. This chapter includes some of the national organizations that provide this type of support. It is not intended to be a comprehensive listing of all organizations that offer these services in the United States, nor does inclusion of any particular organization imply endorsement by the National Cancer Institute, the National Institutes of Health, or the Department of Health and Human Services. The intent of this fact sheet is to provide information useful to individuals nationally. For that reason, it does not include the many local groups that offer valuable assistance to patients and their families in individual states or cities.

Alliance for Lung Cancer Advocacy, Support, and Education (ALCASE)
1601 Lincoln Avenue
Vancouver, WA 98660
Telephone: 360-696-2436; 1-800-298-2436
Fax: 360-735-1305
E-mail: info@alcase.org
Internet Website: http://www.alcase.org

National Organizations That Offer Services to People with Cancer and Their Families, National Cancer Institute Fact Sheet, March 1998.

The ALCASE provides people with lung cancer and their families with programs designed to help improve their quality of life. Programs include education about the disease, psychosocial support, and advocacy about issues concerning lung cancer survivors.

American Brain Tumor Association (ABTA)

Suite 146
2720 River Road
Des Plaines, IL 60018
Telephone: 847-827-9910; 1-800-886-ABTA (1-800-886-2282)
Fax: 847-827-9918
E-mail: info@abta.org
Internet Website: http://www.abta.org

The ABTA supports research, offers printed materials about research and treatment of brain tumors, and provides resource listings of physicians, treatment facilities, and support groups throughout the country.

American Cancer Society (ACS)

1599 Clifton Road NE.
Atlanta, GA 30329
Telephone: 404-320-3333; 1-800-ACS-2345 (1-800-227-2345)
Internet Website: http://www.cancer.org

The ACS is a voluntary organization that offers a variety of services to patients and their families. The ACS also supports research, provides printed materials, and conducts educational programs. A local ACS unit may be listed in the white pages of the telephone directory under "American Cancer Society."

American Cancer Society (ACS) Supported Programs

I Can Cope: I Can Cope is a patient education program that is designed to help patients, families, and friends cope with the day-to-day issues of living with cancer.

International Association of Laryngectomies: This program assists people who have lost their voice as a result of cancer. It provides information on the skills needed by laryngectomies and works toward total rehabilitation of patients,

Look Good ... Feel Better: This program was developed by the Cosmetic, Toiletry, and Fragrance Association Foundation in cooperation with ACS and the National Cosmetology Association. It focuses on techniques that can help people undergoing cancer treatment improve their appearance. For more information, contact a local ACS unit or 1-800-395-LOOK (1-800-395-5665).

Ostomy Rehabilitation Program: The Ostomy Rehabilitation Program provides mutual aid, emotional support, and educational materials to people with ostomies.

Reach to Recovery: The Reach to Recovery Program is a rehabilitation program for women who have or have had breast cancer. The program helps breast cancer patients meet the physical, emotional, and cosmetic needs related to their disease and its treatment.

Association for the Care of Children's Health (ACCH)
PO Box 25707
Alexandria, VA 22313
Telephone: 1-800-808-ACCH (1-800-808-2224)
E-mail: acch@clark.net
Internet Website: http://www.acch.org

The ACCH carries out a variety of programs to promote the health of children. It publishes educational materials on child health of interest to parents, educators, and health professionals.

Cancer Care, Inc.
National Office
275 7th Ave.
New York, NY 10001
Telephone: 212-302-2400; 1-800-813-HOPE (1-800-813-4673)
E-mail: info@cancercare.org
Internet Website: http://www.cancercareinc.org

Cancer Care, Inc., offers counseling, support groups, and financial assistance for nonmedical expenses, home visits by trained volunteers, and referrals to services such as housekeeping, nursing care, and health aids.

Candlelighters Childhood Cancer Foundation (CCCF)
Suite 460
7910 Woodmont Avenue
Bethesda, MD 20814-3015

Telephone: 301-657-8401; 1-800-366-CCCF (1-800-366-2223)
Fax: 301-718-2686
E-mail: info@candlelighters.org
Internet Website: http://www.candlelighters.org

The CCCF is an organization formed by parents of young cancer patients. An important goal of the organization is to help families cope with the emotional stresses of their experiences.

Children's Hospice International
Suite 3C
2202 Mount Vernon Avenue
Alexandria, VA 22301
Telephone: 703-684-0330; 1-800-2-4-CHILD (1-800-242-4453)
Fax: 703-684-0226
E-mail: chiorg@aol.com
Internet Website: http://www.chionline.org

Children's Hospice International provides a network of support for dying children and their families. It serves as a clearinghouse on research programs, support groups, and education and training programs for the care of terminally ill children. It also offers publications on topics such as home care for seriously ill children and pain management.

ENCORE
YWCA Encore Program
YWCA of the USA
Encore Plus Program
Office of Women's Health Advocacy
624 Ninth Street NW, Third Floor
Washington, DC 20001-5303
Telephone: 202-628-3636 1-800-953-PLUS (1-800-953-7587)
Fax: 202-783-7123
E-mail: cgould@ywca.org
Internet Website: http://www.ywca.org

ENCORE is the YWCA's discussion and exercise program for women who have had breast cancer surgery. It is designed to help restore physical strength and emotional well-being. A local branch of the YWCA, listed in the telephone directory, can provide more information about ENCORE.

Hospice Link
Hospice Education Institute
Suite 3-B
190 West Brook Road
Essex, CT 06426-15 11
Telephone: 203-767-1620 (Alaska and Connecticut);
1-800-331-1620

Hospice Link offers information about hospice care and can refer cancer patients and their families to local hospice programs.

Leukemia and Lymphoma Society
Fourth Floor
733 Third Avenue
New York, NY 10016
Telephone:212-573-8484; 1-800-955-4572
E-mail: frankbock@aol.com
Internet Website: http: //www.leukemia.org

The Society is concerned with leukemia, lymphoma, and related diseases. It supports research and provides printed materials and also offers financial assistance and provides information about other resources for patients and their families. Further information may be available by calling a local chapter listed in the white pages of the telephone directory.

National Alliance of Breast Cancer Organizations (NABCO)
10th Floor
Nine East 37th Street
New York, NY 10016
Telephone: 212-719-0154; 1-800-719-9154
E-mail: nabcoinfo@aol.com
Internet Website: http://www.nabco.org

NABCO is a nonprofit organization that provides information about breast cancer and acts as an advocate for the legislative concerns of breast cancer patients and survivors. NABCO provides phone numbers for approximately 350 cancer support groups nationwide. Information on support groups by state can be accessed at http://www.nabco.org/index.html on NABCO's Website.

National Brain Tumor Foundation (NBTF)
414 Thirteenth Street
Suite 700
Oakland, CA 94612-2603
Telephone: 510-839-9777
Fax: 510-839-9779
E-mail: nbtf@braintumor.org
Internet Website: http://www.braintumor.org

NBTF provides patients and families with information to cope with their brain tumors. This organization conducts national and regional conferences; publishes printed materials for patients and family members; provides access to a national network of patient support groups; and assists in answering patient inquiries. NBTF also awards grants to fund research.

National Coalition for Cancer Survivorship (NCCS)
Suite 505
1010 Wayne Avenue
Silver Spring, MD 20910-5600
Telephone:877-622-7937
Fax: 301-565-9670
E-mail: info@cansearch.org
Internet Website: http://www.cansearch.org

NCCS is a network of groups and individuals that offer support to cancer survivors and their loved ones. It provides information and resources on cancer support and quality of life issues.

National Hospice Organization
1700 Diagonal Road, Suite 300
Alexandria, VA 22314
Telephone: 703-243-5900
Fax: 703-525-5762
E-mail: drsnho@cais.com
Internet Website: http://www.nho.org

The National Hospice Organization is an association of groups that provide hospice care. It is designed to increase awareness about hospice services and to champion the rights and issues of terminally ill patients and their family members.

National Kidney Cancer Association
1234 Sherman Avenue
Suite 203
Evanston, IL 60202-1375
Telephone: 847-332-1051; 1-800-850-9132
Fax: 847-332-2978
E-mail: office@nkca.org
Internet Website: http://www.nkca.org

The National Kidney Cancer Association supports research, offers printed materials about the diagnosis and treatment of kidney cancer, sponsors support groups, and provides physician referral information.

National Marrow Donor Program
Suite 500
3433 Broadway Street NE.
Minneapolis, MN 55413
Telephone: 1-800-MARROW-2 (1-800-627-7692)
Internet Website: http://www.marrow.org

The National Marrow Donor Program, which is funded by the Federal Government, was created to improve the effectiveness of the search for bone marrow donors so that a greater number of bone marrow transplantations can be carried out. It keeps a registry of potential bone marrow donors and provides a free packet of information on bone marrow transplantation.

Skin Cancer Foundation
245 Fifth Avenue
New York, NY 10016
Telephone: 212-725-5176; 1-800-SKIN-490 (1-800-754-6490)
Fax: 212-725-5751
E-mail: info@skincancer.org
Internet Website: http://www.skincancer.org

The Skin Cancer Foundation conducts public and medical education programs to help reduce skin cancer. Major goals are to increase public awareness of the importance of taking protective measures against the damaging rays of the sun and to teach people how to recognize the early signs of skin cancer.

United Ostomy Association
Suite 200
19772 MacArthur Blvd.
Irvine, CA 92612-2405
Telephone: 714-660-8624; 1-800-826-0826
E-mail: uoa@deltanet.com
Internet Website: http://www.uoa.org

The United Ostomy Association helps ostomy patients through mutual aid and emotional support. It provides information to patients and the public and sends volunteers to visit with new ostomy patients.

US TOO International, Inc.
Suite 50
930 North York Road
Hinsdale, IL 60521
Telephone: 630-323-1002; 1-800-80-US TOO (1-800-808-7866)
E-mail: ustoo@ustoo.com
Internet Website: http://www.ustoo.com

US TOO is a prostate cancer support group organization. Goals of US TOO are to increase awareness of prostate cancer in the community, educate men newly diagnosed with prostate cancer, offer support groups, and provide the latest information about treatment for this disease.

Y-ME National Breast Cancer Organization, Inc.
212 West Van Buren Street
Chicago, IL 60607-3908
Telephone: 312-294-8597; Hotline:1-800-221-2141
Fax: 312-294-8597
E-mail: info@y-me.org
Internet Website: http://www.y-me.org

Y-ME National Breast Cancer Organization provides information and support to anyone who has been touched by breast cancer. Y-ME serves women with breast cancer and their families through their national hotline, open-door groups, early detection workshops, and support programs. Numerous local chapter offices are located throughout the United States.

Criteria for Inclusion of Organizations in This Chapter

Organizations included in this fact sheet provide services and/or information to cancer patients and their families. They are national non-profit organizations that, like NCI, support scientific research and investigations of new approaches to cancer detection, treatment, and prevention.

Sources of National Cancer Institute Information

Cancer Information Service; Toll-free: 1-800-4-CANCER (1-800-422-6237); TTY: 1-800-332-8615

NCI Online: NCI's main website at http://www.nci.nih.gov or NCI's website for patients, public, and the mass media at http://rex.nci.nih.gov

CancerMail Service: To obtain a contents list, send E-mail to cancermail@icicc.nci.nih.gov with the word "help" in the body of the message.

CancerFax: fax on demand service Dial 301-402-5874 and listen to recorded instructions.

Index

Index

Health Reference Series
COMPLETE CATALOG

AIDS Sourcebook, 1st Edition

Basic Information about AIDS and HIV Infection, Featuring Historical and Statistical Data, Current Research, Prevention, and Other Special Topics of Interest for Persons Living with AIDS

Along with Source Listings for Further Assistance

Edited by Karen Bellenir and Peter D. Dresser. 831 pages. 1995. 0-7808-0031-1. $78.

"One strength of this book is its practical emphasis. The intended audience is the lay reader . . . useful as an educational tool for health care providers who work with AIDS patients. Recommended for public libraries as well as hospital or academic libraries that collect consumer materials."
— *Bulletin of the Medical Library Association, Jan '96*

"This is the most comprehensive volume of its kind on an important medical topic. Highly recommended for all libraries." — *Reference Book Review, '96*

"Very useful reference for all libraries."
— *Choice, Association of College and Research Libraries, Oct '95*

"There is a wealth of information here that can provide much educational assistance. It is a must book for all libraries and should be on the desk of each and every congressional leader. Highly recommended."
— *AIDS Book Review Journal, Aug '95*

"Recommended for most collections."
— *Library Journal, Jul '95*

AIDS Sourcebook, 2nd Edition

Basic Consumer Health Information about Acquired Immune Deficiency Syndrome (AIDS) and Human Immunodeficiency Virus (HIV) Infection, Featuring Updated Statistical Data, Reports on Recent Research and Prevention Initiatives, and Other Special Topics of Interest for Persons Living with AIDS, Including New Antiretroviral Treatment Options, Strategies for Combating Opportunistic Infections, Information about Clinical Trials, and More

Along with a Glossary of Important Terms and Resource Listings for Further Help and Information

Edited by Karen Bellenir. 751 pages. 1999. 0-7808-0225-X. $78.

"Highly recommended."
— *American Reference Books Annual 2000*

"Excellent sourcebook. This continues to be a highly recommended book. There is no other book that provides as much information as this book provides."
— *AIDS Book Review Journal, Dec-Jan 2000*

"Recommended reference source."
— *Booklist, American Library Association, Dec '99*

"A solid text for college-level health libraries."
— *The Bookwatch, Aug '99*

Cited in *Reference Sources for Small and Medium-Sized Libraries, American Library Association, 1999*

Alcoholism Sourcebook

Basic Consumer Health Information about the Physical and Mental Consequences of Alcohol Abuse, Including Liver Disease, Pancreatitis, Wernicke-Korsakoff Syndrome (Alcoholic Dementia), Fetal Alcohol Syndrome, Heart Disease, Kidney Disorders, Gastrointestinal Problems, and Immune System Compromise and Featuring Facts about Addiction, Detoxification, Alcohol Withdrawal, Recovery, and the Maintenance of Sobriety

Along with a Glossary and Directories of Resources for Further Help and Information

Edited by Karen Bellenir. 650 pages. 2000. 0-7808-0325-6. $78.

SEE ALSO Drug Abuse Sourcebook, Substance Abuse Sourcebook

Allergies Sourcebook

Basic Information about Major Forms and Mechanisms of Common Allergic Reactions, Sensitivities, and Intolerances, Including Anaphylaxis, Asthma, Hives and Other Dermatologic Symptoms, Rhinitis, and Sinusitis

Along with Their Usual Triggers Like Animal Fur, Chemicals, Drugs, Dust, Foods, Insects, Latex, Pollen, and Poison Ivy, Oak, and Sumac; Plus Information on Prevention, Identification, and Treatment

Edited by Allan R. Cook. 611 pages. 1997. 0-7808-0036-2. $78.

Alternative Medicine Sourcebook

Basic Consumer Health Information about Alternatives to Conventional Medicine, Including Acupressure, Acupuncture, Aromatherapy, Ayurveda, Bioelectromagnetics, Environmental Medicine, Essence Therapy, Food and Nutrition Therapy, Herbal Therapy, Homeopathy, Imaging, Massage, Naturopathy, Reflexology, Relaxation and Meditation, Sound Therapy, Vitamin and Mineral Therapy, and Yoga, and More

Edited by Allan R. Cook. 737 pages. 1999. 0-7808-0200-4. $78.

"A great addition to the reference collection of every type of library."
— *American Reference Books Annual 2000*

Alzheimer's, Stroke & 29 Other Neurological Disorders Sourcebook, 1st Edition

Basic Information for the Layperson on 31 Diseases or Disorders Affecting the Brain and Nervous System, First Describing the Illness, Then Listing Symptoms, Diagnostic Methods, and Treatment Options, and Including Statistics on Incidences and Causes

Edited by Frank E. Bair. 579 pages. 1993. 1-55888-748-2. $78.

"Nontechnical reference book that provides reader-friendly information."
— Family Caregiver Alliance Update, Winter '96

"Should be included in any library's patient education section." — American Reference Books Annual, 1994

"Written in an approachable and accessible style. Recommended for patient education and consumer health collections in health science center and public libraries." — Academic Library Book Review, Dec '93

"It is very handy to have information on more than thirty neurological disorders under one cover, and there is no recent source like it." — Reference Quarterly, American Library Association, Fall '93

SEE ALSO Brain Disorders Sourcebook

Alzheimer's Disease Sourcebook, 2nd Edition

Basic Consumer Health Information about Alzheimer's Disease, Related Disorders, and Other Dementias, Including Multi-Infarct Dementia, AIDS-Related Dementia, Alcoholic Dementia, Huntington's Disease, Delirium, and Confusional States

Along with Reports Detailing Current Research Efforts in Prevention and Treatment, Long-Term Care Issues, and Listings of Sources for Additional Help and Information

Edited by Karen Bellenir. 524 pages. 1999. 0-7808-0223-3. $78.

"Provides a wealth of useful information not otherwise available in one place. This resource is recommended for all types of libraries."
— American Reference Books Annual 2000

"Recommended reference source."
— Booklist, American Library Association, Oct '99

Arthritis Sourcebook

Basic Consumer Health Information about Specific Forms of Arthritis and Related Disorders, Including Rheumatoid Arthritis, Osteoarthritis, Gout, Polymyalgia Rheumatica, Psoriatic Arthritis, Spondyloarthropathies, Juvenile Rheumatoid Arthritis, and Juvenile Ankylosing Spondylitis

Along with Information about Medical, Surgical, and Alternative Treatment Options, and Including Strategies for Coping with Pain, Fatigue, and Stress

Edited by Allan R. Cook. 550 pages. 1998. 0-7808-0201-2. $78.

"... accessible to the layperson."
— Reference and Research Book News, Feb '99

Asthma Sourcebook

Basic Consumer Health Information about Asthma, Including Symptoms, Traditional and Nontraditional Remedies, Treatment Advances, Quality-of-Life Aids, Medical Research Updates, and the Role of Allergies, Exercise, Age, the Environment, and Genetics in the Development of Asthma

Along with Statistical Data, a Glossary, and Directories of Support Groups and Other Resources for Further Information

Edited by Annemarie S. Muth. 650 pages. 2000. 0-7808-0381-7. $78.

Back & Neck Disorders Sourcebook

Basic Information about Disorders and Injuries of the Spinal Cord and Vertebrae, Including Facts on Chiropractic Treatment, Surgical Interventions, Paralysis, and Rehabilitation

Along with Advice for Preventing Back Trouble

Edited by Karen Bellenir. 548 pages. 1997. 0-7808-0202-0. $78.

"The strength of this work is its basic, easy-to-read format. Recommended."
— Reference and User Services Quarterly, American Library Association, Winter '97

Blood & Circulatory Disorders Sourcebook

Basic Information about Blood and Its Components, Anemias, Leukemias, Bleeding Disorders, and Circulatory Disorders, Including Aplastic Anemia, Thalassemia, Sickle-Cell Disease, Hemochromatosis, Hemophilia, Von Willebrand Disease, and Vascular Diseases

Along with a Special Section on Blood Transfusions and Blood Supply Safety, a Glossary, and Source Listings for Further Help and Information

Edited by Karen Bellenir and Linda M. Shin. 554 pages. 1998. 0-7808-0203-9. $78.

"Recommended reference source."
— Booklist, American Library Association, Feb '99

"An important reference sourcebook written in simple language for everyday, non-technical users. "
— Reviewer's Bookwatch, Jan '99

1056

Brain Disorders Sourcebook

Basic Consumer Health Information about Strokes, Epilepsy, Amyotrophic Lateral Sclerosis (ALS/Lou Gehrig's Disease), Parkinson's Disease, Brain Tumors, Cerebral Palsy, Headache, Tourette Syndrome, and More

Along with Statistical Data, Treatment and Rehabilitation Options, Coping Strategies, Reports on Current Research Initiatives, a Glossary, and Resource Listings for Additional Help and Information

Edited by Karen Bellenir. 481 pages. 1999. 0-7808-0229-2. $78.

"Belongs on the shelves of any library with a consumer health collection." —*E-Streams, Mar '00*

"Recommended reference source."
—*Booklist, American Library Association, Oct '99*

SEE ALSO Alzheimer's, Stroke & 29 Other Neurological Disorders Sourcebook, 1st Edition

Breast Cancer Sourcebook

Basic Consumer Health Information about Breast Cancer, Including Diagnostic Methods, Treatment Options, Alternative Therapies, Help and Self-Help Information, Related Health Concerns, Statistical and Demographic Data, and Facts for Men with Breast Cancer

Along with Reports on Current Research Initiatives, a Glossary of Related Medical Terms, and a Directory of Sources for Further Help and Information

Edited by Edward J. Prucha. 600 pages. 2000. 0-7808-0244-6. $78.

SEE ALSO Cancer Sourcebook for Women, 1st and 2nd Editions, Women's Health Concerns Sourcebook

Burns Sourcebook

Basic Consumer Health Information about Various Types of Burns and Scalds, Including Flame, Heat, Cold, Electrical, Chemical, and Sun Burns

Along with Information on Short-Term and Long-Term Treatments, Tissue Reconstruction, Plastic Surgery, Prevention Suggestions, and First Aid

Edited by Allan R. Cook. 604 pages. 1999. 0-7808-0204-7. $78.

"This key reference guide is an invaluable addition to all health care and public libraries in confronting this ongoing health issue."
—*American Reference Books Annual 2000*

"This is an exceptional addition to the series and is highly recommended for all consumer health collections, hospital libraries, and academic medical centers." —*E-Streams, Mar '00*

"Recommended reference source."
—*Booklist, American Library Association, Dec '99*

SEE ALSO Skin Disorders Sourcebook

Cancer Sourcebook, 1st Edition

Basic Information on Cancer Types, Symptoms, Diagnostic Methods, and Treatments, Including Statistics on Cancer Occurrences Worldwide and the Risks Associated with Known Carcinogens and Activities

Edited by Frank E. Bair. 932 pages. 1990. 1-55888-888-8. $78.

Cited in *Reference Sources for Small and Medium-Sized Libraries, American Library Association, 1999*

"Written in nontechnical language. Useful for patients, their families, medical professionals, and librarians."
—*Guide to Reference Books, 1996*

"Designed with the non-medical professional in mind. Libraries and medical facilities interested in patient education should certainly consider adding the *Cancer Sourcebook* to their holdings. This compact collection of reliable information . . . is an invaluable tool for helping patients and patients' families and friends to take the first steps in coping with the many difficulties of cancer."
—*Medical Reference Services Quarterly, Winter '91*

"Specifically created for the nontechnical reader . . . an important resource for the general reader trying to understand the complexities of cancer."
—*American Reference Books Annual, 1991*

"This publication's nontechnical nature and very comprehensive format make it useful for both the general public and undergraduate students."
—*Choice, Association of College and Research Libraries, Oct '90*

New Cancer Sourcebook, 2nd Edition

Basic Information about Major Forms and Stages of Cancer, Featuring Facts about Primary and Secondary Tumors of the Respiratory, Nervous, Lymphatic, Circulatory, Skeletal, and Gastrointestinal Systems, and Specific Organs; Statistical and Demographic Data; Treatment Options; and Strategies for Coping

Edited by Allan R. Cook. 1,313 pages. 1996. 0-7808-0041-9. $78.

"An excellent resource for patients with newly diagnosed cancer and their families. The dialogue is simple, direct, and comprehensive. Highly recommended for patients and families to aid in their understanding of cancer and its treatment."
—*Booklist Health Sciences Supplement, American Library Association, Oct '97*

"The amount of factual and useful information is extensive. The writing is very clear, geared to general readers. Recommended for all levels."
—*Choice, Association of College and Research Libraries, Jan '97*

1057

Cancer Sourcebook, 3rd Edition

Basic Consumer Health Information about Major Forms and Stages of Cancer, Featuring Facts about Primary and Secondary Tumors of the Respiratory, Nervous, Lymphatic, Circulatory, Skeletal, and Gastrointestinal Systems, and Specific Organs

Along with Statistical and Demographic Data, Treatment Options, Strategies for Coping, a Glossary, and a Directory of Sources for Additional Help and Information

Edited by Edward J. Prucha. 1,069 pages. 2000. 0-7808-0227-6. $78.

Cancer Sourcebook for Women, 1st Edition

Basic Information about Specific Forms of Cancer That Affect Women, Featuring Facts about Breast Cancer, Cervical Cancer, Ovarian Cancer, Cancer of the Uterus and Uterine Sarcoma, Cancer of the Vagina, and Cancer of the Vulva; Statistical and Demographic Data; Treatments, Self-Help Management Suggestions, and Current Research Initiatives

Edited by Allan R. Cook and Peter D. Dresser. 524 pages. 1996. 0-7808-0076-1. $78.

". . . written in easily understandable, non-technical language. Recommended for public libraries or hospital and academic libraries that collect patient education or consumer health materials."
—*Medical Reference Services Quarterly, Spring '97*

"Would be of value in a consumer health library. . . . written with the health care consumer in mind. Medical jargon is at a minimum, and medical terms are explained in clear, understandable sentences."
—*Bulletin of the Medical Library Association, Oct '96*

"The availability under one cover of all these pertinent publications, grouped under cohesive headings, makes this certainly a most useful sourcebook."
—*Choice, Association of College and Research Libraries, Jun '96*

"Presents a comprehensive knowledge base for general readers. Men and women both benefit from the gold mine of information nestled between the two covers of this book. Recommended."
—*Academic Library Book Review, Summer '96*

"This timely book is highly recommended for consumer health and patient education collections in all libraries." —*Library Journal, Apr '96*

SEE ALSO *Breast Cancer Sourcebook, Women's Health Concerns Sourcebook*

Cancer Sourcebook for Women, 2nd Edition

Basic Consumer Health Information about Specific Forms of Cancer That Affect Women, Including Cervical Cancer, Ovarian Cancer, Endometrial Cancer, Uterine Sarcoma, Vaginal Cancer, Vulvar Cancer, and Gestational Trophoblastic Tumor; and Featuring Statistical Information, Facts about Tests and Treatments, a Glossary of Cancer Terms, and an Extensive List of Additional Resources

Edited by Edward J. Prucha. 600 pages. 2000. 0-7808-0226-8. $78.

SEE ALSO *Breast Cancer Sourcebook, Women's Health Concerns Sourcebook*

Cardiovascular Diseases & Disorders Sourcebook, 1st Edition

Basic Information about Cardiovascular Diseases and Disorders, Featuring Facts about the Cardiovascular System, Demographic and Statistical Data, Descriptions of Pharmacological and Surgical Interventions, Lifestyle Modifications, and a Special Section Focusing on Heart Disorders in Children

Edited by Karen Bellenir and Peter D. Dresser. 683 pages. 1995. 0-7808-0032-X. $78.

". . . comprehensive format provides an extensive overview on this subject."
—*Choice, Association of College and Research Libraries, Jun '96*

". . . an easily understood, complete, up-to-date resource. This well executed public health tool will make valuable information available to those that need it most, patients and their families. The typeface, sturdy non-reflective paper, and library binding add a feel of quality found wanting in other publications. Highly recommended for academic and general libraries. "
—*Academic Library Book Review, Summer '96*

SEE ALSO *Healthy Heart Sourcebook for Women, Heart Diseases & Disorders Sourcebook, 2nd Edition*

Communication Disorders Sourcebook

Basic Information about Deafness and Hearing Loss, Speech and Language Disorders, Voice Disorders, Balance and Vestibular Disorders, and Disorders of Smell, Taste, and Touch

Edited by Linda M. Ross. 533 pages. 1996. 0-7808-0077-X. $78.

"This is skillfully edited and is a welcome resource for the layperson. It should be found in every public and medical library." —*Booklist Health Sciences Supplement, American Library Association, Oct '97*

Congenital Disorders Sourcebook

Basic Information about Disorders Acquired during Gestation, Including Spina Bifida, Hydrocephalus, Cerebral Palsy, Heart Defects, Craniofacial Abnormalities, Fetal Alcohol Syndrome, and More

Along with Current Treatment Options and Statistical Data

Edited by Karen Bellenir. 607 pages. 1997. 0-7808-0205-5. $78.

"Recommended reference source."
—*Booklist, American Library Association, Oct '97*

SEE ALSO Pregnancy & Birth Sourcebook

■

Consumer Issues in Health Care Sourcebook

Basic Information about Health Care Fundamentals and Related Consumer Issues, Including Exams and Screening Tests, Physician Specialties, Choosing a Doctor, Using Prescription and Over-the-Counter Medications Safely, Avoiding Health Scams, Managing Common Health Risks in the Home, Care Options for Chronically or Terminally Ill Patients, and a List of Resources for Obtaining Help and Further Information

Edited by Karen Bellenir. 618 pages. 1998. 0-7808-0221-7. $78.

"Both public and academic libraries will want to have a copy in their collection for readers who are interested in self-education on health issues."
—*American Reference Books Annual 2000*

"The editor has researched the literature from government agencies and others, saving readers the time and effort of having to do the research themselves. Recommended for public libraries."
—*Reference and User Services Quarterly, American Library Association, Spring '99*

"Recommended reference source."
—*Booklist, American Library Association, Dec '98*

■

Contagious & Non-Contagious Infectious Diseases Sourcebook

Basic Information about Contagious Diseases like Measles, Polio, Hepatitis B, and Infectious Mononucleosis, and Non-Contagious Infectious Diseases like Tetanus and Toxic Shock Syndrome, and Diseases Occurring as Secondary Infections Such as Shingles and Reye Syndrome

Along with Vaccination, Prevention, and Treatment Information, and a Section Describing Emerging Infectious Disease Threats

Edited by Karen Bellenir and Peter D. Dresser. 566 pages. 1996. 0-7808-0075-3. $78.

Death & Dying Sourcebook

Basic Consumer Health Information for the Layperson about End-of-Life Care and Related Ethical and Legal Issues, Including Chief Causes of Death, Autopsies, Pain Management for the Terminally Ill, Life Support Systems, Insurance, Euthanasia, Assisted Suicide, Hospice Programs, Living Wills, Funeral Planning, Counseling, Mourning, Organ Donation, and Physician Training

Along with Statistical Data, a Glossary, and Listings of Sources for Further Help and Information

Edited by Annemarie S. Muth. 641 pages. 1999. 0-7808-0230-6. $78.

"This book is a definite must for all those involved in end-of-life care." —*Doody's Review Service, '00*

■

Diabetes Sourcebook, 1st Edition

Basic Information about Insulin-Dependent and Non-insulin-Dependent Diabetes Mellitus, Gestational Diabetes, and Diabetic Complications, Symptoms, Treatment, and Research Results, Including Statistics on Prevalence, Morbidity, and Mortality

Along with Source Listings for Further Help and Information

Edited by Karen Bellenir and Peter D. Dresser. 827 pages. 1994. 1-55888-751-2. $78.

". . . very informative and understandable for the layperson without being simplistic. It provides a comprehensive overview for laypersons who want a general understanding of the disease or who want to focus on various aspects of the disease."
—*Bulletin of the Medical Library Association, Jan '96*

■

Diabetes Sourcebook, 2nd Edition

Basic Consumer Health Information about Type 1 Diabetes (Insulin-Dependent or Juvenile-Onset Diabetes), Type 2 (Noninsulin-Dependent or Adult-Onset Diabetes), Gestational Diabetes, and Related Disorders, Including Diabetes Prevalence Data, Management Issues, the Role of Diet and Exercise in Controlling Diabetes, Insulin and Other Diabetes Medicines, and Complications of Diabetes Such as Eye Diseases, Periodontal Disease, Amputation, and End-Stage Renal Disease

Along with Reports on Current Research Initiatives, a Glossary, and Resource Listings for Further Help and Information

Edited by Karen Bellenir. 688 pages. 1998. 0-7808-0224-1. $78.

"This comprehensive book is an excellent addition for high school, academic, medical, and public libraries. This volume is highly recommended."
—*American Reference Books Annual 2000*

"An invaluable reference." —*Library Journal, May '00*

Selected as one of the 250 "Best Health Sciences Books of 1999." — *Doody's Rating Service, Mar-Apr 2000*

"Recommended reference source."
— *Booklist, American Library Association, Feb '99*

". . . provides reliable mainstream medical information . . . belongs on the shelves of any library with a consumer health collection." — *E-Streams, Sep '99*

"Provides useful information for the general public."
— *Healthlines, University of Michigan Health Management Research Center, Sep/Oct '99*

■

Diet & Nutrition Sourcebook, 1st Edition

Basic Information about Nutrition, Including the Dietary Guidelines for Americans, the Food Guide Pyramid, and Their Applications in Daily Diet, Nutritional Advice for Specific Age Groups, Current Nutritional Issues and Controversies, the New Food Label and How to Use It to Promote Healthy Eating, and Recent Developments in Nutritional Research

Edited by Dan R. Harris. 662 pages. 1996. 0-7808-0084-2. $78.

"Useful reference as a food and nutrition sourcebook for the general consumer." — *Booklist Health Sciences Supplement, American Library Association, Oct '97*

"Recommended for public libraries and medical libraries that receive general information requests on nutrition. It is readable and will appeal to those interested in learning more about healthy dietary practices."
— *Medical Reference Services Quarterly, Fall '97*

"An abundance of medical and social statistics is translated into readable information geared toward the general reader." — *Bookwatch, Mar '97*

"With dozens of questionable diet books on the market, it is so refreshing to find a reliable and factual reference book. Recommended to aspiring professionals, librarians, and others seeking and giving reliable dietary advice. An excellent compilation." — *Choice, Association of College and Research Libraries, Feb '97*

SEE ALSO *Digestive Diseases & Disorders Sourcebook, Gastrointestinal Diseases & Disorders Sourcebook*

■

Diet & Nutrition Sourcebook, 2nd Edition

Basic Consumer Health Information about Dietary Guidelines, Recommended Daily Intake Values, Vitamins, Minerals, Fiber, Fat, Weight Control, Dietary Supplements, and Food Additives

Along with Special Sections on Nutrition Needs throughout Life and Nutrition for People with Such Specific Medical Concerns as Allergies, High Blood Cholesterol, Hypertension, Diabetes, Celiac Disease, Seizure Disorders, Phenylketonuria (PKU), Cancer, and Eating Disorders, and Including Reports on Current Nutrition Research and Source Listings for Additional Help and Information

Edited by Karen Bellenir. 650 pages. 1999. 0-7808-0228-4. $78.

"This reference document should be in any public library, but it would be a very good guide for beginning students in the health sciences. If the other books in this publisher's series are as good as this, they should all be in the health sciences collections."
— *American Reference Books Annual 2000*

"Recommended reference source."
— *Booklist, American Library Association, Dec '99*

SEE ALSO *Digestive Diseases & Disorders Sourcebook, Gastrointestinal Diseases & Disorders Sourcebook*

■

Digestive Diseases & Disorders Sourcebook

Basic Consumer Health Information about Diseases and Disorders that Impact the Upper and Lower Digestive System, Including Celiac Disease, Constipation, Crohn's Disease, Cyclic Vomiting Syndrome, Diarrhea, Diverticulosis and Diverticulitis, Gallstones, Heartburn, Hemorrhoids, Hernias, Indigestion (Dyspepsia), Irritable Bowel Syndrome, Lactose Intolerance, Ulcers, and More

Along with Information about Medications and Other Treatments, Tips for Maintaining a Healthy Digestive Tract, a Glossary, and Directory of Digestive Diseases Organizations

Edited by Karen Bellenir. 335 pages. 1999. 0-7808-0327-2. $48.

"Recommended reference source."
— *Booklist, American Library Association, May '00*

SEE ALSO *Diet & Nutrition Sourcebook, 1st and 2nd Editions, Gastrointestinal Diseases & Disorders Sourcebook*

■

Disabilities Sourcebook

Basic Consumer Health Information about Physical and Psychiatric Disabilities, Including Descriptions of Major Causes of Disability, Assistive and Adaptive Aids, Workplace Issues, and Accessibility Concerns

Along with Information about the Americans with Disabilities Act, a Glossary, and Resources for Additional Help and Information

Edited by Dawn D. Matthews. 616 pages. 2000. 0-7808-0389-2. $78.

■

Domestic Violence & Child Abuse Sourcebook

Basic Information about Spousal/ Partner, Child, and Elder Physical, Emotional, and Sexual Abuse, Teen Dating Violence, and Stalking, Including Information about Hotlines, Safe Houses, Safety Plans, and Other Resources for Support and Assistance, Community Ini-

tiatives, and Reports on Current Directions in Research and Treatment

Along with a Glossary, Sources for Further Reading, and Governmental and Non-Governmental Organizations Contact Information

Edited by Helene Henderson. 600 pages. 2000. 0-7808-0235-7. $78.

■

Drug Abuse Sourcebook

Basic Consumer Health Information about Illicit Substances of Abuse and the Diversion of Prescription Medications, Including Depressants, Hallucinogens, Inhalants, Marijuana, Narcotics, Stimulants, and Anabolic Steroids

Along with Facts about Related Health Risks, Treatment Issues, and Substance Abuse Prevention Programs, a Glossary of Terms, Statistical Data, and Directories of Hotline Services, Self-Help Groups, and Organizations Able to Provide Further Information

Edited by Karen Bellenir. 600 pages. 2000. 0-7808-0242-X. $78.

SEE ALSO *Alcoholism Sourcebook, Substance Abuse Sourcebook*

■

Ear, Nose & Throat Disorders Sourcebook

Basic Information about Disorders of the Ears, Nose, Sinus Cavities, Pharynx, and Larynx, Including Ear Infections, Tinnitus, Vestibular Disorders, Allergic and Non-Allergic Rhinitis, Sore Throats, Tonsillitis, and Cancers That Affect the Ears, Nose, Sinuses, and Throat

Along with Reports on Current Research Initiatives, a Glossary of Related Medical Terms, and a Directory of Sources for Further Help and Information

Edited by Karen Bellenir and Linda M. Shin. 576 pages. 1998. 0-7808-0206-3. $78.

"Overall, this sourcebook is helpful for the consumer seeking information on ENT issues. It is recommended for public libraries."
—*American Reference Books Annual, 1999*

"Recommended reference source."
—*Booklist, American Library Association, Dec '98*

■

Endocrine & Metabolic Disorders Sourcebook

Basic Information for the Layperson about Pancreatic and Insulin-Related Disorders Such as Pancreatitis, Diabetes, and Hypoglycemia; Adrenal Gland Disorders Such as Cushing's Syndrome, Addison's Disease, and Congenital Adrenal Hyperplasia; Pituitary Gland Disorders Such as Growth Hormone Deficiency, Acromegaly, and Pituitary Tumors; Thyroid Disorders Such as Hypothyroidism, Graves' Disease, Hashimoto's Disease, and Goiter; Hyperparathyroidism; and Other

Diseases and Syndromes of Hormone Imbalance or Metabolic Dysfunction

Along with Reports on Current Research Initiatives

Edited by Linda M. Shin. 574 pages. 1998. 0-7808-0207-1. $78.

"Omnigraphics has produced another needed resource for health information consumers."
—*American Reference Books Annual 2000*

"Recommended reference source."
—*Booklist, American Library Association, Dec '98*

■

Environmentally Induced Disorders Sourcebook

Basic Information about Diseases and Syndromes Linked to Exposure to Pollutants and Other Substances in Outdoor and Indoor Environments Such as Lead, Asbestos, Formaldehyde, Mercury, Emissions, Noise, and More

Edited by Allan R. Cook. 620 pages. 1997. 0-7808-0083-4. $78.

"Recommended reference source."
—*Booklist, American Library Association, Sep '98*

"This book will be a useful addition to anyone's library." —*Choice Health Sciences Supplement, Association of College and Research Libraries, May '98*

". . . a good survey of numerous environmentally induced physical disorders . . . a useful addition to anyone's library."
—*Doody's Health Sciences Book Reviews, Jan '98*

". . . provide[s] introductory information from the best authorities around. Since this volume covers topics that potentially affect everyone, it will surely be one of the most frequently consulted volumes in the *Health Reference Series*." —*Rettig on Reference, Nov '97*

■

Ethical Issues in Medicine Sourcebook

Basic Information about Controversial Treatment Issues, Genetic Research, Reproductive Technologies, and End-of-Life Decisions, Including Topics Such as Cloning, Abortion, Fertility Management, Organ Transplantation, Health Care Rationing, Advance Directives, Living Wills, Physician-Assisted Suicide, Euthanasia, and More; Along with a Glossary and Resources for Additional Information

Edited by Helene Henderson. 600 pages. 2000. 0-7808-0237-3. $78.

Family Planning Sourcebook

Basic Consumer Health Information about Planning for Pregnancy and Contraception, Including Traditional Methods, Barrier Methods, Permanent Methods, Future Methods, Emergency Contraception, and Birth Control Choices for Women at Each Stage of Life

Along with Statistics, Glossary, and Sources of Additional Information

Edited by Amy Marcaccio Keyzer. 600 pages. 2000. 0-7808-0379-5. $78.

SEE ALSO *Pregnancy & Birth Sourcebook*

■

Fitness & Exercise Sourcebook

Basic Information on Fitness and Exercise, Including Fitness Activities for Specific Age Groups, Exercise for People with Specific Medical Conditions, How to Begin a Fitness Program in Running, Walking, Swimming, Cycling, and Other Athletic Activities, and Recent Research in Fitness and Exercise

Edited by Dan R. Harris. 663 pages. 1996. 0-7808-0186-5. $78.

"A good resource for general readers."
— *Choice, Association of College and Research Libraries, Nov '97*

"The perennial popularity of the topic . . . make this an appealing selection for public libraries."
— *Rettig on Reference, Jun/Jul '97*

■

Food & Animal Borne Diseases Sourcebook

Basic Information about Diseases That Can Be Spread to Humans through the Ingestion of Contaminated Food or Water or by Contact with Infected Animals and Insects, Such as Botulism, E. Coli, Hepatitis A, Trichinosis, Lyme Disease, and Rabies

Along with Information Regarding Prevention and Treatment Methods, and Including a Special Section for International Travelers Describing Diseases Such as Cholera, Malaria, Travelers' Diarrhea, and Yellow Fever, and Offering Recommendations for Avoiding Illness

Edited by Karen Bellenir and Peter D. Dresser. 535 pages. 1995. 0-7808-0033-8. $78.

"Targeting general readers and providing them with a single, comprehensive source of information on selected topics, this book continues, with the excellent caliber of its predecessors, to catalog topical information on health matters of general interest. Readable and thorough, this valuable resource is highly recommended for all libraries."
— *Academic Library Book Review, Summer '96*

"A comprehensive collection of authoritative information."
— *Emergency Medical Services, Oct '95*

Food Safety Sourcebook

Basic Consumer Health Information about the Safe Handling of Meat, Poultry, Seafood, Eggs, Fruit Juices, and Other Food Items, and Facts about Pesticides, Drinking Water, Food Safety Overseas, and the Onset, Duration, and Symptoms of Foodborne Illnesses, Including Types of Pathogenic Bacteria, Parasitic Protozoa, Worms, Viruses, and Natural Toxins

Along with the Role of the Consumer, the Food Handler, and the Government in Food Safety; a Glossary, and Resources for Additional Help and Information

Edited by Dawn D. Matthews. 339 pages. 1999. 0-7808-0326-4. $48.

"This book takes the complex issues of food safety and foodborne pathogens and presents them in an easily understood manner. [It does] an excellent job of covering a large and often confusing topic."
— *American Reference Books Annual 2000*

"Recommended reference source."
— *Booklist, American Library Association, May '00*

■

Forensic Medicine Sourcebook

Basic Consumer Information for the Layperson about Forensic Medicine, Including Crime Scene Investigation, Evidence Collection and Analysis, Expert Testimony, Computer-Aided Criminal Identification, Digital Imaging in the Courtroom, DNA Profiling, Accident Reconstruction, Autopsies, Ballistics, Drugs and Explosives Detection, Latent Fingerprints, Product Tampering, and Questioned Document Examination

Along with Statistical Data, a Glossary of Forensics Terminology, and Listings of Sources for Further Help and Information

Edited by Annemarie S. Muth. 574 pages. 1999. 0-7808-0232-2. $78.

"There are several items that make this book attractive to consumers who are seeking certain forensic data. . . . This is a useful current source for those seeking general forensic medical answers."
— *American Reference Books Annual 2000*

"A wealth of information, useful statistics, references are up-to-date and extremely complete. This wonderful collection of data will help students who are interested in a career in any type of forensic field. It is a great resource for attorneys who need information about types of expert witnesses needed in a particular case. It also offers useful information for fiction and nonfiction writers whose work involves a crime. A fascinating compilation. All levels."
— *Choice, Association of College and Research Libraries, Jan 2000*

Gastrointestinal Diseases & Disorders Sourcebook

Basic Information about Gastroesophageal Reflux Disease (Heartburn), Ulcers, Diverticulosis, Irritable Bowel Syndrome, Crohn's Disease, Ulcerative Colitis, Diarrhea, Constipation, Lactose Intolerance, Hemorrhoids, Hepatitis, Cirrhosis, and Other Digestive Problems, Featuring Statistics, Descriptions of Symptoms, and Current Treatment Methods of Interest for Persons Living with Upper and Lower Gastrointestinal Maladies

Edited by Linda M. Ross. 413 pages. 1996. 0-7808-0078-8. $78.

"... very readable form. The successful editorial work that brought this material together into a useful and understandable reference makes accessible to all readers information that can help them more effectively understand and obtain help for digestive tract problems."
— *Choice, Association of College and Research Libraries, Feb '97*

SEE ALSO *Diet & Nutrition Sourcebook, 1st and 2nd Editions, Digestive Diseases & Disorders Sourcebook*

∎

Genetic Disorders Sourcebook, 1st Edition

Basic Information about Heritable Diseases and Disorders Such as Down Syndrome, PKU, Hemophilia, Von Willebrand Disease, Gaucher Disease, Tay-Sachs Disease, and Sickle-Cell Disease, Along with Information about Genetic Screening, Gene Therapy, Home Care, and Including Source Listings for Further Help and Information on More Than 300 Disorders

Edited by Karen Bellenir. 642 pages. 1996. 0-7808-0034-6. $78.

"Recommended for undergraduate libraries or libraries that serve the public."
— *Science & Technology Libraries, Vol. 18, No. 1, '99*

"Provides essential medical information to both the general public and those diagnosed with a serious or fatal genetic disease or disorder."
— *Choice, Association of College and Research Libraries, Jan '97*

"Geared toward the lay public. It would be well placed in all public libraries and in those hospital and medical libraries in which access to genetic references is limited." — *Doody's Health Sciences Book Review, Oct '96*

∎

Genetic Disorders Sourcebook, 2nd Edition

Basic Consumer Information about Hereditary Diseases and Disorders, Including Cystic Fibrosis, Down Syndrome, Hemophilia, Huntington's Disease, Sickle Cell Anemia, and More

Along with Facts about Genes, Gene Therapy, Genetic Screening, Ethics of Gene Testing, Genetic Counseling,

a Glossary of Genetic Terminology, and a Resource List for Help, Support, and Further Information

Edited by Kathy Massimini. 650 pages. 2000. 0-7808-0241-1. $78.

∎

Head Trauma Sourcebook

Basic Information for the Layperson about Open-Head and Closed-Head Injuries, Treatment Advances, Recovery, and Rehabilitation

Along with Reports on Current Research Initiatives

Edited by Karen Bellenir. 414 pages. 1997. 0-7808-0208-X. $78.

∎

Health Insurance Sourcebook

Basic Information about Managed Care Organizations, Traditional Fee-for-Service Insurance, Insurance Portability and Pre-Existing Conditions Clauses, Medicare, Medicaid, Social Security, and Military Health Care

Along with Information about Insurance Fraud

Edited by Wendy Wilcox. 530 pages. 1997. 0-7808-0222-5. $78.

"Particularly useful because it brings much of this information together in one volume. This book will be a handy reference source in the health sciences library, hospital library, college and university library, and medium to large public library."
— *Medical Reference Services Quarterly, Fall '98*

Awarded "Books of the Year Award"
— *American Journal of Nursing, 1997*

"The layout of the book is particularly helpful as it provides easy access to reference material. A most useful addition to the vast amount of information about health insurance. The use of data from U.S. government agencies is most commendable. Useful in a library or learning center for healthcare professional students."
— *Doody's Health Sciences Book Reviews, Nov '97*

∎

Health Resources Sourcebook

Basic Consumer Health Information about Sources of Medical Assistance, Featuring an Annotated Directory of Private and Public Consumer Health Organizations and Listings of Other Resources, Including Hospitals, Hospices, and State Medical Associations

Along with Guidelines for Locating and Evaluating Health Information

Edited by Dawn D. Matthews. 500 pages. 2000. 0-7808-0328-0. $78.

Healthy Aging Sourcebook

Basic Consumer Health Information about Maintaining Health through the Aging Process, Including Advice on Nutrition, Exercise, and Sleep, Help in Making Decisions about Midlife Issues and Retirement, and Guidance Concerning Practical and Informed Choices in Health Consumerism

Along with Data Concerning the Theories of Aging, Different Experiences in Aging by Minority Groups, and Facts about Aging Now and Aging in the Future; and Featuring a Glossary, a Guide to Consumer Help, Additional Suggested Reading, and Practical Resource Directory

Edited by Jenifer Swanson. 536 pages. 1999. 0-7808-0390-6. $78.

SEE ALSO *Physical & Mental Issues in Aging Sourcebook*

Healthy Heart Sourcebook for Women

Basic Consumer Health Information about Cardiac Issues Specific to Women, Including Facts about Major Risk Factors and Prevention, Treatment and Control Strategies, and Important Dietary Issues

Along with a Special Section Regarding the Pros and Cons of Hormone Replacement Therapy and Its Impact on Heart Health, and Additional Help, Including Recipes, a Glossary, and a Directory of Resources

Edited by Dawn D. Matthews. 336 pages. 2000. 0-7808-0329-9. $48.

SEE ALSO *Cardiovascular Diseases & Disorders Sourcebook, 1st Edition, Heart Diseases & Disorders Sourcebook, 2nd Edition, Women's Health Concerns Sourcebook*

Heart Diseases & Disorders Sourcebook, 2nd Edition

Basic Consumer Health Information about Heart Attacks, Angina, Rhythm Disorders, Heart Failure, Valve Disease, Congenital Heart Disorders, and More, Including Descriptions of Surgical Procedures and Other Interventions, Medications, Cardiac Rehabilitation, Risk Identification, and Prevention Tips

Along with Statistical Data, Reports on Current Research Initiatives, a Glossary of Cardiovascular Terms, and Resource Directory

Edited by Karen Bellenir. 612 pages. 2000. 0-7808-0238-1. $78.

SEE ALSO *Cardiovascular Diseases & Disorders Sourcebook, 1st Edition, Healthy Heart Sourcebook for Women*

Immune System Disorders Sourcebook

Basic Information about Lupus, Multiple Sclerosis, Guillain-Barré Syndrome, Chronic Granulomatous Disease, and More

Along with Statistical and Demographic Data and Reports on Current Research Initiatives

Edited by Allan R. Cook. 608 pages. 1997. 0-7808-0209-8. $78.

Infant & Toddler Health Sourcebook

Basic Consumer Health Information about the Physical and Mental Development of Newborns, Infants, and Toddlers, Including Neonatal Concerns, Nutrition Recommendations, Immunization Schedules, Common Pediatric Disorders, Assessments and Milestones, Safety Tips, and Advice for Parents and Other Caregivers

Along with a Glossary of Terms and Resource Listings for Additional Help

Edited by Jenifer Swanson. 600 pages. 2000. 0-7808-0246-2. $78.

Kidney & Urinary Tract Diseases & Disorders Sourcebook

Basic Information about Kidney Stones, Urinary Incontinence, Bladder Disease, End Stage Renal Disease, Dialysis, and More

Along with Statistical and Demographic Data and Reports on Current Research Initiatives

Edited by Linda M. Ross. 602 pages. 1997. 0-7808-0079-6. $78.

Learning Disabilities Sourcebook

Basic Information about Disorders Such as Dyslexia, Visual and Auditory Processing Deficits, Attention Deficit/Hyperactivity Disorder, and Autism

Along with Statistical and Demographic Data, Reports on Current Research Initiatives, an Explanation of the Assessment Process, and a Special Section for Adults with Learning Disabilities

Edited by Linda M. Shin. 579 pages. 1998. 0-7808-0210-1. $78.

Named "Oustanding Reference Book of 1999."
— *New York Public Library, Feb 2000*

"An excellent candidate for inclusion in a public library reference section. It's a great source of information. Teachers will also find the book useful. Definitely worth reading."
— *Journal of Adolescent & Adult Literacy, Feb 2000*

"Readable . . . provides a solid base of information regarding successful techniques used with individuals who have learning disabilities, as well as practical sug-

gestions for educators and family members. Clear language, concise descriptions, and pertinent information for contacting multiple resources add to the strength of this book as a useful tool."
— *Choice, Association of College and Research Libraries, Feb '99*

"Recommended reference source."
— *Booklist, American Library Association, Sep '98*

"This is a useful resource for libraries and for those who don't have the time to identify and locate the individual publications."
— *Disability Resources Monthly, Sep '98*

◼

Liver Disorders Sourcebook

Basic Consumer Health Information about the Liver and How It Works; Liver Diseases, Including Cancer, Cirrhosis, Hepatitis, and Toxic and Drug Related Diseases; Tips for Maintaining a Healthy Liver; Laboratory Tests, Radiology Tests, and Facts about Liver Transplantation

Along with a Section on Support Groups, a Glossary, and Resource Listings

Edited by Joyce Brennfleck Shannon. 591 pages. 2000. 0-7808-0383-3. $78.

◼

Medical Tests Sourcebook

Basic Consumer Health Information about Medical Tests, Including Periodic Health Exams, General Screening Tests, Tests You Can Do at Home, Findings of the U.S. Preventive Services Task Force, X-ray and Radiology Tests, Electrical Tests, Tests of Blood and Other Body Fluids and Tissues, Scope Tests, Lung Tests, Genetic Tests, Pregnancy Tests, Newborn Screening Tests, Sexually Transmitted Disease Tests, and Computer Aided Diagnoses

Along with a Section on Paying for Medical Tests, a Glossary, and Resource Listings

Edited by Joyce Brennfleck Shannon. 691 pages. 1999. 0-7808-0243-8. $78.

"A valuable reference guide."
— *American Reference Books Annual 2000*

"Recommended for hospital and health sciences libraries with consumer health collections."
— *E-Streams, Mar '00*

"This is an overall excellent reference with a wealth of general knowledge that may aid those who are reluctant to get vital tests performed."
— *Today's Librarian, Jan 2000*

Men's Health Concerns Sourcebook

Basic Information about Health Issues That Affect Men, Featuring Facts about the Top Causes of Death in Men, Including Heart Disease, Stroke, Cancers, Prostate Disorders, Chronic Obstructive Pulmonary Disease, Pneumonia and Influenza, Human Immunodeficiency Virus and Acquired Immune Deficiency Syndrome, Diabetes Mellitus, Stress, Suicide, Accidents and Homicides; and Facts about Common Concerns for Men, Including Impotence, Contraception, Circumcision, Sleep Disorders, Snoring, Hair Loss, Diet, Nutrition, Exercise, Kidney and Urological Disorders, and Backaches

Edited by Allan R. Cook. 738 pages. 1998. 0-7808-0212-8. $78.

"This comprehensive resource and the series are highly recommended."
— *American Reference Books Annual 2000*

"Recommended reference source."
— *Booklist, American Library Association, Dec '98*

◼

Mental Health Disorders Sourcebook, 1st Edition

Basic Information about Schizophrenia, Depression, Bipolar Disorder, Panic Disorder, Obsessive-Compulsive Disorder, Phobias and Other Anxiety Disorders, Paranoia and Other Personality Disorders, Eating Disorders, and Sleep Disorders

Along with Information about Treatment and Therapies

Edited by Karen Bellenir. 548 pages. 1995. 0-7808-0040-0. $78.

"This is an excellent new book . . . written in easy-to-understand language." — *Booklist Health Sciences Supplement, American Library Association, Oct '97*

". . . useful for public and academic libraries and consumer health collections."
— *Medical Reference Services Quarterly, Spring '97*

"The great strengths of the book are its readability and its inclusion of places to find more information. Especially recommended." — *Reference Quarterly, American Library Association, Winter '96*

". . . a good resource for a consumer health library."
— *Bulletin of the Medical Library Association, Oct '96*

"The information is data-based and couched in brief, concise language that avoids jargon. . . . a useful reference source." — *Readings, Sep '96*

"The text is well organized and adequately written for its target audience." — *Choice, Association of College and Research Libraries, Jun '96*

". . . provides information on a wide range of mental disorders, presented in nontechnical language."
— *Exceptional Child Education Resources, Spring '96*

"Recommended for public and academic libraries."
— *Reference Book Review, 1996*

Mental Health Disorders Sourcebook, 2nd Edition

Basic Consumer Health Information about Anxiety Disorders, Depression and Other Mood Disorders, Eating Disorders, Personality Disorders, Schizophrenia, and More, Including Disease Descriptions, Treatment Options, and Reports on Current Research Initiatives

Along with Statistical Data, Tips for Maintaining Mental Health, a Glossary, and Directory of Sources for Additional Help and Information

Edited by Karen Bellenir. 605 pages. 2000. 0-7808-0240-3. $78.

■

Mental Retardation Sourcebook

Basic Consumer Health Information about Mental Retardation and Its Causes, Including Down Syndrome, Fetal Alcohol Syndrome, Fragile X Syndrome, Genetic Conditions, Injury, and Environmental Sources

Along with Preventive Strategies, Parenting Issues, Educational Implications, Health Care Needs, Employment and Economic Matters, Legal Issues, a Glossary, and a Resource Listing for Additional Help and Information

Edited by Joyce Brennfleck Shannon. 642 pages. 2000. 0-7808-0377-9. $78.

■

Obesity Sourcebook

Basic Consumer Health Information about Diseases and Other Problems Associated with Obesity, and Including Facts about Risk Factors, Prevention Issues, and Management Approaches

Along with Statistical and Demographic Data, Information about Special Populations, Research Updates, a Glossary, and Source Listings for Further Help and Information

Edited by Wilma Caldwell. 400 pages. 2000. 0-7808-0333-7. $48.

■

Ophthalmic Disorders Sourcebook

Basic Information about Glaucoma, Cataracts, Macular Degeneration, Strabismus, Refractive Disorders, and More

Along with Statistical and Demographic Data and Reports on Current Research Initiatives

Edited by Linda M. Ross. 631 pages. 1996. 0-7808-0081-8. $78.

■

Oral Health Sourcebook

Basic Information about Diseases and Conditions Affecting Oral Health, Including Cavities, Gum Disease, Dry Mouth, Oral Cancers, Fever Blisters, Canker Sores, Oral Thrush, Bad Breath, Temporomandibular Disorders, and other Craniofacial Syndromes

Along with Statistical Data on the Oral Health of Americans, Oral Hygiene, Emergency First Aid, Information on Treatment Procedures and Methods of Replacing Lost Teeth

Edited by Allan R. Cook. 558 pages. 1997. 0-7808-0082-6. $78.

"Unique source which will fill a gap in dental sources for patients and the lay public. A valuable reference tool even in a library with thousands of books on dentistry. Comprehensive, clear, inexpensive, and easy to read and use. It fills an enormous gap in the health care literature." — Reference and User Services Quarterly, American Library Association, Summer '98

"Recommended reference source."
— Booklist, American Library Association, Dec '97

■

Osteoporosis Sourcebook

Basic Consumer Health Information about Primary and Secondary Osteoporosis, Juvenile Osteoporosis, Related Conditions, and Other Such Bone Disorders as Fibrous Dysplasia, Myeloma, Osteogenesis Imperfecta, Osteopetrosis, and Paget's Disease

Along with Information about Risk Factors, Treatments, Traditional and Non-Traditional Pain Management, and Including a Glossary and Resource Directory

Edited by Allan R. Cook. 600 pages. 2000. 0-7808-0239-X. $78.

SEE ALSO Women's Health Concerns Sourcebook

■

Pain Sourcebook

Basic Information about Specific Forms of Acute and Chronic Pain, Including Headaches, Back Pain, Muscular Pain, Neuralgia, Surgical Pain, and Cancer Pain

Along with Pain Relief Options Such as Analgesics, Narcotics, Nerve Blocks, Transcutaneous Nerve Stimulation, and Alternative Forms of Pain Control, Including Biofeedback, Imaging, Behavior Modification, and Relaxation Techniques

Edited by Allan R. Cook. 667 pages. 1997. 0-7808-0213-6. $78.

"The text is readable, easily understood, and well indexed. This excellent volume belongs in all patient education libraries, consumer health sections of public libraries, and many personal collections."
— American Reference Books Annual, 1999

"A beneficial reference." — Booklist Health Sciences Supplement, American Library Association, Oct '98

"The information is basic in terms of scholarship and is appropriate for general readers. Written in journalistic style . . . intended for non-professionals. Quite thorough in its coverage of different pain conditions and summarizes the latest clinical information regarding pain treatment."
— Choice, Association of College and Research Libraries, Jun '98

"Recommended reference source."
— Booklist, American Library Association, Mar '98

Pediatric Cancer Sourcebook

Basic Consumer Health Information about Leukemias, Brain Tumors, Sarcomas, Lymphomas, and Other Cancers in Infants, Children, and Adolescents, Including Descriptions of Cancers, Treatments, and Coping Strategies

Along with Suggestions for Parents, Caregivers, and Concerned Relatives, a Glossary of Cancer Terms, and Resource Listings

Edited by Edward J. Prucha. 587 pages. 1999. 0-7808-0245-4. $78.

"A valuable addition to all libraries specializing in health services and many public libraries."
— American Reference Books Annual 2000

■

Physical & Mental Issues in Aging Sourcebook

Basic Consumer Health Information on Physical and Mental Disorders Associated with the Aging Process, Including Concerns about Cardiovascular Disease, Pulmonary Disease, Oral Health, Digestive Disorders, Musculoskeletal and Skin Disorders, Metabolic Changes, Sexual and Reproductive Issues, and Changes in Vision, Hearing, and Other Senses

Along with Data about Longevity and Causes of Death, Information on Acute and Chronic Pain, Descriptions of Mental Concerns, a Glossary of Terms, and Resource Listings for Additional Help

Edited by Jenifer Swanson. 660 pages. 1999. 0-7808-0233-0. $78.

"This is a treasure of health information for the layperson." *— Choice Health Sciences Supplement, Association of College & Research Libraries, May 2000*

"Recommended for public libraries."
— American Reference Books Annual 2000

"Recommended reference source."
— Booklist, American Library Association, Oct '99

SEE ALSO *Healthy Aging Sourcebook*

■

Plastic Surgery Sourcebook

Basic Consumer Health Information on Cosmetic and Reconstructive Plastic Surgery, Including Statistical Information about Different Surgical Procedures, Things to Consider Prior to Surgery, Plastic Surgery Techniques and Tools, Emotional and Psychological Considerations, and Procedure-Specific Information

Along with a Glossary of Terms and a Listing of Resources for Additional Help and Information

Edited by M. Lisa Weatherford. 400 pages. 2000. 0-7808-0214-4. $48.

Podiatry Sourcebook

Basic Consumer Health Information about Foot Conditions, Diseases, and Injuries, Including Bunions, Corns, Calluses, Athlete's Foot, Plantar Warts, Hammertoes and Clawtoes, Club Foot, Heel Pain, Gout, and More

Along with Facts about Foot Care, Disease Prevention, Foot Safety, Choosing a Foot Care Specialist, a Glossary of Terms, and Resource Listings for Additional Information

Edited by M. Lisa Weatherford. 600 pages. 2000. 0-7808-0215-2. $78.

■

Pregnancy & Birth Sourcebook

Basic Information about Planning for Pregnancy, Maternal Health, Fetal Growth and Development, Labor and Delivery, Postpartum and Perinatal Care, Pregnancy in Mothers with Special Concerns, and Disorders of Pregnancy, Including Genetic Counseling, Nutrition and Exercise, Obstetrical Tests, Pregnancy Discomfort, Multiple Births, Cesarean Sections, Medical Testing of Newborns, Breastfeeding, Gestational Diabetes, and Ectopic Pregnancy

Edited by Heather E. Aldred. 737 pages. 1997. 0-7808-0216-0. $78.

"A well-organized handbook. Recommended."
— Choice, Association of College and Research Libraries, Apr '98

"Reecommended reference source."
— Booklist, American Library Association, Mar '98

"Recommended for public libraries."
— American Reference Books Annual, 1998

SEE ALSO *Congenital Disorders Sourcebook, Family Planning Sourcebook*

■

Public Health Sourcebook

Basic Information about Government Health Agencies, Including National Health Statistics and Trends, Healthy People 2000 Program Goals and Objectives, the Centers for Disease Control and Prevention, the Food and Drug Administration, and the National Institutes of Health

Along with Full Contact Information for Each Agency

Edited by Wendy Wilcox. 698 pages. 1998. 0-7808-0220-9. $78.

"Recommended reference source."
— Booklist, American Library Association, Sep '98

"This consumer guide provides welcome assistance in navigating the maze of federal health agencies and their data on public health concerns."
— SciTech Book News, Sep '98

Rehabilitation Sourcebook

Basic Consumer Health Information about Rehabilitation for People Recovering from Heart Surgery, Spinal Cord Injury, Stroke, Orthopedic Impairments, Amputation, Pulmonary Impairments, Traumatic Injury, and More, Including Physical Therapy, Occupational Therapy, Speech/ Language Therapy, Massage Therapy, Dance Therapy, Art Therapy, and Recreational Therapy

Along with Information on Assistive and Adaptive Devices, a Glossary, and Resources for Additional Help and Information

Edited by Dawn D. Matthews. 531 pages. 1999. 0-7808-0236-5. $78.

"Recommended reference source."
—Booklist, American Library Association, May '00

■

Respiratory Diseases & Disorders Sourcebook

Basic Information about Respiratory Diseases and Disorders, Including Asthma, Cystic Fibrosis, Pneumonia, the Common Cold, Influenza, and Others, Featuring Facts about the Respiratory System, Statistical and Demographic Data, Treatments, Self-Help Management Suggestions, and Current Research Initiatives

Edited by Allan R. Cook and Peter D. Dresser. 771 pages. 1995. 0-7808-0037-0. $78.

"Designed for the layperson and for patients and their families coping with respiratory illness. . . . an extensive array of information on diagnosis, treatment, management, and prevention of respiratory illnesses for the general reader." *—Choice, Association of College and Research Libraries, Jun '96*

"A highly recommended text for all collections. It is a comforting reminder of the power of knowledge that good books carry between their covers."
—Academic Library Book Review, Spring '96

"A comprehensive collection of authoritative information presented in a nontechnical, humanitarian style for patients, families, and caregivers."
—Association of Operating Room Nurses, Sep/Oct '95

■

Sexually Transmitted Diseases Sourcebook

Basic Information about Herpes, Chlamydia, Gonorrhea, Hepatitis, Nongonoccocal Urethritis, Pelvic Inflammatory Disease, Syphilis, AIDS, and More

Along with Current Data on Treatments and Preventions

Edited by Linda M. Ross. 550 pages. 1997. 0-7808-0217-9. $78.

Skin Disorders Sourcebook

Basic Information about Common Skin and Scalp Conditions Caused by Aging, Allergies, Immune Reactions, Sun Exposure, Infectious Organisms, Parasites, Cosmetics, and Skin Traumas, Including Abrasions, Cuts, and Pressure Sores

Along with Information on Prevention and Treatment

Edited by Allan R. Cook. 647 pages. 1997. 0-7808-0080-X. $78.

". . . comprehensive, easily read reference book."
—Doody's Health Sciences Book Reviews, Oct '97

SEE ALSO Burns Sourcebook

■

Sleep Disorders Sourcebook

Basic Consumer Health Information about Sleep and Its Disorders, Including Insomnia, Sleepwalking, Sleep Apnea, Restless Leg Syndrome, and Narcolepsy

Along with Data about Shiftwork and Its Effects, Information on the Societal Costs of Sleep Deprivation, Descriptions of Treatment Options, a Glossary of Terms, and Resource Listings for Additional Help

Edited by Jenifer Swanson. 439 pages. 1998. 0-7808-0234-9. $78.

"This text will complement any home or medical library. It is user-friendly and ideal for the adult reader."
—American Reference Books Annual 2000

"Recommended reference source."
—Booklist, American Library Association, Feb '99

"A useful resource that provides accurate, relevant, and accessible information on sleep to the general public. Health care providers who deal with sleep disorders patients may also find it helpful in being prepared to answer some of the questions patients ask."
—Respiratory Care, Jul '99

■

Sports Injuries Sourcebook

Basic Consumer Health Information about Common Sports Injuries, Prevention of Injury in Specific Sports, Tips for Training, and Rehabilitation from Injury

Along with Information about Special Concerns for Children, Young Girls in Athletic Training Programs, Senior Athletes, and Women Athletes, and a Directory of Resources for Further Help and Information

Edited by Heather E. Aldred. 624 pages. 1999. 0-7808-0218-7. $78.

"Public libraries and undergraduate academic libraries will find this book useful for its nontechnical language." *—American Reference Books Annual 2000*

"While this easy-to-read book is recommended for all libraries, it should prove to be especially useful for public, high school, and academic libraries; certainly it should be on the bookshelf of every school gymnasium."
—E-Streams, Mar '00

Substance Abuse Sourcebook

Basic Health-Related Information about the Abuse of Legal and Illegal Substances Such as Alcohol, Tobacco, Prescription Drugs, Marijuana, Cocaine, and Heroin; and Including Facts about Substance Abuse Prevention Strategies, Intervention Methods, Treatment and Recovery Programs, and a Section Addressing the Special Problems Related to Substance Abuse during Pregnancy

Edited by Karen Bellenir. 573 pages. 1996. 0-7808-0038-9. $78.

"A valuable addition to any health reference section. Highly recommended."
— *The Book Report, Mar/Apr '97*

". . . a comprehensive collection of substance abuse information that's both highly readable and compact. Families and caregivers of substance abusers will find the information enlightening and helpful, while teachers, social workers and journalists should benefit from the concise format. Recommended."
— *Drug Abuse Update, Winter '96/'97*

SEE ALSO *Alcoholism Sourcebook, Drug Abuse Sourcebook*

■

Traveler's Health Sourcebook

Basic Consumer Health Information for Travelers, Including Physical and Medical Preparations, Transportation Health and Safety, Essential Information about Food and Water, Sun Exposure, Insect and Snake Bites, Camping and Wilderness Medicine, and Travel with Physical or Medical Disabilities

Along with International Travel Tips, Vaccination Recommendations, Geographical Health Issues, Disease Risks, a Glossary, and a Listing of Additional Resources

Edited by Joyce Brennfleck Shannon. 650 pages. 2000. 0-7808-0384-1. $78.

■

Women's Health Concerns Sourcebook

Basic Information about Health Issues That Affect Women, Featuring Facts about Menstruation and Other Gynecological Concerns, Including Endometriosis, Fibroids, Menopause, and Vaginitis; Reproductive Concerns, Including Birth Control, Infertility, and Abortion; and Facts about Additional Physical, Emotional, and Mental Health Concerns Prevalent among Women Such as Osteoporosis, Urinary Tract Disorders, Eating Disorders, and Depression

Along with Tips for Maintaining a Healthy Lifestyle

Edited by Heather E. Aldred. 567 pages. 1997. 0-7808-0219-5. $78.

"Handy compilation. There is an impressive range of diseases, devices, disorders, procedures, and other physical and emotional issues covered . . . well organized, illustrated, and indexed." — *Choice, Association of College and Research Libraries, Jan '98*

SEE ALSO *Breast Cancer Sourcebook, Cancer Sourcebook for Women, 1st and 2nd Editions, Healthy Heart Sourcebook for Women, Osteoporosis Sourcebook*

■

Workplace Health & Safety Sourcebook

Basic Information about Musculoskeletal Injuries, Cumulative Trauma Disorders, Occupational Carcinogens and Other Toxic Materials, Child Labor, Workplace Violence, Histoplasmosis, Transmission of HIV and Hepatitis-B Viruses, and Occupational Hazards Associated with Various Industries, Including Mining, Confined Spaces, Agriculture, Construction, Electrical Work, and the Medical Professions, with Information on Mortality and Other Statistical Data, Preventative Measures, Reproductive Risks, Reducing Stress for Shiftworkers, Noise Hazards, Industrial Back Belts, Reducing Contamination at Home, Preventing Allergic Reactions to Rubber Latex, and More

Along with Public and Private Programs and Initiatives, a Glossary, and Sources for Additional Help and Information

Edited by Chad Kimball. 600 pages. 2000. 0-7808-0231-4. $78.

■

Worldwide Health Sourcebook

Basic Information about Global Health Issues, Including Nutrition, Reproductive Health, Disease Dispersion and Prevention, Emerging Diseases, Health Risks, and the Leading Causes of Death

Along with Global Health Concerns for Children, Women, and the Elderly, Mental Health Issues, Research and Technology Advancements, and Economic, Environmental, and Political Health Implications, a Glossary, and a Resource Listing for Additional Help and Information

Edited by Joyce Brennfleck Shannon. 500 pages. 2000. 0-7808-0330-2. $78.

■

Health Reference Series Cumulative Index 1999

A Comprehensive Index to the Individual Volumes of the Health Reference Series, Including a Subject Index, Name Index, Organization Index, and Publication Index;

Along with a Master List of Acronyms and Abbreviations

Edited by Edward J. Prucha, Anne Holmes, and Robert Rudnick. 990 pages. 2000. 0-7808-0382-5. $78.